Antimicrobial Resistance: Control Mechanism, Regulation and Clinical Implications

Antimicrobial Resistance: Control Mechanism, Regulation and Clinical Implications

Editor: Leona Ahrens

AMERICAN
MEDICAL PUBLISHERS
www.americanmedicalpublishers.com

AMERICAN
MEDICAL PUBLISHERS
www.americanmedicalpublishers.com

Cataloging-in-Publication Data

Antimicrobial resistance : control mechanism, regulation and clinical implications / edited by Leona Ahrens.
p. cm.
Includes bibliographical references and index.
ISBN 978-1-63927-885-5
1. Drug resistance in microorganisms. 2. Drug resistance in microorganisms--Prevention.
3. Anti-infective agents. 4. Communicable Disease--Treatment. 5. Resistance to drugs in microorganisms.
I. Ahrens, Leona.
QR177 .A58 2023
616.904 1--dc23

American Medical Publishers,
41 Flatbush Avenue,
1st Floor, New York,
NY 11217, USA

ISBN 978-1-63927-885-5 (Hardback)

Contents

Preface

Antimicrobial resistance (AMR) refers to the decreased effectiveness of a medication, such as an antineoplastic or antimicrobial, to treat a disease or condition. Resistance among microbes is common due to random mutations. Drug resistance occurs when parasites, fungi, viruses and bacteria transform over time and they do not respond to the medications. The clinical implication of AMR is that it makes the treatment of infections difficult while simultaneously increasing the risk of spreading the diseases. This resistance may develop naturally through sustained exposure to antimicrobials. There are some specific antiviral drugs that are utilized for treating various viral infections, such as hepatitis B, influenza, HIV and herpes. These drugs stop the viruses from reproducing by blocking the key stages of replication cycle in infected cells. Some strains of each virus have developed resistance to the administered drugs. AMR can be prevented and controlled by the consumption of antibiotics only when they are required, modifying and inactivating a drug, and active efflux of a drug. This book elucidates the clinical aspects and innovative models around prospective developments in the study of antimicrobial resistance. It aims to serve as a resource guide for students and experts alike and contribute to the growth of research on the control mechanism, regulation and clinical implications of antimicrobial resistance.

Various studies have approached the subject by analyzing it with a single perspective, but the present book provides diverse methodologies and techniques to address this field. This book contains theories and applications needed for understanding the subject from different perspectives. The aim is to keep the readers informed about the progresses in the field; therefore, the contributions were carefully examined to compile novel researches by specialists from across the globe.

Indeed, the job of the editor is the most crucial and challenging in compiling all chapters into a single book. In the end, I would extend my sincere thanks to the chapter authors for their profound work. I am also thankful for the support provided by my family and colleagues during the compilation of this book.

Editor

1

Repurposing and Revival of the Drugs: A New Approach to Combat the Drug Resistant Tuberculosis

Divakar Sharma[1,2]*, Yogesh K. Dhuriya[3], Nirmala Deo[1] and Deepa Bisht[1]

[1] Department of Biochemistry, National JALMA Institute for Leprosy and Other Mycobacterial Diseases, Agra, India, [2] Interdisciplinary Biotechnology Unit, Aligarh Muslim University, Aligarh, India, [3] Developmental Toxicology Laboratory, Systems Toxicology and Health Risk Assessment Group, CSIR-Indian Institute of Toxicology Research (CSIR-IITR), Lucknow, India

***Correspondence:**
Divakar Sharma
divakarsharma88@gmail.com

Emergence of drug resistant tuberculosis like multi drug resistant tuberculosis (MDR-TB), extensively drug-resistant tuberculosis (XDR-TB) and totally drug resistant tuberculosis (TDR-TB) has created a new challenge to fight against these bad bugs of *Mycobacterium tuberculosis*. Repurposing and revival of the drugs are the new trends/options to combat these worsen situations of tuberculosis in the antibiotics resistance era or in the situation of global emergency. Bactericidal and synergistic effect of repurposed/revived drugs along with the latest drugs bedaquiline and delamanid used in the treatment of MDR-TB, XDR-TB, and TDR-TB might be the choice for future promising combinatorial chemotherapy against these bad bugs.

Keywords: drug resistance tuberculosis, repurposing, revival of drugs, synergistic effect, proteomics and bioinformatics

INTRODUCTION

Current Scenario

Mycobacterium tuberculosis is a deadly infectious pathogen causing tuberculosis (TB) worldwide. According to WHO (2016) 10.4 million new cases with 1.5 million deaths including 0.4 million individuals with HIV-TB co-infection were reported globally (WHO, 2016). Although TB can be cured by chemotherapy, but the emergence of drug resistant tuberculosis [such as multidrug-resistant tuberculosis (MDR-TB), extensively drug-resistant tuberculosis (XDR-TB) and totally drug resistant tuberculosis (TDR-TB)] has created a new challenge to combat the adverse situation of the disease. Since the decade rates of antibiotic resistance to first and second line anti-TB drugs are dramatically increasing (Cambau et al., 2015). Due to various complexities and high burden of HIV-TB co-infection treatments of MDR-TB, XDR-TB, and TDR-TB are problematic. Apart from the genomics studies various proteomics as well as bioinformatics studies regarding to the drug resistance tuberculosis were accumulated in the last decade (Jiang et al., 2007; Zhang and Yew, 2009; Sharma et al., 2010, 2014, 2015a,b, 2016a,b, 2017; Kumar et al., 2013; Lata et al., 2015a,b; Singh et al., 2015; Sharma and Bisht, 2016, 2017a,b,c;) and suggested the novel drug resistance mechanisms/markers/targets for potential therapeutics in near future. Proteomics and bioinformatics play a crucial role in the diagnostics and therapeutics against the emerging bad bug of tuberculosis. Apart from the expression proteomics studies cited above we have reported that Rv0148 (Putative short-chain type dehydrogenase/reductase) and Rv3841 (ferritin protein) have potentially involved in aminoglycosides resistance (Sharma et al., 2015b, 2016a) and could be the potential diagnostics and therapeutics against the second line of drug resistance. To combat these worsened situations (MDR-TB, XDR-TB, and TDR-TB) new and effective drugs and diagnostics are urgently needed. However, as we know that development of new drugs and diagnostics are enormously expensive and time consuming process.

Repurposing and Revival of Drugs: A Chemotherapeutic Option against Drug Resistant Tuberculosis

Repurposing and revival of the drugs are the new trends/options or one of the pharmaceutical strategies to treat the particular disease that are already FDA approved for other diseases (Tsukamura, 1980; Van Deun et al., 2010) and also for tuberculosis earlier, in this antibiotics resistance era or in the situation of global emergency. Many compounds in TB advanced clinical trials are the molecules that were formerly used to treat other infectious diseases/tuberculosis earlier and now they have been repurposed for treatment of TB (Nayer and Steinbach, 1939; Tsukamura, 1980; Van Deun et al., 2010; Hasse et al., 2014).

Sulfonamides and sulphanilamide were first used in 1930s as an anti-TB drug (Nayer and Steinbach, 1939) but its use was discontinued due to its lesser efficacy as compared to first line drugs (streptomycin and isoniazid). Revival of sulfamethoxazole (SMX) in TB was first pointed out by its efficacy to prevent the TB infection in HIV patients whose receiving trimethoprim/sulfamethoxazole (TMP/SMX) to prevent other infection such as *Pneumocystis jirovecii* (Hasse et al., 2014). In a Nigerian trial study on patients of HIV-MDR-TB coinfetion, efficiency of MDR-TB treatment by TMP/SMX confirmed a significantly shorter time to sputum conversion in these patients (Oladimeji et al., 2014). Sulfadiazine is an anti-leprosy drug which is repurposed in the treatment of MDR-TB and XDR-TB. Brouqui et al. (2013) suggested that sulfadiazine regimen is safe and effective against MDR-TB and TDR-TB treatment (Ameen and Drancourt, 2013; Brouqui et al., 2013).

Clofazimine (CZM) is one of the repurposed molecules, has been initially used as an anti-leprosy drug since half the century. It was recently repurposed for managing the treatment of MDR-TB (Van Deun et al., 2010). CZM is recommended as a second-line anti-TB drug and used in combination with other anti-TB drugs for the treatment of drug-resistant tuberculosis. CZM-containing regimen can cure MDR-TB cases in 9–12 months. In *M. tuberculosis,* CZM appears to act as a prodrug, which is reduced by type 2-NADH dehydrogenase, to release reactive oxygen species (ROS) upon reoxidation by oxygen (O_2) (Yano et al., 2011). CZM, exhibits noticeable anti-mycobacterial and anti-inflammatory activity by inhibition of phospholipase and effects on potassium transporters, respectively (Steele et al., 1999; Cholo et al., 2006). Previous published studies have reported that CZM has good quality efficacy and little toxicity against drug-resistant mycobacterial strains in animal models, which suggested, CZM as a promising anti-TB drug for the management of MDR-TB (Van Deun et al., 2010; Cholo et al., 2012). Recently, numerous observational studies have reported that CZM including regimens provided a useful role in the treatment of patients with MDR-TB (Cholo et al., 2006; Van Deun et al., 2010).

Linezolid, an oxazolidinone antibiotic which is used for treatment of gram-positive bacterial infections (Till et al., 2002; Yanagihara et al., 2002), has now potentially repurposed for the treatment of drug resistant TB (MDR-TB and XDR-TB) (Fortún et al., 2005). Linezolid is an effective anti-TB drug for treating MDR-TB and XDR-TB with various side effects such as neurotoxicity and hematologic toxicity (Tang et al., 2015). Schecter et al. (2010) suggested that linezolid had low rates of discontinuation, well tolerated and good efficacy in the treatment of MDR-TB. Most recently in a case study Jaspard et al. (2017) reported, bedaquiline and linezolid drug combination might be safe for XDR-TB in the late third trimester of pregnancy or pregnant woman. Pregnant woman gave birth to a child without abnormalities follow-up of the fetal showed that no fetal toxicities upto 2 years after the delivery (Jaspard et al., 2017).

Minocycline is also one of the repurposed molecules, has been initially used in the treatment of leprosy since the 1980s (Tsukamura, 1980). In 2008 it was repurposed for managing the treatment of XDR-TB patient in Japan (Kawada et al., 2008). Combinatorial therapy of amoxicillin/clavulanic acid along with other second-line drugs has been used in the treatment of MDR-TB. It's cheaper cost and less toxicity has made the drug of choice in WHO group five drugs (Cassir et al., 2014). Recently, combinatorial treatment by amoxicillin/clavulanic acid and carbapenems has reduced the *M. tuberculosis* load (Diacon et al., 2016). Hugonnet et al. (2009) reported the *in vitro* activity of meropenem combined with clavulanate against XDR strains and paying attention to repurpose these beta-lactams as new anti-TB drugs (Hugonnet et al., 2009). However, carbapenems have been used successfully as part of salvage therapies for XDR patients, they have to be administered intravenously (Tiberi et al., 2016). Recently, an early bactericidal activity-Phase II (EBA Phase II) clinical trial has validated the promising potential of a carbapenem combined with amoxicillin and clavulanic acid for TB treatment (Diacon et al., 2016).

Singhal et al. (2014) reported that the FDA-approved antidiabetic drug metformin (MET) inhibits the intracellular mycobacterial growth by inducing mitochondrial ROS production, restricts disease immunopathology, enhances the efficacy of other anti-TB drugs and could be used as combinatorial therapy against the drug resistant tuberculosis. Gupta et al. (2013) suggested that tuberculosis treatment shortening by verapamil as an adjunctive therapy in mice has opened the direction for future research on verapamil and other efflux pump inhibitors in human tuberculosis. Gupta et al. (2014) also reported that efflux inhibition with verapamil tremendously decreases the MIC of bedaquiline and CZM to *M. tuberculosis* and suggested the synergistic effects of verapamil and bedaquiline in an animal model of TB infection. Recently Dutta et al. (2016) reported that statin a lipid-lowering drug (repurposed for TB treatment) when added to the first-line antitubercular drugs, reduces the lung bacillary burden in chronically infected mice.

Host-directed therapies are important adjunctive therapies for tuberculosis treatment that expanded by host immune effector mechanisms. Recently Gupta et al. (2017) showed that denileukin diftitox potentiates standard TB treatment in the mouse model, which might be due to depletion of T-regulatory and myeloid-derived suppressor cells during TB infection.

Synergistic Effects of Repurposed/Revived Drugs: With Others Anti-TB Drugs Used in Treatments of Tuberculosis Bad Bug

Synergistic effect of repurposed/revived drugs with other anti-TB drugs has been used for the future selection of these drugs in the WHO regimen which could be used in the treatment of MDR-TB, XDR-TB, and TDR-TB. In a study Zhang et al. (2015) suggested that CZM in combination with ethambutol (EMB) and moxifloxacin (MOX) may be a potential drug regimen for the treatment of MDR-TB. Synergistic effect of SMX has been reported *in vitro* with rifampicin (Macingwana et al., 2012). Tasneen et al. (2011) suggested CZM was the best third drug in combination with bedaquiline and pyrazinamide for the treatment of MDR-TB and a good example of drug synergism. Partial synergistic effect was oveserved between linezolid and capreomycin and suggested the efficacy of this combinatorial therapy against *M. tuberculosis* (Zhao et al., 2016). Most recently synergistic effect of bedaquiline and linezolid combinatorial therapy has been reported in XDR-TB of pregnant woman which is a good symbol of synergy for the last line of drugs (Jaspard et al., 2017). In a study synergistic effect carbapenems with rifampicin have been reported against *M. tuberculosis* (Kaushik et al., 2015).

CONCLUSION AND FUTURE PERSPECTIVE

On the basis of the reported literature and studies (regarding to proteomics, bioinformatics, and repurposing/revival of drugs) cited above we suggest that proteomics and bioinformatics play a crucial role in the exploration of diagnostics, therapeutics and mechanism of resistance against drug resistance tuberculosis. Repurposing and revival of the drugs is an alternative strategy to combat from this inadequate situation of drug resistance tuberculosis in this antibiotic resistance era. Synergistic effect of repurposed/revived drugs (sulfamethoxazole, sulfadiazine, clofazimine, linezolid, minocycline, amoxicillin/clavulanic acid, and carbapenems like meropenem) along with the latest drugs (bedaquiline and delamanid) used in the treatment of MDR-TB and XDR-TB might be one of the promising combinatorial chemotherapy for the treatment of MDR-TB, XDR-TB, and TDR-TB. Synergistic effect of these repurposed/revived drugs with bedaquiline and delamanid combinatorial therapy could be added a different perspective over the existed literature.

AUTHOR CONTRIBUTIONS

DS design the concept and wrote the manuscript. DS, YD, ND, and DB finalized the manuscript.

ACKNOWLEDGMENTS

The authors are grateful to Director, NJIL & OMD for the support. DS is ICMR-PDFs (ICMR, New Delhi).

REFERENCES

Ameen, S. M., and Drancourt, M. (2013). *In vitro* susceptibility of *Mycobacterium tuberculosis* to trimethoprim and sulfonamides in France. *Antimicrob. Agents Chemother.* 57, 6370–6371. doi: 10.1128/AAC.01683-13

Brouqui, P., Aubry, C., Million, M., Drancourt, M., and Raoult, D. (2013). Totally resistant tuberculosis: Will antileprosy drugs be helpful? *Int. J. Antimicrob. Agents* 42, 584–585. doi: 10.1016/j.ijantimicag.2013.08.004

Cambau, E., Viveiros, M., Machado, D., Raskine, L., Ritter, C., Tortoli, E., et al. (2015). Revisiting susceptibility testing in MDR-TB by a standardized quantitative phenotypic assessment in a European multicentre study. *J. Antimicrob. Chemother.* 70, 686–696. doi: 10.1093/jac/dku438

Cassir, N., Rolain, J. M., and Brouqui, P. (2014). A new strategy to fight antimicrobial resistance: the revival of old antibiotics. *Front. Microbiol.* 5:551. doi: 10.3389/fmicb.2014.00551

Cholo, M., Boshoff, H. I., Steel, H. C., Cockeran, R., Matlola, N. M., Downing, K. J., et al. (2006). Effects of clofazimine on potassium uptake by a Trk-deletion mutant of *Mycobacterium tuberculosis*. *J. Antimicrob. Chemother.* 57, 79–84. doi: 10.1093/jac/dki409

Cholo, M. C., Steel, H. C., Fourie, P. B., Germishuizen, W. A., and Anderson, R. (2012). Clofazimine: current status and future prospects. *J. Antimicrob. Chemother.* 67, 290–298. doi: 10.1093/jac/dkr444

Diacon, A. H., van der Merwe, L., Barnard, M., von Groote-Bidlingmaier, F., Lange, C., García-Basteiro, A. L., et al. (2016). beta-Lactams against Tuberculosis–new trick for an old dog? *N. Engl. J. Med.* 375, 393–394. doi: 10.1056/NEJMc1513236

Dutta, N. K., Bruiners, N., Pinn, M. L., Zimmerman, M. D., Prideaux, B., Dartois, V., et al. (2016). Statin adjunctive therapy shortens the duration of TB treatment in mice. *J. Antimicrob. Chemother.* 71, 1570–1577. doi: 10.1093/jac/dkw014

Fortún, J., Martín-Dávila, P., Navas, E., Pérez-Elías, M. J., Cobo, J., Tato, M., et al. (2005). Linezolid for the treatment of multidrug-resistant tuberculosis. *J. Antimicrob. Chemother.* 56, 180–185. doi: 10.1093/jac/dki148

Gupta, S., Cheung, L., Pokkali, S., Winglee, K., Guo, H., Murphy, J. R., et al. (2017). Suppressor cell-depleting immunotherapy with denileukin diftitox is an effective host-directed therapy for tuberculosis. *J. Infect. Dis.* 215, 1883–1887. doi: 10.1093/infdis/jix208

Gupta, S., Cohen, K. A., Winglee, K., Maiga, M., Diarra, B., and Bishai, W. R. (2014). Efflux inhibition with verapamil potentiates bedaquiline in *Mycobacterium tuberculosis*. *Antimicrob. Agents Chemother.* 58, 574–576. doi: 10.1128/AAC.01462-13

Gupta, S., Tyagi, S., Almeida, D. V., Maiga, M. C., Ammerman, N. C., and Bishai, W. R. (2013). Acceleration of tuberculosis treatment by adjunctive therapy with verapamil as an efflux inhibitor. *Am. J. Respir. Crit. Care Med.* 188, 600–607. doi: 10.1164/rccm.201304-0650OC

Hasse, B., Walker, A. S., Fehr, J., Furrer, H., Hoffmann, M., Battegay, M., et al. (2014). Cotrimoxazole prophylaxis is associated with reduced risk of incident tuberculosis in participants in the Swiss HIV Cohort Study. *Antimicrob. Agents Chemother.* 58, 2363–2368. doi: 10.1128/AAC.01868-13

Hugonnet, J. E., Tremblay, L. W., Boshoff, H. I., Barry, C. E. III, and Blanchard, J. S. (2009). Meropenem-clavulanate is effective against extensively drug-resistant *Mycobacterium tuberculosis*. *Science* 323, 1215–1218. doi: 10.1126/science.1167498

Jaspard, M., Elefant-Amoura, E., Melonio, I., De Montgolfier, I., Veziris, N., and Caumes, E. (2017). Bedaquiline and linezolid for extensively drug-resistant tuberculosis in pregnant woman. *Emerg. Infect. Dis.* 23, 1731–1732. doi: 10.3201/eid2310.161398

Jiang, X., Zhang, W., Gao, F., Huang, Y., Lv, C., and Wang, H. (2007). Comparison of the proteome of isoniazid-resistant and -susceptible strains of *Mycobacterium tuberculosis*. *Microb. Drug Resist.* 12, 231–238. doi: 10.1089/mdr.2006.12.231

Kaushik, A., Makkar, N., Pandey, P., Parrish, N., Singh, U., and Lamichhane, G. (2015). Carbapenems and rifampin exhibit synergy against *Mycobacterium tuberculosis* and *Mycobacterium abscessus*. *Antimicrob. Agents Chemother.* 59, 6561–6567. doi: 10.1128/AAC.01158-15

Kawada, H., Yamazato, M., Shinozawa, Y., Suzuki, K., Otani, S., Ouchi, M., et al. (2008). Achievement of sputum culture negative conversion by minocycline in a case with extensively drug-resistant pulmonary tuberculosis. *Kekkaku* 83, 725–728.

Kumar, B., Sharma, D., Sharma, P., Katoch, V. M., Venkatesan, K., and Bisht, D. (2013). Proteomic analysis of *Mycobacterium tuberculosis* isolates resistant to kanamycin and amikacin. *J. Proteomics* 94, 68–77. doi: 10.1016/j.jprot.2013.08.025

Lata, M., Sharma, D., Deo, N., Tiwari, P. K., Bisht, D., and Venkatesan, K. (2015a). Proteomic analysis of ofloxacin-mono resistant *Mycobacterium tuberculosis* isolates. *J. Proteomics* 127, 114–121. doi: 10.1016/j.jprot.2015.07.031

Lata, M., Sharma, D., Kumar, B., Deo, N., Tiwari, P. K., Bisht, D., et al. (2015b). Proteome analysis of ofloxacin and moxifloxacin induced *Mycobacterium tuberculosis* isolates by proteomic approach. *Protein Pept. Lett.* 22, 362–371.

Macingwana, L., Baker, B., Ngwane, A. H., Harper, C., Cotton, M. F., Hesseling, A., et al. (2012). Sulfamethoxazole enhances the antimycobacterial activity of rifampicin. *J. Antimicrob. Chemother.* 67, 2908–2911. doi: 10.1093/jac/dks306

Nayer, H., and Steinbach, M. (1939). Sulfanilamide in clinical tuberculosis. *Am. Rev. Tuberc.* 40, 470–472.

Oladimeji, O., Isaakidis, P., Obasanya, O. J., Eltayeb, O., Khogali, M., Van den Bergh, R., et al. (2014). Intensive-phase treatment outcomes among hospitalized multidrug-resistant tuberculosis patients: results from a nationwide cohort in Nigeria. *PLOS ONE* 9:e94393. doi: 10.1371/journal.pone.0094393

Schecter, G. F., Scott, C., True, L., Raftery, A., Flood, J., and Mase, S. (2010). Linezolid in the treatment of multidrug-resistant tuberculosis. *Clin. Infect. Dis.* 50, 49–55. doi: 10.1086/648675

Sharma, D., and Bisht, D. (2016). An efficient and rapid lipophilic proteins extraction from *Mycobacterium tuberculosis* H37Rv for two dimensional gel electrophoresis. *Electrophoresis* 37, 1187–1190. doi: 10.1002/elps.201600025

Sharma, D., and Bisht, D. (2017a). Secretory proteome analysis of streptomycin resistant *Mycobacterium tuberculosis* clinical isolates. *SLAS Discov.* 22, 1229–1238. doi: 10.1177/2472555217698428

Sharma, D., and Bisht, D. (2017b). *M. tuberculosis* hypothetical proteins and proteins of unknown function: Hope for exploring novel resistance mechanisms as well as future target of drug resistance. *Front. Microbiol.* 8:465. doi: 10.3389/fmicb.2017.00465

Sharma, D., and Bisht, D. (2017c). Role of bacterioferritin & ferritin in *M. tuberculosis* pathogenesis and drug resistance: a future perspective by interactomic approach. *Front. Cell. Infect. Microbiol.* 7:240. doi: 10.3389/fcimb.2017.00240

Sharma, D., Deo, N., and Bisht, D. (2017). Proteomics and bioinformatics: a modern way to elucidate the resistome in *Mycobacterium tuberculosis*. *J. Proteomics Bioinform.* 10:e33. doi: 10.4172/jpb.1000e33

Sharma, D., Kumar, B., Lata, M., Joshi, B., Venkatesan, K., Shukla, S., et al. (2015a). Comparative proteomic analysis of aminoglycosides resistant and susceptible *Mycobacterium tuberculosis* clinical isolates for exploring potential drug targets. *PLOS ONE* 10:e0139414. doi: 10.1371/journal.pone.0139414

Sharma, D., Lata, M., Faheem, M., Khan, A. U., Joshi, B., Venkatesan, K., et al. (2015b). Cloning, expression and correlation of Rv0148 to amikacin & kanamycin resistance. *Curr. Proteomics* 12, 96–100. doi: 10.2174/157016461202150903113053

Sharma, D., Lata, M., Faheem, M., Khan, A. U., Joshi, B., Venkatesan, K., et al. (2016a). *M. tuberculosis* ferritin (Rv3841): potential involvement in Amikacin (AK) & Kanamycin (KM) resistance. *Biochem. Biophys. Res. Commun.* 478, 908–912. doi: 10.1016/j.bbrc.2016.08.049

Sharma, D., Lata, M., Singh, R., Deo, N., Venkatesan, K., and Bisht, D. (2016b). Cytosolic proteome profiling of aminoglycosides resistant *Mycobacterium tuberculosis* clinical isolates using MALDI-TOF/MS. *Front. Microbiol.* 7:1816. doi: 10.3389/fmicb.2016.01816

Sharma, D., Shankar, H., Lata, M., Joshi, B., Venkatesan, K., and Bisht, D. (2014). Culture filtrate proteome analysis of aminoglycoside resistant clinical isolates of *Mycobacterium tuberculosis*. *BMC Infect. Dis.* 14(Suppl.):60. doi: 10.1186/1471-2334-14-S3-P60

Sharma, P., Kumar, B., Gupta, Y., Singhal, N., Katoch, V. M., Venkatesan, K., et al. (2010). Proteomic analysis of streptomycin resistant and sensitive clinical isolates of *Mycobacterium tuberculosis*. *Proteome Sci.* 8:59. doi: 10.1186/1477-5956-8-59

Singh, A., Gopinath, K., Sharma, P., Bisht, D., Sharma, P., Singh, N., et al. (2015). Comparative proteomic analysis of sequential isolates of *Mycobacterium tuberculosis* from a patient with pulmonary tuberculosis turning from drug sensitive to multidrug resistant. *Indian J. Med. Res.* 141, 27–45. doi: 10.4103/0971-5916.154492

Singhal, A., Jie, L., Kumar, P., Hong, G. S., Leow, M. K., Paleja, B., et al. (2014). Metformin as adjunct antituberculosis therapy. *Sci. Transl. Med.* 6:263ra159. doi: 10.1126/scitranslmed.3009885

Steele, H., Matlola, N. M., and Anderson, R. (1999). Inhibition of potassium transport and growth of mycobacteria exposed to clofazimine and B669 is associated with a calcium-independent increase in microbial phospholipase A2 activity. *J. Antimicrob. Chemother.* 44, 209–216. doi: 10.1093/jac/44.2.209

Tang, S., Yao, L., Hao, X., Zhang, X., Liu, G., Liu, X., et al. (2015). Efficacy, safety and tolerability of linezolid for the treatment of XDR-TB: a study in China. *Eur. Respir. J.* 45, 161–170. doi: 10.1183/09031936.00035114

Tasneen, R., Li, S., Peloquin, C., Taylor, D., Williams, K., Andries, K., et al. (2011). Sterilizing activity of novel TMC207- and PA-824-containing regimens in a murine model of tuberculosis. *Antimicrob. Agents Chemother.* 55, 5485–5492. doi: 10.1128/AAC.05293-11

Tiberi, S., D'Ambrosio, L., De Lorenzo, S., Viggiani, P., Centis, R., Sotgiu, G., et al. (2016). Ertapenem in the treatment of multidrug-resistant tuberculosis: first clinical experience. *Eur. Respir. J.* 47, 333–336. doi: 10.1183/13993003.01278-2015

Till, M., Wixson, R. L., and Pertel, P. E. (2002). Linezolid treatment for osteomyelitis due to vancomycin-resistant *Enterococcus faecium*. *Clin. Infect. Dis.* 34, 1412–1414. doi: 10.1086/340265

Tsukamura, M. (1980). *In-vitro* antimycobacterial activity of minocycline. *Tubercle* 61, 37–38. doi: 10.1016/0041-3879(80)90058-6

Van Deun, A., Maug, A. K., Salim, M. A., Das, P. K., Sarker, M. R., Daru, P., et al. (2010). Short, highly effective, and inexpensive standardized treatment of multidrug-resistant tuberculosis. *Am. J. Respir. Crit. Care Med.* 182, 684–692. doi: 10.1164/rccm.201001-0077OC

WHO (2016). *Global Tuberculosis Control 2016*. Available at: http://www.who.int/tb/publications/global_report/en/

Yanagihara, K., Kaneko, Y., Sawai, T., Miyazaki, Y., Tsukamoto, K., Hirakata, Y., et al. (2002). Efficacy of linezolid against methicillin-resistant or vancomycin-insensitive *Staphylococcus aureus* in a model of hematogenous pulmonary infection. *Antimicrob. Agents Chemother.* 46, 3288–3291. doi: 10.1128/AAC.46.10.3288-3291.2002

Yano, T., Kassovska-Bratinova, S., The, J. S., Winkler, J., Sullivan, K., Isaacs, A., et al. (2011). Reduction of clofazimine by mycobacterial type 2 NADH:quinone oxidoreductase: a pathway for the generation of bactericidal levels of reactive oxygen species. *J. Biol. Chem.* 286, 10276–10287. doi: 10.1074/jbc.M110.200501

Zhang, Y., and Yew, W. W. (2009). Mechanisms of drug resistance in *Mycobacterium tuberculosis*. *Int. J. Tuberc. Lung Dis.* 13, 1320–1330.

Zhang, Z., Li, T., Qu, G., Pang, Y., and Zhao, Y. (2015). In vitro synergistic activity of clofazimine and other antituberculous drugs against multidrug-resistant *Mycobacterium tuberculosis* isolates. *Int. J. Antimicrob. Agents* 45, 71–75. doi: 10.1016/j.ijantimicag.2014.09.012

Zhao, W., Zheng, M., Wang, B., Mu, X., Li, P., Fu, L., et al. (2016). Interactions of linezolid and second-line anti-tuberculosis agents against multidrug-resistant *Mycobacterium tuberculosis* in vitro and in vivo. *Int. J. Infect. Dis.* 52, 23–28. doi: 10.1016/j.ijid.2016.08.027

2

Serotype is Associated with High Rate of Colistin Resistance Among Clinical Isolates of *Salmonella*

*Qixia Luo[1], Yuan Wang[1], Hao Fu[1], Xiao Yu[1], Beiwen Zheng[1], Yunbo Chen[1], Björn Berglund[1,2] and Yonghong Xiao[1]**

[1] State Key Laboratory for Diagnosis and Treatment of Infectious Diseases, National Clinical Research Center for Infectious Diseases, The First Affiliated Hospital, College of Medicine, Zhejiang University, Hangzhou, China, [2] Department of Clinical and Experimental Medicine, Linköping University, Linköping, Sweden

***Correspondence:**
Yonghong Xiao
xiaoyonghong@zju.edu.cn;
xiao-yonghong@163.com

To investigate the prevalence, probable mechanisms and serotype correlation of colistin resistance in clinical isolates of *Salmonella* from patients in China, *Salmonella* isolates were collected from fecal and blood samples of patients. In this study, 42.8% (136/318) clinical isolated *Salmonella* were resistant to colistin. MIC distribution for colistin at serotype level among the two most prevalent serotypes originating from humans in China indicated that *Salmonella* Enteritidis (83.9% resistance, 125/149) were significantly less susceptible than *Salmonella* Typhimurium (15.3% resistance, 9/59, $P < 0.01$). *mcr* genes and mutations in PmrAB confer little for rate of colistin resistant *Salmonella* isolated from human patients. Phylogenetic tree based on core-genome single nucleotide polymorphisms (SNPs) was separately by the serotypes and implied a diffused distribution of MICs in the same serotype isolates. Relatvie expression levels of colistin resistant related *pmr* genes were significantly higher in non-*mcr* colistin resistant *S.* Typhimurium than in colistin sensitive *S.* Typhimurium, but no discernable differences between colistin resistant and sensitive *S.* Enteritidis, indicating a different mechanism between colistin resistant *S.* Typhimurium and *S.* Enteritidis. In conclusion, colistin susceptibility and colistin resistant mechanism of clinical isolated *Salmonella* were closely associated with specific serotypes, at least in the two most prevalent serotype Enteritidis and Typhimurium. We suggest clinical microbiology laboratory interpreting *Salmonella* colistin MIC results in the serotype level.

Keywords: *Salmonella* enterica, serotype, colistin susceptibility, clinical isolates, phylogenetic analysis, *pmr* genes

INTRODUCTION

Polymyxins, which include polymyxin B and colistin, are cyclic polypeptide antibiotics that are synthesized by members of the *Paenibacillus* genus (Olaitan et al., 2014). As an old class of antimicrobials, polymyxins have been increasingly revitalized as a last resort drug to combat infections caused by multidrug-resistant (MDR) and carbapenem-resistant bacteria (Poirel et al., 2017). The target of polymyxins is the outer membrane lipopolysaccharide (LPS) of Gram-negative bacteria. Binding of polymyxin to the LPS increases the permeability of the bacterial membrane, leading to leakage of the cytoplasmic content and ultimately cell death (Olaitan et al., 2014). Resistance to polymyxins can be conferred via mutations in chromosomal genes, such as genes involved in the PmrAB/PhoPQ two-component systems, which promote the expression of LPS modification related genes, such as *pmrC, pmrE*, and *pmrHFJKLM* operon (Olaitan et al., 2014; Poirel et al., 2017). Plasmid-mediated colistin resistance genes (*mcr*) have since discovery in 2015 been frequently observed, and their continued widespread dissemination has became a challenge to public health worldwide (Liu et al., 2016; Luo et al., 2020).

Salmonella is one of the most important causes of foodborne diarrheal disease, even bloodstream infection (Ashton et al., 2017; Mohan et al., 2019). Although colistin is not a standardized option for treating infections caused by *Salmonella* in humans, the increasing reports of MDR and carbapenem-resistant *Salmonella*, in particular strains harboring *mcr*-genes isolated from patients (Kock et al., 2018; Lu et al., 2019; Sun et al., 2020), indicate that these pathogens constitute a public health concern which calls more attention to the epidemic characteristics of colistin resistance. Colistin resistance in *Salmonella* spp. can be conferred by mutations in *pmrAB*, or more rarely, by the colistin resistance gene *mcr* (Cui et al., 2017). Interestingly, our daily experimental results indicated the rate of colistin resistance among clinical isolates of *Salmonella* spp. are considerably higher compared to other Enterobacteriaceae, such as *Escherichia coli* and *Klebsiella pneumoniae* (Zhang et al., 2017). The objective of this study was to investigate the prevalence and probable mechanisms of colistin resistance in clinical isolates of *Salmonella* in China.

MATERIALS AND METHODS

Collection of *Salmonella* Isolates and Serotyping

A total of 318 isolates of *Salmonella* spp. were collected from clinical samples nationwide in China from 2014 to 2018, including 218 isolates from bloodstream infection and 100 isolates from fecal samples that were derived from diarrhea patients (**Supplementary Table 1**). *Salmonella* serotyping was conducted according to the White-Kauffmann-Le Minor scheme (9th Edition) by performing a slide agglutination test (State Serum Institute (SSI), Copenhagen, Denmark).

Colistin Susceptibility Testing

Cation-adjusted Mueller-Hinton Broth (Oxoid, Basingstoke, United Kingdom) dilutions were used for colistin MIC determination according to the CLSI-EUCAST joint recommendations. *E. col* ATCC 25922 was used as a control. The experiment was conducted in duplicate on at least two separate occasions. The higher MIC was accepted for analysis in the duplicative test within one double dilution difference, or a third replicate would be measured (Kulengowski et al., 2019). The results were interpreted according to the EUCAST colistin breakpoint for Enterobacteriaceae (MIC > 2 mg/L, resistant).

Anlaysis of Colistin Resistance Mechanisms

The isolates were screened by using primers targeting *mcr-1* to *mcr-9* from previous studies (Luo et al., 2017; Borowiak et al., 2020). For the colistin-resistant isolates, *pmrA* and *pmrB* were amplified by primers *pmrAB*-F and *pmrAB*-R (**Supplementary Table 2**). The positive PCR products were sequenced with Sanger sequencing for verification. The sequences of *pmrA* and *pmrB* were compared to that of *S.* Typhimurium LT2 (GenBank: GCA_000006945.2), a colistin-susceptible *Salmonella* reference strain.

Whole-Genome Sequencing and Bioinformatic Analysis

Genomic DNA of 136 randomly selected *Salmonella* spp. isolates (including 64 colistin resistant and 72 susceptible isolates) were extracted using Gentra Puregene Yeast/Bact. Kit (Qiaqen, Hilden, Germany). Genomes were sequenced using the Illumina HiSeq 2500-PE150 platform (Illumina, San Diego, CA, United States). Quality-trimmed raw sequence data was assembled by using SPAdes 3.13.0. Annotation was performed by uploading the data to the RAST server (rast.nmpdr.org). All the assembled genomes were deposited in NCBI, the genome accession numbers were listed in **Supplementary Table 1**.

A phylogenetic tree based on SNPs in the core-genome was constructed via kSNP version 3.0 (Gardner et al., 2015). iTOL (V4) was used for the display, manipulation and annotation of phylogenetic trees (Letunic and Bork, 2019). Multi-sequence typing (MLST) were identified using BacWGSTdb (Ruan and Feng, 2016). All whole-genome sequenced *Salmonella* genomes were analyzed by using the SeqSero 1.2 software (Zhang et al., 2015)[1] for serotype prediction. The results from SeqSero were compared to the traditional Kauffman-White serotyping. When the serotype of one isolate from SeqSero 1.2 was inconsistent with the serotyping from the slide agglutination test, the serotype

[1] https://cge.cbs.dtu.dk/services/SeqSero/

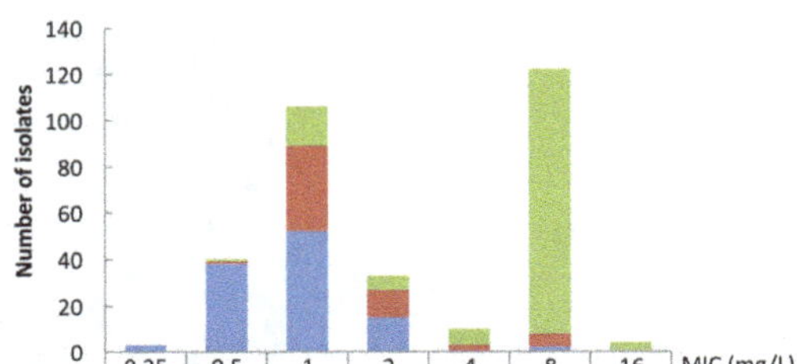

	0.25	0.5	1	2	4	8	16
S.Enteritidis	0	1	17	6	7	114	4
S.Typhimurium	0	1	37	12	3	6	0
other serotypes	3	38	52	15	0	2	0

FIGURE 1 | Number of isolates and MIC distribution of different serotypes of *Salmonella*. "Other serotypes" presents serotypes except for Enteritidis and Typhimurium.

was determined according to the phylogenetic clusters using core-genome SNPs.

Reverse Transcription-Quantitative PCR (qRT-PCR)

Overnight cultures of the target *Salmonella* isolates were diluted 1:100 and subcultured in MH medium for ~4 h at 37°C (OD_{600} ~0.6). Cells were collected at 4°C by centrifuging at 10,000 rpm for 1 min, and RNA was extracted using TRIzol Reagent (Invitrogen). DNase I-treated RNA was obtained using an RNeasy Mini Kit (QIAGEN, No. 75142), and mRNA expression levels of the target genes were examined using real-time PCR primers listed in **Supplementary Table 2**. qRT-PCR was performed using an ABI 7300 96-well system (Applied Biosystems) with SYBR Premix Ex Taq II (cat. no. RR820A; TaKaRa). Expression levels of target genes were normalized against the 16S rRNA gene of *S. enterica* using the standard curve method.

Statistical Analysis

Hypothesis testing was performed by stratifying the analyses for isolates of *Salmonella* Enteritidis and *Salmonella* Typhimurium. Due to the low prevalence of isolates with other serotypes, these were excluded from the analyses. Fisher's exact tests were used to determine if resistant and susceptible phenotypes were equally distributed in S. Enteritidis and S. Typhimurium, and among isolates from blood and intestinal samples. A Mann-Whitney test was performed to determine if MICs were equally distributed among isolates of S. Enteritidis and S. Typhimurium. For the statistical analysis of relative expression levels of *pmr* genes, values are presented as means ± standard deviation (SD). Rank-sum tests were performed for pair-wise

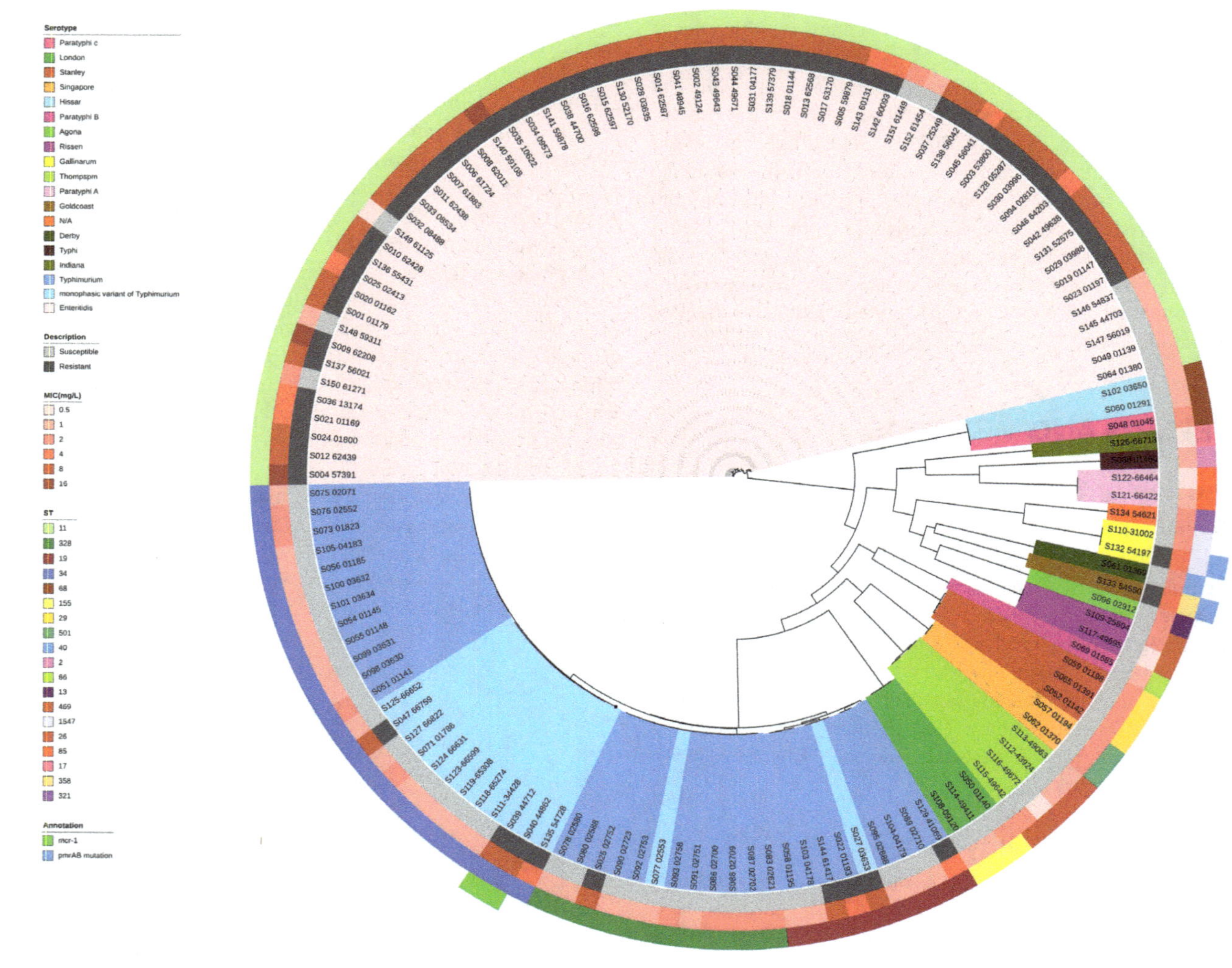

FIGURE 2 | Maximum parsimony tree of the whole-genome sequenced 136 clinical *Salmonella* isolates. MICs (mg/L) and sequence types of colistin among different serotype *Salmonella* isolates were shown. Maximum parsimony tree were generated based on core-genome SNPs by kSNP 3.0. Isolates with different serotypes are indicated in the inner ring with different colors. Colistin MICs in mg/L are shown, along with corresponding *mcr-1* gene and *pmrAB* mutations known to be associated with phenotypic resistance. For the description of colistin susceptibility, resistance corresponds to MIC > 2 mg/L and susceptible corresponds to MIC ≤ 2 mg/L.

comparisons of groups and $P < 0.05$ (two-tailed) was considered significant.

RESULTS

Colistin MICs and Resistance Mechanisms Among *Salmonella* Isolated From Human Patients

The colistin MICs of the tested *Salmonella* spp. isolates ranged from 0.25 mg/L to 16 mg/L (**Figure 1**). The two most prevalent MICs were 8 mg/L (38.4%, 122/318) and 1 mg/L (33.3%, 106/318). 42.8% (136/318) of colistin MICs of the isolates were measured as > 2 mg/L. MIC_{50} and MIC_{90} of the isolates were 2 and 8 mg/L, respectively. 48.6% (106/218) of the bloodstream infection isolates were identified as colistin-resistant, whereas 30% (30/100) of the isolates from intestinal samples were determined as colistin-resistant.

Resistance mechanisms of all the colistin-resistant isolates were investigated by screening for *mcr* genes and sequencing of *pmrA* and *pmrB*. Out of 136 colistin-resistant isolates, two were as *mcr-1* positive (S039-44712 and S040-44862), none had other *mcr* genes, and two had *pmrAB* mutations which affected the amino acid sequence (S132-54197 and S133-54550). The isolates with *pmrAB* mutations carried a missense point mutation in *pmrA* (T89S), and five missense mutations in *pmrB* (M15T, G73S, V74I, I83V, A111T). However, none of the mutations were predicted to affect the protein function.

Relation Between Serotypes and Colistin Susceptibility

18 serotypes were identified among the 318 isolates. *S.* Enteritidis (n = 149) and *S.* Typhimurium (n = 59) were found to be the overall most prevalent. *S.* Enteritidis (122/218) was the most common among isolates from bloodstream infection samples, followed by *S.* Typhimurium (12/218), whereas the inverse was

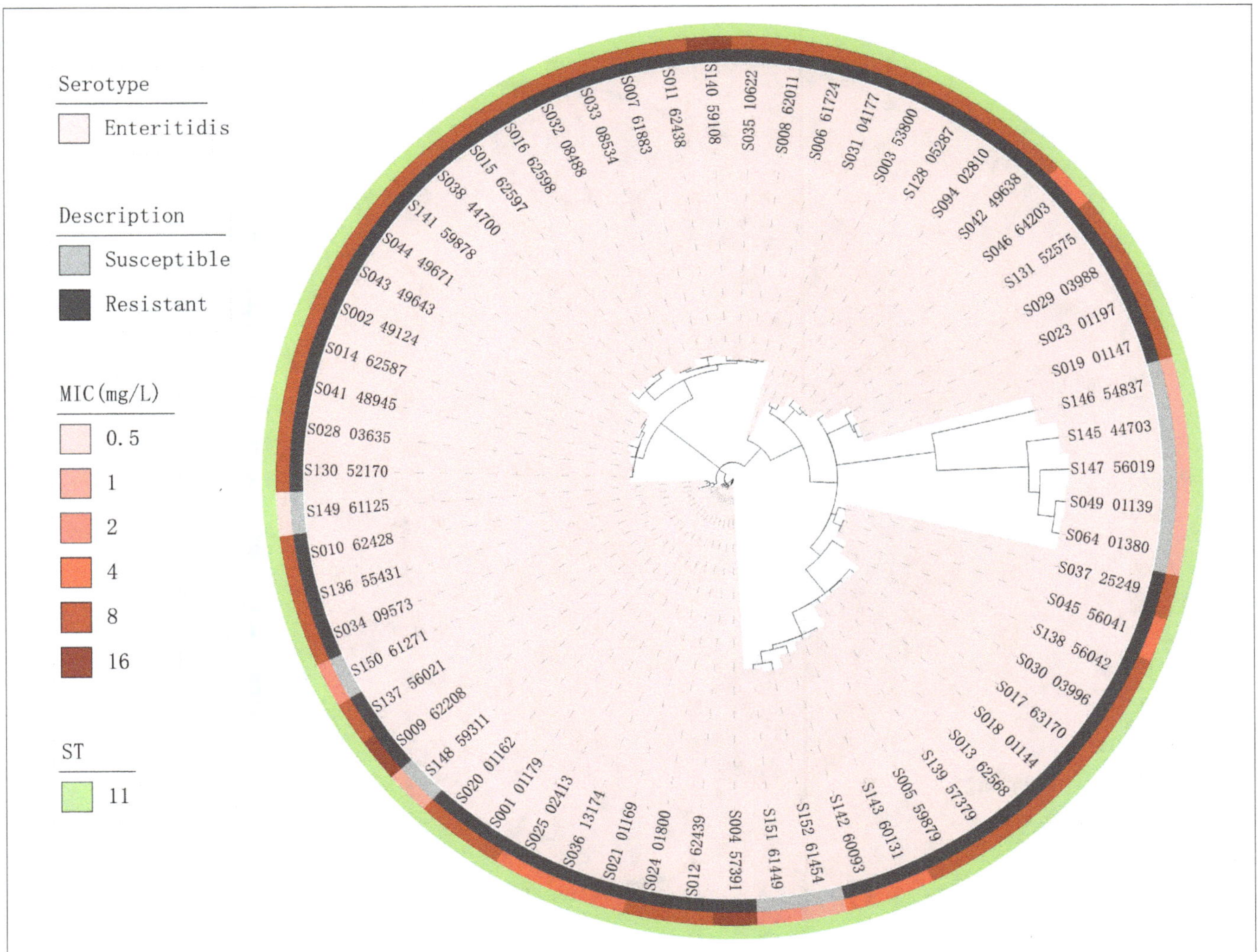

FIGURE 3 | Zoomed-in maximum parsimony tree showing the Enteritidis serotype sub-clade of the clinical *Salmonella* isolates. Colistin MICs in mg/L and sequence types are shown. For the description of colistin susceptibility, resistance corresponds to MIC > 2 mg/L and susceptible corresponds to MIC ≤ 2 mg/L.

true among isolates from patients with intestinal infections, with 27.0% (27/100) *S.* Enteritidis and 47.0% (47/100) *S.* Typhimurium ($P < 0.01$).

The rate of colistin-resistant *S.* Enteritidis and *S.* Typhimurium were 83.9% (125/149) and 15.3% (9/59), respectively. Isolates of *S.* Enteritidis were significantly less susceptible than isolates of *S.* Typhimurium ($P < 0.01$) and had significantly higher MICs ($P < 0.01$). *S.* Enteritidis was most prevalent among the colistin-resistant isolates, representing 91.9% (125/136) of all with the resistance phenotype, followed by *S.* Typhimurium (6.6%, 9/136). All colistin-resistant isolates were *S.* Enteritidis and *S.* Typhimurium, except for the two isolates (S132-54197 and S133-54550) which were identified as *Salmonella* Gallinarum (1/2) and *Salmonella* Goldcoast (1/1), respectively.

Serotype Comparison and Phylogenetic Analysis

In order to discover the relation between *Salmonella* serotypes, phylogenetic evolution and MICs, *Salmonella* serotypes were confirmed and phylogenetic trees based on core-genome SNPs were generated. The whole-genome sequenced isolates were predicted serotypes using SeqSero 1.2 and were compared to the traditional Kauffman-White serotyping. Phylogenetic analysis was employed to confirm the serotyping, by using core-genome SNPs as described above. 63 *S.* Enteritidis, 45 *S.* Typhimurium and 28 isolates of other serotypes were identified from the 136 whole-genome sequenced isolates, and were 98.4% (63/64), 97.8% (45/46), and 92.9% (28/30) identical to the traditional Kauffman-White serotyping, respectively.

Phylogenetic trees based on core-genome SNPs were generated for WGS isolates of all serotypes (**Figure 2**), for all *S.* Enteritidis isolates (**Figure 3**) and for all *S.* Typhimurium isolates (**Figure 4**). The relation between serotypes, sequence types and MICs was inferred in the phylogenetic tree (**Figure 2**). The isolates clustered by serotypes and sequence types in the phylogenetic tree but not by MICs. The *S.* Enteritidis isolates showed little variation in their core genomes. The numbers of SNPs of serotype Enteritidis isolates ranged

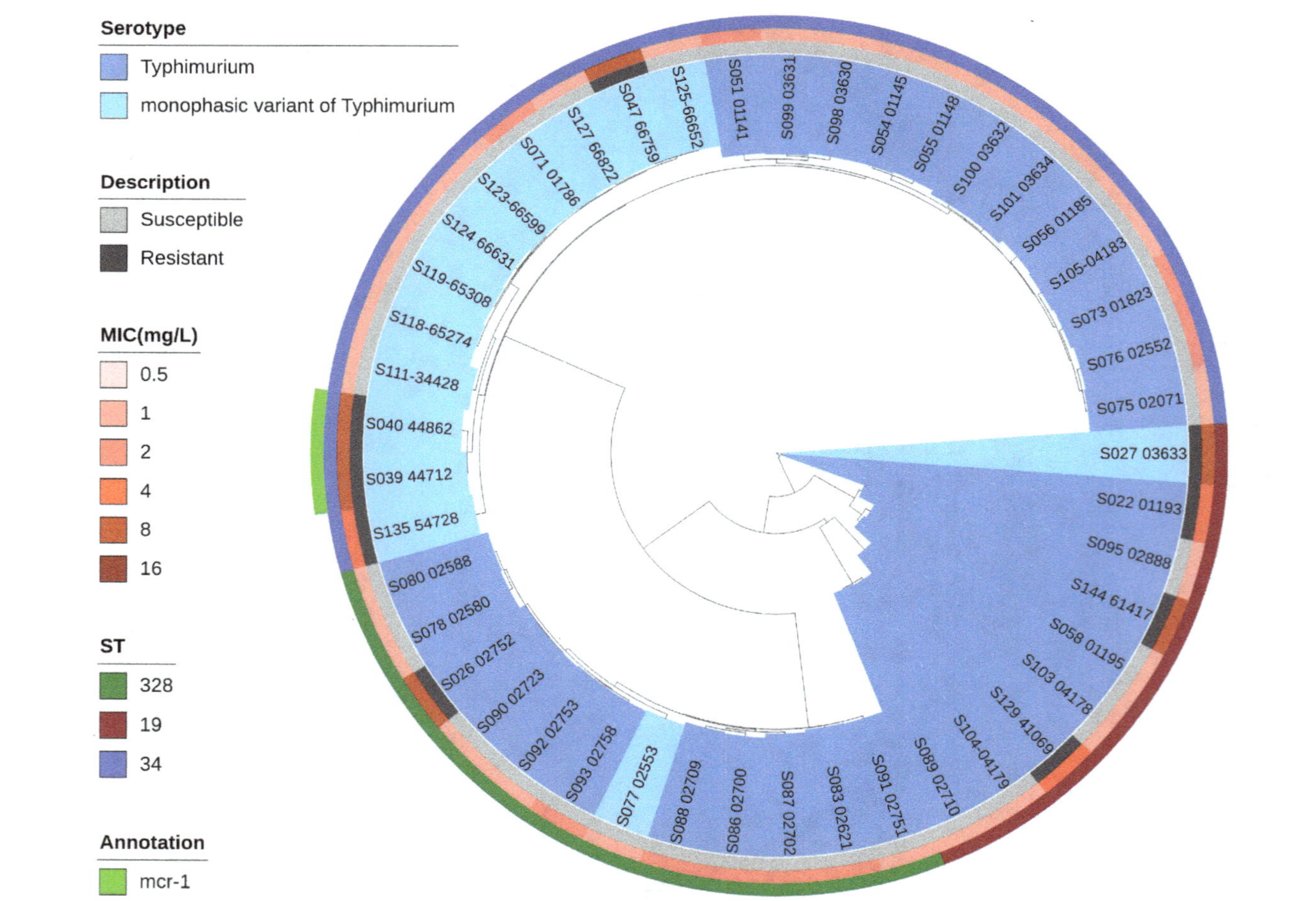

FIGURE 4 | Zoomed-in maximum parsimony tree showing the Typhimurium and monophasic variant of Typhimurium (*Salmonella* 4,[5],12:i:-) serotypes sub-clade of the clinical *Salmonella* isolates. Colistin MICs in mg/L and sequence types are shown. For the description of colistin susceptibility, resistance corresponds to MIC > 2 mg/L and susceptible corresponds to MIC ≤ 2 mg/L.

from 1 to 236, which was very closely in evolution, but did not constitute a single clone. Sequence type of all serotype Enteritidis were ST11 (**Figure 3**). Five colistin-susceptible isolates (S049, S064, S145, S146, S147) clustered together while the remaining five colistin-susceptible isolates (S148, S149, S150, S151, S152) were more diffusely distributed (**Figure 3**). In contrast isolates of *S.* Typhimurium showed a considerable diversity in their core genomes (**Figure 4**). The two *mcr-1* positive *S.* Typhimurium isolates were both monophasic variant of Typhimurium and clustered together, while the other colistin-resistant *S.* Typhimurium isolates were more dispersed.

Comparision of Expression Levels of *pmr* genes in Colistin Resistant and Sensitive *S.* Typhimurium or *S.* Enteritidis

In order to discover if there are different mechanisms between colistin resistant *S.* Typhimurium and *S.* Enteritidis, expression levels of LPS modification related *pmr* genes (*pmrC*, *pmrD*, *pmrE*, and *pmrHFJKLM* operon) in colistin sensitive *S.* Typhimurium or *S.* Enteritidis were compared with non-*mcr* colistin resistant *S.* Typhimurium or *S.* Enteritidis, respectively. Seven isolates of each serotype were colistin resistance (**Supplementary Table 1**) and seven were colistin sensitive (**Supplementary Table 1**). Relatvie expression levels of all *pmr* genes were enhanced in colistin resistant *S.* Typhimurium than in colistin sensitive *S.* Typhimurium ($P < 0.05$) but no discernable differences between colistin resistant and sensitive *S.* Enteritidis (**Figure 5**), indicating a different mechanism between colistin resistant *S.* Typhimurium and *S.* Enteritidis.

DISCUSSION

Previous studies on colistin susceptibility of *Salmonella* spp. utilizing surveillance data from poultry, food and human clinical sources in European countries and the United States, have indicated a correlation between *Salmonella* serotype and colistin MICs (Tyson et al., 2018; Alvarez et al., 2019). Though the occurrence of *Salmonella* serotypes vary from different countries and sources, the inhomogeneity was confirmed in the current study in which the high rate of colistin resistance of *Salmonella* spp. isolated from human patients from China was clearly linked to specific serotypes.

S. Enteritidis and *S.* Typhimurium were the predominant serotypes overall (with *S.* Enteritidis being the most prevalent), however, there was a sizeable and significant difference in colistin susceptibility and MICs between isolates of the two serotypes. Interestingly, the colistin resistance rate of bloodstream infection isolates was significantly higher compared to that of isolates from intestinal samples ($P < 0.01$). This difference was attributable to that *S.* Enteritidis were significantly more common among bloodstream isolates compared to the *S.* Typhimurium ($P < 0.01$). This indicates that not only is *S.* Enteritidis more likely to be colistin-resistant compared to *S.* Typhimurium, but also more frequently cause severe infections in China.

Carriage of *mcr* genes and missense mutations causing amino acid substitutions in PmrAB are the most commonly reported colistin resistance mechanisms in *Salmonella* spp. Surprisingly, in this study, only four isolates were observed with either of these resistance mechanisms, including two *S.* Typhimurium isolates carried *mcr-1* and two isolates had missense mutations in *pmrAB*. According to previous studies in China, *S.* Typhimurium appear to more easily acquire *mcr* genes compared to *S.* Enteritidis (Li et al., 2016; Cui et al., 2017; Luo et al., 2020). This may be because *S.* Typhimurium in general is more susceptible to colistin than *S.* Enteritidis, and so tend to acquire *mcr* genes in order to adapt to colistin selection pressure. No *pmrAB* mutations were found in colistin resistant *S.* Enteritidis, though the high rate of colistin resistance were observed in this serotype. Relatvie expression levels of *pmr* genes were enhanced in colistin resistant *S.* Typhimurium than in colistin sensitive *S.* Typhimurium, but no discernable differences between colistin

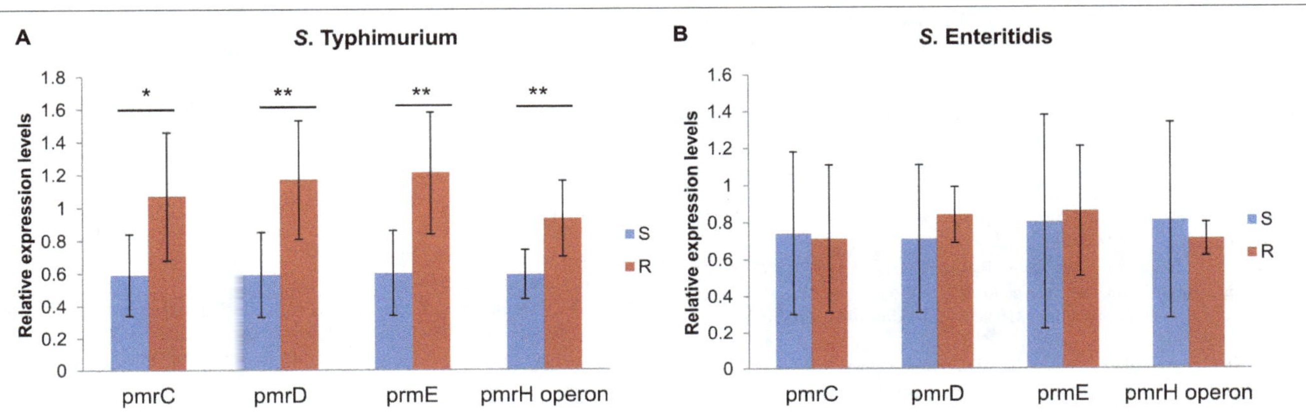

FIGURE 5 | Relative expression levels of *pmrC*, *pmrD*, *pmrE* and *pmrHFJKLM* operon in colistin resistant and sensitive isolates of serotype Typhimurium **(A)** and Enteritidis **(B)**. Gene expression levels of each target gene were identified and compared with 16s rRNA expression levels of each isolates. Relative gene expression levels of colistin sensitive (S) group and colistin resistant (R) group in serotype Typhimurium and Enteritidis were compared using *p*-values calculated by Statistical Package for the Social Sciences (SPSS) using rank-sum tests, respectively (*$P < 0.05$, **$P < 0.01$).

resistant and sensitive *S.* Enteritidis, which indicating a *pmr* related mechanism that confers to colistin resistance to non-*mcr S.* Typhimurium, but a *pmr* unrelated mechanism in colistin resistant *S.* Enteritidis. The large proportion of isolates with unknown resistance mechanisms in the current study indicate that other, as of yet uncharacterized, resistance mechanisms may be more important for *Salmonella* spp.

Aside from that unknown colistin resistance mechanisms could account for the difference in colistin resistance rates of *S.* Enteritidis and *S.* Typhimurium in this study, there could also be intrinsic differences between the serotypes which play an important role. The target of polymyxins is the outer membrane LPS of Gram-negative bacteria. These suggests that the O-antigen (surface LPS of the cell) might play a role in colistin susceptibility. Whether and how different O-antigen confer a different colistin susceptibility phenotype of *Salmonella* needs to be further investigation.

An epidemiological cut-off value for colistin regarding *Salmonella* spp. is lacking in the data presented by EUCAST; currently, only the MIC distribution of *S.* Dublin is presented. The results in this study indicate a very high rate of colistin resistance among *S.* Enteritidis in clinical isolates in China, and this could be associated to elevated wild type MICs compared to other serotypes. Further studies including isolates of *S.* Enteritidis from other countries and other sources are warranted to explore this possibility.

AUTHOR CONTRIBUTIONS

QL and YX conceived and designed the experiments. YW, HF, XY, and YC performed the experiments. QL, BB, and BZ analyzed the data. QL wrote the manuscript. All authors contributed to the article and approved the submitted version.

FUNDING

This work was supported by the National Key R&D Program of China (2017YFC1600100), the National Natural Science Foundation of China (81702040), the National Science Foundation of Zhejiang province, China (LY20H190002), the Swedish Research Council for Environment, Agricultural Sciences and Spatial Planning (Formas) (2016-00640), and the Swedish Foundation for International Cooperate in Research and Higher Education (STINT) (CH2016-6707).

ACKNOWLEDGMENTS

We thank Jinru Ji, Chaoqun Ying, and Yunhui Fang, for the support of technical support and quality control.

REFERENCES

Alvarez, J., Lopez, G., Muellner, P., de Frutos, C., Ahlstrom, C., Serrano, T., et al. (2019*). Identifying emerging trends in antimicrobial resistance using *Salmonella* surveillance data in poultry in Spain. *Transbound. Emerg. Dis.* 67, doi: 10.1111/tbed.13346

Ashton, P. M., Owen, S. V., Kaindama, L., Rowe, W. P. M., Lane, C. R., Larkin, L., et al. (2017). Public health surveillance in the UK revolutionises our understanding of the invasive *Salmonella* typhimurium epidemic in Africa. *Genome Med.* 9:92. doi: 10.1186/s13073-017-0480-487

Borowiak, M., Baumann, B., Fischer, J., Thomas, K., Deneke, C., Hammerl, J. A., et al. (2020). Development of a novel mcr-6 to mcr-9 multiplex PCR and assessment of mcr-1 to mcr-9 occurrence in colistin-resistant *Salmonella enterica* isolates from environment, feed, animals and food (2011-2018) in Germany. *Front. Microbiol.* 11:80. doi: 10.3389/fmicb.2020.00080

Cui, M., Zhang, J., Gu, Z., Li, R., Chan, E. W., Yan, M., et al. (2017). Prevalence and molecular characterization of mcr-1-positive *Salmonella* strains recovered from clinical specimens in China. *Antimicrob Agents Chemother* 61:e02471-16. doi: 10.1128/AAC.02471-2416

Gardner, S. N., Slezak, T., and Hall, B. G. (2015). kSNP3.0: SNP detection and phylogenetic analysis of genomes without genome alignment or reference genome. *Bioinformatics* 31, 2877–2878. doi: 10.1093/bioinformatics/btv271

Kock, R., Daniels-Haardt, I., Becker, K., Mellmann, A., Friedrich, A. W., Mevius, D., et al. (2018). Carbapenem-resistant *enterobacteriaceae* in wildlife, food-producing, and companion animals: a systematic review. *Clin. Microbiol. Infect.* 24, 1241–1250. doi: 10.1016/j.cmi.2018.04.004

Kulengowski, B., Ribes, J. A., and Burgess, D. S. (2019). Polymyxin B EtestR compared with gold-standard broth microdilution in carbapenem-resistant *Enterobacteriaceae* exhibiting a wide range of polymyxin B MICs. *Clin. Microbiol. Infect.* 25, 92–95. doi: 10.1016/j.cmi.2018.04.008

Letunic, I., and Bork, P. (2019). Interactive Tree Of Life (iTOL) v4: recent updates and new developments. *Nucleic Acids Res.* 47, 256–259. doi: 10.1093/nar/gkz239

Li, X. P., Fang, L. X., Song, J. Q., Xia, J., Huo, W., Fang, J. T., et al. (2016). Clonal spread of mcr-1 in PMQR-carrying ST34 *Salmonella* isolates from animals in China. *Sci. Rep.* 6:38511. doi: 10.1038/srep38511

Liu, Y. Y., Wang, Y., Walsh, T. R., Yi, L. X., Zhang, R., Spencer, J., et al. (2016). Emergence of plasmid-mediated colistin resistance mechanism MCR-1 in animals and human beings in China: a microbiological and molecular biological study. *Lancet Infect Dis.* 16, 161–168. doi: 10.1016/s1473-3099(15)00424-427

Lu, X., Zeng, M., Xu, J., Zhou, H., Gu, B., Li, Z., et al. (2019). Epidemiologic and genomic insights on mcr-1-harbouring *Salmonella* from diarrhoeal outpatients in Shanghai. China, 2006–2016. *EBioMedicine* 42, 133–144. doi: 10.1016/j.ebiom.2019.03.006

Luo, Q., Wan, F., Yu, X., Zheng, B., Chen, Y., Gong, C., et al. (2020). MDR *Salmonella enterica* serovar Typhimurium ST34 carrying mcr-1 isolated from cases of bloodstream and intestinal infection in children in China. *J. Antimicrob. Chemotherapy* 75, 92–95. doi: 10.1093/jac/dkz415

Luo, Q., Yu, W., Zhou, K., Guo, L., Shen, P., Lu, H., et al. (2017). Molecular epidemiology and colistin resistant mechanism of mcr-positive and mcr-negative clinical isolated *Escherichia coli*. *Front. Microbiol.* 8:2262. doi: 10.3389/fmicb.2017.02262

Mohan, A., Munusamy, C., Tan, Y. C., Muthuvelu, S., Hashim, R., Chien, S. L., et al. (2019). Invasive *Salmonella* infections among children in Bintulu, Sarawak, Malaysian Borneo: a 6-year retrospective review. *BMC Infect Dis.* 19:330. doi: 10.1186/s12879-019-3963-x

Olaitan, A. O., Morand, S., and Rolain, J. M. (2014). Mechanisms of polymyxin resistance: acquired and intrinsic resistance in bacteria. *Front. Microbiol.* 5:643. doi: 10.3389/fmicb.2014.00643

Poirel, L., Jayol, A., and Nordmann, P. (2017). Polymyxins: antibacterial activity, susceptibility testing, and resistance mechanisms encoded by plasmids or chromosomes. *Clin. Microbiol. Rev.* 30, 557–596. doi: 10.1128/CMR.00064-16

Ruan, Z., and Feng, Y. (2016). BacWGSTdb, a database for genotyping and source tracking bacterial pathogens. *Nucleic Acids Res.* 44, 682–687. doi: 10.1093/nar/gkv1004

Sun, R. Y., Ke, B. X., Fang, L. X., Guo, W. Y., Li, X. P., Yu, Y., et al. (2020). Global clonal spread of mcr-3-carrying MDR ST34 *Salmonella enterica* serotype Typhimurium and monophasic 1,4,[5],12:i:- variants from clinical isolates. *J. Antimicrob Chemother* 75, 1756–1765. doi: 10.1093/jac/dkaa115

Tyson, G. H., Bodeis-Jones, S., Caidi, H., Cook, K., Dessai, U., Haro, J., et al. (2018). Proposed epidemiological cutoff values for ceftriaxone, cefepime, and colistin in *Salmonella*. *Foodborne Pathog Dis.* 15, 701–704. doi: 10.1089/fpd.2018.2490

Zhang, R., Liu, L., Zhou, H., Chan, E. W., Li, J., Fang, Y., et al. (2017). Nationwide surveillance of clinical carbapenem-resistant *Enterobacteriaceae* (CRE) strains in China. *EBioMedicine* 19, 98–106. doi: 10.1016/j.ebiom.2017.04.032

Zhang, S., Yin, Y., Jones, M. B., Zhang, Z., Deatherage Kaiser, B. L., Dinsmore, B. A., et al. (2015). *Salmonella* serotype determination utilizing high-throughput genome sequencing data. *J. Clin. Microbiol.* 53, 1685–1692. doi: 10.1128/JCM.00323-315

3

Efficacy of Colistin and Its Combination With Rifampin *in Vitro* and in Experimental Models of Infection Caused by Carbapenemase-Producing Clinical Isolates of *Klebsiella pneumoniae*

María E. Pachón-Ibáñez[1], Gema Labrador-Herrera[1], Tania Cebrero-Cangueiro[1], Caridad Díaz[2], Younes Smani[1], José P. del Palacio[2], Jesús Rodríguez-Baño[3,4], Alvaro Pascual[3,5], Jerónimo Pachón[1,4] and M. Carmen Conejo[5]*

[1] Clinical Unit of Infectious Diseases, Microbiology, and Preventive Medicine, Institute of Biomedicine of Seville, University Hospital Virgen del Rocío/CSIC/University of Seville, Seville, Spain, [2] Fundacion Centro de Excelencia en Investigación de Medicamentos Innovadores en Andalucía, MEDINA Foundation, Granada, Spain, [3] Clinical Unit of Infectious Diseases, Microbiology, and Preventive Medicine, Institute of Biomedicine of Seville, University Hospital Virgen de Macarena/CSIC/University of Seville, Seville, Spain, [4] Department of Medicine, University of Seville, Seville, Spain, [5] Department of Microbiology, University of Seville, Seville, Spain

***Correspondence:**
María E. Pachón-Ibáñez
mpachon-ibis@us.es

Despite the relevance of carbapenemase-producing *Klebsiella pneumoniae* (CP-Kp) infections there are a scarce number of studies to evaluate *in vivo* the efficacy of combinations therapies. The bactericidal activity of colistin, rifampin, and its combination was studied (time–kill curves) against four clonally unrelated clinical isolates of CP-Kp, producing VIM-1, VIM-1 plus DHA-1(acquired AmpC β-lactamase), OXA-48 plus CTX-M-15 (extended spectrum β-lactamase) and KPC-3, respectively, with colistin MICs of 0.5, 64, 0.5, and 32 mg/L, respectively. The efficacies of antimicrobials in monotherapy and in combination were tested in a murine peritoneal sepsis model, against all the CP-Kp. Their efficacies were tested in the pneumonia model against the OXA-48 plus CTX-M-15 producers. The development of colistin-resistance was analyzed for the colistin-susceptible strains *in vitro* and *in vivo*. *In vitro*, colistin plus rifampin was synergistic against all the strains at 24 h. *In vivo*, compared to the controls, rifampin alone reduced tissue bacterial concentrations against VIM-1 and OXA-48 plus CTX-M-15 strains; CMS plus rifampin reduced tissue bacterial concentrations of these two CP-Kp and of the KPC-3 strain. Rifampin and the combination increased the survival against the KPC-3 strain; in the pneumonia model, the combination also improved the survival. No resistant mutants appeared with the combination. In conclusion, CMS plus rifampin had a low and heterogeneous efficacy in the treatment of severe peritoneal sepsis model due to CP-Kp producing different carbapenemases, increasing survival only against the KPC-3 strain. The combination showed efficacy in the less severe pneumonia model. The combination prevented *in vitro* and *in vivo* the development of colistin resistant mutants.

Keywords: *Klebsiella pneumoniae*, animal models, carbapenemase producers, colistin, rifampin

INTRODUCTION

Carbapenem-resistant *Klebsiella pneumoniae* strains are spreading worldwide, representing an urgent threat to public health, as stressed by the Center for Disease Control and Prevention (CDC) of United States, the European Centre for Disease Prevention and Control (ECDC) and the World Health Organization (WHO). The rapid spread, mostly in hospital settings, is transforming many common health care-associated complications into infections that are sometimes untreatable with the currently available antimicrobials (Nordmann et al., 2012).

The carbapenem resistance *in K. pneumoniae* is mainly due to the production of acquired carbapenemases (Falagas et al., 2014). The most important carbapenemases found in this species may belong to the Ambler classes A (mainly KPC), B (the most frequent are VIM and IMP) and D (OXA-48-like enzymes). Invasive infections by isolates producing VIM and KPC are associated with high death rates (Tzouvelekis et al., 2012). The information about infections caused by OXA-48-producers is scarce, mostly because of its difficult identification (Nordmann et al., 2011; Canton et al., 2012; Tzouvelekis et al., 2012). Nevertheless, OXA-48 is the most frequent carbapenemase produced by Enterobacteriaceae isolated in many European countries (Canton et al., 2012; Palacios-Baena et al., 2016; De Laveleye et al., 2017).

Although the hydrolysis spectrum of these enzymes may vary, they hydrolyze most beta-lactams, including carbapenems. Moreover, carbapenemase producers often show co-resistance to other antimicrobial agents, leaving very few treatment options, such as tigecycline, colistin, and some aminoglycosides (de Oliveira et al., 2015). So, in an attempt to improve the poor clinical efficacy of the available drugs, combination therapy is often used as definitive therapy for infections caused by carbapenemase-producing *K. pneumoniae* (CP-Kp). To date, recommendations are based on few retrospective clinical studies and *in vitro* studies (Tzouvelekis et al., 2012). In addition, a scarce number of *in vivo* studies have assessed the efficacy of antimicrobial combinations against CP-Kp (Tzouvelekis et al., 2012). Clinical studies have reported favorable outcomes for patients treated with combinations of colistin and a carbapenem, tigecycline, fosfomycin, or an aminoglycoside (Michalopoulos et al., 2010; Lee and Burgess, 2012; Munoz-Price et al., 2013; Daikos et al., 2014). However, little data exists on which combination therapy is superior.

Several studies have reported synergistic activity of colistin and rifampin against colistin-resistant and colistin-susceptible KPC-producing *K. pneumoniae* clinical strains, using the checkerboard method. Similarly, studies based on time-kill experiments detected synergy with this combination against colistin-resistant KPC or NDM producers clinical strains, but no synergistic effect against VIM producers. To our knowledge, there is no data regarding the efficacy of this combination against *K. pneumoniae* producing OXA-48, nor *in vivo* studies to validate the *in vitro* results previously mentioned (Elemam et al., 2010; Tascini et al., 2013; Nastro et al., 2014; Tangden et al., 2014). Thus, the aim of this study was to evaluate the *in vitro* and *in vivo* efficacy of CMS plus rifampin against CP-Kp clinical strains producing different carbapenemases.

MATERIALS AND METHODS

Bacterial Strains, Beta-lactamase Characterization and Molecular Typing

Four genetically unrelated clinical isolates of CP-Kp were studied: Kp07, a VIM-1 ST 1603 clone producer (Miro et al., 2013); Kp21, which co-produced VIM-1 and the acquired AmpC type beta-lactamase DHA-1 ST 11 clone (Miro et al., 2013); Kp28, co-producing OXA-48 ST11 clone and the extended spectrum beta-lactamase (ESBL) CTX-M-15 (Oteo et al., 2015); and Kp29, co-producing KPC-3 ST512 clone with the broad spectrum beta-lactamases TEM-1 and SHV-11 (Lopez-Cerero et al., 2014), thereinafter VIM-1, VIM-1/DHA-1, OXA-48 plus CTX-M-15, and KPC-3 producers, respectively. Identification of these isolates was confirmed by a Microflex LT-MALDI Biotyper mass spectrometer (Bruker Daltonics GmbH, Bremen, Germany). The presence of carbapenemase genes, and genes coding for other beta-lactamases was confirmed by PCR and sequencing as described previously. The absence of genetic relation among the isolates was confirmed by PFGE analysis of chromosomal restriction fragments obtained after *Xba*I cleavage following the criteria of Tenover et al. (1995). Two of the strains, KPC-3 and VIM-1 (DHA-1) were multidrug-resistant while the other two were not. The antibiotic susceptibility profiles are included in the Supplementary Information.

Antimicrobials

For the *in vitro* assays, antimicrobials, colistin sulfate salt and rifampin, were used as standard laboratory powders (Sigma-Aldrich, Madrid, Spain). For *in vivo* experiments, clinical formulations were used: colistimethate sodium (CMS) (Genéricos Españoles S.A., Madrid, Spain) and rifampin (Sanofi-Aventis, Madrid, Spain).

In Vitro Studies

Antimicrobial Susceptibility Testing

MICs of antibiotics were determined by broth microdilution as recommended by the Clinical and Laboratory Standards Institute [CLSI] (2012), using Mueller Hinton broth II (MHB) (Becton Dickinson & Co., Sparks, MD, United States) and agar dilution method for fosfomycin. MIC results were interpreted according to the European Committee on Antimicrobial Susceptibility Testing [EUCAST] (2016)[1] breakpoints. Studies were performed in triplicate.

Time-Kill Curves

The concentrations of colistin used for susceptible strains corresponded to the MIC value obtained by microdilution,

[1] http://www.eucast.org/clinical_breakpoints/

whereas the concentration used for resistant strains was 2 mg/L, the susceptibility breakpoint recommended by European Committee on Antimicrobial Susceptibility Testing [EUCAST] (2016). Rifampin was used at a fixed concentration of 2 mg/L. Experiments were carried out with a starting inoculum of 1×10^6 cfu/mL and the antibiotics alone or in combination. Tubes were incubated at 37°C, with shaking, and samples were taken at 0, 1, 3, 6, and 24 h, serially diluted and plated using a spiral platter (Eddy Jet, IUL S.A., Barcelona, Spain). Bacterial colonies were counted using an automatic counter (Flash & Go, IUL S.A., Barcelona, Spain) (Pournaras et al., 2011; Souli et al., 2011). Experiments were performed three times on separate occasions. Synergy was defined as a decrease $\geq$ 2 $\log_{10}$ cfu/mL for the antimicrobial combination compared with the most active single agent. Bactericidal activities of single antibiotics or combination were defined as a decrease $\geq$ 3 $\log_{10}$ cfu/mL from the starting inoculum (Souli et al., 2009). Studies were performed in triplicate.

Animals

Immunocompetent C57BL/6 female mice weighing approximately 20 g (Production and Experimentation Animal Center, University of Seville, Seville, Spain) were used; they had a sanitary status of murine pathogen free and were assessed for genetic authenticity. Mice were housed in an individually ventilated cage system under specific pathogen-free conditions, and water and food supplied *ad libitum*. This study was carried out following the recommendations in the Guide for the Care and Use of Laboratory Animals (Souli et al., 2011). Experiments were approved by the Committee on the Ethics of Animal Experiments of the University Hospital Virgen Macarena, Seville, Spain (CI 1961). All procedures were performed under sodium thiopental (B. Braun Medical S.A., Spain) anesthesia, and all efforts were made to minimize suffering.

Pharmacokinetic/Pharmacodynamic Analysis

Serum antibiotic concentrations were determined in healthy mice after a single intraperitoneal (ip) administration of CMS (20 mg/kg) or rifampin (25 mg/kg). In sets of three anesthetized mice, blood samples from the periorbital plexus were obtained at different time points after the administration of CMS and rifampin. Blood samples were immediately centrifuged (4500 rpm, 15 min at 4°C), and serum samples stored at −80°C until the analysis. Both serum free and total antibiotic concentrations were measured using HPLC-tandem mass spectrometry (LC-MS/MS) (Waters et al., 2008; Gobin et al., 2010). Free fractions of the drugs were calculated as described previously (Waters et al., 2008; Gonzalez et al., 2013; Cheah et al., 2015).

Maximum concentration of drug in serum (C_{max}), elimination half-life ($t_{1/2}$), area under the concentration-time curve from 0 to 24 h (AUC_{0-24}), free AUC_{0-24} ($fAUC_{0-24}$), AUC_{0-24}/MIC and $fAUC_{0-24}$/MIC ratios were calculated using the PKSOLVER program (Zhang et al., 2010). The pharmacodynamic targets to assess the efficacy were $fAUC_{0-24}$/MIC and AUC_{0-24}/MIC for CMS and rifampin, respectively.

Experimental Models

Peritoneal Sepsis Model

A previously described murine peritoneal sepsis model was used (Parra Millan et al., 2016). Briefly, groups of un-anesthetized C57BL/6 mice were infected by ip injection of 0.5 mL of the Minimal Lethal Dose (MLD) of each strain, corresponding to ($\log_{10}$ cfu/mL): 8.97, 8.94 9.35, and 8.38 for VIM-1, VIM-1/DHA-1, OXA-48 plus CTX-M-15, and KPC-3 strains, respectively. Treatments were initiated 4 h post-inoculation. For each one of the strains, mice were randomly included into four different therapeutic groups: (1) controls (untreated), (2) CMS, 20 mg/kg/8 h/ip, (3) rifampin, 25 mg/kg/6 h/ip, and (4) CMS plus rifampin, using the same dosing schedule as in monotherapy. The sample size for the combination groups and CMS monotherapy for the colistin-susceptible strains (VIM-1 and OXA-48 plus CTX-M-15) was 15 mice; nevertheless, for the monotherapies in case of resistance to colistin (VIM-1/DHA-1 and KPC-3) and for rifampin, the sample size was 10 to accomplish the 3Rs (Replacement, Reduction and Refinement) rules for performing animal research. Afterward, mice were treated and monitored for 72 h. The antimicrobial dosages were based on the PK/PD data, and their proven efficacy, alone and in combination, in previous experimental murine models of infection (Pachon-Ibanez et al., 2010). Samples were extracted and processed immediately after the death of mice; the survivor mice were sacrificed (sodium thiopental) at the 72 h. Aseptic thoracotomies were carried out, and blood samples were obtained for qualitative blood cultures; results were expressed as positive ($\geq$1 cfu present in the plate) or negative. Spleens were aseptically extracted, weighed, and homogenized in sterile saline (Stomacher 80; Tekmar Co., Cincinnati, OH, United States) before quantitative cultures ($\log_{10}$ cfu/g) in Columbia agar with 5% sheep blood plates.

Pneumonia Model

A previously characterized murine pneumonia model was used (Pachon-Ibanez et al., 2010; Docobo-Perez et al., 2012; Parra Millan et al., 2016) with the OXA-48 plus CTX-M-15 strain, as OXA-48 is the most prevalent carbapenemase in Spain nowadays (Palacios-Baena et al., 2016). Anesthetized mice were infected intratracheally, using 50 μl of a final inoculum of 8.18 $\log_{10}$ cfu/mL. Therapies were initiated 4 h post-infection and treatment groups and dosages were the same as in the peritoneal sepsis model. Mice were treated and monitored over 72 h. After death or sacrifice of the mice at 72 h, blood and lungs samples were aseptically obtained and processed as detailed above.

In Vitro and *in Vivo* Selection of Colistin-Resistant and Rifampin-Resistant Mutants

Up to 10 colonies, of colistin-susceptible strains exposed during 24 h to colistin at the MIC, alone or in combination with rifampin, in time-kill curves, and from controls (non-exposed to the antimicrobials), were sub-cultured twice in antimicrobial free medium and frozen at −80°C until MIC testing.

In the experimental murine pneumonia model, after processing the lungs as described above, the remaining homogenized tissue was vortexed and centrifuged, and the pellet was resuspended in 2 mL of sterile saline. All the volume was spread on agar and incubated for 48 h at 37°C. A maximum of ten colonies recovered from each lung were selected, sub cultured in antibiotic free medium twice and frozen at −80°C until MIC testing.

MICs determinations of colistin and rifampin were carried out in triplicate.

Statistical Analysis

Mortality and bacteremia rates are expressed as percentages and bacterial tissue concentrations ($\log_{10}$ cfu/g) as means ± *SD*. The two-tailed Fisher's test, analysis of variance (ANOVA), and the Dunnet and Tukey *post hoc* tests were used. A $P < 0.05$ was considered significant. The SPSS v22.0 statistical package was used (SPSS Inc).

RESULTS

In Vitro Results

Antimicrobial Susceptibility Testing

MICs of each antibiotic for the four clinical isolates are shown in **Table 1**. Two strains were resistant to colistin (VIM-1/DHA-1 and KPC-3 producers).

Time-Kill Curves

The results are shown in **Figure 1**. Colistin was bactericidal at 3 h against the VIM-1 producer, but an important regrowth at 24 h. In addition, colistin reduced bacterial concentration (2.5 $\log_{10}$ decrease in cfu/mL) of the OXA-48 plus CTX-M-15-producing isolate, again with an important regrowth at 24 h. Colistin did not display any bactericidal activity against the colistin-resistant isolates (VIM-1/DHA-1 and KPC-3 producers). Rifampin did not show bactericidal activity against any strain. The combination was synergistic against all the strains at 24 h, but achieving only a bacteriostatic effect against the VIM-1, VIM-1/DHA-1, and OXA-48 plus CTX-M-15 isolates; on the contrary, the combination was bactericidal against the KPC-3 isolate.

TABLE 1 | MICs of colistin and rifampin for the four carbapenemase-producing *K. pneumoniae* clinical strains.

Strains	MIC (mg/L) [SIR]	
	Colistin	Rifampin
VIM-1	0.5 [*]	32 [***]
VIM-1/DHA-1	64 [**]	>128 [***]
OXA-48/CTX-M-15	0.5 [*]	32 [***]
KPC-3	32 [**]	64 [***]

**Susceptible, MIC ≤ 2 mg/L. **Resistant, MIC > 2 mg/L. ***Breakpoints are not defined (intrinsically resistant).*

Pharmacokinetics and Pharmacodynamics

Pharmacokinetic parameters of each antimicrobial are shown in **Table 2**. Pharmacodynamics profiles are shown in **Tables 3, 4**.

In Vivo Results: Peritoneal Sepsis Model

The efficacies of the antimicrobials are shown in **Table 3**. Mortality, bacterial clearance on spleen and bacteremia, are analyzed immediately after the death of mice or at the end of the experiment (72 h of treatment).

Mortality

Mortality in all control groups (non-treated) was 100% within the first 24 h post-infection. Rifampin and its combination with CMS reduced mortality in animals infected with the KPC-3 strain to a 66.67% and a 40%, respectively, but not CMS alone. There was no reduction of mortality with any treatment when the peritoneal sepsis was produced by the other strains.

Bacterial Clearance From Spleen

Rifampin alone improved significantly the clearance of bacteria from spleen (CFU/g of tissue) compared with the control and the CMS groups in mice infected with either of the two colistin-susceptible strains producing VIM-1 (7.14 ± 0.48 vs. 8.92 ± 0.46 and 7.14 ± 0.48 vs. 8.60 ± 0.30, respectively) or OXA-48 plus CTX-M-15 (8.24 ± 0.76 vs. 9.56 ± 0.47, and 8.24 ± 0.76 vs. 9.52 ± 0.55, respectively). CMS plus rifampin reduced the bacterial concentration compared with the controls for both colistin-susceptible strains, producing VIM-1 or OXA-48 plus CTX-M-15 and for the colistin-resistant strain producing KPC-3, (6.01 ± 1.77 vs. 8.92 ± 0.46, 7.06 ± 2.50 vs. 9.56 ± 0.47, and 6.76 ± 2.48 vs. 10.19 ± 0.29, respectively). The combination was also better than CMS alone for both colistin-susceptible strains (6.01 ± 1.77 vs. 8.60 ± 0.30, 7.06 ± 2.50 vs. 9.52 ± 0.55, respectively).

Bacteremia

CMS plus rifampin showed the best effect among all the treatment groups in sterilizing blood cultures of mice infected with any of the four strains. Nevertheless, this reduction was only significant in mice infected with the VIM-1 producer (53.33% vs. 100%).

Pneumonia Model Results

Table 4 summarizes the results for the pneumonia model.

Mortality

The severity of this model was lower, with a mortality of 40% at the end of the experiment (72 h) using the MLD in the control group. Only the combination therapy decreased significantly mortality compared with the control group (6.26% vs. 40%; $P < 0.05$).

Bacterial Clearance From Lungs

Rifampin alone and its combination with CMS decreased significantly bacterial lung concentration compared with the

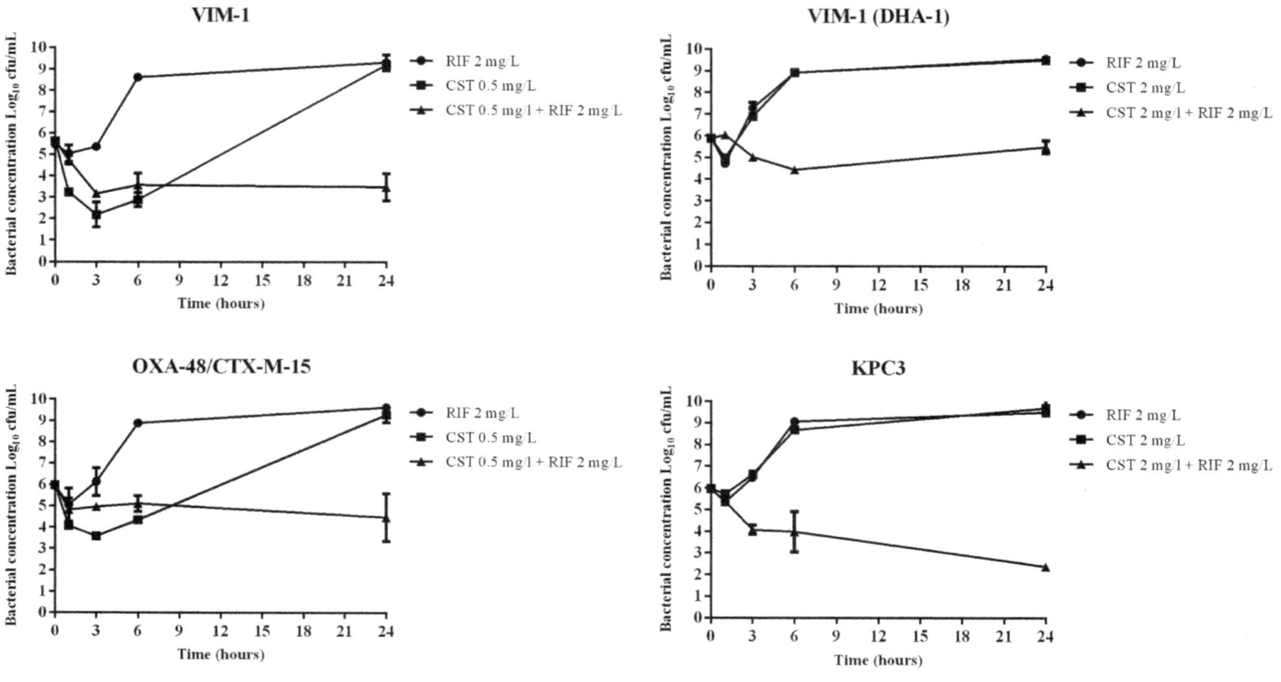

FIGURE 1 | Time-kill curves for colistin (CST) and rifampin (RIF) alone and in combination against four clinical strains of carbapenemase producing strains (VIM-1, VIM-1/DHA-1, OXA-48/CTX-M-15 and KPC3). The CST concentration used for colistin-susceptible strains corresponded to the value of their MICs (colistin 0.5 mg/L for VIM-1 and OXA-48/CTX-M-15); for colistin-resistant isolates the concentration of CST was that corresponding to the susceptibility breakpoint recommended by EUCAST (colistin 2 mg/L for VIM-1/DHA-1 and KPC-3). The RIF concentration used for all strains was 2 mg/L. RIF, filled circles; CST, filled squares; combination of both antimicrobials, filled triangles.

control (3.07 ± 1.63 vs. 8.05 ± 2.36, and 2.99 ± 1.36 vs. 8.05 ± 2.36, respectively).

Bacteremia

None of the antimicrobial treatments achieved a significant reduction of the bacteremia in comparison with the control group.

In Vitro and *in Vivo* Selection of Colistin-Resistant Mutants and Rifampin-Resistant Mutants

Colistin MICs of colonies recovered from susceptible strains (producing VIM-1 or OXA-48 plus CTX-M-15) after exposure at the MIC during 24 h in time-kill curves increased from 0.5 mg/L to > 8 mg/L. No mutants resistant to colistin were detected when these strains were exposed to the combination of colistin plus rifampin.

The MIC of rifampin for the colonies recovered from the lungs of mice challenged with OXA-48 plus CTX-M-15 producer and treated with rifampin alone increased from 16 to > 256 mg/L (16-folds) and the MIC of colistin from the colonies recovered from the lungs of mice treated with CMS as monotherapy increased from 1 to > 32 mg/L (32-folds). Nevertheless, the MICs of rifampin and colistin remained unchanged for those recovered from the control and the combination group.

DISCUSSION

The results of this study show that CMS alone has no significant efficacy in terms of bacterial clearance either from tissue and blood or in the survival rate in the peritoneal sepsis model, even in animals infected with strains susceptible to this antimicrobial. To investigate whether these disappointing results were due to a model effect, additional experiments were made in a less severe murine pneumonia model using the strain producing OXA-48 plus CTX-M-15. Once again, the bacterial lung and blood concentrations as well as mortality were no different from those

TABLE 2 | Pharmacokinetic profiles of CMS and rifampin in mice serum.

Antimicrobial (dose [mg/kg], route of administration)	Drug	C_{max} (mg/L)	$t_{1/2}$ (h)	AUC_{0-24} (mg·h/L)
CST (20, ip)	*t*CST	2.87	3.82	13.65
	*f*CST	0.24	3.82	1.15
RIF (25, ip)	*t*RIF	72.58	19.33	1103.58
	*f*RIF	2.90	19.33	44.14

CST, colistin; RIF, rifampin; ip, intraperitoneal; tCST, total colistin; fCST, free colistin; tRIF, total rifampin; fRIF, free rifampin; ip., intraperitoneal; C_{max}, maximum concentration of drug in serum; $t_{1/2}$, half-life; AUC_{0-24}, area under the concentration-time curve from 0 to 24 h; $fAUC_{0-24}$, the unbound fraction AUC_{0-24}.

TABLE 3 | *In vivo* efficacy and pharmacodynamics of CMS and rifampin, alone and in combination, for the experimental peritoneal sepsis model.

Strain	Treatment group	*n*	Log_{10} cfu/g spleen (mean ± *SD*)	Bacteremia (%)	Mice mortality (%)	AUC_{0-24}/MIC^*	$fAUC_{0-24}/MIC^*$
VIM-1	CTL	9	8.92 ± 0.46	100	100	NA	NA
	CST	15	8.60 ± 0.30	100	93.33	NA	2.30
	RIF	8	7.14 ± 0.48[a]	100	100	34.50	NA
	CST + RIF	15	6.01 ± 1.77[a]	53.33[b]	93.33	NA	NA
VIM-1/DHA-1	CTL	10	9.46 ± 0.32	100	100	NA	NA
	CST	6	9.54 ± 0.34	100	100	NA	0.04
	RIF	8	9.68 ± 0.09	100	100	8.60	NA
	CST+RIF	15	7.64 ± 3.02	73.33	73.33	NA	NA
OXA-48 plus CTX- M-15	CTL	10	9.56 ± 0.47	100	100	NA	NA
	CST	15	9.52 ± 0.55	100	100	NA	2.30
	RIF	10	8.24 ± 0.76[c]	100	100	34.50	NA
	CST+RIF	15	7.06 ± 2.50[c]	87.67	73.33	NA	NA
KPC-3	CTL	10	10.19 ± 0.29	100	100	NA	NA
	CST	8	9.19 ± 1.85	100	75	NA	0.02
	RIF	9	7.20 ± 2.96	88.88	66.67[d]	17.20	NA
	CST+RIF	15	6.76 ± 2.48[d]	77	40[d]	NA	NA

*CTL, control (no antimicrobial treatment); CST, colistin; RIF, rifampin; cfu, colony-forming unit; AUC_{0-24}, area under the concentration-time curve from 0 to 24 h; $fAUC_{0-24}$, the unbound fraction AUC_{0-24}. *PD parameters were determined in healthy mice after CMS or rifampin injection. [a]$P \leq 0.02$ compared to CTL and CST groups. [b]$P < 0.05$ compared to CTL, CST, and RIF groups. [c]$P < 0.05$ compared to CTL and CST groups. [d]$P < 0.05$ compared to CTL group.*

TABLE 4 | *In vivo* efficacy and pharmacodynamics of CMS and rifampin, alone and in combination, for the experimental pneumonia model.

Strain	Treatment group	*n*	Log_{10} cfu/g lung (mean ± *SD*)	Bacteremia (%)	Mice mortality (%)	AUC_{0-24}/MIC^*	$fAUC_{0-24}/MIC^*$
OXA-48 plus CTX- M-15	CTL	15	8.05 ± 2.36	53.30	40	NA	NA
	CST	15	5.14 ± 3.78	40	26.70	NA	2.30
	RIF	15	3.07 ± 1.63[a]	20	13.30	34.50	NA
	CST+RIF	16	2.99 ± 1.36[a]	31.25	6.26[a]	NA	NA

*CTL, control (no antimicrobial treatment); CST, colistin; RIF, rifampin; cfu, colony-forming unit, AUC_{0-24}, area under the concentration-time curve from 0 to 24 h; $fAUC_{0-24}$, the unbound fraction AUC_{0-24}. *PD parameters were determined in healthy mice after CMS or rifampin injection. [a]$P < 0.05$ compared to CTL group.*

of the control group. We believe that these results are related with the development of colistin resistance during the CMS monotherapy found in the pneumonia model.

The CMS dosage used in this study has been proven to be effective in several murine experimental studies using clinical multidrug-resistant (MDR) *Acinetobacter baumannii* strains susceptible to colistin (MIC = 0.5 mg/L) (Pachon-Ibanez et al., 2010; Docobo-Perez et al., 2012; Parra Millan et al., 2016). Nevertheless, when this CMS dosage was used in a murine pneumonia model by a NDM-1-producing *K. pneumoniae* clinical strain, CMS monotherapy was not effective as we found in the present study (Docobo-Perez et al., 2012). Similar results were reported by de Oliveira et al. (2015) in a retrospective clinical study, observing suboptimal efficacy of polymyxins in the treatment of KPC-producing Enterobacteriaceae infections, even in combination with imipenem or meropenem.

One possible explanation to the lack of efficacy found with CMS alone, could be that the PD parameter predictive of colistin efficacy, $fAUC_{0-24}/MIC$ ratio (Cheah et al., 2015), has been described in infections caused by other Gram-negative bacilli, such as *Pseudomonas aeruginosa* and *A. baumannii*. So, the present results would suggest that the described $fAUC_{0-24}/MIC$ values to achieve various magnitudes of bacterial killing in these Gram-negative bacilli are not the appropriate for the treatment of CP-Kp infections, even for isolates with the same MIC values. However, in these studies the end-point to define the $fAUC_{0-24}/MIC$ values predicting colistin efficacy was to achieve a 2 log_{10} decrease in bacterial concentrations in lungs or thigh, but not to evaluate the mice survival rates.

Colistimethate sodium monotherapy did not reduce significantly the bacterial lung and blood results or the survival in the less severe pneumonia model by the strain producing OXA-48 plus CTX-M-15. However, it is noteworthy that CMS achieved a bacterial lung decrease of 2.91 log_{10} cfu/g, a value defined as optimal for *P. aeruginosa* and *A. baumannii* (Cheah et al., 2015), although the wide *SD* precluded the significance of these data.

In addition, the results in the pneumonia model demonstrate that the severity of the chosen animal model is important when studying the efficacy of antimicrobial treatments. Thus, new colistin $fAUC_{0-24}$/MIC values have to be defined for CP-Kp and, in our opinion, for the treatment of other Gram-negative bacilli infections.

The activity of rifampin in monotherapy in the peritoneal sepsis model was also limited, reducing only bacterial spleen concentration compared to control and CMS groups, infected with VIM-1 or OXA-48 plus CTX-M-15 strains, for which an $AUC_{0-24\ h}$/MIC = 34.5, predictor of efficacy was achieved. In the case of animals infected with the KPC-3 strain, rifampin did not decrease significantly the bacterial load in spleen or blood, but reduced the mortality. However, the survival mice conditions suggested that if the experiment were longer than 72 h, all animals included in this treatment group would have died shortly after. Moreover, a huge increase in MIC of rifampin was observed after rifampin *in vivo* monotherapy. In the less severe pneumonia model by OXA-48 plus CTX-M-15 strain, rifampin monotherapy increased significantly the bacterial clearing from lungs and blood, and also increased the mice survival. The efficacy of rifampin against other Gram-negative bacteria has been showed in experimental pneumonia models in mice (Wolff et al., 1999; Montero et al., 2004; Pachon-Ibanez et al., 2010, 2011). Nevertheless, rifampin alone cannot be an alternative due to the generation of rifampin-resistant mutants (Pachon-Ibanez et al., 2006).

Colistimethate sodium in combination with rifampin demonstrated *in vitro* a synergistic effect against the four strains, but the effect was bactericidal only against KPC-3 strain. These results are in accordance with other studies showing synergy of this combination against KPC-producing *K. pneumoniae* strains. Nastro et al. (2014) reported a synergistic effect at 24 h against 27 colistin-resistant KPC-2-producing *K. pneumoniae* clinical strains. Similarly, Elemam et al. (2010) found synergy with polymyxin B plus rifampin against 12 KPC-producing *K. pneumoniae* clinical strains. Tascini et al. (2013) also reported that CMS plus rifampin exhibited synergy against 13 colistin-resistant KPC-producing *K. pneumoniae* clinical strains, moreover being bactericidal against the 62%. On the contrary, in the case of *K. pneumoniae* producing VIM-1 the results of the present study differ from those by Tangden et al. (2014), where CMS plus rifampin did not exhibit synergy against two colistin-susceptible VIM-1-producing *K. pneumoniae* clinical strains.

With regard to the *in vivo* efficacy of CMS plus rifampin in the experimental murine peritoneal sepsis model by the colistin-susceptible VIM-1, the combination was better than the control and CMS groups taking into account the bacterial clearance from spleen and blood. When using the colistin-susceptible OXA-48 plus CTX-M-15 strain, the combination only reduced the bacterial spleen concentration. For these two colistin-susceptible strains, CMS and rifampin achieved the pharmacodynamic values described as optimal, $fAUC_{0-24}$/MIC and AUC_{0-24}/MIC, respectively (Jayaram et al., 2003; Gumbo et al., 2007; Landersdorfer et al., 2017). Nevertheless, is worth mentioning that the efficacy of the combination for both colistin-susceptible strains was not optimal, if we consider that mortality rates remained 93.3 and 73.3%, respectively.

Against the colistin-resistant KPC-3 strain, this combination reduced the bacterial spleen concentration and mortality, in accordance with the *in vitro* synergy studies. Nastro et al. (2014) reported a favorable outcome in five patients with colistin-resistant KPC-2-producing *K. pneumoniae* infections when treated with a combination of CMS plus rifampin. Against the other colistin-resistant strain, producing VIM-1/DHA-1, this combination was not efficacious, in contrast with the synergy observed in the time-kill studies.

In the pneumonia model caused by the OXA-48 plus CTX-M-15 strain, the activity of CMS plus rifampin was similar to that of rifampin in monotherapy, decreasing the bacterial lung concentration and increasing the mice survival compared with the control group. This combination has been successfully used against other Gram-negative bacilli (Pachon-Ibanez et al., 2010). In this pneumonia model, the strain of *K. pneumoniae* developed colistin resistance and a considerable increase in the MIC of rifampin when used as monotherapies, which was prevented with the combination. This prevention of colistin resistant mutant with this combination have been reported previously as in the *in vitro* study published by Rodriguez et al. (2010) in which they proved that the association of colistin plus rifampin was synergistic against heteroresistant *A. baumannii* isolates and prevented the development of colistin-resistant mutants (Rodriguez et al., 2010).

Limitations of the study have to be done, first that even though we wanted to evaluate the *in vitro* and *in vivo* effect of colistin plus rifampin combination against clonally unrelated clinical isolates of *K. pneumoniae* producing other carbapenemases, the number of the tested strains is low. Moreover, the less severe pneumonia model was only performed with one of the strains, and we believe it will be very interesting to do it with all of the strains.

In summary, the results obtained suggest that CMS plus rifampin has a low and heterogeneous efficacy in the treatment of severe infections, such as a peritoneal sepsis infection, caused by different CP-Kp strains, increasing only the mice survival in the infection caused by the KPC-3 strain. CMS plus rifampin combination prevents *in vivo* the development of mutants resistant to colistin. Because of the lack of available alternatives for these colistin-resistant KPC-3-producing strains, the combination of CMS and rifampin might be considered for further evaluation. Moreover, this combination showed efficacy in the less severe pneumonia model by the OXA-48 plus CTX-M-15 strain. Finally, an optimal PD index value for CMS efficacy needs to be defined for *K. pneumoniae.* Overall, the results of the present study suggest that the efficacy of CMS plus rifampin depends on the class of carbapenemase produced by *K. pneumoniae* and on the severity of the infection.

AUTHOR CONTRIBUTIONS

MP-I has planned and coordinated the experiments, analyzed the results, and written the manuscript. GL-H and TC-C had performed the *in vitro* and *in vivo* experiments. CD and JPP had performed the antibiotic concentrations studies by HPLC-tandem mass spectrometry (LC-MS/MS). YS had reviewed the manuscript and the experiments. JR-B, AP, and JP had reviewed the manuscript and the experiments. MCC obtained the funds to perform the studies and wrote the project, contributed to the performance of the *in vitro* experiment, and reviewed the results and the manuscript.

FUNDING

This study was supported by the Consejería de Salud of the Junta de Andalucía (PI-0622-2012) and supported by Plan Nacional de I+D+i and Instituto de Salud Carlos III, Subdirección General de Redes y Centros de Investigación Cooperativa, Ministerio de Economía y Competitividad, Spanish Network for Research in Infectious Diseases (REIPI RD12/0015/0001) – co-financed by European Development Regional Fund "A way to achieve Europe" ERDF. The MEDINA authors disclosed the receipt of financial support from Fundación MEDINA, a public-private partnership of Merck Sharp & Dohme de España S.A./Universidad de Granada/Junta de Andalucía.

REFERENCES

Canton, R., Akova, M., Carmeli, Y., Giske, C. G., Glupczynski, Y., Gniadkowski, M., et al. (2012). Rapid evolution and spread of carbapenemases among *Enterobacteriaceae* in Europe. *Clin. Microbiol. Infect.* 18, 413–431. doi: 10.1111/j.1469-0691.2012.03821.x

Cheah, S. E., Wang, J., Nguyen, V. T., Turnidge, J. D., Li, J., and Nation, R. L. (2015). New pharmacokinetic/pharmacodynamic studies of systemically administered colistin against *Pseudomonas aeruginosa* and *Acinetobacter baumannii* in mouse thigh and lung infection models: smaller response in lung infection. *J. Antimicrob. Chemother.* 70, 3291–3297. doi: 10.1093/jac/dkv267

Clinical and Laboratory Standards Institute [CLSI] (2012). *Methods for Dilution Antimicrobial Susceptibility Tests for Bacteria That Grow Aerobically; Approved Standard—Ninth Edition. CLSI Document M07-A9.* Wayne, PA: Clinical and Laboratory Standards Institute.

Daikos, G. L., Tsaousi, S., Tzouvelekis, L. S., Anyfantis, I., Psichogiou, M., Argyropoulou, A., et al. (2014). Carbapenemase-producing *Klebsiella pneumoniae* bloodstream infections: lowering mortality by antibiotic combination schemes and the role of carbapenems. *Antimicrob. Agents Chemother.* 58, 2322–2328. doi: 10.1128/AAC.02166-13

De Laveleye, M., Huang, T. D., Bogaerts, P., Berhin, C., Bauraing, C., Sacre, P., et al. (2017). Increasing incidence of carbapenemase-producing *Escherichia coli* and *Klebsiella pneumoniae* in Belgian hospitals. *Eur. J. Clin. Microbiol. Infect. Dis.* 36, 139–146. doi: 10.1007/s10096-016-2782-x

de Oliveira, M. S., De Assis, D. B., Freire, M. P., Boas Do Prado, G. V., Machado, A. S., Abdala, E., et al. (2015). Treatment of KPC-producing *Enterobacteriaceae*: suboptimal efficacy of polymyxins. *Clin. Microbiol. Infect.* 21, 179.e1–179.e7. doi: 10.1016/j.cmi.2014.07.010

Docobo-Perez, F., Nordmann, P., Dominguez-Herrera, J., Lopez-Rojas, R., Smani, Y., Poirel, L., et al. (2012). Efficacies of colistin and tigecycline in mice with experimental pneumonia due to NDM-1-producing strains of *Klebsiella pneumoniae* and *Escherichia coli*. *Int. J. Antimicrob. Agents* 39, 251–254. doi: 10.1016/j.ijantimicag.2011.10.012

Elemam, A., Rahimian, J., and Doymaz, M. (2010). In vitro evaluation of antibiotic synergy for polymyxin B-resistant carbapenemase-producing *Klebsiella pneumoniae*. *J. Clin. Microbiol.* 48, 3558–3562. doi: 10.1128/JCM.01106-10

European Committee on Antimicrobial Susceptibility Testing [EUCAST] (2016). *European Society of Clinical Microbiology and Infectious Diseases. Clinical Breakpoints.* Bochum: EUCAST.

Falagas, M. E., Tansarli, G. S., Karageorgopoulos, D. E., and Vardakas, K. Z. (2014). Deaths attributable to carbapenem-resistant *Enterobacteriaceae* infections. *Emerg. Infect. Dis.* 20, 1170–1175. doi: 10.3201/eid2007.121004

Gobin, P., Lemaitre, F., Marchand, S., Couet, W., and Olivier, J. C. (2010). Assay of colistin and colistin methanesulfonate in plasma and urine by liquid chromatography-tandem mass spectrometry. *Antimicrob. Agents Chemother.* 54, 1941–1948. doi: 10.1128/AAC.01367-09

Gonzalez, D., Schmidt, S., and Derendorf, H. (2013). Importance of relating efficacy measures to unbound drug concentrations for anti-infective agents. *Clin. Microbiol. Rev.* 26, 274–288. doi: 10.1128/CMR.00092-12

Gumbo, T., Louie, A., Deziel, M. R., Liu, W., Parsons, L. M., Salfinger, M., et al. (2007). Concentration-dependent *Mycobacterium tuberculosis* killing and prevention of resistance by rifampin. *Antimicrob. Agents Chemother.* 51, 3781–3788. doi: 10.1128/AAC.01533-06

Jayaram, R., Gaonkar, S., Kaur, P., Suresh, B. L., Mahesh, B. N., Jayashree, R., et al. (2003). Pharmacokinetics-pharmacodynamics of rifampin in an aerosol infection model of tuberculosis. *Antimicrob. Agents Chemother.* 47, 2118–2124. doi: 10.1128/AAC.47.7.2118-2124.2003

Landersdorfer, C. B., Nguyen, T. H., Lieu, L. T., Nguyen, G., Bischof, R. J., Meeusen, E. N., et al. (2017). Substantial targeting advantage achieved by pulmonary administration of colistin methanesulfonate in a large-animal model. *Antimicrob. Agents Chemother.* 61:e01934-16. doi: 10.1128/AAC.01934-16

Lee, G. C., and Burgess, D. S. (2012). Treatment of *Klebsiella pneumoniae* carbapenemase (KPC) infections: a review of published case series and case reports. *Ann. Clin. Microbiol. Antimicrob.* 11:32. doi: 10.1186/1476-0711-11-32

Lopez-Cerero, L., Egea, P., Gracia-Ahufinger, I., Gonzalez-Padilla, M., Rodriguez-Lopez, F., Rodriguez-Bano, J., et al. (2014). Characterisation of the first ongoing outbreak due to KPC-3-producing *Klebsiella pneumoniae* (ST512) in Spain. *Int. J. Antimicrob. Agents* 44, 538–540. doi: 10.1016/j.ijantimicag.2014.08.006

Michalopoulos, A., Virtzili, S., Rafailidis, P., Chalevelakis, G., Damala, M., and Falagas, M. E. (2010). Intravenous fosfomycin for the treatment of nosocomial infections caused by carbapenem-resistant *Klebsiella pneumoniae* in critically ill patients: a prospective evaluation. *Clin. Microbiol. Infect.* 16, 184–186. doi: 10.1111/j.1469-0691.2009.02921.x

Miro, E., Aguero, J., Larrosa, M. N., Fernandez, A., Conejo, M. C., Bou, G., et al. (2013). Prevalence and molecular epidemiology of acquired AmpC β-lactamases and carbapenemases in *Enterobacteriaceae* isolates from 35 hospitals in Spain. *Eur. J. Clin. Microbiol. Infect. Dis.* 32, 253–259. doi: 10.1007/s10096-012-1737-0

Montero, A., Ariza, J., Corbella, X., Domenech, A., Cabellos, C., Ayats, J., et al. (2004). Antibiotic combinations for serious infections caused by carbapenem-resistant *Acinetobacter baumannii* in a mouse pneumonia model. *J. Antimicrob. Chemother.* 54, 1085–1091. doi: 10.1093/jac/dkh485

Munoz-Price, L. S., Poirel, L., Bonomo, R. A., Schwaber, M. J., Daikos, G. L., Cormican, M., et al. (2013). Clinical epidemiology of the global expansion of *Klebsiella pneumoniae* carbapenemases. *Lancet Infect. Dis.* 13, 785–796. doi: 10.1016/S1473-3099(13)70190-7

Nastro, M., Rodriguez, C. H., Monge, R., Zintgraff, J., Neira, L., Rebollo, M., et al. (2014). Activity of the colistin-rifampicin combination against colistin-resistant, carbapenemase-producing Gram-negative bacteria. *J. Chemother.* 26, 211–216. doi: 10.1179/1973947813Y.0000000136

Nordmann, P., Dortet, L., and Poirel, L. (2012). Carbapenem resistance in *Enterobacteriaceae*: here is the storm! *Trends Mol. Med.* 18, 263–272. doi: 10.1016/j.molmed.2012.03.003

Nordmann, P., Naas, T., and Poirel, L. (2011). Global spread of Carbapenemase-producing *Enterobacteriaceae*. *Emerg. Infect. Dis.* 17, 1791–1798. doi: 10.3201/eid1710.110655

Oteo, J., Ortega, A., Bartolome, R., Bou, G., Conejo, C., Fernandez-Martinez, M., et al. (2015). Prospective multicenter study of carbapenemase-producing *Enterobacteriaceae* from 83 hospitals in Spain reveals high in vitro susceptibility to colistin and meropenem. *Antimicrob. Agents Chemother.* 59, 3406–3412. doi: 10.1128/AAC.00086-15

Pachon-Ibanez, M. E., Docobo-Perez, F., Jimenez-Mejias, M. E., Ibanez-Martinez, J., Garcia-Curiel, A., Pichardo, C., et al. (2011). Efficacy of rifampin, in monotherapy and in combinations, in an experimental murine pneumonia model caused by panresistant *Acinetobacter baumannii* strains. *Eur. J. Clin. Microbiol. Infect. Dis.* 30, 895–901. doi: 10.1007/s10096-011-1173-6

Pachon-Ibanez, M. E., Docobo-Perez, F., Lopez-Rojas, R., Dominguez-Herrera, J., Jimenez-Mejias, M. E., Garcia-Curiel, A., et al. (2010). Efficacy of rifampin and its combinations with imipenem, sulbactam, and colistin in experimental models of infection caused by imipenem-resistant *Acinetobacter baumannii*. *Antimicrob. Agents Chemother.* 54, 1165–1172. doi: 10.1128/AAC.00367-09

Pachon-Ibanez, M. E., Fernandez-Cuenca, F., Docobo-Perez, F., Pachon, J., and Pascual, A. (2006). Prevention of rifampicin resistance in *Acinetobacter baumannii* in an experimental pneumonia murine model, using rifampicin associated with imipenem or sulbactam. *J. Antimicrob. Chemother.* 58, 689–692. doi: 10.1093/jac/dkl303

Palacios-Baena, Z. R., Oteo, J., Conejo, C., Larrosa, M. N., Bou, G., Fernandez-Martinez, M., et al. (2016). Comprehensive clinical and epidemiological assessment of colonisation and infection due to carbapenemase-producing *Enterobacteriaceae* in Spain. *J. Infect.* 72, 152–160. doi: 10.1016/j.jinf.2015.10.008

Parra Millan, R., Jimenez Mejias, M. E., Sanchez Encinales, V., Ayerbe Algaba, R., Gutierrez Valencia, A., Pachon Ibanez, M. E., et al. (2016). Efficacy of lysophosphatidylcholine in combination with antimicrobial agents against *Acinetobacter baumannii* in experimental murine peritoneal sepsis and pneumonia models. *Antimicrob. Agents Chemother.* 60, 4464–4470. doi: 10.1128/AAC.02708-15

Pournaras, S., Vrioni, G., Neou, E., Dendrinos, J., Dimitroulia, E., Poulou, A., et al. (2011). Activity of tigecycline alone and in combination with colistin and meropenem against *Klebsiella pneumoniae* carbapenemase (KPC)-producing *Enterobacteriaceae* strains by time-kill assay. *Int. J. Antimicrob. Agents* 37, 244–247. doi: 10.1016/j.ijantimicag.2010.10.031

Rodriguez, C. H., De Ambrosio, A., Bajuk, M., Spinozzi, M., Nastro, M., Bombicino, K., et al. (2010). In vitro antimicrobials activity against endemic *Acinetobacter baumannii* multiresistant clones. *J. Infect. Dev. Ctries.* 4, 164–167. doi: 10.3855/jidc.604

Souli, M., Galani, I., Boukovalas, S., Gourgoulis, M. G., Chryssouli, Z., Kanellakopoulou, K., et al. (2011). In vitro interactions of antimicrobial combinations with fosfomycin against KPC-2-producing *Klebsiella pneumoniae* and protection of resistance development. *Antimicrob. Agents Chemother.* 55, 2395–2397. doi: 10.1128/AAC.01086-10

Souli, M., Rekatsina, P. D., Chryssouli, Z., Galani, I., Giamarellou, H., and Kanellakopoulou, K. (2009). Does the activity of the combination of imipenem and colistin in vitro exceed the problem of resistance in metallo-β-lactamase-producing *Klebsiella pneumoniae* isolates? *Antimicrob. Agents Chemother.* 53, 2133–2135. doi: 10.1128/AAC.01271-08

Tangden, T., Hickman, R. A., Forsberg, P., Lagerback, P., Giske, C. G., and Cars, O. (2014). Evaluation of double- and triple-antibiotic combinations for VIM- and NDM-producing *Klebsiella pneumoniae* by in vitro time-kill experiments. *Antimicrob. Agents Chemother.* 58, 1757–1762. doi: 10.1128/AAC.00741-13

Tascini, C., Tagliaferri, E., Giani, T., Leonildi, A., Flammini, S., Casini, B., et al. (2013). Synergistic activity of colistin plus rifampin against colistin-resistant KPC-producing *Klebsiella pneumoniae*. *Antimicrob. Agents Chemother.* 57, 3990–3993. doi: 10.1128/AAC.00179-13

Tenover, F. C., Arbeit, R. D., Goering, R. V., Mickelsen, P. A., Murray, B. E., Persing, D. H., et al. (1995). Interpreting chromosomal DNA restriction patterns produced by pulsed-field gel electrophoresis: criteria for bacterial strain typing. *J. Clin. Microbiol.* 33, 2233–2239.

Tzouvelekis, L. S., Markogiannakis, A., Psichogiou, M., Tassios, P. T., and Daikos, G. L. (2012). Carbapenemases in *Klebsiella pneumoniae* and other *Enterobacteriaceae*: an evolving crisis of global dimensions. *Clin. Microbiol. Rev.* 25, 682–707. doi: 10.1128/CMR.05035-11

Waters, N. J., Jones, R., Williams, G., and Sohal, B. (2008). Validation of a rapid equilibrium dialysis approach for the measurement of plasma protein binding. *J. Pharm. Sci.* 97, 4586–4595. doi: 10.1002/jps.21317

Wolff, M., Joly-Guillou, M. L., Farinotti, R., and Carbon, C. (1999). In vivo efficacies of combinations of beta-lactams, beta-lactamase inhibitors, and rifampin against *Acinetobacter baumannii* in a mouse pneumonia model. *Antimicrob. Agents Chemother.* 43, 1406–1411.

Zhang, Y., Huo, M., Zhou, J., and Xie, S. (2010). PKSolver: an add-in program for pharmacokinetic and pharmacodynamic data analysis in Microsoft Excel. *Comput. Methods Programs Biomed.* 99, 306–314. doi: 10.1016/j.cmpb.2010.01.007

4

Enlarging the Toolbox Against Antimicrobial Resistance: Aptamers and CRISPR-Cas

*Higor Sette Pereira†, Thaysa Leite Tagliaferri† and Tiago Antônio de Oliveira Mendes**

Laboratory of Synthetic Biology and Modelling of Biological Systems, Department of Biochemistry and Molecular Biology, Universidade Federal de Viçosa, Viçosa, Brazil

***Correspondence:**
Tiago Antônio de Oliveira Mendes
tiagoaomendes@ufv.br

†These authors share first authorship

In the post-genomic era, molecular treatments and diagnostics have been envisioned as powerful techniques to tackle the antimicrobial resistance (AMR) crisis. Among the molecular approaches, aptamers and CRISPR-Cas have gained support due to their practicality, sensibility, and flexibility to interact with a variety of extra- and intracellular targets. Those characteristics enabled the development of quick and onsite diagnostic tools as well as alternative treatments for pan-resistant bacterial infections. Even with such potential, more studies are necessary to pave the way for their successful use against AMR. In this review, we highlight those two robust techniques and encourage researchers to refine them toward AMR. Also, we describe how aptamers and CRISPR-Cas can work together with the current diagnostic and treatment toolbox.

Keywords: antimicrobial resistance, molecular diagnostic, alternative treatments, aptamer, CRISPR-Cas

ANTIBIOTIC RESISTANCE CRISIS

Despite antimicrobials' impact on modern medicine since their introduction in the first part of the 19th century (Powers, 2004; CDC, 2019), resistant bacteria quickly emerged throughout the decades. Drug resistance to all available antibiotics has been detected in clinical bacteria, threatening all advances achieved within the antibiotic era and urging for alternative treatments (CDC, 2019).

Abbreviations: ALISA, Aptamer-linked immobilized sorbent assay; AMR, Antimicrobial resistance; ARG, Antimicrobial resistance genes; CRISPR-Cas, Clustered regularly interspaced short palindromic repeats, CRISPR-associated enzymes; crRNA, CRISPR RNA; COVID-19, Coronavirus disease 2019; DNA, Deoxyribonucleic acid; FDA, Food and Drug Administration; HIV, Human immunodeficiency virus; KPC, *Klebsiella pneumoniae* carbapenemase; LAMP, Loop-mediated isothermal amplification; MALDI-TOF MS, Matrix-assisted laser desorption/ionization time-of-flight mass spectrometry; MRSA, Methicillin-resistant *Staphylococcus aureus*; NDM, New Delhi metallo-β-lactamase; NGS, Next-generation sequencing; PAM, Protospacer adjacent motif; PBP, Penicillin-binding protein; RNA, Ribonucleic acid; RNP, Ribonucleoprotein; RT-qPCR, quantitative reverse transcription PCR; SARS, Severe acute respiratory syndrome; SARS-CoV-2, Severe acute respiratory syndrome coronavirus 2; SELEX, Systematic evolution of ligands by exponential enrichment; sgRNA, single-guide RNA; siRNA, Small interfering RNA; SNP, Single-nucleotide polymorphism; TALEN, Transcription activator-like effector nucleases; tracrRNA, trans-activating CRISPR RNA.

Bacteria have developed resistance mechanisms to avoid, disrupt, eject, or resist the currently used antimicrobials (**Box 1**). They can be intrinsically resistant to antibiotics by using structural or functional inherent bacterial features or acquire resistance via genetic mutations or by horizontal transference of genetic elements (Blair et al., 2015; Munita and Arias, 2016).

The spread of bacterial resistance mechanisms has been much faster than the development of new treatments. New investments on antimicrobial research have been discouraged due to their elevated production costs and long-term development process (Adams and Brantner, 2010). On top of that, the misuse and over-prescription of antibiotics, which stem from uncertainties in diagnosis, contribute to the antimicrobial resistance (AMR) crisis escalation (Llor and Bjerrum, 2014; Malik and Bhattacharyya, 2019). The lack of rapid diagnostic tools directly affects initial treatment decisions, which might lead to empirical treatment guided only by clinical presentation (Fischer et al., 2004; Leekha et al., 2011).

Phenotypic-based diagnostics are currently considered as gold standards in AMR assessment. The "catch-all" resistance characteristic of phenotypic tests enables the evaluation of microbial susceptibility in a relatively unbiased way (Mitsakakis et al., 2018). Although efforts have been made to provide quick phenotypic tests (~7 h) (Pancholi et al., 2018) to better guide antibiotic treatment, the most used techniques still require microorganism culture, with a turnaround time of around 18 h. This delays the availability of the AMR profiles, which might be accessible up to 72 h after sample collection (Leekha et al., 2011). Besides time-to-result limitation, phenotypic tests generally require laboratory structure (Mitsakakis et al., 2018). Therefore, quicker and accessible diagnostic tools are imperative to guide the first medical decisions regarding antimicrobial therapy prescription worldwide.

MOLECULAR APPROACHES

The search for more precise molecular diagnostic tools with quicker turnaround times has been encouraged to better guide clinical practice and public health policies. The recent global SARS-CoV-2 (severe acute respiratory syndrome coronavirus 2) outbreak has shown that in a matter of weeks, diagnostic centers have been overloaded with patients' samples and quick result release is required for viral spread control. So far, until 21 December 2020, SARS-CoV-2 virus infected 75,704,857 individuals, with 1,690,061 deaths worldwide[1]. We dare to draw here a parallel between SARS-CoV-2 and the AMR crisis. Currently, AMR infections cause around 700,000 deaths per year (O'Neil, 2016). In both cases, an early diagnosis would give trustworthy information for discrimination and contention of the causative agent. With alarming death numbers, the exploration of alternative treatments and diagnostics comes into the spotlight as an attempt to revert the current scenario caused by AMR.

Different molecular tools have been employed as a diagnostic to identify infectious disease agents and their resistance profile. RT-qPCR (quantitative reverse transcription PCR) and NGS (Next-Generation Sequencing) have been currently playing a key role in the diagnostics of the SARS-CoV-2, different from what happened in the 2002 SARS outbreak (Sheridan, 2020). qPCR is also an outstanding tool for the molecular detection of antimicrobial resistance genes (ARGs) (Waseem et al., 2019) directly from patient samples such as urine, blood, and cerebrospinal fluid (Singh et al., 2017). In addition to qPCR, metagenomic, LAMP (Loop-mediated isothermal amplification), and whole genome sequencing approaches not only characterize pathogens at the species level but also detect ARGs (Zankari et al., 2012; Dekker, 2018; Ota et al., 2019).

The molecular diagnostic tools described above offer an abundant panel to recognize DNA and RNA of infectious microorganisms. Complementarily, proteomics- and metabolomics-based techniques have been gaining momentum into the clinical molecular diagnostic field, for instance, MALDI-TOF MS (Matrix-Assisted Laser Desorption/Ionization Time-of-Flight Mass Spectrometry) (Patrinos et al., 2017). However, these tools require expensive equipment and laboratory structure, hampering their wide implementation as *in loco* diagnostic tools.

Aptamers and CRISPR-Cas (clustered repetitive interspaced short palindromic repeats, CRISPR-associated enzymes) systems have been slowly gaining support in clinical diagnosis and treatment of infectious diseases. Both can be employed as an onsite diagnostic tool with a quick turnaround time, which makes them more interesting than other methods targeting proteins or nucleic acids. Therefore, reviewing these two robust techniques attempts to encourage molecular biologist researchers to develop and refine clinical molecular tools against ARGs. Those methods do not necessarily intend to substitute the already implemented diagnostic approaches, but to stimulate their combination to circumvent antibiotic misuse. Also, their application in therapy will be reviewed to help paving the way for their use as treatments against multidrug-resistant agents.

APPLICATION OF APTAMERS INTO DETECTION AND NEUTRALIZATION OF AMR FACTORS

A substantial boost in aptamer application in research and clinical institutes has been noted worldwide (McKeague et al., 2015). Also called chemical antibodies (Toh et al., 2015), most aptamers interact with their targets in a constant equilibrium with binding affinities up to 1 pM (Ha et al., 2017). They offer a cheap large-scale production with chemical modifications, low or no immunogenicity, small size (close to 3 nm), flexibility in tridimensional structure, and great stability in different conditions of pH, temperature, and organic solvents (Yoon and Rossi, 2018). Also, aptamers interact with high sensitivity toward their targets, being able to discriminate a single amino acid mutation (Chen et al., 2015). Due to their small size, aptamers reach cavities that are often not accessible to monoclonal antibodies and, therefore, penetrate cell tissues more easily (Xiang et al., 2015). In this process, intracellular

[1] https://covid19.who.int/

BOX 1 | Antimicrobial resistance mechanism.

Resistance mechanisms date back to thousands of years and have been probably used to endure the presence of toxic compounds present in nature—including antimicrobials derived from different microorganisms, while they also provide alternative cellular functions (Allen et al., 2010; D'costa et al., 2011). Bacteria can evade antimicrobials via reduction of drug intracellular concentration either by low membrane permeability or through antibiotic efflux; target modification by genetic mutation or post-translational modification; and inactivation of the antibiotic by hydrolysis or its modification (Blair et al., 2015). With the introduction and constant presence of antimicrobials in medical care, agriculture and animal health, the spread of resistant microorganisms and the evolution of their defense strategies have been accelerated (**Figure 1**; CDC, 2019). From all resistance mechanisms, genes responsible for antibiotic inactivation and target alteration (**Figure 1** I and III, respectively) are commonly spread by plasmids and phage transduction (Munita and Arias, 2016; Calero-Caceres et al., 2019). Antibiotic inactivation is a usual strategy adopted for instance against beta-lactams and aminoglycosides. Beta-lactams can be hydrolyzed by enzymes encoded by the *bla* genes (beta-lactamase genes), such as bla_{TEM}, bla_{KPC} and bla_{OXA}. Aminoglycosides, by its turn, are chemically inactivated by mainly three biochemical reaction, named adenylation, acetylation, and phosphorylation catalyzed by the enzymes nucleotidyltransferases (ANT), acetyltransferases (AAC), and phosphotransferases (APH), respectively (Doi et al., 2016; Munita and Arias, 2016; Bush and Bradford, 2019). An advantage of the hydrolysis over the chemical alteration strategy is the requirement of water instead of chemical compounds as a co-substrate, which ease enzyme activity outside the cell. Target alteration can be achieved by four main strategies, affecting several antimicrobials (not limited to the examples), as follows: (i) Target protection. One of the best-studied examples involves the determinants Tet(M) and Tet(O), which confers resistance to tetracycline. They interact with the ribosome and dislodge the drug from its binding site. (ii) Mutation of the antimicrobial target site. The development of mutations in the chromosomal genes *gyrA-gyrB* and *parC-parE* codifying for DNA gyrase and topoisomerase IV, respectively, promotes resistance against fluoroquinolones. (iii) Enzymatic alteration. Macrolide resistance is acquired by *erm* genes (erythromycin ribosomal methylation), which codify enzymes responsible for 50S ribosomal subunit methylation. This alteration weakens the binding of the erythromycin to the ribosome. (iv) Replacement/bypass of the target. Beta-lactam resistance is frequently acquired by Gram-positive microorganisms via *mecA* gene. The gene encodes an exogen penicillin-binding protein (PBP2a) that has low affinity for the beta-lactams, opposite to what happens to endogen PBPs (Munita and Arias, 2016).

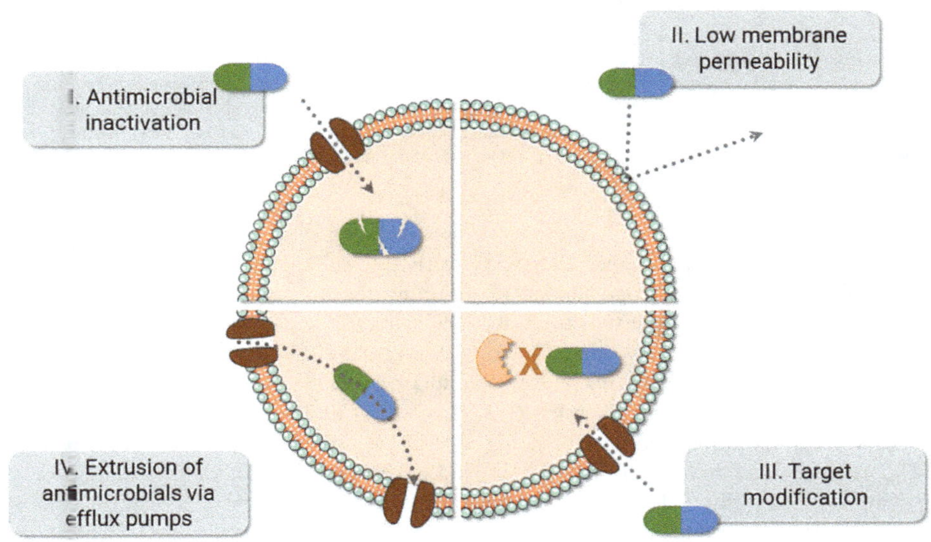

FIGURE 1 | Bacteria fight back antimicrobials. The main bacterial resistance mechanisms are displayed above. Of note, resistance against one class of antibiotics can be achieved using different strategies. For instance, resistance against beta-lactams can be caused by PBP2a (III), beta-lactamase (I), or by a combination of different mechanisms, i.e., reduction of porins (II) and the use of beta-lactamase (I). Also, efflux pumps can expel several antibiotic classes (IV) and are frequently present in multidrug resistance bacteria.

aptamers could be internalized by either a clathrin-dependent or -independent mechanism and co-localized in subcellular compartments, directly associated to its target, as reviewed in Yoon and Rossi (2018; **Figure 2**).

Single-stranded oligonucleotides can assume several secondary conformations such as hairpin, loop, pseudoknot, and G-quadruplex, which assure a unique folding for each sequence and allow interaction with specific sites (Yunn et al., 2015). DNA and RNA aptamers have similar binding characteristics, although DNA nucleotides have lower operating cost and offer greater stability than RNA, which in turn have greater versatility in their three-dimensional structures that directly affect target affinity.

Aptamer selection commonly occurs via a randomized process of systematic evolution of ligands by exponential enrichment (SELEX), firstly reported in 1990 (Ellington and Szostak, 1990; Tuerk and Gold, 1990). SELEX is based on iterative rounds of incubation of the oligonucleotide pool with the target, frequently divided into four stages: incubation, partition, recovery, and amplification. Also, aptamer–target affinity slowly increases alongside the rounds until the most specific aptamer is selected. SELEX allows greater versatility of binding conditions, which favors the adaptation of selected oligonucleotides to different cellular and non-cellular environments (McKeague et al., 2015).

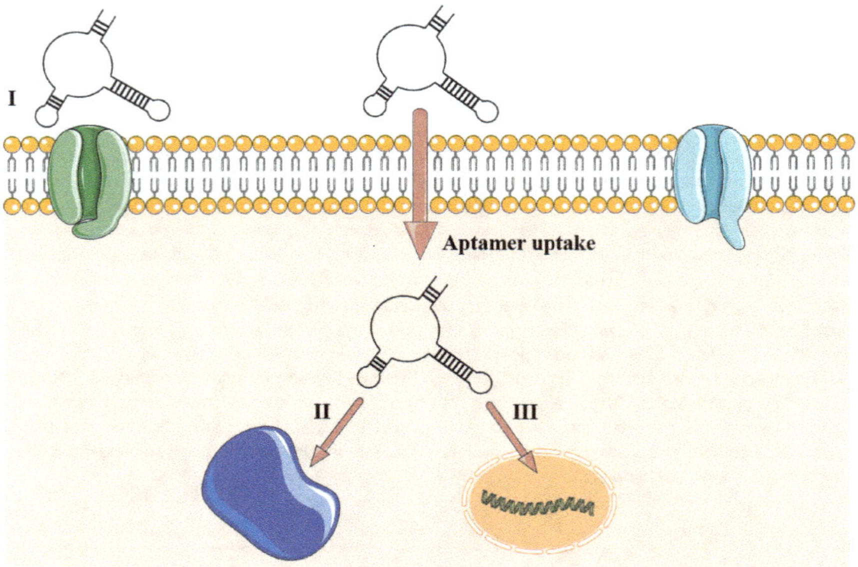

FIGURE 2 | Aptamer–target interactions in extra- and intracellular environments. (I) Aptamer recognizing cell membrane receptor or surface protein. The aptamer is uptaken into the cellular environment and can be located in some subcellular compartments such as lysosome, mitochondria, Golgi, and endoplasmic reticulum or guided to the nucleus in eukaryotic cells (Yoon and Rossi, 2018) or be stored into the cytoplasm of prokaryotic cells. (II) Cytosolic intracellular aptamers recognizing circulating proteins. (III) Nuclear intramers interacting directly with genetic elements. Aptamers' uptake is mediated to the intracellular environment by a clathrin-dependent mechanism. Clathrin is a group of proteins present in membrane cavities that assist in membrane vesicle formation during the molecule internalization by endocytosis.

Aptamer selection against many biological and chemical targets has been described (Qiao et al., 2018; Dalirirad and Steckl, 2020), along with its use in drug development (Esposito et al., 2018), bioimaging (Kim et al., 2019), food inspection (Duan et al., 2016), genetic modulation (Mol et al., 2019), and as a delivery vehicle (Zhuang et al., 2020). In antiviral therapy, G-3 aptamer dually inhibits HIV-1 cell replication both by blocking virus entrance via CCR5 receptor and by delivering a siRNA that decreases HIV-1 cytoplasmatic traffic (Zhou et al., 2015). Also, aptamers blocked quorum sensing and inhibited biofilm formation in *Pseudomonas aeruginosa* infections (Zhao et al., 2019). Even with many progresses, there is currently only one aptamer approved for clinical use, named pegaptanib. It is the main component of Macugen®, released by the FDA in 2004 to treat age-related macular degeneration (Gragoudas et al., 2004). Recently, there have been 10 therapeutic aptamers at different stages of clinical trials (Kaur et al., 2018), most of them employed to inhibit protein–protein interaction or act as antagonist (Yunn et al., 2015). To date, there is no aptamer currently approved by FDA for diagnostic purposes, even though they fit the quality standards of the diagnostic industry: affordable, sensitive, specific, user-friendly, and robust.

Different diagnostic devices based on aptamers have been proposed, including Aptamer-Linked Immobilized Sorbent Assay (ALISA), dot-blot, lateral-flow strips conjugated to nanomaterials, and the promising aptamer-based sensors (Stoltenburg et al., 2016; Shin et al., 2018; Su et al., 2018; Xiong et al., 2020). Aptasensors can be conjugated to a wide diversity of reporter molecules without modification of their activity (McKeague et al., 2015). Signal transducers commonly conjugated to aptasensors include but are not limited to colorimetric, electrochemical, and fluorescent approaches (Bai et al., 2017; Bayrac et al., 2017; Cai et al., 2019). Linking aptamer-based biosensors with nanomaterials can increase specificity and sensitivity of target binding up to 10-fold and offers a platform for rapid point-of-care diagnostic (<1 h) (Dalirirad and Steckl, 2020). Aptasensors have well-established protocols of chemical conjugation of aptamers with color or signal-transductor molecules, such as gold, silver, platinum, iron oxide nanoparticles, or carbon nanotubes and graphene oxide (Duan et al., 2016; Dehghani et al., 2018; Gao et al., 2018; Hua et al., 2018; Das et al., 2019a; Fan et al., 2020). The application of aptasensors for disease diagnosis has been tested in different samples, e.g., plasma and spiked nasal swab (Qiao et al., 2018), cultured bacteria (Maldonado et al., 2020), and urine and serum samples (Su et al., 2018). A lateral-flow paper strip conjugated with a gold nanoparticle aptamer-based sensor was developed to onsite detection of dopamine in urine samples (Dalirirad and Steckl, 2020).

When repurposed to bacteria, aptamers could recognize them by binding to antigens or cell surface receptors, or interacting with the whole cell through unknown targets (Tang et al., 2016; Song M. Y. et al., 2017; Shin et al., 2019). Although there are uncertainties concerning the mechanisms of aptamer uptake in bacteria, a report indicates that aptamers could traffic inside bacterial cells (Afrasiabi et al., 2020), similarly to what is shown in **Figure 2**. From 2016 to 2020, several papers have reported the use of aptamers applied to diagnostics of bacterial infections

(**Table 1**). Nearly all studies employed biosensors based on DNA aptamers, which indicates that for diagnostic purposes, the DNA stability overcomes the advantage of tridimensional possibilities of RNA. It is worth mentioning that only three of these studies targeted resistant bacteria or products of ARGs. First, Fan et al. (2020) made a graphene-oxide aptasensor based on peroxidase-like activity for the detection of purified PBP2a protein, encoded by the *mec*A gene. Also, Maldonado et al. (2020) employed a fast and label-free photonic pegylated aptasensor that recognizes both pure PBP2a protein and methicillin-resistant *Staphylococcus aureus* (MRSA)-infected cells in culture. Finally, Qiao et al. (2018) detected PBP2a in *S. aureus* cells collected in clinical plasma and spiked nasal swab samples infected with MRSA strains using a single bacterial lysis step. Predominantly, the diagnostic approach using aptamer has been focusing on the detection of the whole cell instead of its biological specific components, such as proteins or toxins. Therefore, due to the well-established protein-SELEX approach, there is still room for finding highly specific aptamers that bind to proteins associated with ARGs and enrich the diagnostic toolbox.

CRISPR-CAS AS A TOOL AGAINST ANTIMICROBIAL-RESISTANT PATHOGENS

CRISPR-Cas is a ribonucleoprotein (RNP) prokaryotic complex present in 50% of the bacteria and in most archaea that behaves as a prokaryotic adaptive immune system (Makarova et al., 2015). The system confers protection against mobile genetic elements, i.e., bacteriophages, plasmids, and transposons in three coordinated phases: adaptation, CRISPR RNA (crRNA) biogenesis, and interference (Hille et al., 2018). Nearly all CRISPR-Cas system counts on an ingenious mechanism to prevent self-targeting. This includes the recognition of a short sequence called protospacer adjacent motif (PAM) during adaptation and interference stages, present only in foreign nucleic acids (Mojica et al., 2009; Marraffini and Sontheimer, 2010).

Based mainly on the signature *Cas* genes, the new classification of CRISPR-Cas systems includes two different classes, six types, and 33 subtypes (Makarova et al., 2020). The most widespread class 1 CRISPR-Cas comprises types I, III, and IV. It is characterized by effector complexes with multiple Cas proteins responsible for a coordinated action from pre-crRNA processing to target cleavage. By its turn, class 2 consists of types II, V, and VI, which contains a single-protein effector module able to recognize and cleave the targeting nucleic acid (**Table 2**; Makarova et al., 2020).

Upon unraveling the CRISPR-Cas potential of gene editing in an easier, cheaper, and flexible way compared to previously established tools [for instance, TALENs (transcription activator-like effector nucleases) and Zinc-finger nucleases], the systems have been quickly repurposed to the biomedical and biotechnology fields (Chen and Gao, 2014; Liu et al., 2018; Zhang et al., 2019; Li et al., 2020). Class 2 CRISPR-Cas has been an attractive option for gene editing as a result of the effector module's simpler architecture when compared to class 1 (Makarova et al., 2020). Target specificity and cutting activity of the nucleases can be virtually programmed to any gene of interest by means of the short-length crRNA sequence. The engineering of a single-guide RNA (sgRNA) by fusing Cas9 crRNA and tracrRNA was a benchmark for gene editing (Jinek et al., 2012), but off-target effects still hold back CRISPR-Cas full potential. Several studies have tried to overcome this drawback by employing a plethora of modifications to increase the system specificity for gene editing (Kleinstiver et al., 2016; Slaymaker et al., 2016; Chen et al., 2017; Casini et al., 2018; Lee et al., 2018). Similarly, collateral effects of some Cas enzymes, i.e., the ability to indiscriminately (*trans-*) cleave ssDNA/ssRNA unleashed by site-specific DNA/RNA (*cis-*) bound by the crRNA, may also be a limitation for gene editing. However, here, this feature has been exploited for diagnostic purposes.

The collateral effect of Cas12 and Cas13 has been used as a key step to create several diagnostic platforms, such as DETECTR, HOLMES (both using Cas12), SHERLOCK, and CARMEN-Cas13 (the last two using Cas13) (Gootenberg et al., 2017; Chen et al., 2018; Li S. Y. et al., 2018; Ackerman et al., 2020). All platforms have similar diagnostic strategies, which involve the incubation of Cas enzymes (Cas12/Cas13) along with the target nucleic acid and fluorescent ssDNA/ssRNA reporters. By detecting the target nucleic acid, the Cas enzymes *trans*-cleave the quenched-fluorescent ssDNA/ssRNA reporters inserted into the platform, generating a robust fluorescent signal from around 1-h incubation (**Figure 3**) with a good correlation with PCR-based methods (Gootenberg et al., 2017; Chen et al., 2018; Gootenberg et al., 2018). In order to achieve attomolar sensitivity, the nucleic acid detection platforms were coupled to DNA amplification steps (i.e., PCR, recombinase polymerase amplification, and loop-mediated amplification) or reverse transcriptase combined with a DNA amplification step and T7 transcription for RNA targets (Gootenberg et al., 2017; Chen et al., 2018; Gootenberg et al., 2018; Li S. Y. et al., 2018; Ackerman et al., 2020; Broughton et al., 2020). To further enhance signal sensitivity, CRISPR type III effector nuclease Csm6, responsible for non-specific RNA degradation, can be combined with Cas13 activity (Gootenberg et al., 2018).

CARMEN-Cas13 and SHERLOCK have also been explored for multiplexing assays. The first one was specifically developed for this purpose and uses droplets containing either sample or detection solution, arranged pairwise. CARMEN can test more than 4500 crRNA–target pairs on a single microfluidic chip, which represents a simultaneous detection of around 170 agents (Ackerman et al., 2020). SHERLOCK, however, explored different *trans*-cleavage ssRNA preferences of Cas13 orthologs to develop a four-channel single-reaction multiplexing (Gootenberg et al., 2018). A different multiplexing strategy is employed by FLASH, a platform that uses Cas9 to enrich low-abundance targets from complex backgrounds (including clinical specimens) before NGS (**Figure 3**; Quan et al., 2019). Both CARMEN-Cas13 and FLASH offered an important multiplexing capacity but rely on robust laboratory structure, which may impar its implementation in less developed regions. SHERLOCK, however, has demonstrated its feasibility also as a paper-based test, which

TABLE 1 | Report of literature aptamers applied in the diagnostic of bacterial infections from 2016 to 2020.

Target	Oligo	Binding affinity or LOD	References
Acinetobacter baumannii isolates	DNA	7.547 ± 1.353 pM	Rasoulinejad and Gargari, 2016
Bacillus subtilis, Citrobacter freundii, Escherichia coli, Enterobacter aerogenes, Klebsiella pneumoniae, and Staphylococcus epidermidis cells	DNA	9.22–38.5 nM	Song M. Y. et al., 2017
Campylobacter jejuni cells	DNA	100 CFU ml−1	Dehghani et al., 2018
Escherichia coli and *Staphylococcus aureus* pathogenic cells	DNA	100 CFU ml−1	Xu et al., 2018
Escherichia coli ATCC cells	DNA	11.97 ± 2.94 nM	Marton et al., 2016
Escherichia coli cells	DNA	3 CFU ml−1	Jin et al., 2017
Escherichia coli cells	DNA	0.66 CFU ml−1	Hua et al., 2018
Escherichia coli O157 cells	DNA	107.6 ± 67.8 pM	Amraee et al., 2017
Escherichia coli O157:H7 cells	DNA	1.46 × 103 CFU ml−1	Yu et al., 2018
Escherichia coli whole cells	RNA	2 × 104 CFU ml−1	Dua et al., 2016
Escherichia coli whole-cells	DNA	102 CFU ml−1	Wu et al., 2017
Glycolipid antigen of *Mycobacterium tuberculosis*	DNA	668 ± 159 nM	Tang et al., 2016
Gram-negative outer membrane vesicles	DNA	25 ng/ml	Shin et al., 2019
HspX protein in tuberculous meningitis	DNA	10 pg	Das et al., 2019b
Listeria monocytogenes cells	DNA	2.5 CFU ml−1	Suh et al., 2018
Methicillin-resistant *Staphylococcus aureus* strains	DNA	1.38 × 103 CFU ml−1	Qiao et al., 2018
MPT64 antigen of *Mycobacterium tuberculosis*	DNA	0.2 fg ml−1	Bai et al., 2017
MPT64 antigen of *Mycobacterium tuberculosis*	DNA	100 CFU ml−1	Li N. et al., 2018
Mycobacterium tuberculosis cells	DNA	100 CFU ml−1	Zhang et al., 2017
Mycobacterium tuberculosis H37Ra cells	DNA	5.09 ± 1.43 nM	Mozioglu et al., 2016
Mycolactone in Buruli ulcer	RNA	1.59–73.0 μM	Sakyi et al., 2016
Mycoplasma-infected cells	DNA	Not informed	Liu et al., 2019
Neisseria meningitidis serogroup B	DNA	28.3–39.1 pM	Mirzakhani et al., 2017
PBP2a detection	DNA	20 nM	Fan et al., 2020
PBP2a in nosocomial infections	DNA	29 CFU ml^{-1}	Maldonado et al., 2020
Protein A of *Staphylococcus aureus*	DNA	11.3 nM	Stoltenburg et al., 2016
Protein A of *Staphylococcus aureus*	DNA	10 CFU ml^{-1}	Reich et al., 2017
Pseudomonas aeruginosa cells	DNA	100 CFU ml^{-1}	Gao et al., 2018
Pseudomonas aeruginosa cells	DNA	60 CFU ml^{-1}	Das et al., 2019a
Salmonella enterica serovar *typhimurium* in milk samples	DNA	3.37×10^2 CFU ml^{-1}	Zhang et al., 2018
Salmonella enteritidis cells	DNA	0.309 μM	Bayrac and Oktem, 2017
Salmonella enteritis cells	DNA	25 CFU ml^{-1}	Chinnappan et al., 2017
Salmonella typhimurium cells	DNA	10 CFU ml^{-1}	Duan et al., 2016
Salmonella typhimurium cells	DNA	123 ± 23 nM	Lavu et al., 2016
Salmonella Typhimurium cells	DNA	1 CFU ml^{-1}	Ren et al., 2019
Salmonella Typhimurium cells	DNA	80 CFU ml^{-1}	Wang et al., 2020
Salmonella Typhimurium cells	DNA	10 CFU ml^{-1}	Appaturi et al., 2020
Shigella sonnei cells	DNA	15.89 ± 1.77 nM	Song M. S. et al., 2017
Staphylococcus aureus and *Escherichia coli* cells	DNA	10–2,000 CFU ml^{-1}	Shen et al., 2016
Staphylococcus aureus cells	DNA	16 CFU ml^{-1}	Kurt et al., 2016
Staphylococcus aureus cells	DNA	10^3 CFU ml^{-1}	Bayrac et al., 2017
Staphylococcus aureus cells	DNA	39 CFU ml^{-1}	Cai et al., 2019
Streptococcus pyogenes cells	DNA	7 nM	Hamula et al., 2016
Streptococcus pyogenes serotype M3 cell	DNA	7.47 ± 1.72 pM	Alfavian et al., 2017
Vibrio parahaemolyticus cells	DNA	$2.04e^{-9} \pm 0.12$ M	Ahn et al., 2018
Vibrio parahaemolyticus cells	DNA	10 CFU ml^{-1}	Sun et al., 2019

Papers recovered on the PUBMED NCBI website. Binding affinity and Limit of Detection (LOD) were represented by K_d and CFU counting, respectively.

amplifies its potential to become a widely spread quick-and-cheap ($0.61 per test) diagnostic method (Gootenberg et al., 2017). The addition of an extra step called HUDSON before SHERLOCK protocol enabled the viral detection directly from bodily fluids, contributing to the creation of a field-deployable diagnostic platform (Myhrvold et al., 2018). Its efficiency to detect bacteria directly from patient samples, however, is yet to be defined. Also, SHERLOCK might benefit from Cas13 engineering

TABLE 2 | General features of CRISPR-Cas systems based on the most well-characterized subtypes.

Type	Multisubunity RNP complex	Single protein	Signature enzyme	Seed sequence	Most common substrates		Cleavage
					RNA	DNA	
I	X		Cas3	1–5 nt and 7–8 nt		X	Single-stranded DNA cleavage
II		X	Cas9	10–12 nt		X	Blunt double-stranded DNA break
III	X		Cas10	Not defined*	X	X	Specific and non-specific ssRNA cleavage. Double-stranded DNA break
IV	Defective CRISPR-Cas loci typically lacking the effector nuclease and the adaptation module						
V		X	Cas12	~18 nt		X	Double-stranded DNA break with staggered overhangs, non-specific ssDNA break
VI		X	Cas13	Not defined#	X		Specific and non-specific ssRNA cleavage

*Seed sequence: PAM-proximal sequence in which full complementarity is required for CRISPR-Cas interference. As (i) some CRISPR-Cas subtypes have promiscuous PAM sequences, (ii) the site sequence varies among the subtypes; the PAM sequences have not been displayed in this table. Gleditzsch et al. (2019) review the PAM recognition strategies for all CRISPR-Cas types and engineering approaches to change the PAM recognition sequence. *Inconsistent conclusions regarding the seed region of CRISPR type III: absence of seed or its presence in the 5′ end (Cao et al., 2016) or 3′ end (Peng et al., 2015). #Central seed region proposed for Cas13a (Abudayyeh et al., 2016; Liu et al. 2017). Table based on Semenova et al. (2011); Chen et al. (2018), Hille et al. (2018), and Makarova et al. (2020).*

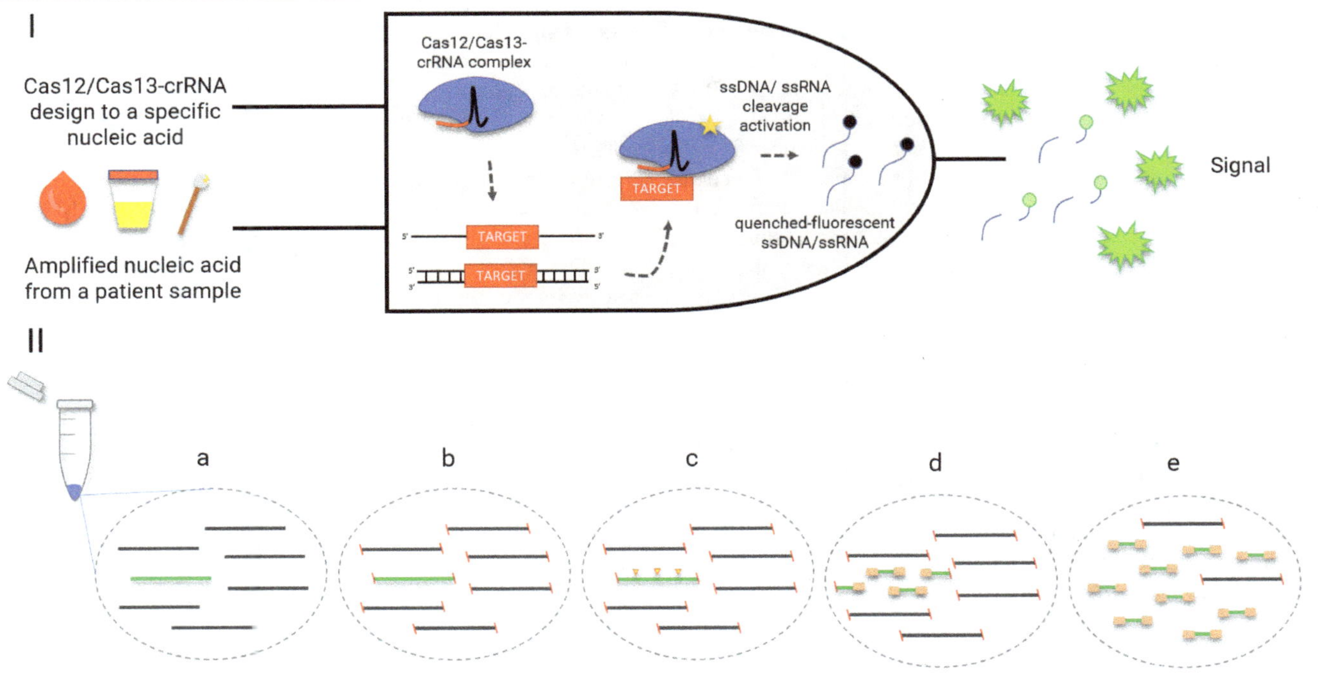

FIGURE 3 | CRISPR-Cas-based diagnostics. (I) A logic gate type "AND" of CRISPR-Cas12/13-based diagnostics. Amplified nucleic acid from patient samples can be used as input. Attomolar concentrations of RNA extracted from serum or urine samples could be detected. Without purification, Cas13 could detect RNA in samples containing up to 2% serum. The diagnostic could be performed also in cfDNA liquid biopsy samples and DNA extracted from anal swabs (Gootenberg et al., 2017; Chen et al., 2018; Gootenberg et al., 2018). A specific crRNA design to match a desired target, for instance, an antimicrobial resistance gene, is coupled with the Cas12/Cas13 as a second necessary input for the diagnostic. Once the target-positive sample is identified by the Cas12/Cas13-crRNA complex, the fluorescent output is generated. The fluorescent signal is a result of a collateral *trans*-cleavage of the quenched-fluorescent ssDNA/ssRNA by Cas12/Cas13, respectively. (II) CRISPR-Cas9 enrichment for NGS detection (Quan et al., 2019). (a) DNA or cDNA sequences containing the gene of interest (green); (b) blockage of DNA extremities; (c) CRISPR-Cas9 cleaves the target gene into fragments appropriately sized for NGS (yellow arrows); (d) ligation of universal sequencing adapters; (e) enrichment of the target sequence, which is now ready for NGS.

in order to increase target preference options and therefore the multiplexing panel.

When focusing on ARGs, *Klebsiella pneumoniae* carbapenemase (KPC) and New Delhi metallo-β-lactamase (NDM) were precisely detected and distinguished from five clinical isolates of *K. pneumoniae* (Gootenberg et al., 2017). Also, HIV drug resistance mutations from 22 patient samples could be identified (Ackerman et al., 2020). As an advantage, these platforms offer a highly specific detection of single-nucleotide polymorphisms (SNPs), which can be valuable to precisely distinguish any desired resistance gene variant (Li S. Y. et al., 2018; Myhrvold et al., 2018).

Of note, the power of the platforms to face real-world challenges has been demonstrated with the detection of SARS-CoV-2 during the COVID-19 pandemic (Ackerman et al., 2020; Broughton et al., 2020) and with the FDA emergency authorization for CRISPR SARS-CoV-2 Rapid Diagnostic using SHERLOCK platform (Guglielmi, 2020).

When employed against AMR, CRISPR-Cas9, Cas3, and Cas13 have been explored as a powerful sequence-specific antimicrobial. Cell death is an expected outcome when sgRNA is directed to genes on the chromosome or plasmids containing a toxin–antitoxin system. For vectors without toxin–antitoxin, plasmid clearance or drastic copy number reduction can be achieved when targeting plasmids up to 300 copies/cell (Bikard et al., 2014; Citorik et al., 2014; Yosef et al., 2015; Kiga et al., 2020; Tagliaferri et al., 2020). Consequently to plasmid clearance in clinical isolates, other non-targeting ARGs harbored on the target vector were also eliminated, and antibiotic reusability could be confirmed in a *Galleria mellonella* infection model (Tagliaferri et al., 2020). Several variants or sub-variants of the resistance gene can be covered with one sgRNA/crRNA directed to a conserved genetic region (Kim et al., 2016; Tagliaferri et al., 2020), while selecting a sequence from a variable region may be a strategy to achieve a narrow-spectrum effect. CRISPR-Cas-mediated interference can also be fine-tuned according to the delivery approach. CRISPR-Cas delivery can be mediated by bacteriophages, and the specificity of phage–host interactions is an advantage when the target is placed in complex environments, such as microbiota (Bikard et al., 2014; Citorik et al., 2014; Yosef et al., 2015). Alternatively, the CRISPR-Cas system can be delivered via conjugative plasmid (Citorik et al., 2014; Rodrigues et al., 2019; Ruotsalainen et al., 2019). Opposite to the phage-mediated approach, lack of specific receptors for plasmid uptake during conjugation is considered as an advantage over phage delivery, as mutations in the receptors may lead to phage resistance. On the other hand, the conjugation rate is slower when compared to transduction (Ruotsalainen et al., 2019).

DISCUSSION AND FUTURE DIRECTIONS

Even with eminent demand, little has been explored of CRISPR-Cas and aptamer potential toward treatment of bacterial infection. As for CRISPR-Cas approach, Cas9 immunogenicity must be considered (Crudele and Chamberlain, 2018), as well as the definition of the most appropriate delivery method to optimize CRISPR-Cas effect in targeting bacteria within complex microbial communities. Environmental assessments may be required to evaluate risks involved on plasmid clearance and bacterial death, which can affect the frequency of non-targeting bacterial species and non-targeting plasmids. Also, with the ordinary or induced death of the targeting bacteria, CRISPR-Cas nucleic acid will naturally be released into the environment and strategies to prevent spread and horizontal transference of CRISPR-Cas system still need to be developed.

Important limitations of *in vivo* use of aptamers stem from their susceptibility to nuclease degradation and rapid elimination due to renal filtration, but chemical adjustments to the oligonucleotide structure have contributed to decrease those shortcomings (Rohloff et al., 2014). As an FDA-approved aptamer-based therapy is already a reality, we believe that the extension of this technology to other fields, including AMR, is a matter of time.

In contrast to treatment application, CRISPR-Cas-mediated diagnostic has been recently FDA-approved for detecting SARS-CoV-2, paving the way for further applications. Its high scalability and multiplexing properties are of great value for the detection and surveillance of the wide varieties of ARGs. A limitation of this approach is the target of either DNA or RNA, which confirms the presence but not the functionality of the ARGs. Aptamers by their turn target ARG products, but in order to be used as an independent diagnostic tool, increased sensitivity to attomolar levels may be required to bacterial detection in bloodstream (Kelley, 2017). As a counterpoint, the target flexibility of CRISPR-Cas, its simplicity, and the rational design of sgRNA/crRNA can be an advantage over the more complex and randomized process of aptamer selection.

We envisioned that, in the near future, CRISPR-Cas and aptamers can be combined to treat and/or diagnose resistant bacterial infections due to their aforementioned complementary characteristics. Together, those strategies have already shown to reduce CRISPR-Cas-related off-target effects in the HEK293 cell line (Zhao et al., 2020) and to increase the delivery selectivity in liver cells (Zhuang et al., 2020), and the combination was a powerful and reliable molecular sensor able to detect nasopharyngeal carcinoma biomarkers (Li et al., 2021). Whether their combined characteristics will also be beneficial for AMR diagnostics and for treating infections caused by resistant bacteria is yet to be determined. A recent study developed a strategy to recognize surface proteins on MRSA strains by aptamer and CRISPR-Cas12a-assisted rolling circle amplification (Xu et al., 2020). Still, there is a gallery of CRISPR-Cas/aptamer combinations and target bacteria to be tested, as well as further optimizations to achieve attomolar sensitivity.

Studies employing aptamer and CRISPR-Cas for diagnostics have demonstrated their ability to provide shorter turnaround time results than the gold standard AMR phenotypic tests, which can take up to 72 h to be released. This, along with the possibility of developing paper-based diagnostics, highlights the techniques' potential to be employed as a first guidance to clinical decisions related to antimicrobial use. Altogether, the molecular approaches may offer a suitable solution to circumvent antibiotic misuse in the first antibiotic prescription, currently guided only by empirical decisions.

AUTHOR CONTRIBUTIONS

HP, TT, and TM designed and wrote the manuscript. HP and TT analyzed the data. All authors contributed to the article and approved the submitted version.

FUNDING

The group received funding from Conselho Nacional de Desenvolvimento Científico e Tecnológico (CNPq), Coordenação de Aperfeiçoamento de Pessoal de Nível Superior (CAPES), Fundação de Amparo à Pesquisa do Estado de Minas Gerais (FAPEMIG), Fundação Arthur Bernardes, and the Bill and Melinda Gates Foundation (Grant No. OPP1193112). HP was supported by CNPq Ph.D. Fellowship. TT was supported by CNPq Postdoc Fellowship—Brazil (160598/2019-2).

REFERENCES

Abudayyeh, O. O., Gootenberg, J. S., Konermann, S., Joung, J., Slaymaker, I. M., Cox, D. B., et al. (2016). C2c2 is a single-component programmable RNA-guided RNA-targeting CRISPR effector. *Science* 353:aaf5573. doi: 10.1126/science.aaf5573

Ackerman, C. M., Myhrvold, C., Thakku, S. G., Freije, C. A., Metsky, H. C., Yang, D. K., et al. (2020). Massively multiplexed nucleic acid detection using Cas13. *Nature* 582, 277–282. doi: 10.1038/s41586-020-2279-8

Adams, C. P., and Brantner, V. V. (2010). Spending on new drug development1. *Health Econ.* 19, 130–141. doi: 10.1002/hec.1454

Afrasiabi, S., Pourhajibagher, M., Raoofian, R., Tabarzad, M., and Bahador, A. (2020). Therapeutic applications of nucleic acid aptamers in microbial infections. *J. Biomed. Sci.* 27:6.

Ahn, J. Y., Lee, K. A., Lee, M. J., Sekhon, S. S., Rhee, S. K., Cho, S. J., et al. (2018). Surface plasmon resonance aptamer biosensor for discriminating pathogenic bacteria vibrio parahaemolyticus. *J. Nanosci. Nanotechnol.* 18, 1599–1605. doi: 10.1166/jnn.2018.14212

Alfavian, H., Mousavi Gargari, S. L., Rasoulinejad, S., and Medhat, A. (2017). Development of a DNA aptamer that binds specifically to group a streptococcus serotype M3. *Can. J. Microbiol.* 63, 160–168. doi: 10.1139/cjm-2016-0495

Allen, H. K., Donato, J., Wang, H. H., Cloud-Hansen, K. A., Davies, J., and Handelsman, J. (2010). Call of the wild: antibiotic resistance genes in natural environments. *Nat. Rev. Microbiol.* 8, 251–259. doi: 10.1038/nrmicro2312

Amraee, M., Oloomi, M., Yavari, A., and Bouzari, S. (2017). DNA aptamer identification and characterization for *E. coli* O157 detection using cell based SELEX method. *Anal. Biochem.* 536, 36–44. doi: 10.1016/j.ab.2017.08.005

Appaturi, J. N., Pulingam, T., Thong, K. L., Muniandy, S., Ahmad, N., and Leo, B. F. (2020). Rapid and sensitive detection of Salmonella with reduced graphene oxide-carbon nanotube based electrochemical aptasensor. *Anal. Biochem.* 589:113489. doi: 10.1016/j.ab.2019.113489

Bai, L., Chen, Y., Bai, Y., Chen, Y., Zhou, J., and Huang, A. (2017). Fullerene-doped polyaniline as new redox nanoprobe and catalyst in electrochemical aptasensor for ultrasensitive detection of *Mycobacterium tuberculosis* MPT64 antigen in human serum. *Biomaterials* 133, 11–19. doi: 10.1016/j.biomaterials.2017.04.010

Bayrac, C., and Oktem, H. A. (2017). Evaluation of *Staphylococcus aureus* DNA aptamer by enzyme-linked aptamer assay and isothermal titration calorimetry. *J. Mol. Recognit.* 30, 1–9.

Bayrac, C., Eyidogan, F., and Avni Oktem, H. (2017). DNA aptamer-based colorimetric detection platform for *Salmonella Enteritidis*. *Biosens. Bioelectron.* 98, 22–28. doi: 10.1016/j.bios.2017.06.029

Bikard, D., Euler, C. W., Jiang, W., Nussenzweig, P. M., Goldberg, G. W., Duportet, X., et al. (2014). Exploiting CRISPR-Cas nucleases to produce sequence-specific antimicrobials. *Nat. Biotechnol.* 32, 1146–1150. doi: 10.1038/nbt.3043

Blair, J. M., Webber, M. A., Baylay, A. J., Ogbolu, D. O., and Piddock, L. J. (2015). Molecular mechanisms of antibiotic resistance. *Nat. Rev. Microbiol.* 13, 42–51.

Broughton, J. P., Deng, X., Yu, G., Fasching, C. L., Servellita, V., Singh, J., et al. (2020). CRISPR-Cas12-based detection of SARS-CoV-2. *Nat Biotechnol.* 38, 870–874.

Bush, K., and Bradford, P. A. (2019). Interplay between beta-lactamases and new beta-lactamase inhibitors. *Nat. Rev. Microbiol.* 17, 295–306. doi: 10.1038/s41579-019-0159-8

Cai, R., Yin, F., Zhang, Z., Tian, Y., and Zhou, N. (2019). Functional chimera aptamer and molecular beacon based fluorescent detection of *Staphylococcus aureus* with strand displacement-target recycling amplification. *Anal. Chim. Acta* 1075, 128–136. doi: 10.1016/j.aca.2019.05.014

Calero-Caceres, W., Ye, M., and Balcazar, J. L. (2019). Bacteriophages as environmental reservoirs of antibiotic resistance. *Trends Microbiol.* 27, 570–577. doi: 10.1016/j.tim.2019.02.008

Cao, L., Gao, C. H., Zhu, J., Zhao, L., Wu, Q., Li, M., et al. (2016). Identification and functional study of type III-A CRISPR-Cas systems in clinical isolates of *Staphylococcus aureus*. *Int. J. Med. Microbiol.* 306, 686–696. doi: 10.1016/j.ijmm.2016.08.005

Casini, A., Olivieri, M., Petris, G., Montagna, C., Reginato, G., Maule, G., et al. (2018). A highly specific SpCas9 variant is identified by in vivo screening in yeast. *Nat. Biotechnol.* 36, 265–271. doi: 10.1038/nbt.4066

CDC, (2019). *Antibiotic Resistance Threats in the United States*. Atlanta: CDC.

Chen, J. S., Dagdas, Y. S., Kleinstiver, B. P., Welch, M. M., Sousa, A. A., Harrington, L. B., et al. (2017). Enhanced proofreading governs CRISPR-Cas9 targeting accuracy. *Nature* 550, 407–410. doi: 10.1038/nature24268

Chen, J. S., Ma, E., Harrington, L. B., Da Costa, M., Tian, X., Palefsky, J. M., et al. (2018). CRISPR-Cas12a target binding unleashes indiscriminate single-stranded DNase activity. *Science* 360, 436–439. doi: 10.1126/science.aar6245

Chen, K., and Gao, C. (2014). Targeted genome modification technologies and their applications in crop improvements. *Plant Cell Rep.* 33, 575–583. doi: 10.1007/s00299-013-1539-6

Chen, L., Rashid, F., Shah, A., Awan, H. M., Wu, M., Liu, A., et al. (2015). The isolation of an RNA aptamer targeting to p53 protein with single amino acid mutation. *Proc. Natl. Acad. Sci. U.S.A.* 112, 10002–10007. doi: 10.1073/pnas.1502159112

Chinnappan, R., Alamer, S., Eissa, S., Rahamn, A. A., Abu Salah, K. M., and Zourob, M. (2017). Fluorometric graphene oxide-based detection of *Salmonella enteritis* using a truncated DNA aptamer. *Mikrochim. Acta* 185:61.

Citorik, R. J., Mimee, M., and Lu, T. K. (2014). Sequence-specific antimicrobials using efficiently delivered RNA-guided nucleases. *Nat. Biotechnol.* 32, 1141–1145. doi: 10.1038/nbt.3011

Crudele, J. M., and Chamberlain, J. S. (2018). Cas9 immunity creates challenges for CRISPR gene editing therapies. *Nat. Commun.* 9:3497.

Dalirirad, S., and Steckl, A. J. (2020). Lateral flow assay using aptamer-based sensing for on-site detection of dopamine in urine. *Anal. Biochem.* 596:113637. doi: 10.1016/j.ab.2020.113637

Das, R., Dhiman, A., Kapil, A., Bansal, V., and Sharma, T. K. (2019a). Aptamer-mediated colorimetric and electrochemical detection of *Pseudomonas aeruginosa* utilizing peroxidase-mimic activity of gold NanoZyme. *Anal. Bioanal. Chem.* 411, 1229–1238. doi: 10.1007/s00216-018-1555-z

Das, R., Dhiman, A., Mishra, S. K., Haldar, S., Sharma, N., Bansal, A., et al. (2019b). Structural switching electrochemical DNA aptasensor for the rapid diagnosis of tuberculous meningitis. *Int. J. Nanomed.* 14, 2103–2113. doi: 10.2147/ijn.s189127

D'costa, V. M., King, C. E., Kalan, L., Morar, M., Sung, W. W., Schwarz, C., et al. (2011). Antibiotic resistance is ancient. *Nature* 477, 457–461.

Dehghani, Z., Hosseini, M., Mohammadnejad, J., Bakhshi, B., and Rezayan, A. H. (2018). Colorimetric aptasensor for *Campylobacter jejuni* cells by exploiting the peroxidase like activity of Au@Pd nanoparticles. *Mikrochim. Acta* 185:448.

Dekker, J. P. (2018). Metagenomics for clinical infectious disease diagnostics steps closer to reality. *J. Clin. Microbiol.* 56:e00850-18.

Doi, Y., Wachino, J. I., and Arakawa, Y. (2016). Aminoglycoside resistance: the emergence of acquired 16S ribosomal RNA methyltransferases. *Infect. Dis. Clin. North Am.* 30, 523–537.

Dua, P., Ren, S., Lee, S. W., Kim, J. K., Shin, H. S., Jeong, O. C., et al. (2016). Cell-SELEX based identification of an RNA aptamer for *Escherichia coli* and its use in various detection formats. *Mol. Cells* 39, 807–813. doi: 10.14348/molcells.2016.0167

Duan, N., Xu, B., Wu, S., and Wang, Z. (2016). Magnetic nanoparticles-based aptasensor using gold nanoparticles as colorimetric probes for the detection of *Salmonella typhimurium*. *Anal. Sci.* 32, 431–436. doi: 10.2116/analsci.32.431

Ellington, A. D., and Szostak, J. W. (1990). In vitro selection of RNA molecules that bind specific ligands. *Nature* 346, 818–822. doi: 10.1038/346818a0

Esposito, C. L., Nuzzo, S., Catuogno, S., Romano, S., De Nigris, F., and De Franciscis, V. (2018). STAT3 gene silencing by aptamer-siRNA chimera as selective therapeutic for glioblastoma. *Mol. Ther. Nucleic Acids* 10, 398–411. doi: 10.1016/j.omtn.2017.12.021

Fan, Y., Cui, M., Liu, Y., Jin, M., and Zhao, H. (2020). Selection and characterization of DNA aptamers for constructing colorimetric biosensor for detection of PBP2a. *Spectrochim. Acta A Mol. Biomol. Spectrosc.* 228:117735. doi: 10.1016/j.saa.2019.117735

Fischer, J. E., Harbarth, S., Agthe, A. G., Benn, A., Ringer, S. A., Goldmann, D. A., et al. (2004). Quantifying uncertainty: physicians' estimates of infection in critically ill neonates and children. *Clin. Infect. Dis.* 38, 1383–1390. doi: 10.1086/420741

Gao, R., Zhong, Z., Gao, X., and Jia, L. (2018). Graphene oxide quantum dots assisted construction of fluorescent aptasensor for rapid detection of *Pseudomonas aeruginosa* in food samples. *J. Agric. Food Chem.* 66, 10898–10905. doi: 10.1021/acs.jafc.8b02164

Gleditzsch, D., Pausch, P., Muller-Esparza, H., Ozcan, A., Guo, X., Bange, G., et al. (2019). PAM identification by CRISPR-Cas effector complexes: diversified mechanisms and structures. *RNA Biol.* 16, 504–517. doi: 10.1080/15476286.2018.1504546

Gootenberg, J. S., Abudayyeh, O. O., Kellner, M. J., Joung, J., Collins, J. J., and Zhang, F. (2018). Multiplexed and portable nucleic acid detection platform with Cas13. Cas12a, and Csm6. *Science* 360, 439–444. doi: 10.1126/science.aaq0179

Gootenberg, J. S., Abudayyeh, O. O., Lee, J. W., Essletzbichler, P., Dy, A. J., Joung, J., et al. (2017). Nucleic acid detection with CRISPR-Cas13a/C2c2. *Science* 356, 438–442. doi: 10.1126/science.aam9321

Gragoudas, E. S., Adamis, A. P., Cunningham, E. T. Jr., Feinsod, M., and Guyer, D. R. (2004). Pegaptanib for neovascular age-related macular degeneration. *N. Engl. J. Med.* 351, 2805–2816.

Guglielmi, G. (2020). First CRISPR test for the coronavirus approved in the United States. *Nature* doi: 10.1038/d41586-020-01402-9 Online ahead of print.

Ha, N. R., Jung, I. P., La, I. J., Jung, H. S., and Yoon, M. Y. (2017). Ultra-sensitive detection of kanamycin for food safety using a reduced graphene oxide-based fluorescent aptasensor. *Sci. Rep.* 7:40305.

Hamula, C. L., Peng, H., Wang, Z., Tyrrell, G. J., Li, X. F., and Le, X. C. (2016). An improved SELEX technique for selection of DNA aptamers binding to M-type 11 of *Streptococcus pyogenes*. *Methods* 97, 51–57. doi: 10.1016/j.ymeth.2015.12.005

Hille, F., Richter, H., Wong, S. P., Bratovic, M., Ressel, S., and Charpentier, E. (2018). The biology of CRISPR-Cas: backward and forward. *Cell* 172, 1239–1259. doi: 10.1016/j.cell.2017.11.032

Hua, R., Hao, N., Lu, J., Qian, J., Liu, Q., Li, H., et al. (2018). A sensitive Potentiometric resolved ratiometric Photoelectrochemical aptasensor for *Escherichia coli* detection fabricated with non-metallic nanomaterials. *Biosens. Bioelectron.* 106, 57–63. doi: 10.1016/j.bios.2018.01.053

Jin, B., Wang, S., Lin, M., Jin, Y., Zhang, S., Cui, X., et al. (2017). Upconversion nanoparticles based FRET aptasensor for rapid and ultrasenstive bacteria detection. *Biosens. Bioelectron.* 90, 525–533. doi: 10.1016/j.bios.2016.10.029

Jinek, M., Chylinski, K., Fonfara, I., Hauer, M., Doudna, J. A., and Charpentier, E. (2012). A programmable dual-RNA-guided DNA endonuclease in adaptive bacterial immunity. *Science* 337, 816–821. doi: 10.1126/science.1225829

Kaur, H., Bruno, J. G., Kumar, A., and Sharma, T. K. (2018). Aptamers in the therapeutics and diagnostics pipelines. *Theranostics* 8, 4016–4032. doi: 10.7150/thno.25958

Kelley, S. O. (2017). What are clinically relevant levels of cellular and biomolecular analytes? *ACS Sens.* 2, 193–197. doi: 10.1021/acssensors.6b00691

Kiga, K., Tan, X. E., Ibarra-Chavez, R., Watanabe, S., Aiba, Y., Sato'o, Y., et al. (2020). Development of CRISPR-Cas13a-based antimicrobials capable of sequence-specific killing of target bacteria. *Nat. Commun.* 11:2934.

Kim, H. J., Park, J. Y., Lee, T. S., Song, I. H., Cho, Y. L., Chae, J. R., et al. (2019). PET imaging of HER2 expression with an 18F-fluoride labeled aptamer. *PLoS One* 14:e0211047. doi: 10.1371/journal.pone.0211047

Kim, J. S., Cho, D. H., Park, M., Chung, W. J., Shin, D., Ko, K. S., et al. (2016). CRISPR/Cas9-mediated re-sensitization of antibiotic-resistant *Escherichia coli* harboring extended-spectrum beta-lactamases. *J. Microbiol. Biotechnol.* 26, 394–401. doi: 10.4014/jmb.1508.08080

Kleinstiver, B. P., Pattanayak, V., Prew, M. S., Tsai, S. Q., Nguyen, N. T., Zheng, Z., et al. (2016). High-fidelity CRISPR-Cas9 nucleases with no detectable genome-wide off-target effects. *Nature* 529, 490–495. doi: 10.1038/nature16526

Kurt, H., Yuce, M., Hussain, B., and Budak, H. (2016). Dual-excitation upconverting nanoparticle and quantum dot aptasensor for multiplexed food pathogen detection. *Biosens. Bioelectron.* 81, 280–286. doi: 10.1016/j.bios.2016.03.005

Lavu, P. S., Mondal, B., Ramlal, S., Murali, H. S., and Batra, H. V. (2016). Selection and characterization of aptamers using a modified whole cell bacterium SELEX for the detection of *Salmonella enterica* serovar Typhimurium. *ACS Comb. Sci.* 18, 292–301. doi: 10.1021/acscombsci.5b00123

Lee, J. K., Jeong, E., Lee, J., Jung, M., Shin, E., Kim, Y. H., et al. (2018). Directed evolution of CRISPR-Cas9 to increase its specificity. *Nat. Commun.* 9:3048.

Leekha, S., Terrell, C. L., and Edson, R. S. (2011). General principles of antimicrobial therapy. *Mayo Clin. Proc.* 86, 156–167. doi: 10.4065/mcp.2010.0639

Li, H., Xing, S., Xu, J., He, Y., Lai, Y., Wang, Y., et al. (2021). Aptamer-based CRISPR/Cas12a assay for the ultrasensitive detection of extracellular vesicle proteins. *Talanta* 221:121670. doi: 10.1016/j.talanta.2020.121670

Li, H., Yang, Y., Hong, W., Huang, M., Wu, M., and Zhao, X. (2020). Applications of genome editing technology in the targeted therapy of human diseases: mechanisms, advances and prospects. *Signal Transduct. Target. Ther.* 5:1.

Li, N., Huang, X., Sun, D., Yu, W., Tan, W., Luo, Z., et al. (2018). Dual-aptamer-based voltammetric biosensor for the *Mycobacterium tuberculosis* antigen MPT64 by using a gold electrode modified with a peroxidase loaded composite consisting of gold nanoparticles and a Zr(IV)/terephthalate metal-organic framework. *Mikrochim. Acta* 185:543.

Li, S. Y., Cheng, Q. X., Wang, J. M., Li, X. Y., Zhang, Z. L., Gao, S., et al. (2018). CRISPR-Cas12a-assisted nucleic acid detection. *Cell Discov.* 4:20.

Liu, H. L. C., Zhao, Y., Han, X., Zhou, Z., Wang, C., Li, R., et al. (2018). Comparing successful gene knock-in efficiencies of CRISPR/Cas9 with ZFNs and TALENs gene editing systems in bovine and dairy goat fetal fibroblasts. *J. Integr. Agric.* 17, 406–414. doi: 10.1016/s2095-3119(17)61748-9

Liu, L., Li, X., Ma, J., Li, Z., You, L., Wang, J., et al. (2017). The molecular architecture for RNA-guided RNA cleavage by cas13a. *Cell* 170:e710.

Liu, Y., Jiang, W., Yang, S., Hu, J., Lu, H., Han, W., et al. (2019). Rapid detection of mycoplasma-infected cells by an ssDNA aptamer probe. *ACS Sens.* 4, 2028–2038. doi: 10.1021/acssensors.9b00582

Llor, C., and Bjerrum, L. (2014). Antimicrobial resistance: risk associated with antibiotic overuse and initiatives to reduce the problem. *Ther. Adv. Drug Saf.* 5, 229–241. doi: 10.1177/2042098614554919

Makarova, K. S., Wolf, Y. I., Alkhnbashi, O. S., Costa, F., Shah, S. A., Saunders, S. J., et al. (2015). An updated evolutionary classification of CRISPR-Cas systems. *Nat. Rev. Microbiol.* 13, 722–736.

Makarova, K. S., Wolf, Y. I., Iranzo, J., Shmakov, S. A., Alkhnbashi, O. S., Brouns, S. J. J., et al. (2020). Evolutionary classification of CRISPR-Cas systems: a burst of class 2 and derived variants. *Nat. Rev. Microbiol.* 18, 67–83. doi: 10.1038/s41579-019-0299-x

Maldonado, J., Estevez, M. C., Fernandez-Gavela, A., Gonzalez-Lopez, J. J., Gonzalez-Guerrero, A. B., and Lechuga, L. M. (2020). Label-free detection of nosocomial bacteria using a nanophotonic interferometric biosensor. *Analyst* 145, 497–506. doi: 10.1039/c9an01485c

Malik, B., and Bhattacharyya, S. (2019). Antibiotic drug-resistance as a complex system driven by socio-economic growth and antibiotic misuse. *Sci. Rep.* 9:9788.

Marraffini, L. A., and Sontheimer, E. J. (2010). Self versus non-self discrimination during CRISPR RNA-directed immunity. *Nature* 463, 568–571. doi: 10.1038/nature08703

Marton, S., Cleto, F., Krieger, M. A., and Cardoso, J. (2016). Isolation of an Aptamer that Binds Specifically to *E. coli*. *PLoS One* 11:e0153637. doi: 10.1371/journal.pone.0153637

McKeague, M., De Girolamo, A., Valenzano, S., Pascale, M., Ruscito, A., Velu, R., et al. (2015). Comprehensive analytical comparison of strategies used for small molecule aptamer evaluation. *Anal. Chem.* 87, 8608–8612. doi: 10.1021/acs.analchem.5b02102

Mirzakhani, K., Mousavi Gargari, S. L., Rasooli, I., and Rasoulinejad, S. (2017). Development of a DNA Aptamer for screening *Neisseria meningitidis* serogroup B by cell selex. *Iran Biomed. J.* 22, 193–201.

Mitsakakis, K., Kaman, W. E., Elshout, G., Specht, M., and Hays, J. P. (2018). Challenges in identifying antibiotic resistance targets for point-of-care diagnostics in general practice. *Future Microbiol.* 13, 1157–1164. doi: 10.2217/fmb-2018-0084

Mojica, F. J. M., Diez-Villasenor, C., Garcia-Martinez, J., and Almendros, C. (2009). Short motif sequences determine the targets of the prokaryotic CRISPR defence system. *Microbiology* 155, 733–740. doi: 10.1099/mic.0.023960-0

Mol, A. A., Groher, F., Schreiber, B., Ruhmkorff, C., and Suess, B. (2019). Robust gene expression control in human cells with a novel universal TetR aptamer splicing module. *Nucleic Acids Res.* 47:e132. doi: 10.1093/nar/gkz753

Mozioglu, E., Gokmen, O., Tamerler, C., Kocagoz, Z. T., and Akgoz, M. (2016). Selection of Nucleic acid aptamers specific for *Mycobacterium tuberculosis*. *Appl. Biochem. Biotechnol.* 17 , 849–864. doi: 10.1007/s12010-015-1913-7

Munita, J. M., and Arias, C. A. (2016). Mechanisms of antibiotic resistance. *Microbiol. Spectr.* 4, 1–24.

Myhrvold, C., Freije, C. A., Gootenberg, J. S., Abudayyeh, O. O., Metsky, H. C., Durbin, A. F., et al. (2018). Field-deployable viral diagnostics using CRISPR-Cas13. *Science* 360, 444–448. doi: 10.1126/science.aas8836

O'Neil, J. (2016). *Tackling Drug-Resistant Infections Globally: Final Report and Recommendations [Online]*. Available online at: http://amr-review.org (accessed July 19, 2020).

Ota, Y., Furuhashi, K., Nanba, T., Yamanaka, K., Ishikawa, J., Nagura, O., et al. (2019). A rapid and simple detection method for phenotypic antimicrobial resistance in *Escherichia coli* by loop-mediated isothermal amplification. *J. Med. Microbiol.* 68, 169–177. doi: 10.1099/jmm.0.000903

Pancholi, P., Carroll, K. C., Buchan, B. W., Chan, R. C., Dhiman, N., Ford, B., et al. (2018). Multicenter evaluation of the accelerate phenotest BC kit for rapid identification and phenotypic antimicrobial susceptibility testing using morphokinetic cellular analysis. *J. Clin. Microbiol.* 56:e01329-17.

Patrinos, G. P., Danielson, P. B., and Ansorge, W. J. (2017). "Molecular diagnostics: past, present, and future," in *Molecular Diagnostic* ed. G.P. Patrinos, (Amsterdam: Elsevier), 520.

Peng, W., Feng, M., Feng, X., Liang, Y. X., and She, Q. (2015). An archaeal CRISPR type III-B system exhibiting distinctive RNA targeting features and mediating dual RNA and DNA interference. *Nucleic Acids Res.* 43, 406–417. doi: 10.1093/nar/gku1302

Powers, J. H. (2004). Antimicrobial drug development–the past, the present, and the future. *Clin. Microbiol. Infect* 10(Suppl. 4), 23–31. doi: 10.1111/j.1465-0691.2004.1007.x

Qiao, J., Meng, X., Sun, Y., Li, Q., Zhao, R., Zhang, Y., et al. (2018). Aptamer-based fluorometric assay for direct identification of methicillin-resistant *Staphylococcus aureus* from clinical samples. *J. Microbiol. Methods* 153, 92–98. doi: 10.1016/j.mimet.2018.09.011

Quan, J., Langelier, C., Kuchta, A., Batson, J., Teyssier, N., Lyden, A., et al. (2019). FLASH: a next-generation CRISPR diagnostic for multiplexed detection of antimicrobial resistance sequences. *Nucleic Acids Res.* 47:e83. doi: 10.1093/nar/gkz418

Rasoulinejad, S., and Gargari, S. L. M. (2016). Aptamer-nanobody based ELASA for specific detection of *Acinetobacter baumannii* isolates. *J. Biotechnol.* 231, 46–54. doi: 10.1016/j.jbiotec.2016.05.024

Reich, P., Stoltenburg, R., Strehlitz, B., Frense, D., and Beckmann, D. (2017). Development of an impedimetric aptasensor for the detection of *Staphylococcus aureus*. *Int. J. Mol. Sci.* 18:2484. doi: 10.3390/ijms18112484

Ren, J., Liang, G., Man, Y., Li, A., Jin, X., Liu, Q., et al. (2019). Aptamer-based fluorometric determination of *Salmonella Typhimurium* using Fe3O4 magnetic separation and CdTe quantum dots. *PLoS One* 14:e0218325. doi: 10.1371/journal.pone.0218325

Rodrigues, M., Mcbride, S. W., Hullahalli, K., Palmer, K. L., and Duerkop, B. A. (2019). Conjugative delivery of CRISPR-Cas9 for the selective depletion of antibiotic-resistant enterococci. *Antimicrob. Agents Chemother.* 63:e01454-9.

Rohloff, J. C., Gelinas, A. D., Jarvis, T. C., Ochsner, U. A., Schneider, D. J., Gold, L., et al. (2014). Nucleic acid ligands with protein-like side chains: modified aptamers and their use as diagnostic and therapeutic agents. *Mol. Ther. Nucleic Acids* 3:e201. doi: 10.1038/mtna.2014.49

Ruotsalainen, P., Penttinen, R., Mattila, S., and Jalasvuori, M. (2019). Midbiotics: conjugative plasmids for genetic engineering of natural gut flora. *Gut Microbes* 10, 643–653. doi: 10.1080/19490976.2019.1591136

Sakyi, S. A., Aboagye, S. Y., Otchere, I. D., Liao, A. M., Caltagirone, T. G., and Yeboah-Manu, D. (2016). RNA aptamer that specifically binds to mycolactone and serves as a diagnostic tool for diagnosis of buruli ulcer. *PLoS Negl. Trop Dis.* 10:e0004950. doi: 10.1371/journal.pntd.0004950

Semenova, E., Jore, M. M., Datsenko, K. A., Semenova, A., Westra, E. R., Wanner, B., et al. (2011). Interference by clustered regularly interspaced short palindromic repeat (CRISPR) RNA is governed by a seed sequence. *Proc. Natl. Acad. Sci. U.S.A.* 108, 10098–10103.

Shen, H., Wang, J., Liu, H., Li, Z., Jiang, F., Wang, F. B., et al. (2016). Rapid and selective detection of pathogenic bacteria in bloodstream infections with aptamer-based recognition. *ACS Appl. Mater Interfaces* 8, 19371–19378. doi: 10.1021/acsami.6b06671

Sheridan, C. (2020). Coronavirus and the race to distribute reliable diagnostics. *Nat. Biotechnol.* 38, 382–384. doi: 10.1038/d41587-020-00002-2

Shin, H. S., Gedi, V., Kim, J. K., and Lee, D. K. (2019). Detection of gram-negative bacterial outer membrane vesicles using DNA aptamers. *Sci. Rep.* 9:13167.

Shin, W. R., Sekhon, S. S., Rhee, S. K., Ko, J. H., Ahn, J. Y., Min, J., et al. (2018). Aptamer-based paper strip sensor for detecting vibrio fischeri. *ACS Comb Sci.* 20, 261–268. doi: 10.1021/acscombsci.7b00190

Singh, R. K., Dhama, K., Karthik, K., Tiwari, R., Khandia, R., Munjal, A., et al. (2017). Advances in diagnosis, surveillance, and monitoring of Zika virus: an update. *Front. Microbiol.* 8:2677.

Slaymaker, I. M., Gao, L., Zetsche, B., Scott, D. A., Yan, W. X., and Zhang, F. (2016). Rationally engineered Cas9 nucleases with improved specificity. *Science* 351, 84–88. doi: 10.1126/science.aad5227

Song, M. S., Sekhon, S. S., Shin, W. R., Kim, H. C., Min, J., Ahn, J. Y., et al. (2017). Detecting and discriminating Shigella sonnei using an aptamer-based fluorescent biosensor platform. *Molecules* 22:825. doi: 10.3390/molecules22050825

Song, M. Y., Nguyen, D., Hong, S. W., and Kim, B. C. (2017). Broadly reactive aptamers targeting bacteria belonging to different genera using a sequential toggle cell-SELEX. *Sci. Rep.* 7:43641.

Stoltenburg, R., Krafcikova, P., Viglasky, V., and Strehlitz, B. (2016). G-quadruplex aptamer targeting protein a and its capability to detect *Staphylococcus aureus* demonstrated by Elona. *Sci. Rep.* 6:33812.

Su, Y., Shao, C., Huang, X., Qi, J., Ge, R., Guan, H., et al. (2018). Extraction and detection of bisphenol a in human serum and urine by aptamer-functionalized magnetic nanoparticles. *Anal. Bioanal. Chem.* 410, 1885–1891. doi: 10.1007/s00216-017-0801-0

Suh, S. H., Choi, S. J., Dwivedi, H. P., Moore, M. D., Escudero-Abarca, B. I., and Jaykus, L. A. (2018). Use of DNA aptamer for sandwich type detection of *Listeria monocytogenes*. *Anal. Biochem.* 557, 27–33. doi: 10.1016/j.ab.2018.04.009

Sun, Y., Duan, N., Ma, P., Liang, Y., Zhu, X., and Wang, Z. (2019). Colorimetric aptasensor based on truncated aptamer and trivalent DNAzyme for *Vibrio parahemolyticus* determination. *J. Agric. Food Chem.* 67, 2313–2320. doi: 10.1021/acs.jafc.8b06893

Tagliaferri, T. L., Guimaraes, N. R., Pereira, M. P. M., Vilela, L. F. F., Horz, H. P., Dos Santos, S. G., et al. (2020). Exploring the potential of CRISPR-Cas9 under challenging conditions: facing high-copy plasmids and counteracting beta-lactam resistance in clinical strains of *Enterobacteriaceae*. *Front. Microbiol.* 11:578.

Tang, X. L., Wu, S. M., Xie, Y., Song, N., Guan, Q., Yuan, C., et al. (2016). Generation and application of ssDNA aptamers against glycolipid antigen ManLAM of *Mycobacterium tuberculosis* for TB diagnosis. *J. Infect.* 72, 573–586. doi: 10.1016/j.jinf.2016.01.014

Toh, S. Y., Citartan, M., Gopinath, S. C., and Tang, T. H. (2015). Aptamers as a replacement for antibodies in enzyme-linked immunosorbent assay. *Biosens. Bioelectron.* 64, 392–403. doi: 10.1016/j.bios.2014.09.026

Tuerk, C., and Gold, L. (1990). Systematic evolution of ligands by exponential enrichment: RNA ligands to bacteriophage T4 DNA polymerase. *Science* 249, 505–510. doi: 10.1126/science.2200121

Wang, L., Huo, X., Qi, W., Xia, Z., Li, Y., and Lin, J. (2020). Rapid and sensitive detection of *Salmonella Typhimurium* using nickel nanowire bridge for electrochemical impedance amplification. *Talanta* 211:120715. doi: 10.1016/j.talanta.2020.120715

Waseem, H., Jameel, S., Ali, J., Saleem, Ur Rehman, H., Tauseef, I., et al. (2019). Contributions and challenges of high throughput qPCR for determining antimicrobial resistance in the environment: a critical review. *Molecules* 24:163. doi: 10.3390/molecules24010163

Wu, G., Dai, Z., Tang, X., Lin, Z., Lo, P. K., Meyyappan, M., et al. (2017). Graphene field-effect transistors for the sensitive and selective detection of *Escherichia coli* Using Pyrene-tagged DNA aptamer. *Adv. Healthc Mater* 6:1700736.

Xiang, D., Zheng, C., Zhou, S. F., Qiao, S., Tran, P. H., Pu, C., et al. (2015). Superior Performance of aptamer in tumor penetration over antibody: implication of aptamer-based theranostics in solid tumors. *Theranostics* 5, 1083–1097. doi: 10.7150/thno.11711

Xiong, Y., Zhang, J., Yang, Z., Mou, Q., Ma, Y., Xiong, Y., et al. (2020). Functional DNA regulated CRISPR-Cas12a sensors for point-of-care diagnostics of non-nucleic-acid targets. *J. Am. Chem. Soc.* 142, 207–213. doi: 10.1021/jacs.9b09211

Xu, L., Dai, Q., Shi, Z., Liu, X., Gao, L., Wang, Z., et al. (2020). Accurate MRSA identification through dual-functional aptamer and CRISPR-Cas12a assisted rolling circle amplification. *J. Microbiol. Methods* 173:105917. doi: 10.1016/j.mimet.2020.105917

Xu, Y., Wang, H., Luan, C., Liu, Y., Chen, B., and Zhao, Y. (2018). Aptamer-based hydrogel barcodes for the capture and detection of multiple types of pathogenic bacteria. *Biosens. Bioelectron.* 100, 404–410. doi: 10.1016/j.bios.2017.09.032

Yoon, S., and Rossi, J. J. (2018). Aptamers: uptake mechanisms and intracellular applications. *Adv. Drug Deliv. Rev.* 134, 22–35. doi: 10.1016/j.addr.2018.07.003

Yosef, I., Manor, M., Kiro, R., and Qimron, U. (2015). Temperate and lytic bacteriophages programmed to sensitize and kill antibiotic-resistant bacteria. *Proc. Natl. Acad. Sci. U.S.A.* 112, 7267–7272. doi: 10.1073/pnas.1500107112

Yu, X., Chen, F., Wang, R., and Li, Y. (2018). Whole-bacterium SELEX of DNA aptamers for rapid detection of *E.coli* O157:H7 using a QCM sensor. *J. Biotechnol.* 266, 39–49. doi: 10.1016/j.jbiotec.2017.12.011

Yunn, N. O., Koh, A., Han, S., Lim, J. H., Park, S., Lee, J., et al. (2015). Agonistic aptamer to the insulin receptor leads to biased signaling and functional selectivity through allosteric modulation. *Nucleic Acids Res.* 43, 7688–7701. doi: 10.1093/nar/gkv767

Zankari, E., Hasman, H., Cosentino, S., Vestergaard, M., Rasmussen, S., Lund, O., et al. (2012). Identification of acquired antimicrobial resistance genes. *J. Antimicrob. Chemother.* 67, 2640–2644. doi: 10.1093/jac/dks261

Zhang, J., Liu, J., Yang, W., Cui, M., Dai, B., Dong, Y., et al. (2019). Comparison of gene editing efficiencies of CRISPR/Cas9 and TALEN for generation of MSTN knock-out cashmere goats. *Theriogenology* 132, 1–11. doi: 10.1016/j.theriogenology.2019.03.029

Zhang, X., Feng, Y., Yao, Q., and He, F. (2017). Selection of a new *Mycobacterium tuberculosis* H37Rv aptamer and its application in the construction of a SWCNT/aptamer/Au-IDE MSPQC H37Rv sensor. *Biosens. Bioelectron.* 98, 261–266. doi: 10.1016/j.bios.2017.05.043

Zhang, Y., Luo, F., Zhang, Y., Zhu, L., Li, Y., Zhao, S., et al. (2018). A sensitive assay based on specific aptamer binding for the detection of *Salmonella enterica* serovar Typhimurium in milk samples by microchip capillary electrophoresis. *J. Chromatogr. A* 1534, 188–194. doi: 10.1016/j.chroma.2017.12.054

Zhao, J., Inomata, R., Kato, Y., and Miyagishi, M. (2020). Development of aptamer-based inhibitors for CRISPR/Cas system. *Nucleic Acids Res.* doi: 10.1093/nar/gkaa865 Online ahead of print.

Zhao, M., Li, W., Liu, K., Li, H., and Lan, X. (2019). C4-HSL aptamers for blocking qurom sensing and inhibiting biofilm formation in *Pseudomonas aeruginosa* and its structure prediction and analysis. *PLoS One* 14:e0212041. doi: 10.1371/journal.pone.0212041

Zhou, J., Satheesan, S., Li, H., Weinberg, M. S., Morris, K. V., Burnett, J. C., et al. (2015). Cell-specific RNA aptamer against human CCR5 specifically targets HIV-1 susceptible cells and inhibits HIV-1 infectivity. *Chem. Biol.* 22, 379–390. doi: 10.1016/j.chembiol.2015.01.005

Zhuang, J., Tan, J., Wu, C., Zhang, J., Liu, T., Fan, C., et al. (2020). Extracellular vesicles engineered with valency-controlled DNA nanostructures deliver CRISPR/Cas9 system for gene therapy. *Nucleic Acids Res.* 48, 8870–8882. doi: 10.1093/nar/gkaa683

5

Prevention of Dermal Abscess Formation Caused by *Staphylococcus aureus* Using Phage JD007 in Nude Mice

Bingyu Ding[1,2], Qingtian Li[2], Mingquan Guo[3], Ke Dong[3], Yan Zhang[3], Xiaokui Guo[3], Qingzhong Liu[1], Li Li[1]* and Zelin Cui[1]*

[1] Department of Laboratory Medicine, Shanghai General Hospital, Shanghai Jiao Tong University School of Medicine, Shanghai, China, [2] Department of Laboratory Medicine, Ruijin Hospital, Shanghai Jiao Tong University School of Medicine, Shanghai, China, [3] Department of Immunology and Microbiology, Shanghai Jiao Tong University School of Medicine, Shanghai, China

***Correspondence:**
Li Li
annylish@126.com
Zelin Cui
czl_phage@126.com;
czl@sjtu.edu.cn

Aim: In this study, *Staphylococcus* phage JD007 bactericidal activity and induced immune responses during treatment were assessed in a dermal abscess model.

Materials and Methods: Dermal abscesses in nude mice were established by injecting a clinical isolate of *S. aureus* SA325 isolated from the back under-dermal abscess of an in-patient.

Results: Phage JD007 was able to inhibit the growth of *S. aureus* SA325 at MOI = 1 or 10, significantly preventing the formation of dermal abscesses. Moderate immune responses were observed in the prevention group through detection of cytokines.

Conclusion: Phage JD007 inhibits the formation of dermal abscesses caused by a clinical *S. aureus* strain in nude mice without robust immune responses.

Keywords: *Staphylococcus aureus*, dermal abscess, inhibition, nude mouse, phage JD007

INTRODUCTION

With the increasing prevalence antibiotic resistant infections, including MRSA (methicillin-resistant *Staphylococcus aureus*) and the emergence of VRSA (vancomycin-resistant *S. aureus*) (Xiao et al., 2013; Limbago et al., 2014), innovative treatments are urgently needed. Recently, there has been renewed interest in phage therapy (Thiel, 2004; Salmond and Fineran, 2015), which has been proposed as a potential antimicrobial therapy as far back as the 1920's (Salmond and Fineran, 2015). Advances in biotechnology have led to the identification of numerous classes of bacteriophages with different host specificities such as K, GH15, Twort, phiIPLA-RODI, and phiIPLA-C1C (O'Flaherty et al., 2004; Kwan et al., 2005; Gu et al., 2012b; Gutierrez et al., 2015). Furthermore, whole genome sequences of these phages enables us to understand their biology at a much deeper level (Cui et al., 2017b).

Phages have been used to treat infectious disease in various animal models. A single dose of phage MR10 exhibited efficacy similar to linezolid in resolving the course of hindpaw infection in diabetic animals, suggesting this approach could serve as an effective strategy in treating MRSA mediated foot infections in diabetic individuals (Chhibber et al., 2013). Phage LS2a has been shown to prevent abscess formation in rabbits when injected simultaneously with *S. aureus* into the subcutaneous site (Wills et al., 2005). Phage Kpn5 could potentially be used as stand-alone therapy for the *Klebsiella pneumoniae* induced burn wound infection, effective even against antibiotic-resistant strains (Kumari et al., 2009). Additionally, in clinical trials, phage products have showed efficacy according to some reports (Marza et al., 2006).

Phage host specificity narrows their use with lysing efficacies that can vary significantly depending on the phage strain. Reports have also documented failures of phage therapy *in vivo* (Sarker and Brussow, 2016), so, it is necessary to evaluate phages' bacteria killing efficacy both *in vitro* and in an animal model. *Staphylococcus* phage JD007, which belongs to family of *Myoviridae* was identified in 2012 and has been shown to have wide host range (Cui et al., 2012), capable of killing *S. aureus* of different MLST Types (Cui et al., 2017a). The aim of this study is to evaluate the treatment efficacy of JD007 in dermal abscesses caused by a clinical strain of MRSA and the immune responses elicited during therapy.

MATERIALS AND METHODS

Animals

BALB/c nude mice (WT, Shanghai Super B&K laboratory animal Corp. Ltd., [SCXK(HU)2005—0001], Shanghai, China) were used in this study. Dermal abscesses were stereo tactically induced as described previously (Capparelli et al., 2007). Uninfected mice served as controls. Mice were euthanized on days 1, 3 and 10 after infection. Ethics eligibility of this study was approved by the Shanghai General Hospital Ethics Committee (Shanghai Jiao Tong University School of Medicine). All experiments were performed in accordance with the national animal protection guidelines approved by the local animal ethics committee. Fifty mice were randomly divided into five groups, 10 mice in each group, including control group (no treatment), phage JD007 group (injected with purified phage JD007), infection group (infected by *S. aureus* SA325), prevention group (phage JD007 were injected 1 h before mice was infected by *S. aureus* SA325), and treatment group (phage JD007 was injected 1 h after mice were infected by *S. aureus* SA325).

Bacteriophage Purification

High-titre phage stocks were obtained through amplification in liquid LB (Luria-Bertani) medium supplemented with 10 μM $MgCl_2$ and 5 μM $CaCl_2$. In culture, *S. aureus* SA325 was infected phage JD007 at a MOI of 0.1 and incubated at 37°C overnight. The visible bacterial lysate in liquid culture were obtained, and then incubated with chloroform (final concentration was 2%) for 30 min with gentle shaking to kill residual bacteria. Remaining bacterial products were removed by centrifugation at 6,500 rpm (Beckman, JA18.0, United States) for 15 min. Phage contained in the supernatant was enriched at 4°C overnight using polyethylene glycol (PEG) 8000 (final concentration 10% w/v), and precipitated at 8,500 rpm for 20 min (Beckman, JA18.0, United States). Afterwards, the pellet was dissolved in TM buffer [(Tris-Mg^{2+} Buffer) 10 mM Tris-HCl (pH 7.2–7.5), 100 mM NaCl, 10 mM $MgCl_2$.5 mM $CaCl_2$] and vortexed. PEG 8000 was removed by adding the same volume of chloroform after vortexing. The solution was centrifuged at 4,000 *g*/min for 10 min, and the supernatant containing the phage was

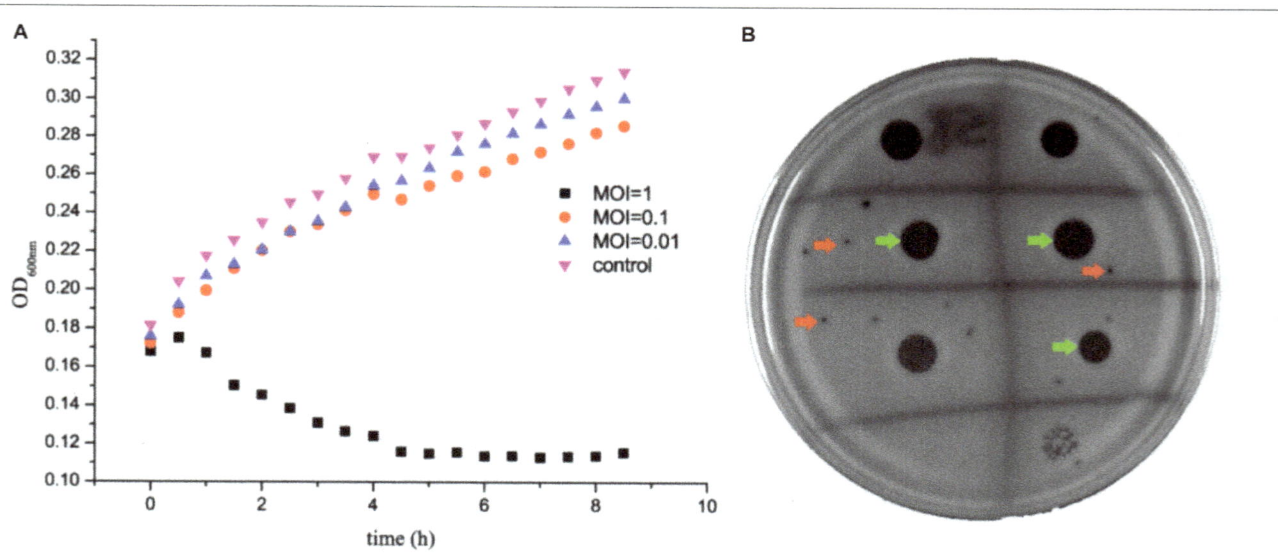

FIGURE 1 | *Staphylococcus aureus* SA325 growth was inhibited by phage JD007 *in vitro*. **(A)** Phage JD007 could inhibit the growth of SA325 at MOI = 1. **(B)** Inhibition zones and plaques were formed by phage JD007 in two-layer agar plate of SA325 and were marked using green and red arrows, respectively.

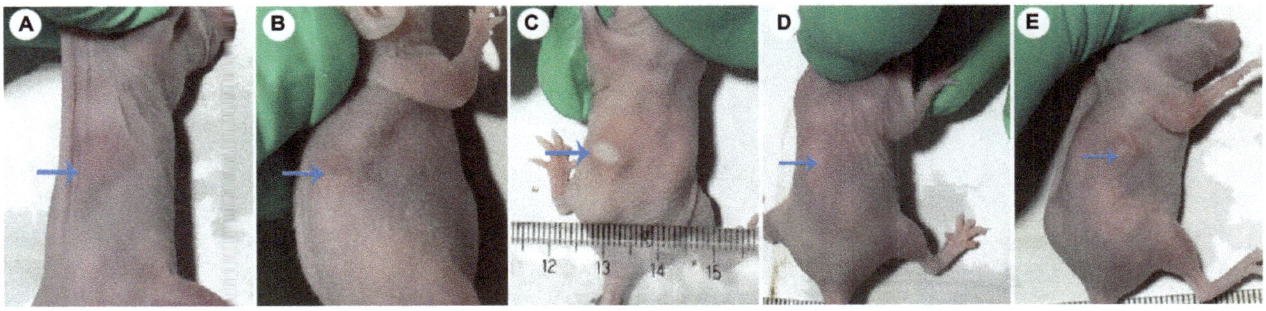

FIGURE 2 | Photos of dermal abscesses in nude BALB/c mice using phage JD007. **(A–E)** Represented the dermal abscesses of mice individually in control group, phage group, infection group, prevention group, and treatment group. The blue arrows showed the skin sites injected with *S. aureus* SA325.

isolated. CsCl was added at a concentration of 0.5 g per 1 mL, and the phages were purified by discontinuous centrifugation in a CsCl gradient (1.35, 1.45, 1.50, and 1.70g/cm^3) in TM buffer in Ultra-Clear tubes (Beckman Coulter, Inc., Fullerton, CA, United States) by centrifuging at 35000 rpm/min for 4 h. Finally, the layer with enriched phage was obtained with a syringe, dialyzed against TM buffer and stored at 4°C (Boulanger, 2009).

S. aureus Strain and Culture Condition

Staphylococcus aureus strain SA325 (MRSA, confirmed by antibiotic resistant profile was isolated from an in-patient with a re-occurring back under-dermal abscess due to long-term bed rest. SA325 concentration was calculated by serial dilutions when grown to $OD_{600\,nm}$ = 0.4, and plated uniformly using the glass spreading rod, and cultured overnight at 37°C, the value of SA325 per $OD_{600\,nm}$ was 9.5 × 10[illegible] CPU/mL.

S. aureus Growth Inhibition Assay

Drop tests were conducted using two-layer agar plates. *S. aureus* SA325 was cultured to $OD_{600\,nm}$ = 0.4 in TSB (Tryptic soy broth) supplemented with 10 μM $MgCl_2$ and 5 μM $CaCl_2$. Bacteria grown to logarithmic phase were mixed with 0.7% agar LB and then poured on the plate of LB agar (1.5%) uniformly, incubating at room temperature for 30 min. Finally, 3 μL of serial dilutions of phage JD007 was dropped on the plate. The inhibition zones were observed after an overnight culture.

The inhibition growth curves for phage JD007 infected *S. aureus* SA325 were determined using MOIs of 0, 0.01, 0.1, and 1 inoculated in 96 well plates separately and incubated at 37°C. $OD_{600\,nm}$ of these cultures was measured every 30 min extending for 8 h. Assay was performed three times (n = 3) with three biological replicates.

Mice Dermal Abscess Infection Model

Staphylococcus aureus was prepared by culturing at 37°C in TSB to exponential phase at which time the bacteria was collected and washed twice with PBS with immediate centrifugation. SA325 was re-suspended at final concentration of 1 × 10^9 CFUs/100μL, and kept on ice before injecting nude mice intradermally.

All animal experiments were approved by the Shanghai General Hospital Ethics Committee (Shanghai Jiao Tong University, China), and conducted according to the Chinese Law for Animal Protection. To investigate the antimicrobial efficacy of phage JD007 for subcutaneous abscesses, BALB/c nude mice (6–8 weeks old) were anesthetized by intraperitoneal injection of a saline solution containing fentanyl (0.05 mg/kg), midazolam (5 mg/kg), and medetomidine (0.5 mg/kg). The backs of the animals were disinfected with 70% ethanol, and 50 μL suspension containing 5 × 10^8 CFU *S. aureus* SA325 in PBS were inoculated subcutaneously; 50 μL of phage JD007 was injected into the infected region. Mice were weighed before inoculation. Weight and abscess formation were measured daily extending for 10 days. The length (L) and width (W) of abscesses were determined using a caliper. The size of the abscesses was then calculated with the standard formula for area: $V = [\pi/2] \times L \times W$ (Weinandy et al., 2014).

Immune Response During Treatment Using *Staphylococcus* Phage JD007

Three mice in each described above were randomly enrolled and euthanized on the third day of the experimental protocol. Serum from each mouse was obtained, and immune cytokines

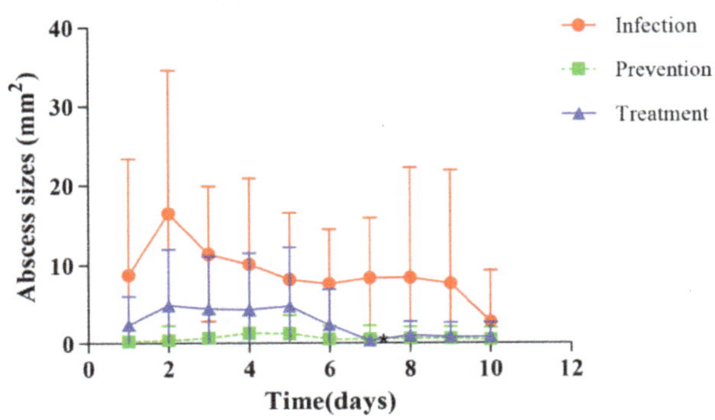

FIGURE 3 | Changes of dermal abscesses sizes formed in nude BALB/c mice during phage therapy. There are no abscesses formed in control and phage groups during the whole procession of observation periods.

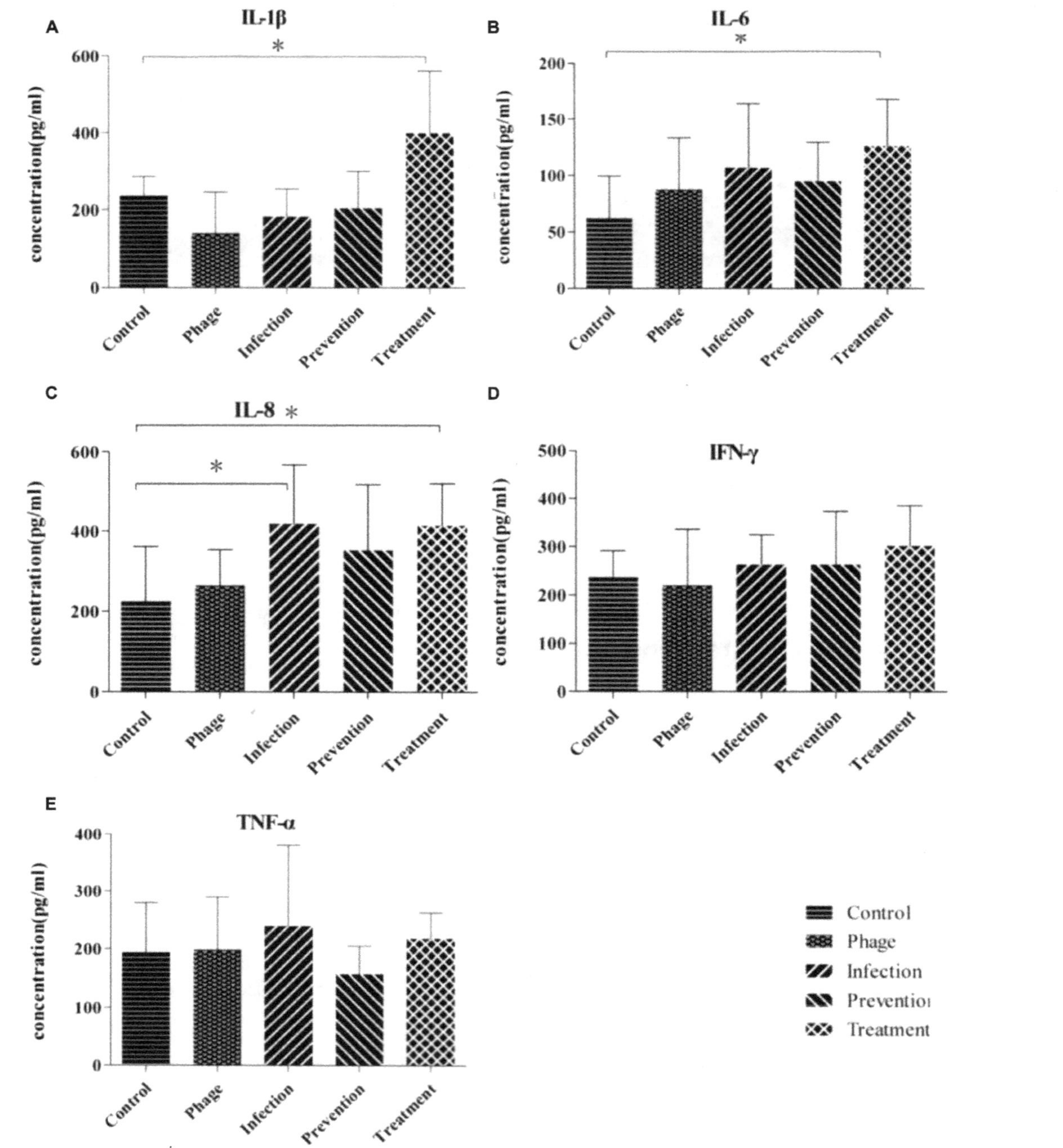

FIGURE 4 | Inflammatory cytokines responses in nude BALB/c mice during phage therapy. **(A–E)** Are separately represents the sera level of IL-1β, IL-6, IL-8, IFN-γ, and TNF-α of mice from different groups, $^{*}p < 0.05$.

(IL-1β, IL-6, IL-8, IFN-γ, and TNF-α) were measured using ELISA (Beijing 4A Biotech Co., Ltd.).

Statistical Analysis

A two-tailed unpaired Student's *t*-test was used for statistical analysis with GraphPad Prism Software. *P*-values of less than 0.05 were considered significant unless specifically indicated otherwise.

RESULTS

S. aureus SA325 Growth Is Inhibited by Phage JD007 *in Vitro*

Staphylococcus aureus SA325 was co-cultured with phage JD007 at 37°C with co-culture $OD_{600\,nm}$ measurements made at 30 min intervals for 8 h. Results showed that phage JD007 inhibited the

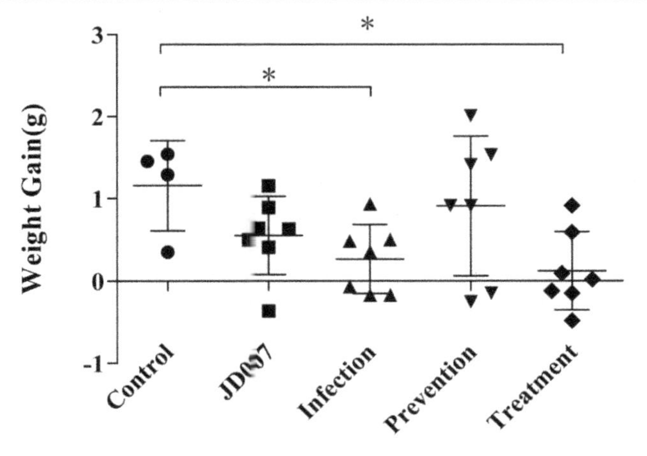

FIGURE 5 | Weights gains in nude BALB/c mice during phage therapy. Body weights gain were calculated by subtracting original body weight from weights on the 10th day. Body weights gains in groups of infection and treatment were significantly lower than that in control group, $*p < 0.05$.

growth of *S. aureus* SA325 as early as 1 h after co-incubation at MOI = 1 (**Figure 1**). Whereas, *S. aureus* SA325 grew normally when infected by phage JD007 at lowers MOIs = 0.1 and 0.01. The drop test results showed that phage JD007 formed clear inhibition zones in two-layer agar plates.

Phage JD007 Prevents *S. aureus* SA325-Mediated Dermal Abscess Formation in Nude BALB/c Mice *in Vivo*

Dermal abscess formation was established in the back of nude mice and observed daily for 10 days. Results showed that the maximum sizes of dermal abscesses were achieved on the second day following infection. On the seventh day, all of the abscesses were scarred. As shown in **Figures 2, 3**, we could see no visible dermal abscesses formed in control group, phage group, and prevention group during the entire observation period. On the third day, the abscess sizes tended to decrease in size, and mice's dermal abscess size in the treatment group were significantly smaller than those in the infection group ($p < 0.05$).

Inflammatory Cytokines Responses of Nude BALB/c Mice During Phage Therapy

Cytokines of IL-1β, IL-6, IL-8, IFN-γ, and TNF-α in the sera were measured using ELISA on the third day. As shown in **Figure 4**, there were no significant differences between IFN-γ and TNF-α among those groups. IL-1β, IL-6, and IL-8 in treatment groups were higher than those in control group, whereas there were no significant differences between the negative control and prevention groups.

Weight of Nude BALB/c Mice During Phage Therapy

Weights of mice in each group were measured daily, encompassing the entire observation period. Body weights gain were calculated by subtracting original body weight from weights on the tenth day. As shown in **Figure 5**, weight gains in infection group and phage treatment were much lower than that compared with control group. The weight gain in the prevention and phage JD007 groups had no significant difference compared with the PBS control group during treatment.

DISCUSSION

Staphylococcus aureus SA325 was isolated from a re-occurring back under-dermal abscess of an in-patient with long-term bed rest. *In vitro* bactericidal activity tests showed that phage JD007 could form a clear inhibition zones using a two-layer soft agar plate assay, and could inhibit growth of SA325 at MOI = 1 or 10.

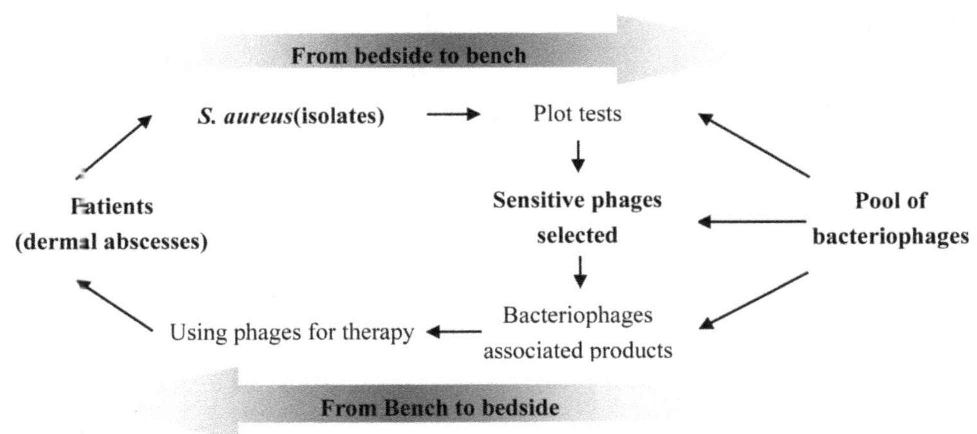

FIGURE 6 | Proposed scheme of selecting phages for therapy. The success of phage therapy needs the pool of phages and their susceptibility to the definite infectious bacterial pathogen at infection sites should be tested previously; the products containing of different phages were produced firstly and the sensitive phages would be chosen for therapy.

In order to evaluate the ability of phage JD007 to prevent or treat of abscesses caused by *S. aureus*, a dermal abscess model was established in nude mice model using clinical isolate SA325, as reported previously (Malachowa et al., 2013). In this study, we successfully established the dermal abscess infection in nude BALB/c mice using *S. aureus* SA325. Furthermore, the efficacies of treatment of the abscesses using phage JD007 were evaluated. There were no observed abscess formation in the prevention group. The average abscess sizes of phage treatment group were smaller than those of the infection group. The results indicate that phage JD007 prevents formation of abscess. Also, it supports earlier observations on phage M^{Sa} inhibition *S. aureus* dermal abscess formation (Capparelli et al., 2007).

To evaluate the response of mice during prevention and treatment after phage JD007 inoculation, the weight changes were observed during the whole process. As bacteriophages are viruses containing nucleic acid and proteins, they may bring some risk to humans when used for the treatment of bacteremia, as the complex composition of the phage may induce unpredictable immune responses when administered to the blood. The average weights gains in the infection and treatment groups were significantly lower than those in the control, PBS, phage JD007, and prevention groups. Furthermore, immune responses of the mice during treatment were evaluated, mice sera was taken on the third day, and the inflammatory cytokines of IL-1β, IL-6, IL-8, IFN-γ, and TNF-α in serum were measured using ELISA. The cytokines IL-1β and IL-6 both belong to endogenous pyrogens, and they can be applied to the hypothalamus regulating center to cause fever. IL-1β and IL-6 levels were significantly higher in the treatment group, while there were no significant differences among prevention, infection, or control groups, indicating that phage JD007 treatment may destroy the cells of *S. aureus* robustly, leading to increase of IL-1β and IL-6 that may cause fever. It's reported that TRIM29 could negatively regulate the proinflammatory cytokine IL-6 and TNF-α production in response to LPS and bacteria *Haemophilus influenzae* (Xing et al., 2016). Whether *S. aureus* infection suppresses the TRIM 29 expression and leads to increased expression of IL-6 should be further examined. IL-8 was significantly elevated in infection and treatment groups. IL-8 can signal chemotactic neutrophil leukocytes and activate T cells in the infection sites, clearing the pathogen. IFN-γ and TNF-α can activate mononuclear macrophages, which can enhance the phagocytosis and killing functions; TNF-α can directly kill the cell infected by virus. There were no significant changes in any of these groups.

The specificity of bacteriophages is one of important reason hindering clinical use of phage for therapy, though cocktails may overcome this fault (Gu et al., 2012a; Mendes et al., 2014). There are numerous public reports describing the success of phage therapy inhibiting infectious diseases caused by dermal associated infections (Vieira et al., 2012; Trigo et al., 2013). We postulate that phage therapy could become an important choice for the treatment of wound infections. As shown in **Figure 6**, the pool of different phages should be established before using them for therapy; at the same time, the bacteria causing infection should be isolated and its sensitivity to the phages in the pool confirmed. The formula of sensitive phages must be prepared at first; once the bacteria causing the infection is confirmed to be sensitive to phages in the pool, the formula containing the sensitive phage should be chosen for treatment of the infections. The success of phage therapy depends upon the pool of different kinds of bacteriophages.

In summary, phage JD007 could inhibit the growth of *S. aureus* both *in vitro* and *in vivo*. Phage JD007 can prevent abscess formation caused by *S. aureus* isolated from an in-patient's abscess samples through under-dermal injection, and can also significantly reduce the severity of dermal abscess caused by *S. aureus*. In conclusion, phage JD007 is a promising candidate phage for use in preventing dermal abscess.

AUTHOR CONTRIBUTIONS

ZC, QTL, and BD carried out the experiments and drafted the manuscript. QTL, KD, BD, QZL, YZ, and MG participated in the mice model experiments. ZC, QTL, XG, and LL participated in the design of the study and performed the statistical analysis. ZC, QTL, and LL conceived the study, participated in its design, and coordinated to help draft the manuscript.

FUNDING

This work was sponsored in part by the National Natural Science Foundation of China (No. 31500154), the fund of Shanghai Health and Family Planning Committee (No. 201440289), and the outstanding medical youth program A of Shanghai General Hospital (No. 06N1702002).

ACKNOWLEDGMENTS

Thanks Luis J. Cocka for suggestions of modification manuscript.

REFERENCES

Boulanger, P. (2009). Purification of bacteriophages and SDS-PAGE analysis of phage structural proteins from ghost particles. *Methods Mol. Biol.* 502, 227–238. doi: 10.1007/978-1-60327-565-1_13

Capparelli, R., Parlato, M., Borriello, G., Salvatore, P., and Iannelli, D. (2007). Experimental phage therapy against *Staphylococcus aureus* in mice. *Antimicrob. Agents Chemother.* 51, 2765–2773. doi: 10.1128/AAC.015 13-06

Chhibber, S., Kaur, T., and Sandeep, K. (2013). Co-therapy using lytic bacteriophage and linezolid: effective treatment in eliminating methicillin resistant *Staphylococcus aureus* (MRSA) from diabetic foot infections. *PLoS One* 8:e56022. doi: 10.1371/journal.pone.0056022

Cui, Z., Feng, T., Gu, F., Li, Q., Dong, K., Zhang, Y., et al. (2017a). Characterization and complete genome of the virulent *Myoviridae* phage JD007 active against a variety of *Staphylococcus aureus* isolates from different hospitals in Shanghai, China. *Virol. J.* 14:26. doi: 10.1186/s12985-017-0701-0

Cui, Z., Guo, X., Dong, K., Zhang, Y., Li, Q., Zhu, Y., et al. (2017b). Safety assessment of *Staphylococcus* phages of the family *Myoviridae* based on complete genome sequences. *Sci. Rep.* 7:41259. doi: 10.1038/srep41259

Cui, Z., Song, Z., Wang, Y., Zeng, L., Shen, W., Wang, Z., et al. (2012). Complete genome sequence of wide-host-range *Staphylococcus aureus* phage JD007. *J. Virol.* 86, 13880–13881. doi: 10.1128/JVI.02728-12

Gu, J., Liu, X., Li, Y., Han, W., Lei, L., Yang, Y., et al. (2012a). A method for generation phage cocktail with great therapeutic potential. *PLoS One* 7:e31698. doi: 10.1371/journal.pone.0031698

Gu, J., Liu, X., Lu, R., Li, Y., Song, J., Lei, L., et al. (2012b). Complete genome sequence of *Staphylococcus aureus* bacteriophage GH15. *J. Virol.* 86, 8914–8915. doi: 10.1128/JVI.01313-12

Gutierrez, D., Vandenheuvel, D., Martinez, B., Rodriguez, A., Lavigne, R., and Garcia, P. (2015). Two phages, phiIPLA-RODI and phiIPLA-C1C, lyse mono- and dual-staphylococcal biofilms. *Appl. Environ. Microbiol.* 81, 3336–3348. doi: 10.1128/AEM.03560-14

Kumari, S., Harjai, K., and Chhibber, S. (2009). Efficacy of bacteriophage treatment in murine burn wound infection induced by *Klebsiella pneumoniae*. *J. Microbiol. Biotechnol.* 19, 622–628.

Kwan, T., Liu, J., DuBow, M., Gros, P., and Pelletier, J. (2005). The complete genomes and proteomes of 27 *Staphylococcus aureus* bacteriophages. *Proc. Natl. Acad. Sci. U.S.A.* 102, 5174–5179. doi: 10.1073/pnas.0501140102

Limbago, B. M., Kallen, A. J., Zhu, W., Eggers, P., McDougal, L. K., and Albrecht, V. S. (2014). Report of the 13th vancomycin-resistant *Staphylococcus aureus* isolate from the United States. *J. Clin. Microbiol.* 52, 998–1002. doi: 10.1128/JCM.02187-13

Malachowa, N., Kobayashi, S. D., Braughton, K. R., and DeLeo, F. R. (2013). Mouse model of *Staphylococcus aureus* skin infection. *Methods Mol. Biol.* 1031, 109–116. doi: 10.1007/978-1-62703-481-4_14

Marza, J. A., Soothill, J. S., Boydell, P., and Collyns, T. A. (2006). Multiplication of therapeutically administered bacteriophages in *Pseudomonas aeruginosa* infected patients. *Burns* 32, 642–646. doi: 10.1016/j.burns.2006.02.012

Mendes, J. J., Leandro, C., Mottola, C., Barbosa, R., Silva, F. A., Oliveira, M., et al. (2014). In vitro design of a novel lytic bacteriophage cocktail with therapeutic potential against organisms causing diabetic foot infections. *J. Med. Microbiol.* 63, 1055–1065. doi: 10.1099/jmm.0.071753-0

O'Flaherty, S., Coffey, A., Edwards, R., Meaney, W., Fitzgerald, G. F., and Ross, R. P. (2004). Genome of staphylococcal phage K: a new lineage of *Myoviridae* infecting gram-positive bacteria with a low G+C content. *J. Bacteriol.* 186, 2862–2871. doi: 10.1128/JB.186.9.2862-2871.2004

Salmond, G. P., and Fineran, P. C. (2015). A century of the phage: past, present and future. *Nat. Rev. Microbiol.* 13, 777–786. doi: 10.1038/nrmicro3564

Sarker, S. A., and Brussow, H. (2016). From bench to bed and back again: phage therapy of childhood *Escherichia coli* diarrhea. *Ann. N. Y. Acad. Sci.* 1372, 42–52. doi: 10.1111/nyas.13087

Thiel, K. (2004). Old dogma, new tricks–21st Century phage therapy. *Nat. Biotechnol.* 22, 31–36. doi: 10.1038/nbt0104-31

Trigo, G., Martins, T. G., Fraga, A. G., Longatto-Filho, A., Castro, A. G., Azeredo, J., et al. (2013). Phage therapy is effective against infection by *Mycobacterium ulcerans* in a murine footpad model. *PLoS Negl. Trop. Dis.* 7:e2183. doi: 10.1371/journal.pntd.0002183

Vieira, A., Silva, Y. J., Cunha, A., Gomes, N. C., Ackermann, H. W., and Almeida, A. (2012). Phage therapy to control multidrug-resistant *Pseudomonas aeruginosa* skin infections: in vitro and ex vivo experiments. *Eur. J. Clin. Microbiol. Infect. Dis.* 31, 3241–3249. doi: 10.1007/s10096-012-1691-x

Weinandy, F., Lorenz-Baath, K., Korotkov, V. S., Bottcher, T., Sethi, S., Chakraborty, T., et al. (2014). A beta-lactone-based antivirulence drug ameliorates *Staphylococcus aureus* skin infections in mice. *ChemMedChem* 9, 710–713. doi: 10.1002/cmdc.201300325

Wills, Q. F., Kerrigan, C., and Soothill, J. S. (2005). Experimental bacteriophage protection against *Staphylococcus aureus* abscesses in a rabbit model. *Antimicrob. Agents Chemother.* 49, 1220–1221. doi: 10.1128/AAC.49.3.1220-1221.2005

Xiao, M., Wang, H., Zhao, Y., Mao, L. L., Brown, M., Yu, Y. S., et al. (2013). National surveillance of methicillin-resistant *Staphylococcus aureus* in China highlights a still-evolving epidemiology with 15 novel emerging multilocus sequence types. *J. Clin. Microbiol.* 51, 3638–3644. doi: 10.1128/JCM.01375-13

Xing, J., Weng, L., Yuan, B., Wang, Z., Jia, L., Jin, R., et al. (2016). Identification of a role for TRIM29 in the control of innate immunity in the respiratory tract. *Nat. Immunol.* 17, 1373–1380. doi: 10.1038/ni.3580

6

Efficiency of Biosynthesized Silver and Zinc Nanoparticles Against Multi-Drug Resistant Pathogens

Kapil Punjabi[1], Sourabh Mehta[2], Rujuta Chavan[3], Vidushi Chitalia[1], Dhanashree Deogharkar[1] and Sunita Deshpande[1]*

[1] *Department of Clinical Pathology, Haffkine Institute for Training, Research and Testing, Mumbai, India,* [2] *National Centre for Nanoscience and Nanotechnology, University of Mumbai, Mumbai, India,* [3] *Department of Microbiology, Guru Nanak Khalsa College, Mumbai, India*

Correspondence:
Kapil Punjabi
kapil9372@gmail.com

Biosynthesis of metallic nanoparticles has acquired particular attention due to its economic feasibility, low toxicity, and simplicity of the process. In this study, extracellular synthesis of silver and zinc nanoparticle was carried out by *Pseudomonas hibiscicola* isolated from the effluent of an electroplating industry in Mumbai. Characterization studies revealed synthesis of 40 and 60 nm nanoparticles of silver (AgNP) and zinc (ZnNP), respectively, with distinct morphology as observed in TEM and its crystalline nature confirmed by XRD. DLS, zeta potential, NTA, and FTIR studies further characterized nanoparticles giving data about its size, stability, and functional groups. Considering the toxicity of nanoparticles the evaluation of antimicrobial activity was studied in the range of non-toxic concentration for normal cell lines. Silver nanoparticles were found to be the most effective antimicrobial against all tested strains and drug-resistant clinical isolates of MRSA, VRE, ESBL, MDR, *Pseudomonas aeruginosa* with MIC in the range of 1.25–5 mg/ml. Zinc nanoparticles were found to be specifically active against Gram-positive bacteria like *Staphylococcus aureus* including its drug-resistant variant MRSA. Both AgNP and ZnNP were found to be effective against *Mycobacterium tuberculosis* and its MDR strain with MIC of 1.25 mg/ml. The synergistic action of nanoparticles assessed in combination with a common antibiotic gentamicin (590 μg/mg) used for the treatment of various bacterial infections by Checker board assay. Silver nanoparticles profoundly exhibited synergistic antimicrobial activity against drug-resistant strains of MRSA, ESBL, VRE, and MDR *P. aeruginosa* while ZnNP were found to give synergism with gentamicin only against MRSA. The MRSA, ESBL, and *P. aeruginosa* strains exhibited MIC of 2.5 mg/ml except VRE which was 10 mg/ml for both AgNPs and ZnNPs. These results prove the great antimicrobial potential of AgNP and ZnNP against drug-resistant strains of community and hospital-acquired infections and opens a new arena of antimicrobials for treatment, supplementary prophylaxis, and prevention therapy.

Keywords: silver nanoparticles, zinc nanoparticles, *Pseudomonas hibiscicola*, MRSA, VRE, MDR-TB

INTRODUCTION

New-age researchers are dedicated to upgrading the current world to a better and easier habitation. To achieve this, nanotechnology will play an important role in newer and improved materials that are robust, economic, and sources of renewable energy and pollution-free environment. The future doctors will use devices made up of such enhanced materials to not only ease the process of diagnostics but also considerably reduce the time and help treatment at early stages. Simpler and faster diagnosis coupled with efficient and reliable treatments will help to cure cancer, diabetes, and various infections. This may seem easy but a difficult road-map lies in front of these researchers, but certainly leads with help of nanotechnology makes it look possible and a revolution seems to be around the corner (Bhattacharyya et al., 2009).

With many arms of nanotechnology being shaped, one major domain is the biomedical application. The biomedical applications of nanotechnology comprise of many sub areas predominantly therapeutic and diagnostic areas have received considerable attention. Different nanoparticles and nanomaterials owing to their small size can easily interact with biomolecules at cellular as well as sub cellular levels. This greatly enhances the signaling of markers in case of diagnostics and improved specificity for targeted therapeutics (Conde et al., 2012).

Multiple applications of nanotechnology across fields like medical, chemical, environmental, agricultural, industrial, energy sciences, and information technology. This attracts major attention from various organizations in both developed and developing nations throughout the world (Roco, 2007).

Many approaches for the synthesis of nanoparticles have been proposed principally categorized into three classes namely – physical, chemical, and biological. Both physical and chemical methods are the major source of nanoparticles in the current period. While these methods ensure continuous supply they also have price to pay in terms of high energy requirements, toxic by-products. This highlights the requirement of sustainable and eco-friendly mode of synthesis. This brings into picture the biological methods with microorganisms playing a significant role. Thus, microbiologists around the world try to identify microorganisms for this capability and develop a simple and cost-effective method to synthesize nanoparticles of constant size, shape, and mono-dispersity (Babu et al., 2011; Horikoshi and Serpone, 2013).

Biosynthesized nanoparticles are ideal candidates for medical applications as they are biocompatible and naturally stable. One of the important property of such nanoparticles is antimicrobial activity. Many green silver nanoparticles have been reported for antibacterial and antibiofilm activity through mechanisms like ROS generation (Qayyum et al., 2017). Also supportive studies on plant derived silver nanoparticles conclude that biogenic nanomaterials are biocompatible and an effective therapeutic agent against bacterial, fungal infections, and cancer treatment (Oves et al., 2018).

Although nanoparticles are considered as future to many areas of science and technology, its probable environmental toxicity is a matter of concern. Thus, in this study, we synthesized nanoparticle, using bacteria isolated from a challenged environment like soil and effluent of electroplating industry and characterized to check potential therapeutic applications if rendered usable by evaluation of its *in vitro* toxicity.

MATERIALS AND METHODS

Synthesis and Characterization of Nanoparticles

The synthesis and characterization of AgNP was followed by our previously reported work using the bacterial culture of *Pseudomonas hibiscicola* isolated from effluent of an electroplating industry. The culture inoculated in sterile nutrient broth and incubated at 37°C for 24 h in an orbital shaker. After incubation, it was centrifuged till clear supernatant was achieved. The supernatant was subjected to 1 mM concentration of silver nitrate AgNO3 (Sigma-Aldrich, United States) and incubated on a shaker with similar conditions. The bio-reduction of silver ions was monitored by visual observation and measuring absorption spectrum of samples using UV–vis Spectrophotometer Thermo scientific Nanodrop – 1000 v3.7 scanning range from 200 to 800 nm (Punjabi et al., 2017). For synthesis of ZnNP, similar procedure was followed; briefly the culture supernatant of *P. hibiscicola* was challenged with 10 mM zinc acetate $[Zn(O_2CCH_3)_2]$ (Himedia labs Pvt. Ltd., India) in 1:2 v/v ratio and incubated in similar conditions. After 24 h of incubation, precipitate formation and turbidity indicated presence of ZnNP in the reaction mixture. Reduction of metal ion to nanoparticle was confirmed by observing plasmon peak in the range of 320–380 nm in UV–Vis spectra (Waghmare et al., 2011).

To determine the size, morphology, and other characters of synthesized ZnNPs, characterization studies were undertaken. Suspension of zinc nanoparticles was subjected to UV–Vis spectroscopy, nanoparticle tracking, and analysis (NTA), DLS – particle size analyzer, and zeta potential analysis of the liquid suspension was done using NanoPlus DLS (Micromeritics Instrument Corporation). While powdered material was used for X-ray diffraction (XRD) patterns that were recorded on normal focus diffractometer (Regaku Miniflex, Japan) at voltage of 30 kV and current 15 mA with scan rate of 3°/min. The data were recorded in the range of 20°–50° and analyzed using Jade 6.0 software. Fourier transform infrared (FTIR) spectra obtained on a JASCO spectrometer (6100 type-A) instrument in the range of 400–4000 cm^{-1} were identified spectroscopy and TEM analysis on a Philips CEM 200 Microscope (Pattanayak, 2013).

Toxicity of Nanoparticles

Toxicity of nanoparticles was assessed on Vero cell line (Monkey kidney cell line). The cell line, Vero passage number 27 was obtained from National Centre for Cell Sciences, Pune, India, in Dulbecco's Modified Essential Medium (DMEM) supplemented with 10% fetal bovine serum (FBS) (complete medium).

To evaluate the effect of AgNP and ZnNP on cell toxicity colorimetric MTT (3-(4, 5-dimethylthiazol-2)-2, 5 diphenyl tetrazolium bromide) assay was performed. The MTT assay is a colorimetric technique wherein amount of absorbance is directly proportional to number of living cells. The MTT tetrazolium compound is reduced by viable cells into an intensely colored formazan precipitate that subsequently is solubilized into a uniformly colored solution with a second procedural step before absorbance is measured using a plate reading spectrophotometer (Freshney, 2010).

Known number (1×10^4 cells) of cells was seeded into tissue culture grade 96-well plates (Riss et al., 2011). Cells were treated with various concentrations (10.0–0.6 mg/ml) of nanoparticles for 24 h and treated with 0. 5% MTT (HiMedia Laboratories Pvt. Ltd., India).

After 4 h, all the contents of wells were removed and 100 μl of dimethyl sulfoxide (DMSO) was added. The absorbance of colored solution was measured on the Multimode reader (Synergy HTX Multimode reader, BIOTEK, India) using a test wavelength of 490 nm (Freshney, 2010; Satyavani et al., 2011). Percentage toxicity was estimated for each concentration, and the IC_{50} value was calculated for both nanoparticles (Freshney, 2005).

Antimicrobial Activity of Nanoparticles

Bacterial Strains

Gram-negative bacteria

Proteus mirabilis ATCC 21100, *Escherichia coli* ATCC 25922, *Klebsiella pneumoniae* ATCC 10031, *K. pneumoniae* ATCC 700603 (extended spectrum β lactamases producer, ESBL), *Pseudomonas aeruginosa* ATCC 27853, *Enterobacter aerogenes* ATCC 13048, *Salmonella typhimurium* ATCC 14028, *Salmonella abony* ATCC 6017, and *Shigella boydii* ATCC 8700.

Gram-positive bacteria

Staphylococcus aureus ATCC 25923, *Bacillus subtillis* ATCC 6633, *S. aureus* ATCC 43300 (methicillin-resistant *S. aureus*, MRSA), *S. aureus* ATCC 6538 *Enterococcus faecalis* ATCC 51299 (vancomycin-resistant *Enterococci*, VRE), *Staphylococcus epidermidis* ATCC 12228, and *Bacillus cereus* ATCC 11778.

Mycobacteria

Mycobacterium tuberculosis H37Rv.

Clinical strains

MDR *P. aeruginosa* and MDR *M. tuberculosis.*

ATCC strains were procured from Clinical Pathology department, Haffkine Institute, microbial culture collection (MCC) Pune, India, and Himedia laboratories Pvt. Ltd., Mumbai, India. The MDR strains of clinical isolates were procured from tertiary care hospital in Mumbai. The drug resistance of the isolates was confirmed before use in the study as per standard protocols of Clinical and Laboratory Standards Institute [CLSI] (2012).

Minimum Inhibitory Concentration

Antimicrobial activity of the nanoparticles synthesized was determined by broth dilution method and confirmation by growth on solid media (Wiegand et al., 2008; Ataee et al., 2011). For determining the minimum concentration of nanoparticles required for the inhibition of bacterial growth, broth dilution method was used according to standard broth microdilution method M07 A9 of Clinical and Laboratory Standards Institute [CLSI] (2012). This method facilitates the testing of inhibitory activity at various nanoparticle concentrations (Clinical and Laboratory Standards Institute [CLSI], 2012).

Anti-mycobacterial Activity – Broth Dilution Method

The minimum inhibitory concentrations (MICs) of silver and zinc nanoparticles were assessed by broth dilution method against *M. tuberculosis* H37Rv and MDR strain. Tenfold serial dilutions of the inoculum suspension were made in M7H9 broth supplemented with Middlebrook OADC enrichment. The stock concentrations of nanoparticles were serially diluted to obtain concentrations in the range 1.25–10 mg/ml. The prepared bacilli suspension (500 μl) was added to all tubes except the control tubes, all the tubes were incubated at 37°C for 7 days, which is physiological temperature favorable for growth of pathogenic strains. To determine the MIC, 10 μl of each tube was transferred to Lowenstein Jensen Medium (LJ medium) and incubated at 37°C for 3 weeks. After incubation, growth on LJ media was analyzed for each concentration of both nanoparticles. The observations were recorded and MIC values were determined (Andrews, 2001; Jadaun et al., 2007).

Synergistic Activity of Gentamicin and Nanoparticles

Disk Diffusion Test for Gentamicin

Antibiotic susceptibility test (AST) against gentamicin (10 μg) and high-level gentamicin (120 μg) (HiMedia labs Pvt. Ltd.) was performed by the Kirby–Bauer disk diffusion test to study the drug-resistant pattern of the aforementioned organisms (Bauer et al., 1966; Clinical and Laboratory Standards Institute [CLSI], 2012).

E-Test

To determine the MIC of gentamicin for these isolates EzyMIC™ Strip (GEN) (0.016–256 mcg/ml) and EzyMIC™ Strip (HLG) (0.064–1024 mcg/ml) (HiMedia labs Pvt. Ltd.) were used. The test was performed on Mueller Hinton agar (HiMedia labs Pvt. Ltd.) swabbing a sterile cotton-swab soaked in inoculum prepared by comparing the turbidity of direct colony suspension to standard 0.5 McFarland. The EzyMIC™ Strip were placed at the center of the agar plate and incubated at 37°C for 24 h. After incubation, the plates were read at the point of complete inhibition of all growth, including hazes, micro-colonies, and isolated colonies as indicated (Nachnani et al., 1992).

MIC of Gentamicin

To determine the MIC of gentamicin, broth dilution method was used according to standard broth microdilution method M07 A9 of Clinical and Laboratory Standards Institute [CLSI] (2012).

Checkerboard Assay

The stock solutions of gentamicin used ranged 2.5 to 160 μg/ml. The stock solutions of silver and zinc nanoparticles used ranged from 0.3 to 20 mg/ml. Double dilutions of both the antibiotic as well as the nanoparticles was used for the assay according to the recommendations of CLSI. A total of 50 μl of sterile nutrient

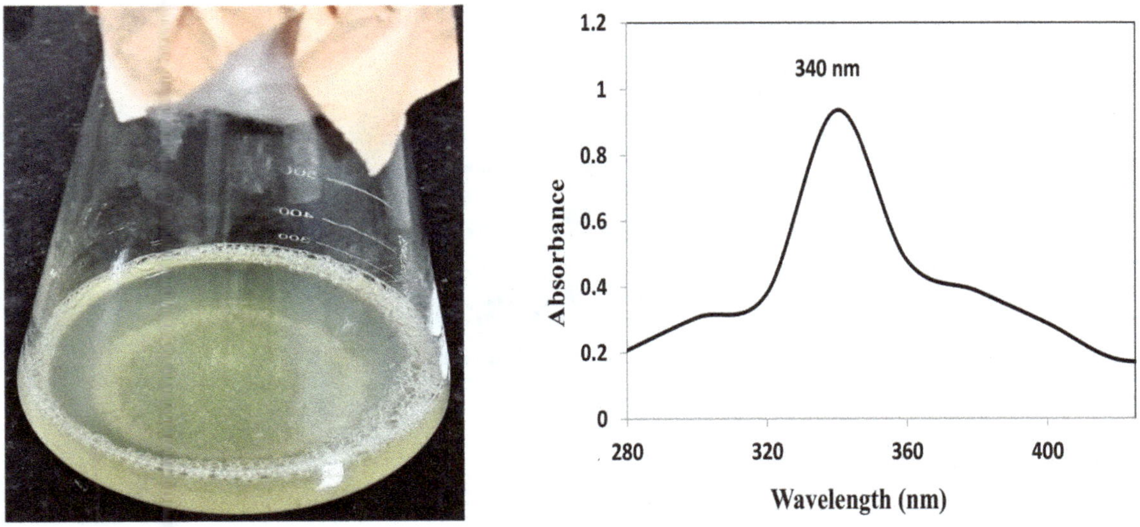

FIGURE 1 | Typical precipitate formation and UV–Vis spectra of the synthesized zinc nanoparticles.

broth was distributed aseptically in all the sterile microtiter plate (96-well plate). The antibiotic gentamicin was serially diluted along the abscissa, while the nanoparticle was diluted along the ordinate. An inoculum equal to 0.5 McFarland turbidity standards was prepared for each culture in sterile saline. Each well was inoculated with 10 µl of the culture. The microtiter plate was incubated at 37°C for 24 h. After incubation, the growth was observed by streaking a loopful from each well in sterile nutrient agar plates. The plates were incubated at 37°C for 24 h. The plates were observed for growth of the test organism. The combination of the drugs in which the growth is completely inhibited was considered as effective MIC for the combination (Breitinger, 2010).

The ΣFICs (fractional inhibitory concentrations) were calculated as follows:

$$\Sigma FIC = FIC\ A + FIC\ B$$

where FIC A is the MIC of drug A (gentamicin) in the combination/MIC of drug A (gentamicin) alone, and FIC B is the MIC of drug B (nanoparticle) in the combination/MIC of drug B (nanoparticle) alone. The combination is considered synergistic when the ΣFIC is ≤ 0.5, indifferent when the ΣFIC is >0.5 to <2, and antagonistic when the ΣFIC is ≥ 2 (Rabadia et al., 2013). The overall study period was 12 months from material synthesis to performing all *in vitro* activities.

RESULTS

Synthesis and Characterization of Nanoparticles

Synthesis of AgNP and ZnNP was achieved extracellularly using *P. hibiscicola* isolated from effluent of electroplating industry. Polydispersed silver nanoparticles of average 40 nm in size were obtained as mentioned in the previous work. In case of ZnNP, typical white precipitate formation as seen in **Figure 1** indicated the synthesis of zinc nanoparticles. The UV–Vis spectra (**Figure 1**) confirm the synthesis of zinc nanoparticles in the reaction mixture.

Further characterization studies gave details about the nanoparticle size, morphology, surface charge, and crystalline nature. The dynamic light scattering (DLS) and zeta potential of the zinc nanoparticles (**Figure 2**) indicated synthesis of stable nanoparticles of size 110 nm and polydispersity index of −0.2. The zeta potential of the zinc nanoparticles was found to be 24.64 mV.

Fourier transform infrared **Figure 3** shows absorption bands at 3513, 2931, and 1020 cm^{-1} indicating the presence of capping agent with the nanoparticles. The spectra correspond to secondary alcohol, alkane, and amine regions. These functional groups have a role in stability/capping of nanoparticles. XRD pattern **Figure 4** shows 2θ values at 31.96°, 34.58°, 36.38°, 47.5°, 56.6°, 62.8°, and 67.9°. All evident peaks could be indexed as the zinc oxide wurtzite structure (JCPDS Data Card No: 36-1451), which confirms the synthesized nanoparticles were free of impurities as it does not contain any characteristics XRD peaks other than zinc oxide peaks.

Nanoparticle tracking and analysis of AgNP and ZnNP (**Figure 5**) shows the particle size distribution which was in the range of 10–70 nm for silver nanoparticles while the mean size was found to be 39 nm with concentration of 3.79×10^8 particles/ml; whereas for ZnNP, the particle size distribution was in the range of 5–90 nm, and mean size was 62 nm with concentration of 4.72×10^8 particles/ml.

The size and morphology of silver nanoparticles synthesized were observed in TEM with average size of 40 nm and most of the population consisting of single crystalline nanoparticles. Spherical zinc nanoparticles of varying size were observed with average size of 60 nm (**Figure 6**).

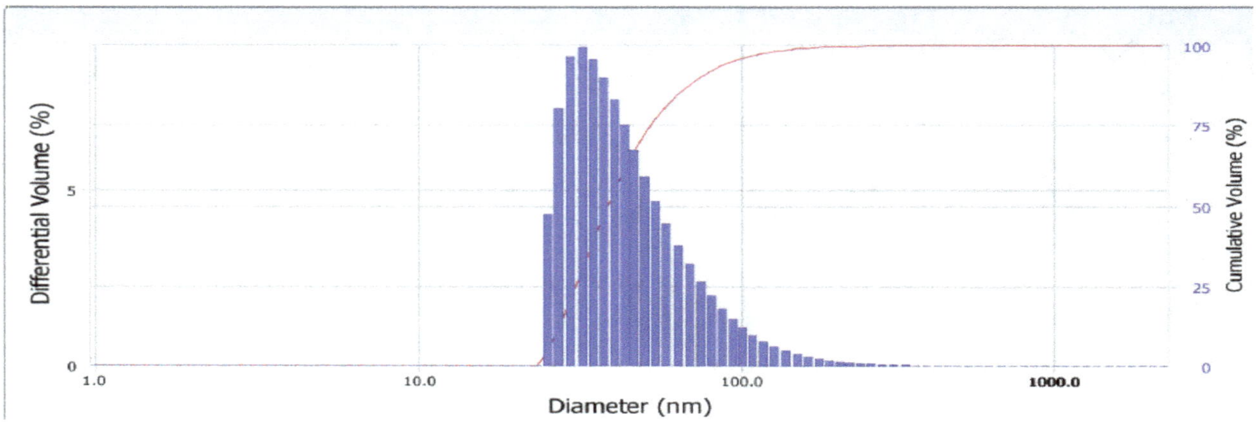

FIGURE 2 | DLS of synthesized zinc nanoparticles.

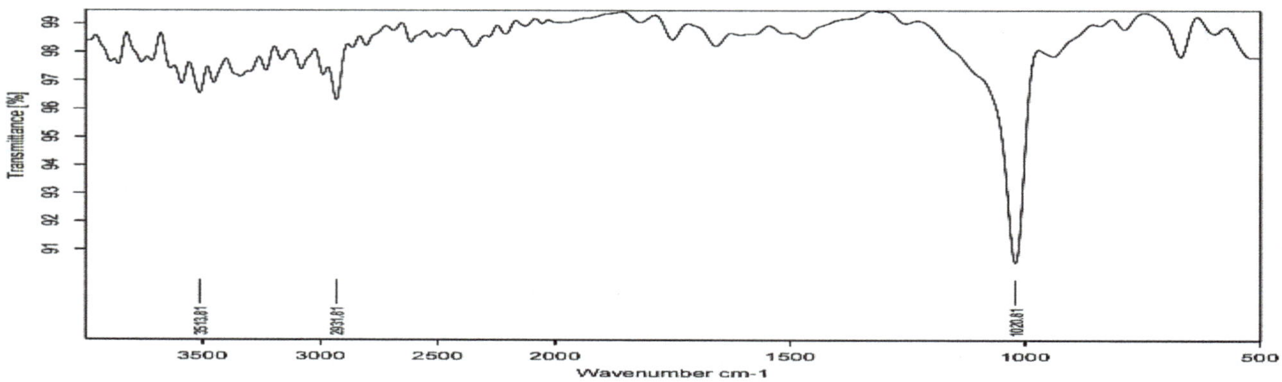

FIGURE 3 | FTIR spectra of zinc nanoparticles.

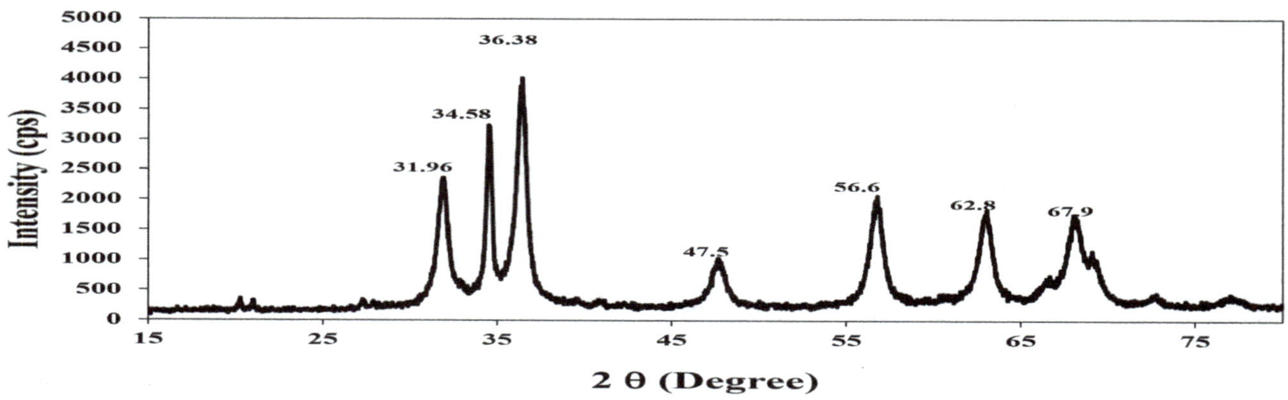

FIGURE 4 | XRD pattern of zinc nanoparticles.

Toxicity of Nanoparticles

Cytotoxicity was evaluated in the range of 0.3 to 10 mg/ml concentration of nanoparticles. Toxicity of a compound is calculated by determining the IC_{50} value, which is that concentration at which growth of cells is inhibited by 50%. The percentage cytotoxicity is plotted against the concentration of nanoparticle as seen in **Figure 7**.

Based on toxicity of nanoparticles to Vero cell line, the IC_{50} values for silver and zinc nanoparticles were found to be 5.54 and 6.24 mg/ml, respectively.

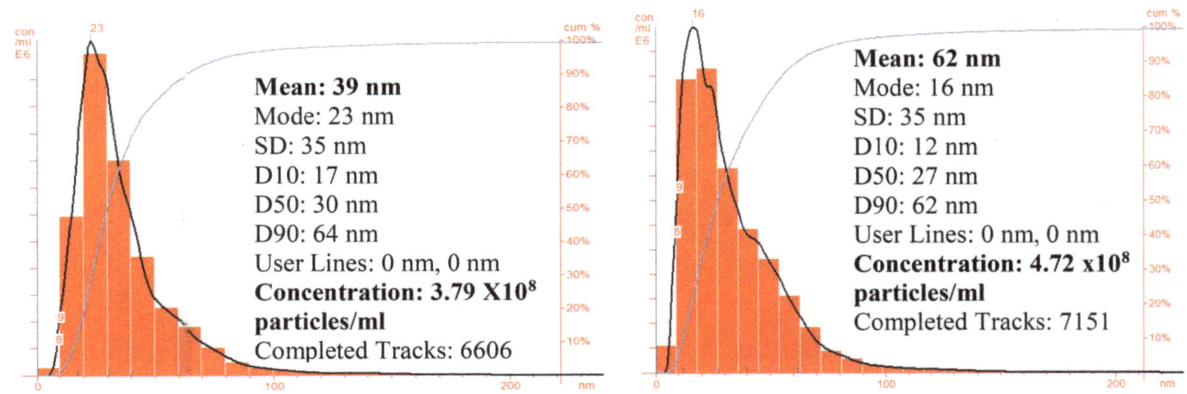

FIGURE 5 | NTA of silver and zinc nanoparticles.

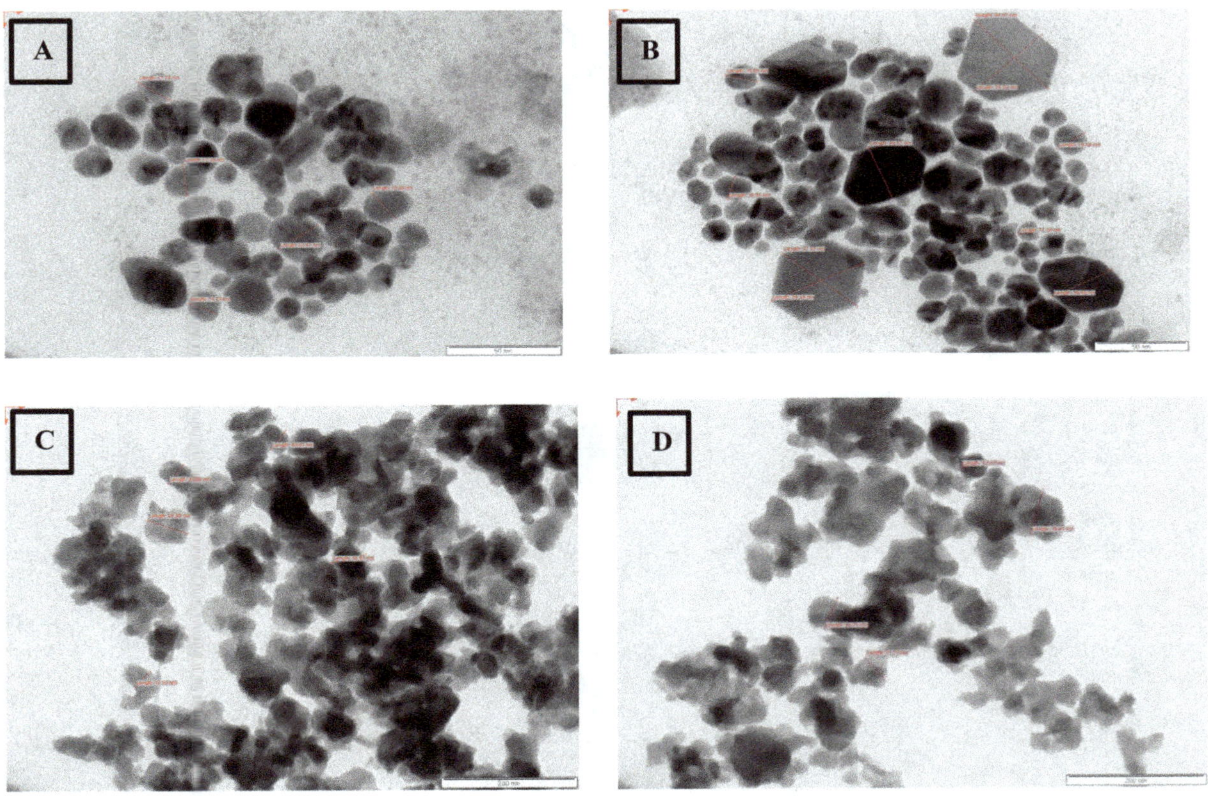

FIGURE 6 | TEM of silver nanoparticles **(A,B)** and zinc nanoparticles **(C,D)**.

Antimicrobial Activity of Nanoparticles

Minimum Inhibitory Concentration

Antimicrobial activity was assessed up to 10 mg/ml concentration of nanoparticle, which is almost double the concentration of cell toxicity to normal cells. For therapeutic consideration as an antimicrobial for synthesized nanoparticles only activity obtained at 5 mg/ml or below was considered. The MIC of both nanoparticles against range pathogenic bacterial strains is as mentioned in **Table 1**.

Anti-mycobacterial Activity – Broth Dilution Method

Table 2 shows the MICs obtained for standard strain and MDR strain of *M. tuberculosis* against both nanoparticles.

Synergistic Activity of Gentamicin and Nanoparticles

Nanoparticles were estimated for its synergistic action with gentamicin against MDR strains. For which susceptibility and MIC of gentamicin were checked, and results of that were

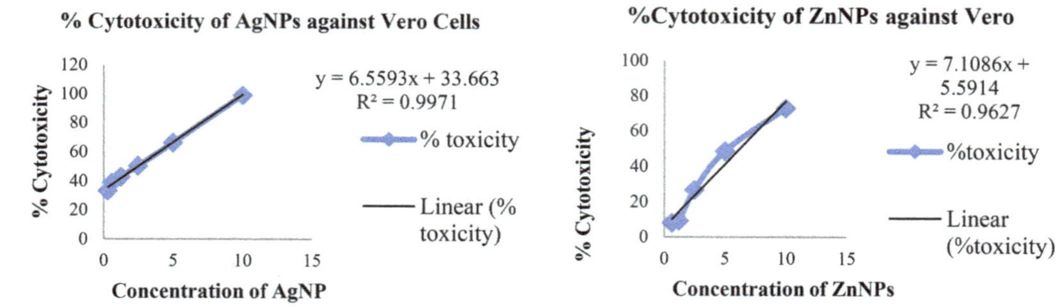

FIGURE 7 | Plot of cytotoxicity vs concentration of nanoparticles.

TABLE 1 | MIC of nanoparticles against range of pathogenic bacteria.

Sr. No.	Organism	ATCC No.	MIC mg/ml	
			AgNPs	ZnNPs
Gram-Negative Bacteria				
1.	*E. coli*	25922	2.5	10
2.	*E. aerogenes*	13048	0.6	>10
3.	*K. pneumoniae* (ESBL)	700603	2.5	>10
4.	*K. pneumoniae*	10031	5	10
5.	*S. typhimurium*	14028	2.5	5
6.	*S. abony*	6017	2.5	>10
7.	*S. boydii*	8700	2.5	>10
8.	*P. mirabilis*	21100	10	1.25
9.	*P. aeruginosa*	27853	2.5	>10
Gram-Positive Bacteria				
10.	*S. aureus*	25923	5	2.5
11.	*S. aureus*	6538	5	5
12.	*S. aureus* (MRSA)	43300	2.5	2.5
13.	*S. epidermidis*	12228	5	5
14.	*E. faecalis* (VRE)	51299	10	>10
15.	*B. subtilis*	6633	>10	>10
16.	*B. cereus*	11778	5	10

TABLE 2 | MIC of nanoparticles against standard and MDR strain of *Mycobacterium tuberculosis*.

Sr. No.	Organism	MIC (mg/ml)	
		AgNPs	ZnNPs
1.	*M. tuberculosis* (H37RV)	1.25	1.25
2.	*M. tuberculosis* (MDR – Clinical isolate)	1.25	1.25

as summarized in **Tables 3, 4**. Representative images in the **Supplementary Material.**

MIC of Gentamicin

The MIC of gentamicin by microbroth dilution method was evaluated up to 320 µg/ml, considering the limit and toxicity of gentamicin. **Table 5** shows the MICs obtained for each test strain.

TABLE 3 | Susceptibility for gentamicin.

Sr. No.	Organism	Diameter of Zone of Inhibition (mm)	
		Gentamicin (10 µg)	High-Level Gentamicin (120 µg)
1.	*S. aureus* ATCC 43300 (MRSA)	6 (R)	12 (R)
2.	*K. pneumoniae* ATCC 700603 (ESBL)	18 (S)	24 (S)
3.	*P. aeruginosa* ATCC 27853	25 (R)	32 (R)
4.	*E. faecalis* ATCC 51299 (VRE)	6 (R)	6 (R)
5.	*P. aeruginosa* (MDR) Clinical isolate	6 (R)	6 (R)

R, resistant; S, susceptible (Clinical and Laboratory Standards Institute [CLSI], 2014).

TABLE 4 | *E*-test MIC for gentamicin.

Sr. No.	Organism	EZY-MIC	
		Gentamicin (0.016–256 mg)	High-Level Gentamicin (0.064–1024 mg)
1.	*S. aureus* ATCC 43300 (MRSA)	256 (R)	1024 (R)
2.	*K. pneumoniae* ATCC 700603 (ESBL)	3 (S)	4 (S)
3.	*P. aeruginosa* ATCC 27853	1 (S)	1.5 (S)
4.	*E. faecalis* ATCC 51299 (VRE)	256 (R)	1024 (R)
5.	*P. aeruginosa* (MDR) clinical isolate	256 (R)	1024 (R)

R, resistant; S, susceptible (Clinical and Laboratory Standards Institute [CLSI], 2014).

Checkerboard Assay

For determination of synergistic activity of synthesized nanoparticles with gentamicin against test strains checkerboard

TABLE 5 | MIC for gentamicin – microbroth dilution method.

Sr. No.	Organism	MIC of Gentamicin (μg/ml)
1.	*S. aureus* ATCC 43300 (MRSA)	20
2.	*K. pneumoniae* ATCC 700603 (ESBL)	2.5
3.	*P. aeruginosa* ATCC 27853	<0.6
4.	*E. faecalis* ATCC 51299 (VRE)	>320
5.	*P. aeruginosa* (MDR) clinical isolate	>320

TABLE 6 | Synergistic activity of nanoparticles and gentamicin.

Sr. No.	Organism	ΣFIC Value	Result
1.	*S. aureus* ATCC 43300 (MRSA)	0.5	Synergistic (with AgNPs)
2.	*K. pneumoniae* ATCC 700603 (ESBL)	0.3	Synergistic (with AgNPs)
3.	*P. aeruginosa* (MDR) clinical isolate	0.2–0.5	Synergistic (with AgNPs)
4.	*S. aureus* ATCC 43300 (MRSA)	0.5	Synergistic (with ZnNPs)

AgNPS, silver nanoparticles; ZnNPs, zinc nanoparticles.

assay was performed. The FIC values and interpretation of synergism are as shown in **Table 6**.

DISCUSSION

Bacterial synthesis of silver nanoparticles by *P. hibiscicola* was first reported in our previous work (Punjabi et al., 2017). Silver nanoparticles synthesized were characterized by various spectral and microscopic techniques to specifically confirm the synthesis and determine the details of synthesized nanoparticles.

In this study, the NTA revealed the average size of AgNP ranged 10 to 70 nm, but the mean size of synthesized silver nanoparticles was found to be 39 nm. This is in accordance to similar studies with biosynthesis of nanoparticles and its measurement by NTA. Birla et al. (2013) report the size distribution of nanoparticles obtained on a particle-by-particle basis in case of NTA which enables particle population, size, intensity of nanoparticle in suspension, and simultaneously determining their Brownian motion. The NTA calculates the particles size by distance traveled by them, and calculation is based on Stokes–Einstein equation. The average size distribution of silver nanoparticles synthesized by *Fusarium oxysporum* in their study was 41 nm (Birla et al., 2013). TEM revealed an average size of 40.0 nm, which is in accordance with results obtained by NTA. The TEM analysis indicated that the particles were crystalline in nature.

The extracellular biosynthesis of silver and zinc oxide nanoparticles was investigated using *Pichia fermentans* JA2 by Chauhan et al. (2015). The biosynthesized silver nanoparticles were found to inhibit most Gram-negative clinical pathogens used in the study, while zinc oxide nanoparticles only inhibited *P. aeruginosa*. The silver and zinc oxide nanoparticles synthesized using *Pichia fermentans* JA2 had potent antibacterial effect that leads to notable contribution to pharmaceutical associations.

The above report boosts the idea of synthesizing zinc nanoparticles by *P. hibiscicola*. Thus, studies were undertaken to synthesize, optimize, and characterize zinc nanoparticles, which were found to be of variable shapes and the average size of 60 nm. Although DLS reports 110 nm, NTA shows 62 nm final size of nanoparticles was only considered as obtained in TEM micrographs, which were 60 nm. In most case, synthesis of zinc oxide nanoparticles often takes place which could highly be possible in this case as well. This could be alleged on basis of the spectra in UV–Vis spectrophotometer and XRD pattern, which does indicate the presence of oxide specific peaks. Different functional groups identified as secondary alcohols, amines, and alkanes by FTIR analysis, which could mainly be due to biological synthesis.

Jayaseelan et al. (2012) present a work for biosynthesis of zinc oxide nanoparticles (ZnONPs) using bacteria, *Aeromonas hydrophila*. The ZnO NPs were characterized, and a peak at 374 nm in the UV–vis spectrum was observed. Further, XRD confirmed the crystalline nature of the nanoparticles and AFM exhibited the morphology of the nanoparticle to be spherical, oval with an average size of 57.72 nm. The FTIR peaks summarized as alkynes, alkanes, alkenes, primary amines, alcohols, acetate, ethers, and carboxyl compounds. The results of zinc nanoparticles synthesized by *P. hibiscicola* are highly compatible with this study. It could well be said so that synthesis of zinc oxide nanoparticles formation takes place by *P. hibiscicola* also.

The most vital parameter to determine the therapeutic feasibility is toxicity of the material. Therefore, *in vitro* cytotoxicity of both nanoparticles synthesized were assessed on animal tissue. The technique employed to do so was MTT assay, which is a colorimetric estimation of living cells determined by absorbance values upon treatment with the drug for a stipulated amount of time. The cell line used to evaluate the toxicity of nanoparticles was Vero a non-cancerous epithelial cell line commonly used for the said purpose.

In one of the reports, use of AgNP as a therapeutic agent is limited due to its cytotoxicity against mammalian cells. Wherein cytotoxicity of *P. putida* synthesized silver nanoparticles against HEp-2 cells was determined by MTT assay. No significant cytotoxic effect at 25 μg/ml concentration was found, which was lethal for the bacteria tested for antibacterial efficacy (Gopinath et al., 2017). This study highlights and supports the results obtained for nanoparticles synthesized by *P. hibiscicola* although the range of concentration varies mainly due to the presence of protein in the nanomaterial. The purification of nanoparticles was not carried out and freeze-dried powders of as-synthesized nanoparticle were used for cytotoxicity and other activities, leading to the larger amount of material.

One of the most important ailments affecting thousands around the world is microbial infections and more to concern is its drug resistance happening at a rapid pace. Special emphasis needs to be given to drug-resistant infections of bacteria in the community and hospital-acquired infections like ESBL, MRSA, VRE, MDR, *P. aeruginosa* infections, and MDR *M. tuberculosis* infections. The resistance development has been concerning, and world organizations have been raising alarms at regular intervals. This has also lead to screening a vast number of agents from both biological as well as the chemical cluster for antimicrobial potential. Nanoparticles have potentially all the requisites for qualification as an antimicrobial agent. Not only can nanoparticles have efficiency against this infection causing etiological agents but can also prevent the current therapeutic agents from being rendered useless due to resistance, by alternative or supplementary therapies with nanoparticles along with regular antibiotics. Thus, an interesting aspect was to evaluate nanoparticles synthesized by *P. hibiscicola* for its antimicrobial activity.

Only activity obtained at or below 5 mg/ml was considered suitable for antimicrobial potential against the test strain considering the toxicity of nanoparticles at higher concentrations. Zinc nanoparticle gave activity only against two Gram-negative and four Gram-positive strains, importantly against MRSA at 2.5 mg/ml. Silver nanoparticles were the most potent antimicrobial with activity against most bacteria. In case of the drug-resistant variants for both ESBL and MRSA, activity was observed at 2.5 mg/ml. Both AgNP and ZnNP had anti-TB activity at 1.25 mg/ml for both strains. These results definitely imply that nanoparticles synthesized by *P. hibiscicola* have great antimicrobial potential. This is encouraging to do further evaluations and assess its practical application with more specific *in vivo* studies.

Abd-Elnaby et al. (2016) reported an excellent antibacterial activity against Gram-negative and Gram-positive bacterial pathogens by microbiologically synthesized AgNPs. Mostafa et al. (2015) report activity of chemically synthesized silver nanoparticles against *P. aeruginosa*, *S. aureus*, *Streptococcus pyogenes*, and *S. typhi*. A report stating anti-tuberculosis activity of biosynthesized silver nanoparticles-mentioned spherical-shaped silver nanoparticles with the average particle size of 5 nm, had anti-mycobacterial activity against *M. tuberculosis* and clinical isolates of multi-drug resistant *M. tuberculosis* (MDR-TB) (Banu and Rathod, 2013).

Arrays of pathogens causing different infections were inhibited with the synthesized nanoparticles suggesting its efficiency in controlling infections. This also recommends for assessment of these nanoparticles for synergistic activity with common antibiotics. Thus, synergistic activity against drug-resistant strains was evaluated with antibiotic gentamicin. Gentamicin is an aminoglycoside and commonly used antibiotic against both Gram-positive and Gram-negative bacteria. Currently, gentamicin is susceptible to some and resistant to some bacterial isolates, but it could fast be completely resistant if measures to control resistance are not in place soon. Thus, hypothetically nanoparticles could rescue this situation with its potential synergistic efficiency if found.

Antibacterial susceptibility against gentamicin was assessed by disk diffusion method followed by MIC of gentamicin by *E* – test and micro broth dilution method. The results of disk diffusion and *E*-test identify all the isolates as resistant to gentamicin as per CLSI guidelines of 2014. The MIC of gentamicin by micro broth dilution method was evaluated with a maximum concentration of 320 μg/ml, which is reportedly a toxic concentration. Synergistic activity of nanoparticles and gentamicin was evaluated by Checkerboard method, considering the MICs and toxicity of both gentamicin and nanoparticles.

Promising results were obtained for synergistic activity, zinc nanoparticles exhibited synergism with gentamicin in case of MRSA, so did silver nanoparticles for MRSA, ESBL, and MDR *P. aeruginosa*. A study on the fugal-mediated synthesis of silver nanoparticles reports synergistic activity of silver nanoparticles with amikacin, kanamycin, and streptomycin against *E. coli*, *S. aureus*, and *P. aeruginosa*. The report concluded synergistic action of antimicrobial agent can significantly curtail side effects by reducing dosages. Thus, use of nanoparticles combined with antibiotics can improve their efficacy against various pathogenic microbes (Barapatre et al., 2016). The results of synergistic activity of nanoparticles synthesized by *P. hibiscicola* are in accordance with this report and rightly suggested nanoparticles can indeed be one of the most effective agents in combating serious infections that are rendered untreatable with available antibiotics. There are limited studies with this extent of antimicrobial activity, with qualitative as well as quantitative data against wide range of ATCC and clinical strains. Further to this, determining the mode of action will be an important aspect. But it is well known that most metallic nanoparticles cause oxidative damage to microbes due to excessive generation of reactive oxygen species (ROS), this can be extended to the nanoparticles synthesized.

The extensive potential of silver and zinc nanoparticles against drug-resistant strains of community and hospital-acquired infections opens a new arena of antimicrobials for treatment, supplementary prophylaxis, and prevention therapy. Biologically synthesized nanoparticles can become future anti-infectives and prove to be one of the most potential therapeutic agents.

CONCLUSION

This study covers certain major areas of nanoscience like biological synthesis, characterization, and biomedical application. It provides an extremely potential isolate capable of synthesizing silver and zinc nanoparticles. Characterization studies revealed synthesis of stable nanoparticles of average size 50 nm for silver and 60 nm for zinc nanoparticles. The cytotoxicity studies of nanoparticles against normal cells (non – cancerous) revealed the toxic concentrations for both. Toxicity is the most important factor for therapeutic application. Efficiency of these nanoparticles against drug-resistant pathogen makes it a viable candidate for therapeutics. Thus, biologically synthesized nanoparticles can become future anti-infective agents and can be formulated for drugs or topical agents.

AUTHOR CONTRIBUTIONS

KP conceptualized and executed the entire experiment as well as the writing of this work. SM helped with the characterization studies, mainly the XRD analysis. RC, VC, and DD helped with the experimental work, including microbial assays and toxicity analysis. VC also helped write and format the manuscript. SD managed the successful completion of the entire project and played an instrumental role in the manuscript.

REFERENCES

Abd-Elnaby, H. M., Abo-Elala, G. M., Abdel-Raouf, U. M., and Hamed, M. M. (2016). Antibacterial and anticancer activity of extracellular synthesized silver nanoparticles from marine *Streptomyces rochei* MHM13. *Egypt. J. Aquat. Res.* 42, 301–312. doi: 10.1016/j.ejar.2016.05.004

Andrews, J. M. (2001). Determination of minimum inhibitory concentrations. *J. Antimicrob. Chemother.* 48(Suppl. 1), 5–16. doi: 10.1093/jac/48.suppl_1.5

Ataee, R., Derakhshanpour, J., Mehrabi Tavana, A., and Eydi, A. (2011). Antibacterial effect of calcium carbonate nanoparticles on *Agrobacterium tumefaciens*. *J. Mil. Med.* 13, 65–70.

Babu, M. M., Sridhar, J., and Gunasekaran, P. (2011). Global transcriptome analysis of *Bacillus cereus* ATCC 14579 in response to silver nitrate stress. *J. Nanobiotechnol.* 9:49. doi: 10.1186/1477-3155-9-49

Banu, A., and Rathod, V. (2013). Biosynthesis of monodispersed silver nanoparticles and their activity against *Mycobacterium tuberculosis*. *Int. J. Biomed. Nanosci. Nanotechnol.* 3, 211–220. doi: 10.1504/IJBNN.2013.054507

Barapatre, A., Aadil, K. R., and Jha, H. (2016). Synergistic antibacterial and antibiofilm activity of silver nanoparticles biosynthesized by lignin-degrading fungus. *Bioresour. Bioprocess.* 3:8. doi: 10.1186/s40643-016-0083-y

Bauer, A., Kirby, W., Sherris, J. C., and Turck, M. (1966). Antibiotic susceptibility testing by a standardized single disk method. *Am. J. Clin. Pathol.* 45, 493–496. doi: 10.1093/ajcp/45.4_ts.493

Bhattacharyya, D., Singh, S., Satnalika, N., Khandelwal, A., and Jeon, S. H. (2009). Nanotechnology, big things from a tiny world: a review. *Nanotechnology* 2, 29–38.

Birla, S. S., Gaikwad, S. C., Gade, A. K., and Rai, M. K. (2013). Rapid synthesis of silver nanoparticles from *Fusarium oxysporum* by optimizing physicocultural conditions. *Sci. World J.* 2013:796018. doi: 10.1155/2013/796018

Breitinger, H. (2010). "Drug synergy–mechanisms and methods of analysis," in *Toxicity and Drug Testing*, ed. B. Acree (London: InTech), 143–166.

Chauhan, R., Reddy, A., and Abraham, J. (2015). Biosynthesis of silver and zinc oxide nanoparticles using *Pichia* fermentans JA2 and their antimicrobial property. *Appl. Nanosci.* 5, 63–71. doi: 10.1007/s13204-014-0292-7

Clinical and Laboratory Standards Institute [CLSI] (2012). *Performance Standards for Antimicrobial Susceptibility Testing; Twenty-Second Informational Supplement. CLSI Document M100-S22.* Wayne, PA: Clinical and Laboratory Standards Institute.

Clinical and Laboratory Standards Institute [CLSI] (2014). *Performance Standards for Antimicrobial Susceptibility Testing: Twenty-Fourth Informational Supplement, M100-S24*, Vol. 34. Wayne, PA: Clinical and Laboratory Standards Institute.

Conde, J., Doria, G., and Baptista, P. (2012). Noble metal nanoparticles applications in cancer. *J. Drug Deliv.* 2012:751075. doi: 10.1155/2012/751075

Freshney, R. I. (2005). *Culture of Animal Cells: A Manual of Basic Technique.* New York, NY: John Wiley and Sons, Inc. doi: 10.1002/9780471747598

Freshney, R. I. (2010). *Culture of Animal Cells.* New York, NY: John Wiley and Sons. doi: 10.1002/9780470649367

Gopinath, V., Priyadarshini, S., Loke, M. F., Arunkumar, J., Marsili, E., MubarakAli, D., et al. (2017). Biogenic synthesis, characterization of antibacterial silver nanoparticles and its cell cytotoxicity. *Arab. J. Chem.* 10, 1107–1117. doi: 10.1016/j.arabjc.2015.11.011

Horikoshi, S., and Serpone, N. (2013). *Introduction to Nanoparticles.* Weinheim: Wiley-VCH Verlag GmbH and Co. KGaA.

Jadaun, G. P., Agarwal, C., Sharma, H., Ahmed, Z., Upadhyay, P., Faujdar, J., et al. (2007). Determination of ethambutol MICs for *Mycobacterium tuberculosis* and *Mycobacterium avium* isolates by resazurin microtitre assay. *J. Antimicrob. Chemother.* 60, 152–155. doi: 10.1093/jac/dkm117

Jayaseelan, C., Rahuman, A. A., Kirthi, A. V., Marimuthu, S., Santhoshkumar, T., Bagavan, A., et al. (2012). Novel microbial route to synthesize ZnO nanoparticles using *Aeromonas hydrophila* and their activity against pathogenic bacteria and fungi. *Spectrochim. Acta A Mol. Biomol. Spectrosc.* 90, 78–84. doi: 10.1016/j.saa.2012.01.006

Mostafa, A. A., Sayed, S. R., Solkamy, E. N., Khan, M., Shaik, M. R., Al-Warthan, A., et al. (2015). Evaluation of biological activities of chemically synthesized silver nanoparticles. *J. Nanomater.* 16:443. doi: 10.1155/2015/789178

Nachnani, S., Scuteri, A., Newman, M. G., Avanessian, A. B., and Lomeli, S. L. (1992). E-test: a new technique for antimicrobial susceptibility testing for periodontal microorganisms. *J. Periodontol.* 63, 576–583. doi: 10.1902/jop.1992.63.7.576

Oves, M., Aslam, M., Rauf, M. A., Qayyum, S., Qari, H. A., Khan, M. S., et al. (2018). Antimicrobial and anticancer activities of silver nanoparticles synthesized from the root hair extract of *Phoenix dactylifera*. *Mater. Sci. Eng. C* 89, 429–443. doi: 10.1016/j.msec.2018.03.035

Pattanayak, U. (2013). *Green Synthesis of Zinc Nano Particle By Microbes.* Doctoral thesis, National Institute of technology, Rourkela.

Punjabi, K., Yedurkar, S., Shah, S., Deshapnde, S., and Vaidya, S. (2017). Biosynthesis of silver nanoparticles by *Pseudomonas* spp isolated from effluent of an electroplating industry. *IET Nanobiotechnol.* 11, 584–590. doi: 10.1049/iet-nbt.2016.0172

Qayyum, S., Oves, M., and Khan, A. U. (2017). Obliteration of bacterial growth and biofilm through ROS generation by facilely synthesized green silver nanoparticles. *PLoS One* 12:e0181363. doi: 10.1371/journal.pone.0181363

Rabadia, A., Kamat, S., and Kamat, D. (2013). Study of synergistic action of cefotaxime and *Terminalia chebula* on *Acinetobacter baumannii* using checkerboard assay. *Int. J. Pharm. Pharm. Sci.* 5, 830–832.

Riss, T. L., Moravec, R. A., and Niles, A. L. (2011). Cytotoxicity testing: measuring viable cells, dead cells, and detecting mechanism of cell death. *Methods Mol. Biol.* 740, 103–114. doi: 10.1007/978-1-61779-108-6_12

Roco, M. C. (2007). "National nanotechnology initiative-past, present, future," in *Handbook on Nanoscience, Engineering and Technology*, eds W. A. Goddard, D. Brenner, S. E. Lyshevski, and G. J. Iafrate (Boca Raton, FL: CRC Press).

Satyavani, K., Gurudeeban, S., Ramanathan, T., and Balasubramanian, T. (2011). Biomedical potential of silver nanoparticles synthesized from calli cells of *Citrullus colocynthis* (L.) schrad. *J. Nanobiotechnol.* 9:43. doi: 10.1186/1477-3155-9-43

Waghmare, S., Deshmukh, A., Kulkarni, S., and Oswaldo, L. (2011). Biosynthesis and characterization of manganese and zinc nanoparticles. *Univ. J. Environ. Res. Technol.* 1, 64–69.

Wiegand, I., Hilpert, K., and Hancock, R. E. (2008). Agar and broth dilution methods to determine the minimal inhibitory concentration (MIC) of antimicrobial substances. *Nat. Protoc.* 3, 163–175. doi: 10.1038/nprot.2007.521

7

Co-Harboring of Novel bla_{KPC-2} Plasmid and Integrative and Conjugative Element Carrying Tn*6203* in Multidrug-Resistant *Pseudomonas aeruginosa*

Heng Cai[1,2,3], Yiwei Zhu[1,2,3], Dandan Hu[1,2,3], Yue Li[1,2,3], Sebastian Leptihn[1,4], Belinda Loh[4], Xiaoting Hua[1,2,3] and Yunsong Yu[1,2,3]**

[1]Department of Infectious Diseases, Sir Run Run Shaw Hospital, Zhejiang University School of Medicine, Hangzhou, China, [2]Key Laboratory of Microbial Technology and Bioinformatics of Zhejiang Province, Hangzhou, China, [3]Regional Medical Center for National Institute of Respiratory Diseases, Sir Run Run Shaw Hospital, Zhejiang University School of Medicine, Hangzhou, China, [4]Zhejiang University-University of Edinburgh Institute, Zhejiang University, Haining, China

***Correspondence:**
Yunsong Yu
yvys119@zju.edu.cn
Xiaoting Hua
xiaotinghua@zju.edu.cn*

Many strains of the opportunistic pathogen *Pseudomonas aeruginosa* have acquired resistance to multiple antibiotics. Carbapenem-resistant *P. aeruginosa* poses a global healthcare problem due to limited therapeutic options for the treatment of infections. Plasmids and integrative and conjugative elements (ICEs) are the major vectors of antibiotic-resistance gene transfer. In our study, four carbapenem-resistant strains of *P. aeruginosa* were isolated from the same patient in a tertiary referral hospital in China, one of these was resistant to gentamicin and tobramycin. In this strain P33, we observed a non-transferable plasmid, pP33-2, carrying a novel bla_{KPC-2} gene segment (IS*Kpn27*-bla_{KPC-2}-IS*Kpn6*-*korC*-ORF-*klcA*-IS*26*), which we concluded to have been formed by IS*26*-mediated gene cluster translocation. In addition, by comparing the chromosomes of the *P. aeruginosa* strains that belong to the same sequence type, we identified an ICE, ICEP33, adjacent to a prophage. The *att*L site of ICEP33 is identical to the terminal part of the *att*R site of the prophage. The ICEP33 element contains the transposon Tn*6203*, which encodes antibiotic and metal resistance genes. The insertion of ICEP33 in the chromosome mediates resistance to multiple antibiotics. Our study contributes to the understanding of the acquisition of antibiotic resistance in *P. aeruginosa* facilitated by mobile genetic elements.

Keywords: plasmid, KPC-2, integrative and conjugative element, prophage, *Pseudomonas aeruginosa*

INTRODUCTION

Multidrug-resistant (MDR) *Pseudomonas aeruginosa* poses a threat to human health, causing severe acute and chronic infections in hospitalized and immunocompromised patients (Horcajada et al., 2019). Due to the increasing resistance levels globally, the World Health Organization has listed this bacteria as a "critical" pathogen of which research and development for new antibiotics are urgently required (Tacconelli et al., 2018). While carbapenems are currently one of the most important classes of antibiotics for the treatment of MDR *P. aeruginosa* strains, they are ineffective in nearly 30% of clinical cases in China (Hu et al., 2019a).

The acquisition of carbapenemase genes is one of the main mechanisms of resistance to carbapenems (van Duin and Doi, 2017). *Klebsiella pneumoniae* carbapenemases (KPCs), belonging to Ambler's class A beta-lactamases, have spread extensively and are often horizontally transferred *via* plasmids (Munoz-Price et al., 2013; Chen et al., 2014b). The previous reports have documented KPC-2-producing *P. aeruginosa* ST463 in Hangzhou, China, and typically, the bla_{KPC-2} genes were plasmid located (Hu et al., 2015b, 2019b). In addition to intrinsic resistances and chromosomal mutations, mobile genetic elements, such as plasmids and integrative and conjugative elements (ICEs), are responsible for spreading resistance genes to *P. aeruginosa* strains (Botelho et al., 2019).

Integrative and conjugative elements are key players in transmitting antibiotic resistance by conjugation like plasmids and then integrating into the chromosome and being replicated as part of the host genome like bacteriophage (Carraro and Burrus, 2015). They carry certain genes that are required for excision, maintenance, conjugative transfer, and integration into the host genome. ICEs may also carry cargo genes that confer diverse phenotypes on the organisms including pathogenicity islands containing virulence-associated genes (Wurdemann and Tummler, 2007; Kung et al., 2010; Roy Chowdhury et al., 2017).

In this study, we found a clinical *P. aeruginosa* isolate carrying a novel bla_{KPC-2} plasmid, pP33-2, markedly different from the bla_{KPC-2} carrying plasmids reported previously. This strain also harbored an ICE, ICEP33 containing a Tn*6203* transposon with several resistance genes.

MATERIALS AND METHODS

Clinical Isolates and Identification

Four isolates, P20, P22, P23, and P33, were cultured from a patient's rectal and throat swabs and tracheotomy tube using Pseudomonas Isolation Agar (Peptone 20 g/l, $MgCl_2$ 1.4 g/l, K_2SO_4 10 g/l, Triclosan 25 mg/l, Agar 13.6 g/l, and Glycerol 20 ml/l.). Bacterial species were identified by the matrix-assisted laser desorption ionization-time of flight mass spectrometry (MALDI-TOF MS; Bruker Daltonik GmbH, Bremen, Germany) and 16S rRNA gene sequencing.

Antimicrobial Susceptibility Testing

Antimicrobial susceptibility testing was performed by broth microdilution. Antibiotics included: piperacillin; piperacillin-tazobactam; ceftazidime; ceftazidime-avibactam; cefepime; aztreonam; imipenem; meropenem; gentamicin; tobramycin; amikacin; ciprofloxacin; levofloxacin; and colistin. The results were interpreted according to Clinical and Laboratory Standards Institute guidelines (CLSI; M100, 30th Edn.; CLSI, 2020). *P. aeruginosa* strain ATCC 27853 was used as the quality control.

Genome Sequencing and Analysis

Genomic DNA was extracted by the QIAamp DNA Mini Kit (Qiagen, Germany) and sequenced by HiSeq (Illumina, San Diego, CA, United States). The paired-end reads were assembled by CLC genomics workbench (version 12). Multilocus sequence typing was identified by the PubMLST[1] (Jolley et al., 2018). Antibiotic resistance genes were identified by the ResFinder 4.1[2] (Zankari et al., 2012) and were further confirmed by PCR. The genomic DNA of P23 and P33 was additionally prepared by the Gentra Puregene Yeast/Bact. Kit (Qiagen) and Nanopore sequencing was performed by a MinION sequencer (Oxford Nanopore Technologies, Oxford, United Kingdom). *De novo* assembly of the Illumina and Nanopore reads was performed using the Unicycler v0.4.8 (Wick et al., 2017). The genome sequence was annotated by Prokka[3] (Seemann, 2014) and manually refined by NCBI Blast (Camacho et al., 2009). The nucleotide polymorphism (SNP) tree was built by snippy-multi and FastTree,[4] visualized by ggtree v2.0.4 (Yu, 2020). Conjugative apparatus was predicted by oriTfinder[5] and MOBscan (Li et al., 2018; Garcillan-Barcia et al., 2020). ICEs were predicted by ICEfinder[6] (Liu et al., 2019).

Conjugation

Conjugation assays were conducted using rifampicin-resistant *Escherichia coli* EC600 and a spontaneous rifampicin-resistant mutant of *P. aeruginosa* PAO1 as the recipient strain. Strain P33 was used as the donor. The selective Mueller-Hinton agar plates contained rifampicin (300 μg/ml) combined with meropenem (0.5 μg/ml) or meropenem (4 μg/ml). Each conjugation experiment was repeated at least three times.

Accession Numbers

The complete sequences of the chromosomes and plasmids from *P. aeruginosa* strain P23 and P33 have been deposited in the GenBank nucleotide database under accession numbers CP065417-CP065418 and CP065412-CP065416, respectively. The genome sequences of *P. aeruginosa* strains P20 and P22 have been deposited in the GenBank database under accession numbers JAEMVM000000000 and JAEMVL000000000, respectively.

RESULTS AND DISCUSSION

Case Report

In August 2019, a 69-year-old man was hospitalized in Sir Run Run Shaw Hospital (Mayo Clinic Care Network) in Hangzhou, China. The patient had been suffering from a severe cough with expectoration for 5 months, in addition to fever and hypotension that began approximately 1 month

[1]https://pubmlst.org/organisms/pseudomonas-aeruginosa
[2]https://cge.cbs.dtu.dk/services/ResFinder/
[3]https://github.com/tseemann/prokka
[4]https://github.com/tseemann/snippy
[5]https://tool-mml.sjtu.edu.cn/oriTfinder
[6]https://db-mml.sjtu.edu.cn/ICEfinder

before hospitalization. The patient's medical history included hypertension, cerebral infarction, and multiple pulmonary infections. Several months before hospitalization, the patient suffered from a bloodstream infection by *P. aeruginosa*. After this renewed hospitalization, the patient's symptoms were controlled by antibiotics and other supportive treatment, such as mechanical ventilation and fluid therapy. The course of antibiotics used is listed in chronological order as follows: cefoperazone-sulbactam, cefuroxime, piperacillin-tazobactam, and cefuroxime. After 1 month, his condition improved and he was discharged. Four *P. aeruginosa* strains P20, P22, P23, and P33 were isolated from different anatomical locations or at different time points during hospitalization (**Table 1**). Specifically, P20 was isolated from the rectal swab on the day of admission; P22 and P23 were isolated from the rectal swab and throat swab on the fifth day after admission, respectively; and P33 was isolated from the tracheotomy tube on the twelfth day.

Results of Antimicrobial Susceptibility Testing

The four *P. aeruginosa* isolates were all resistant to penicillins, β-lactam/β-lactamase inhibitor combination agents, cephems, monobactams, carbapenems, and fluoroquinolones and intermediate to colistin. P20, P22, and P23 were susceptible to aminoglycosides while P33 was susceptible to amikacin but resistant to gentamicin and tobramycin (**Table 1**).

Genetic Relationship and Antibiotic Resistance Genes of the Strains

P20, P22, P23, and P33 were all identified as ST463. An analysis based on SNP showed that P33 was more genetically distant from the other three strains (**Figure 1**). P33 differed from P20 in 315 SNPs, from P22 in 314 SNPs, and from P23 in 306 SNPs. Taking the large number of varied SNPs into consideration, it seems that P33 unlikely evolved from the other three strains recently, i.e., during the hospitalization.

The antimicrobial resistance genes of P33 were different from the other isolates. The genome of P33 contained genes that conferred resistance to β-lactams ($bla_{CARB\text{-}2}$), aminoglycosides (*aac(6')–IIa*, *ant(2")–Ia*), and sulfonamide (*sul1*), which were absent in P20, P22, and P23. While P33 lacked $bla_{OXA\text{-}468}$, the other three strains contained the gene. All of four strains had *aph(3')–IIb*, bla_{KPC-2}, $bla_{PDC-374}$, *catB7*, *crpP*, and *fosA* (**Figure 1**). The genes *aac(6')–IIa* and *ant(2")–Ia* are likely to confer the resistance in P33 to gentamicin and tobramycin. Nanopore sequencing and subsequent analysis showed that the carbapenem-resistant gene bla_{KPC-2} is located in a plasmid found in P23 and P33, respectively. Sequence analysis indicated that P20, P22, and P23 carry a closely related bla_{KPC-2} plasmid, while the one in the P33 is different. The nucleotide sequence of the bla_{KPC-2} plasmid in P33 is about in 30% identical to those in others.

The observations of our study reveal differences in SNP and antimicrobial susceptibility among the strains of the same sequence type (ST463). We speculate that the P33 strain could have acquired the mobile elements carrying the relevant antibiotic resistance genes by exchanging genes with other bacteria in the host microbiome during the long-term repeated infection.

Characterization of Plasmids in P33

Employing Nanopore sequencing, we were able to identify four plasmids in P33, named pP33-1, pP33-2, pP33-3, and pP33-4. Plasmid pP33-1 is 49,654 bp long with an average GC content of 59% and 58 predicted open reading frames (ORFs). Plasmid pP33-2 has a length of 48,306 bp, with an average GC content of 59%. Sequence annotation predicted 64 ORFs. Plasmid pP33-3 is smaller with 3,014 bp, an average GC content of 61% and only three predicted ORFs. Finally, pP33-4 was predicted to contain three ORFs on a similarly sized plasmid (2,953 bp) with an average GC content of 65%.

The genetic structure of pP33-2 can be divided into the general maintenance and the bla_{KPC-2} segment. The general maintenance includes the replication initiation (*repA*), partitioning

TABLE 1 | Summary of antimicrobial susceptibility testing for four strains.

	Antibiotics	P20 (rectal swab, day 0)	P22 (rectal swab, day 5)	P23 (throat swab, day 5)	P33 (tracheotomy tube, day 12)
MIC (μg/ml)	Piperacillin	>256 (R)	>256 (R)	>256 (R)	>256 (R)
	Piperacillin-tazobactam	>256/4 (R)	>256/4 (R)	>256/4 (R)	>256/4 (R)
	Ceftazidime-avibactam	32/4 (R)	16/4 (R)	16/4 (R)	16/4 (R)
	Ceftazidime	256 (R)	256 (R)	256 (R)	128 (R)
	Cefepime	>256 (R)	>256 (R)	>256 (R)	>256 (R)
	Aztreonam	>128 (R)	>128 (R)	>128 (R)	>128 (R)
	Imipenem	>128 (R)	>128 (R)	>128 (R)	>128 (R)
	Meropenem	>128 (R)	>128 (R)	>128 (R)	>128 (R)
	Colistin	0.5 (I)	0.5 (I)	0.5 (I)	0.5 (I)
	Gentamicin	1 (S)	1 (S)	1 (S)	>64 (R)
	Tobramycin	0.5 (S)	0.5 (S)	0.5 (S)	>64 (R)
	Amikacin	4 (S)	4 (S)	4 (S)	8 (S)
	Ciprofloxacin	16 (R)	16 (R)	16 (R)	16 (R)
	Levofloxacin	>64 (R)	>64 (R)	>64 (R)	>64 (R)

S, sensitive; I, intermediate; and R, resistant.

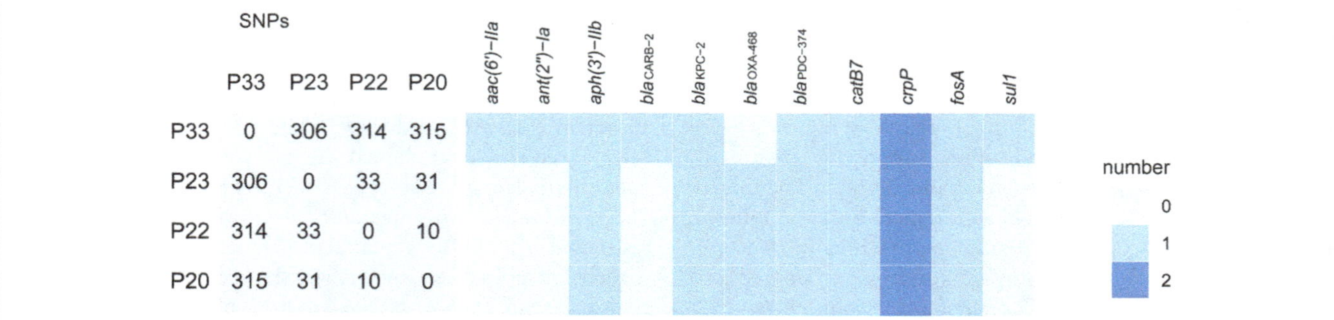

FIGURE 1 | SNP difference matrix and heat map of predicted antibiotic resistance genes of four *Pseudomonas aeruginosa* strains. The numbers in the matrix are the number of variant SNPs between the strains. The indicator denotes the cope number of genes by different color.

(*parAB*), and genes for plasmid maintenance. The plasmid pP33-2 is classified as an unidentified incompatibility (Inc.) type. BLAST analysis showed that pP33-2 is similar to plasmid ID40_1 (LR700249.1), pPA7790 (CP015000.1), pPB353_1 (CP025052.1), pPB354_1 (CP025054.1), pMS14403A (CP049162.1), pJUPA4295 (LC586269.1), and an unnamed plasmid in strain AR_0230 (CP027175.1), with query coverage ranging from 59 to 78% and an identity of 95.24–98.51%. After removing the $bla_{\text{KPC-2}}$ cluster, pP33-2 shares 97–100% coverage with the plasmid sequences mentioned above. Thus, while these plasmids share similar backbones, only pP33-2 carries the $bla_{\text{KPC-2}}$ gene, indicating that pP33-2 is a novel $bla_{\text{KPC-2}}$ plasmid in *P. aeruginosa*.

Plasmid pP33-1 encodes four components of a conjugative apparatus: an origin of transfer (oriT), a relaxase (R), a type IV coupling protein (T4CP), and a type IV secretion system (T4SS; Smillie et al., 2010), while pP33-2 was predicted to harbor only a MOB_C family relaxase and part of T4SS. Although pP33-1 was included as a conjugative helper, conjugation experiments with pP33-2 failed several times, suggesting that pP33-2 might be not transferable.

Evolution of the $bla_{\text{KPC-2}}$ Gene Cluster Within the Strains

Strain P23 harbors the $bla_{\text{KPC-2}}$ gene-containing plasmid pP23, which is very similar to plasmid YLH6_p3 (MK882885.1) and pPA1101 (MH734334.1; Hu et al., 2019b). The accessory modules of $bla_{\text{KPC-2}}$ were different in pPA1101, pP23, and pP33-2 (**Figure 2**). In pPA1101, there was a core module Tn3-IS*Kpn27*-$bla_{\text{KPC-2}}$-IS*Kpn6*-*korC*-ORF-*klcA*-ORF-ORF with two inverted IS*26* elements at both ends. The core module Tn3-IS*Kpn27*-$bla_{\text{KPC-2}}$-IS*Kpn6* was frequently identified as the $bla_{\text{KPC-2}}$ gene cluster in China (Shen et al., 2009; Cai et al., 2014; Chen et al., 2014a; Li et al., 2015). Occasionally, the core module was observed to be interrupted by the IS*26*-based composite transposons (Chen et al., 2014c). When comparing pP23 to pPA1101, a part of the core module appeared to be reversed (**Figure 2**). Due to the intramolecular replicative transposition in inverse orientation, the segment between the original IS*26* and the targeted site on *tnp*A was reversed. An indication that supports our interpretation is that we observed 8-bp sequences (5'-CGATATTT-3') reverse complements of each other that flank the two IS*26* copies (Harmer et al., 2014; He et al., 2015; Partridge et al., 2018).

Unlike sequences reported previously, IS*Kpn27*-$bla_{\text{KPC-2}}$-IS*Kpn6*-*korC*-ORF-*klcA*-IS*26* was found in the KPC module of pP33-2. The gene cluster *korC*-ORF-*klcA* is commonly connected with the core module IS*Kpn27*-$bla_{\text{KPC-2}}$-IS*Kpn6* as mentioned above (Shen et al., 2009; Dai et al., 2016; Shi et al., 2018). However, unilateral IS*26* element insertion is rarely observed. A possible explanation for this is if IS*26* and the adjacent region that included IS*Kpn27*-$bla_{\text{KPC-2}}$-IS*Kpn6*-*korC*-ORF-*klcA*, formed a transferable unit (TU). This TU might then have inserted into another plasmid. Normally, the integration results in two copies IS*26* in direct orientation, one at each boundary between the two participating molecules (Harmer et al., 2014; Harmer and Hall, 2015; Varani et al., 2021). However, we observe only one IS*26* in pP33-2; the other might possibly have been lost through a deletion event.

Blast search results identified plasmid pPA7790 (Nascimento et al., 2016), which was isolated from a patient in Brazil, as being most similar to pP33-2 with 78% query coverage and 98.51% identity. Comparing pP33-2 to pPA7790, the backbone is similar, yet the $bla_{\text{KPC-2}}$ segment in pP33-2 substituted a part of T4SS module in pPA7790 (**Figure 2**).

The mechanism of how the $bla_{\text{KPC-2}}$-carrying plasmid originated has not been completely established. However, it is very plausible that the IS*26* facilitated the spread of KPC among different plasmids in *P. aeruginosa*. The *P. aeruginosa* strain with novel $bla_{\text{KPC-2}}$ plasmid described here might become an important regional epidemic clone.

Integration of ICEP33 Brings Resistance Genes

Among the four clinical isolates, P23 and P33 have the closest genetic relationship (**Figure 1**). A comparison of the chromosomes of P23 and P33 showed there is an 110,131-bp-long insertion downstream of the gene encoding the integrase family protein on the P33 chromosome (**Figure 3**). ICEfinder predicted it to be a putative ICE, hereafter named ICEP33. Within this element, we found the aminoglycosides-resistant genes *aac(6')-IIa* and *ant(2")-Ia* together with $bla_{\text{CARB-2}}$ and *sul1*, which were only found in P33.

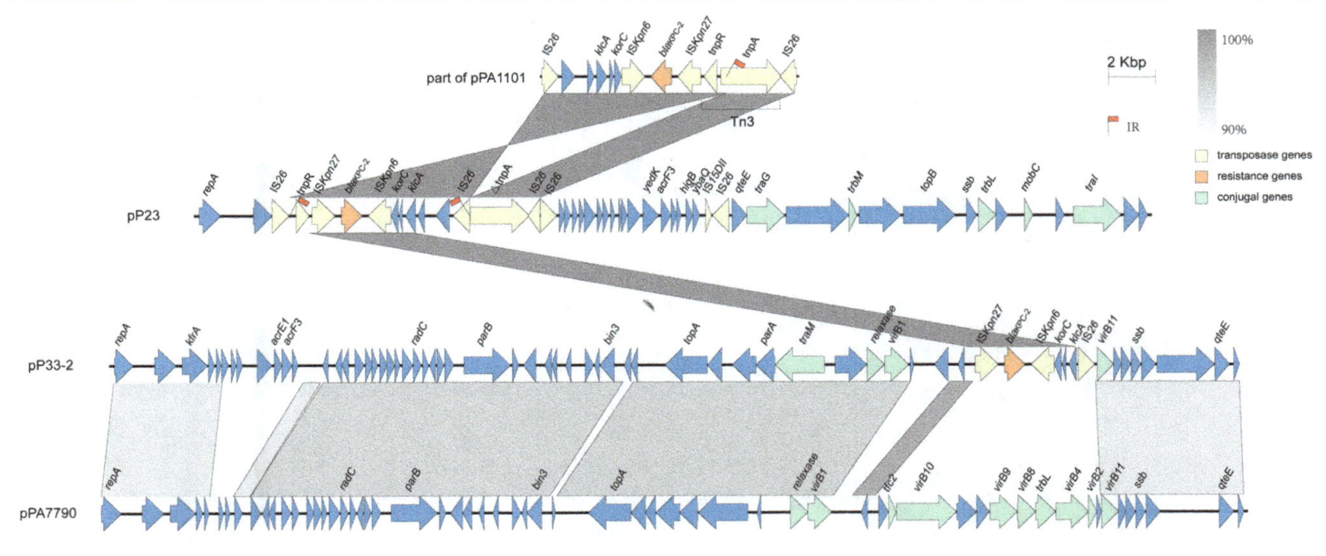

FIGURE 2 | Detailed structure and comparison of the bla_{KPC-2} gene cluster within the strains. Yellow, orange, and green arrows represent transposase, resistance, and conjugal genes, respectively. Arrows indicate the translation orientation of the coding genes. Red flags highlight the positions of inverted repeats.

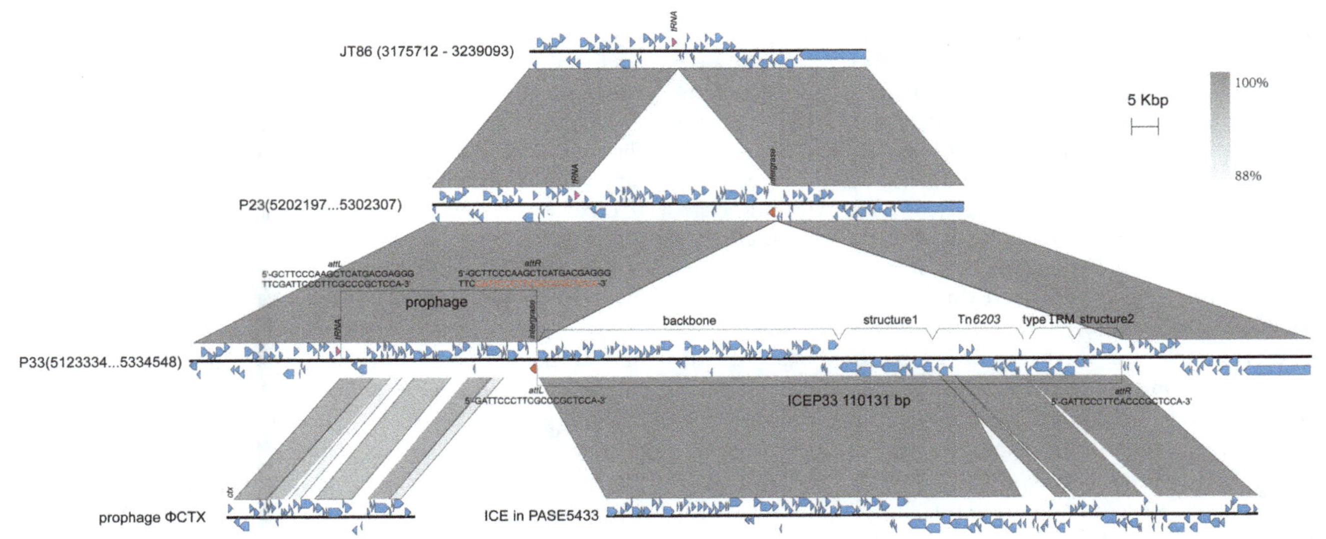

FIGURE 3 | Comparison of partial chromosomes. A prophage integrated into the chromosome first, and then an ICE integrated next to the prophage. The *attL* and *attR* of prophage and ICE are, respectively, labeled. The overlapping att site is marked red. Red arrows represent the genes which ICE and prophage integrate adjacent to. The ICE is divided into four parts.

The antimicrobial resistance genes are organized within a single class I integron integrated in transposon Tn*6203*. In addition, there is a Tn*4378*-like transposon carrying a mercury resistance operon (*mer*) in Tn*6203*. With the exception of the resistance segment, ICEP33 could roughly be divided into four parts: backbone, structure 1, type I restriction and modification (RM) system, and structure 2 (**Figure 3**). The backbone contains genes encoding a bacteriophage P4-like integrase, conjugative apparatuses, and genes for DNA processing and replication. The type I RM is possibly required for ICE self-maintenance (Hu et al., 2015a). Structure 1 and structure 2 contain genes encoding proteins, such as cold shock domain-containing protein, S8 family peptidase and LysR family transcriptional regulator. These structures might be acquired through multiple recombination events during the ICE evolution.

The insertion of ICE is flanked by two attachment (*att*) sites at both ends of the sequence (*att*L and *att*R; Bellanger et al., 2011; Johnson and Grossman, 2015). In P33, the *att*L is 5'-GATTCCCTTCGCCCGCTCCA-3' and the *att*R is 5'-GATTCCCTTCACCCGCTCCA-3'. These site-specific integrations mediated by the bacteriophage P4-like integrase are typically found within the tRNA gene

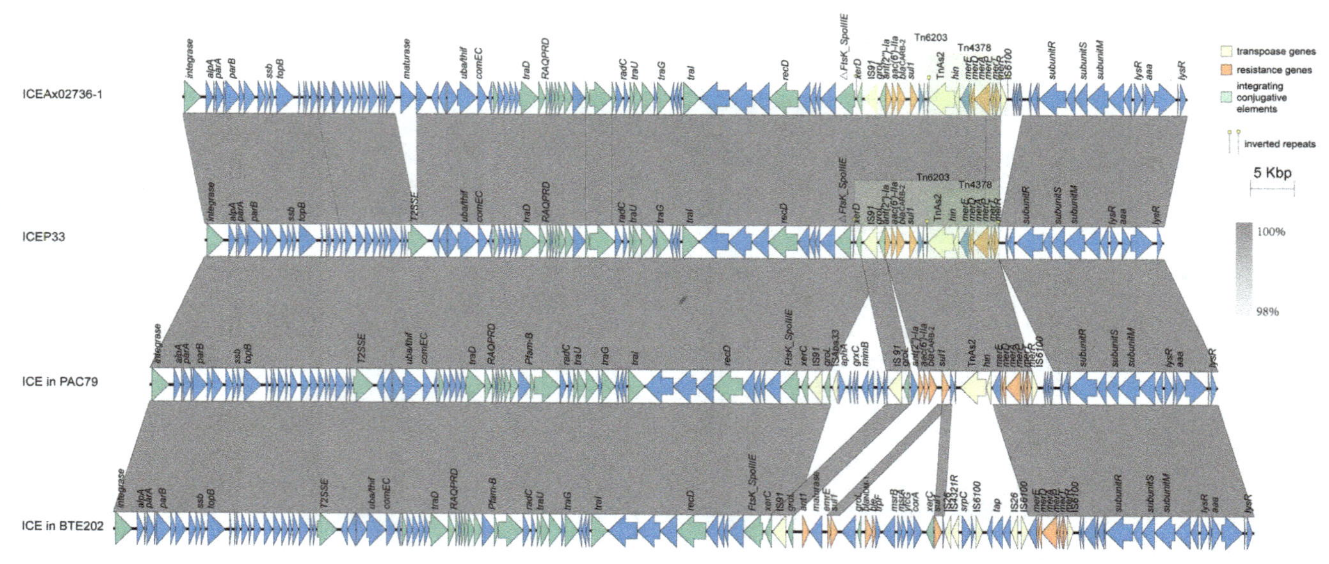

FIGURE 4 | Detailed structure and comparison of similar ICEs. Yellow, orange, and green arrows represent transposase genes, resistance genes, and integrating conjugative elements, respectively. Arrows indicate the translation orientation of the coding genes. Two green shades denote Tn*6203* and Tn*4378*.

(Ravatn et al., 1998a,b; Wozniak and Waldor, 2010; Johnson and Grossman, 2015). However, ICEP33 is integrated approximately 37-kb downstream of tRNA^{Gly}. We found an intact prophage sequence inserted next to the tRNA^{Gly} causing 46 bp direct repeats, which contain the *att* site of ICEP33 (**Figure 3**). This prophage is 36.7 kb in length with an average GC content of 63.8% and 48 predicted ORFs. The prophage encodes 42 phage proteins and 33 of them are similar to P2-like phage ΦCTX (AB008550.1). Compared to ΦCTX, the prophage in P33 lacks the cytotoxin gene (*ctx*) and contains a different integrase gene. We propose that the evolution of this genetic section of the bacterial chromosome happened in succession, with integration of the prophage into the chromosome similar to JT86 (CP062219.1) occurring first, forming the genomic organization that is also observed in P23. In a second step, an ICE integrated next to the prophage and eventually leading to the structure observed in P33 (**Figure 3**). ICEs with bacteriophage P4-like integrase are often found adjacent to phages that target the same *att* site (Botelho et al., 2018). Our study provides a possible order of their insertion. However, whether there is an interaction in integration between ICE and prophage is unclear.

ICEP33 Belongs to *clc*-Like Family

Two large families of ICEs exist in *P. aeruginosa*, the pKLC102 family and the *clc*-like family, which includes *clc* (AJ617740), PAGI-2 (AF440523), and PAGI-3 (AF440524; Kung et al., 2010). ICEP33 is similar to PAGI-15 (KX196168.1) and PAGI-16 (KX196169.1), which were defined as *clc*-like ICEs (Hong et al., 2016), indicating that ICEP33 belongs to the same family. These ICEs all share a similar bipartite structure: the conserved part adjacent to the integration site as backbone and the variable part that consisted of unique cargo ORFs (Kung et al., 2010). ICEP33-like ICEs were also found in other bacteria, such as *Achromobacter xylosoxidans* strain X02736 (GCA_000517225.1; Hu et al., 2015a), *Bordetella trematum* strain E202 (CP049957.1), *P. aeruginosa* strain SE5443 (CP046405.1), and C79 (CP040684.1; **Figures 3, 4**). The antibiotic resistance genetic load is the main difference between them. Compared to the most similar sequence ICEAx02736-1, they both carry the same resistance genes embedded in Tn*6203* modules. In P33, the right end of Tn*6203* was truncated by IS6100 and four predicted ORFs, which led to the loss of an inverted or direct repeat. In addition, it appears that a gene encoding group II intron reverse transcriptase/maturase had inserted into the middle of the gene encoding a DEAD/DEAH box helicase. Interestingly, these ICEs in **Figures 3, 4** are found in different bacterial species in China, indicating that this type of ICE is present in a variety of hosts and may be an important molecular mechanism for the dissemination of resistance genes in the country.

CONCLUSION

In this study, four *P. aeruginosa* strains were isolated from a single patient in an intensive care unit. The horizontal transmission of the antibiotic resistance genes in those strains was hypothesized to be mediated by mobile elements IS*26* and ICEs. In this work, a novel plasmid pP33-2 encoding bla_{KPC-2} is described, which likely originates from an IS*26*-mediated insertion into the position of T4SS; subsequently, a deletion of the IS*26* and a partial removal of the T4SS occurred during evolution. In addition, the resistance genes embedded in the transposon Tn*6203* became part of ICEP33 that was found in the same strain. ICEP33, which belongs to *clc*-like family is integrated adjacent to a prophage sequence. The appearance of the novel bla_{KPC-2}

plasmid and the integration of the ICE has created a new type of MDR *P. aeruginosa* strain, which creates a high risk of a regional epidemic carbapenem-resistant clone, bringing more challenges to the clinical treatment of infections caused by *P. aeruginosa*.

AUTHOR CONTRIBUTIONS

XH, YY, and HC designed the study. HC, YZ, DH, and YL performed the experiments. HC and YZ analyzed the data. HC drafted the article. XH, YY, SL, and BL revised the article. All authors have approved the final article.

FUNDING

This study was supported by the National Natural Science Foundation of China (grant no. 81830069).

ACKNOWLEDGMENTS

We thank Dr. Mark Toleman, Cardiff University, School of Medicine for critically reading the manuscript.

REFERENCES

Bellanger, X., Morel, C., Gonot, F., Puymege, A., Decaris, B., and Guedon, G. (2011). Site-specific accretion of an integrative conjugative element together with a related genomic island leads to cis mobilization and gene capture. *Mol. Microbiol.* 81, 912–925. doi: 10.1111/j.1365-2958.2011.07737.x

Botelho, J., Roberts, A. P., Leon-Sampedro, R., Grosso, F., and Peixe, L. (2018). Carbapenemases on the move: it's good to be on ICEs. *Mob. DNA* 9:37. doi: 10.1186/s13100-018-0141-4

Botelho, J., Grosso, F., and Peixe, L. (2019). Antibiotic resistance in *Pseudomonas aeruginosa* – mechanisms, epidemiology and evolution. *Drug Resist. Updat.* 44:100640. doi: 10.1016/j.drup.2019.07.002

Cai, J. C., Zhang, R., Hu, Y. Y., Zhou, H. W., and Chen, G. X. (2014). Emergence of *Escherichia coli* sequence type 131 isolates producing KPC-2 carbapenemase in China. *Antimicrob. Agents Chemother.* 58, 1146–1152. doi: 10.1128/AAC.00912-13

Camacho, C., Coulouris, G., Avagyan, V., Ma, N., Papadopoulos, J., Bealer, K., et al. (2009). BLAST+: architecture and applications. *BMC Bioinf.* 10:421. doi: 10.1186/1471-2105-10-421

Carraro, N., and Burrus, V. (2015). The dualistic nature of integrative and conjugative elements. *Mob. Genet. Ele.* 5, 98–102. doi: 10.1080/2159256X.2015.1102796

Chen, L., Hu, H., Chavda, K. D., Zhao, S., Liu, R., Liang, H., et al. (2014a). Complete sequence of a KPC-producing IncN multidrug-resistant plasmid from an epidemic *Escherichia coli* sequence type 131 strain in China. *Antimicrob. Agents Chemother.* 58, 2422–2425. doi: 10.1128/AAC.02587-13

Chen, L., Mathema, B., Chavda, K. D., DeLeo, F. R., Bonomo, R. A., and Kreiswirth, B. N. (2014b). Carbapenemase-producing *Klebsiella pneumoniae*: molecular and genetic decoding. *Trends Microbiol.* 22, 686–696. doi: 10.1016/j.tim.2014.09.003

Chen, Y. T., Lin, J. C., Fung, C. P., Lu, P. L., Chuang, Y. C., Wu, T. L., et al. (2014c). KPC-2-encoding plasmids from Escherichia coli and *Klebsiella pneumoniae* in Taiwan. *J. Antimicrob. Chemother.* 69, 628–631. doi: 10.1093/jac/dkt409

CLSI (2020). *Performance Standards for Antimicrobial Susceptibility Testing.* 30th Edn CLSI supplement M100. Wayne, PA, USA: Clinical and Laboratory Standards Institute.

Dai, X., Zhou, D., Xiong, W., Feng, J., Luo, W., Luo, G., et al. (2016). The IncP-6 plasmid p10265-KPC from *Pseudomonas aeruginosa* carries a novel DeltaISEc33-associated bla KPC-2 gene cluster. *Front. Microbiol.* 7:310. doi: 10.3389/fmicb.2016.00310

Garcillan-Barcia, M. P., Redondo-Salvo, S., Vielva, L., and de la Cruz, F. (2020). MOBscan: automated annotation of MOB relaxases. *Methods Mol. Biol.* 2075, 295–308. doi: 10.1007/978-1-4939-9877-7_21

Harmer, C. J., and Hall, R. M. (2015). IS26-mediated precise excision of the IS26-aphA1a translocatable unit. *MBio* 6:e01866-01815. doi: 10.1128/mBio.01866-15

Harmer, C. J., Moran, R. A., and Hall, R. M. (2014). Movement of IS26-associated antibiotic resistance genes occurs via a translocatable unit that includes a single IS26 and preferentially inserts adjacent to another IS26. *MBio* 5, e01801–e01814. doi: 10.1128/mBio.01801-14

He, S., Hickman, A. B., Varani, A. M., Siguier, P., Chandler, M., Dekker, J. P., et al. (2015). Insertion sequence IS26 reorganizes plasmids in clinically isolated multidrug-resistant bacteria by replicative transposition. *MBio* 6:e00762. doi: 10.1128/mBio.00762-15

Hong, J. S., Yoon, E. J., Lee, H., Jeong, S. H., and Lee, K. (2016). Clonal dissemination of *Pseudomonas aeruginosa* sequence type 235 isolates carrying blaIMP-6 and emergence of blaGES-24 and blaIMP-10 on novel genomic islands PAGI-15 and -16 in South Korea. *Antimicrob. Agents Chemother.* 60, 7216–7223. doi: 10.1128/AAC.01601-16

Horcajada, J. P., Montero, M., Oliver, A., Sorli, L., Luque, S., Gomez-Zorrilla, S., et al. (2019). Epidemiology and treatment of multidrug-resistant and extensively drug-resistant *Pseudomonas aeruginosa* infections. *Clin. Microbiol. Rev.* 32:e00031-19. doi: 10.1128/CMR.00031-19

Hu, F., Guo, Y., Yang, Y., Zheng, Y., Wu, S., Jiang, X., et al. (2019a). Resistance reported from China antimicrobial surveillance network (CHINET) in 2018. *Eur. J. Clin. Microbiol. Infect. Dis.* 38, 2275–2281. doi: 10.1007/s10096-019-03673-1

Hu, Y., Zhu, Y., Ma, Y., Liu, F., Lu, N., Yang, X., et al. (2015a). Genomic insights into intrinsic and acquired drug resistance mechanisms in *Achromobacter xylosoxidans*. *Antimicrob. Agents Chemother.* 59, 1152–1161. doi: 10.1128/AAC.04260-14

Hu, Y. Y., Gu, D. X., Cai, J. C., Zhou, H. W., and Zhang, R. (2015b). Emergence of KPC-2-producing *Pseudomonas aeruginosa* sequence type 463 isolates in Hangzhou, China. *Antimicrob. Agents Chemother.* 59, 2914–2917. doi: 10.1128/AAC.04903-14

Hu, Y. Y., Wang, Q., Sun, Q. L., Chen, G. X., and Zhang, R. (2019b). A novel plasmid carrying carbapenem-resistant gene bla KPC-2 in *Pseudomonas aeruginosa*. *Infect. Drug Resist.* 12, 1285–1288. doi: 10.2147/IDR.S196390

Johnson, C. M., and Grossman, A. D. (2015). Integrative and conjugative elements (ICEs): what they do and how they work. *Annu. Rev. Genet.* 49, 577–601. doi: 10.1146/annurev-genet-112414-055018

Jolley, K. A., Bray, J. E., and Maiden, M. C. J. (2018). Open-access bacterial population genomics: BIGSdb software, the PubMLST.org website and their applications. *Wellcome Open Res.* 3:124. doi: 10.12688/wellcomeopenres.14826.1

Kung, V. L., Ozer, E. A., and Hauser, A. R. (2010). The accessory genome of *Pseudomonas aeruginosa*. *Microbiol. Mol. Biol. Rev.* 74, 621–641. doi: 10.1128/MMBR.00027-10

Li, G., Zhang, Y., Bi, D., Shen, P., Ai, F., Liu, H., et al. (2015). First report of a clinical, multidrug-resistant Enterobacteriaceae isolate coharboring fosfomycin resistance gene fosA3 and carbapenemase gene blaKPC-2 on the same transposon, Tn1721. *Antimicrob. Agents Chemother.* 59, 338–343. doi: 10.1128/AAC.03061-14

Li, X., Xie, Y., Liu, M., Tai, C., Sun, J., Deng, Z., et al. (2018). oriTfinder: a web-based tool for the identification of origin of transfers in DNA sequences of bacterial mobile genetic elements. *Nucleic Acids Res.* 46, W229–W234. doi: 10.1093/nar/gky352

Liu, M., Li, X., Xie, Y., Bi, D., Sun, J., Li, J., et al. (2019). ICEberg 2.0: an updated database of bacterial integrative and conjugative elements. *Nucleic Acids Res.* 47, D660–D665. doi: 10.1093/nar/gky1123

Munoz-Price, L. S., Poirel, L., Bonomo, R. A., Schwaber, M. J., Daikos, G. L., Cormican, M., et al. (2013). Clinical epidemiology of the global expansion of *Klebsiella pneumoniae* carbapenemases. *Lancet Infect. Dis.* 13, 785–796. doi: 10.1016/S1473-3099(13)70190-7

Nascimento, A. P., Ortiz, M. F., Martins, W. M., Morais, G. L., Fehlberg, L. C., Almeida, L. G., et al. (2016). Intraclonal genome stability of the metallo-beta-lactamase SPM-1-producing *Pseudomonas aeruginosa* ST277, an endemic clone disseminated in Brazilian hospitals. *Front. Microbiol.* 7:1946. doi: 10.3389/fmicb.2016.01946

Partridge, S. R., Kwong, S. M., Firth, N., and Jensen, S. O. (2018). Mobile genetic elements associated with antimicrobial resistance. *Clin. Microbiol. Rev.* 31:e00088-17. doi: 10.1128/CMR.00088-17

Ravatn, R., Studer, S., Springael, D., Zehnder, A. J., and van der Meer, J. R. (1998a). Chromosomal integration, tandem amplification, and deamplification in *Pseudomonas putida* F1 of a 105-kilobase genetic element containing the chlorocatechol degradative genes from *Pseudomonas* sp. strain B13. *J. Bacteriol.* 180, 4360–4369. doi: 10.1128/JB.180.17.4360-4369.1998

Ravatn, R., Studer, S., Zehnder, A. J., and van der Meer, J. R. (1998b). Int-B13, an unusual site-specific recombinase of the bacteriophage P4 integrase family, is responsible for chromosomal insertion of the 105-kilobase clc element of *Pseudomonas* sp. strain B13. *J. Bacteriol.* 180, 5505–5514. doi: 10.1128/JB.180.21.5505-5514.1998

Roy Chowdhury, P., Scott, M. J., and Djordjevic, S. P. (2017). Genomic islands 1 and 2 carry multiple antibiotic resistance genes in *Pseudomonas aeruginosa* ST235, ST253, ST111 and ST175 and are globally dispersed. *J. Antimicrob. Chemother.* 72, 620–622. doi: 10.1093/jac/dkw471

Seemann, T. (2014). Prokka: rapid prokaryotic genome annotation. *Bioinformatics* 30, 2068–2069. doi: 10.1093/bioinformatics/btu153

Shen, P., Wei, Z., Jiang, Y., Du, X., Ji, S., Yu, Y., et al. (2009). Novel genetic environment of the carbapenem-hydrolyzing beta-lactamase KPC-2 among Enterobacteriaceae in China. *Antimicrob. Agents Chemother.* 53, 4333–4338. doi: 10.1128/AAC.00260-09

Shi, L., Liang, Q., Feng, J., Zhan, Z., Zhao, Y., Yang, W., et al. (2018). Coexistence of two novel resistance plasmids, blaKPC-2-carrying p14057A and tetA(A) -carrying p14057B, in *Pseudomonas aeruginosa*. *Virulence* 9, 306–311. doi: 10.1080/21505594.2017.1372082

Smillie, C., Garcillan-Barcia, M. P., Francia, M. V., Rocha, E. P., and de la Cruz, F. (2010). Mobility of plasmids. *Microbiol. Mol. Biol. Rev.* 74, 434–452. doi: 10.1128/MMBR.00020-10

Tacconelli, E., Carrara, E., Savoldi, A., Harbarth, S., Mendelson, M., Monnet, D. L., et al. (2018). Discovery, research, and development of new antibiotics: the WHO priority list of antibiotic-resistant bacteria and tuberculosis. *Lancet Infect. Dis.* 18, 318–327. doi: 10.1016/S1473-3099(17)30753-3

van Duin, D., and Doi, Y. (2017). The global epidemiology of carbapenemase-producing Enterobacteriaceae. *Virulence* 8, 460–469. doi: 10.1080/21505594.2016.1222343

Varani, A., He, S., Siguier, P., Ross, K., and Chandler, M. (2021). The IS6 family, a clinically important group of insertion sequences including IS26. *Mob. DNA* 12:11. doi: 10.1186/s13100-021-00239-x

Wick, R. R., Judd, L. M., Gorrie, C. L., and Holt, K. E. (2017). Unicycler: resolving bacterial genome assemblies from short and long sequencing reads. *PLoS Comput. Biol.* 13:e1005595. doi: 10.1371/journal.pcbi.1005595

Wozniak, R. A., and Waldor, M. K. (2010). Integrative and conjugative elements: mosaic mobile genetic elements enabling dynamic lateral gene flow. *Nat. Rev. Microbiol.* 8, 552–563. doi: 10.1038/nrmicro2382

Wurdemann, D., and Tummler, B. (2007). In silico comparison of pKLC102-like genomic islands of *Pseudomonas aeruginosa*. *FEMS Microbiol. Lett.* 275, 244–249. doi: 10.1111/j.1574-6968.2007.00891.x

Yu, G. (2020). Using ggtree to visualize data on tree-like structures. *Curr. Protoc. Bioinformatics* 69:e96. doi: 10.1002/cpbi.96

Zankari, E., Hasman, H., Cosentino, S., Vestergaard, M., Rasmussen, S., Lund, O., et al. (2012). Identification of acquired antimicrobial resistance genes. *J. Antimicrob. Chemother.* 67, 2640–2644. doi: 10.1093/jac/dks261

8

Bactericidal Property of Oregano Oil Against Multidrug-Resistant Clinical Isolates

Min Lu[1], *Tianhong Dai*[1*], *Clinton K. Murray*[2] *and Mei X. Wu*[1*]

[1] Wellman Center for Photomedicine, Massachusetts General Hospital, Harvard Medical School, Boston, MA, United States, [2] First Area Medical Laboratory, JBSA-Fort Sam Houston, Houston, TX, United States

***Correspondence:**
Tianhong Dai
TDAI@mgh.harvard.edu
Mei X. Wu
MWU5@mgh.harvard.edu

Development of non-antibiotic alternatives to treat infections caused by multidrug-resistant (MDR) microbes represents one of the top priorities in healthcare and community settings, especially in the care of combat trauma-associated wound infections. Here, we investigate efficacy of oregano oil against pathogenic bacteria including MDR isolates from the combat casualties *in vitro* and in a mouse burn model. Oregano oil showed a significant anti-bacterial activity against 11 MDR clinical isolates including four *Acinetobacter baumannii*, three *Pseudomonas aeruginosa*, and four methicillin-resistant *Staphylococcus aureus* (MRSA) obtained from combat casualties and two luminescent strains of PA01 and MRSA USA300, with a MIC ranging from 0.08 mg/ml to 0.64 mg/ml. Oregano oil also effectively eradicated biofilms formed by each of the 13 pathogens above at similar MICs. Transmission electron microscopy (TEM) and scanning electron microscopy (SEM) revealed that oregano oil damaged bacterial cells and altered the morphology of their biofilms. While efficiently inactivating bacteria, there was no evidence of resistance development after up to 20 consecutive passages of representative bacterial strains in the presence of sublethal doses of oregano oil. *In vivo* study using the third-degree burn wounds infected with PA01 or USA300 demonstrated that oregano oil, topically applied 24 h after bacterial inoculation, sufficiently reduced the bacterial load in the wounds by 3 log_{10} in 1 h, as measured by drastic reduction of bacterial bioluminescence. This bactericidal activity of oregano oil concurred with no significant side effect on the skin histologically or genotoxicity after three topical applications of oregano oil at 10 mg/ml for three consecutive days. The investigation suggests potentials of oregano oil as an alternative to antibiotics for the treatment of wound-associated infections regardless of antibiotic susceptibility.

Keywords: oregano oil, *Pseudomonas aeruginosa*, *Acinetobacter baumannii*, MRSA, biofilms, burn wound, mouse model, bioluminescence imaging

INTRODUCTION

Skin wound infection is a widespread problem in both civilian and military healthcare settings. Skin wounds are particularly prone to bacterial infections because the wounds provide an ideal medium for bacterial proliferation and a portal of entry into the bloodstream and are direct exposure to the "dirty" environment. The infections can be readily treated with a variety of antibiotics if the bacteria involved are susceptible. However, there are only extremely limited or no treatment options when antibiotic resistant strains are involved in the wound infections, which occurs at a worrying speed. If the wound infection cannot be eliminated in a timely fashion, the infection would alter cellular metabolisms and induce persistent inflammation systemically that can predispose the patients to various complications and life-threatening sepsis (Fitzwater et al., 2003; Wang et al., 2018). For instance, burn wound infection outbreaks caused by multidrug-resistant (MDR) organisms emerged as a serious problem early in the course of Iraq military operations despite that the United States military has provided rapid and highly effective care for wounded soldiers (Scott et al., 2007; Vento et al., 2013). As a matter of fact, skin infections caused by MDR bacteria are the most common cause of morbidity and mortality in patients infected with MDR microbes and represent almost 61% of deaths of this infected population (Gomez et al., 2009).

Extensive uses of broad spectrum antibiotics are the single most important factor in evolution of bacterial resistance (Hampton, 2013). A number of studies have shown that the most frequently identified MDR strains of bacteria in nosocomial infections and on the battlefield are Gram-negative bacteria *Acinetobacter baumannii* and *Pseudomonas aeruginosa*, and Gram-positive bacterium methicillin-resistant *Staphylococcus aureus* (MRSA) (Scott et al., 2007; Calhoun et al., 2008; Li et al., 2014; Levin-Reisman et al., 2017). In addition, bacterial biofilms formed by MDR bacteria are the major obstacles in treatment of burn wounds (Bloemsma et al., 2008; Jiang et al., 2017). Bacteria within biofilms can be as much as 1,000 times more resistant to antibiotics and are responsible for recurrent antibiotic-resistant infections elsewhere in the body upon dissemination from the site of the biofilm (Ceri et al., 1999; Caraher et al., 2007). Currently, the only effective treatments available to fight these infections are older drugs like colistin, which are highly toxic and detrimental to the overall health of the patients (Crane et al., 2009). There is a pressing need for the development of non-antibiotic approaches to combat MDR microbes.

Essential oils (EOs) are a mixture of volatile constituents produced by aromatic plant/herbs. There are about 3,000 well-recognized EOs, of which 300 are generally recognized as safe (GRAS) to humans by the United States Food and Drug Administration (U.S. FDA) and have broad applications in food preservation, additives, and favors, perfume, cosmetic industries, antiseptic oral solutions, toothpastes, cleaner, and air fresheners for centuries (Pandey et al., 2017; Sakkas and Papadopoulou, 2017). These natural products are of particular interest as "green" antimicrobial agents because of their low-cost, biocompatibility, potential antibiofilm properties, and friendly to eukaryote cells and environment (Burt, 2004; Nostro et al., 2007; Kavanaugh and Ribbeck, 2012). Among these safe EOs, oregano oil has been shown to have a variety of activities such as antioxidant (Yan et al., 2016), anti-inflammatory (Ocana-Fuentes et al., 2010; Shen et al., 2010), anti-fungal (Akgul and Kivanc, 1988; Soylu et al., 2007), and anti-allergic (Benito et al., 1996). Its antimicrobial effect has been demonstrated *in vitro* cell culture, food systems studies (Lopez-Reyes et al., 2010; Soylu et al., 2010; Munhuweyi et al., 2017), and *in vivo* systemic infections (Manohar et al., 2001; Preuss et al., 2005). In the present study, we investigate effectiveness of oregano oil in inactivation of MDR bacteria isolated from combat casualties *in vitro* and bioluminescent strains of *P. aeruginosa* (PA01) and MRSA (USA300) in mouse burn wounds. Our study showed that oregano oil effectively inactivated various pathogenic bacteria and their biofilms irrespective of their antibiotic susceptibility. The study is the first *in vivo* attempt on the use of oregano oil for the treatment of burn wounds infected with clinically important MDR bacteria.

MATERIALS AND METHODS

Chemical Constituents of Oregano Oil

Oregano oil was purchased from Bulk Apothecary (Aurora, OH, United States) and used throughout the study. To define the constituents of oregano oil, gas chromatography/mass spectrometry (GC-MS) analyses were carried out using an Agilent 6980 GC coupled to an Agilent 5973N MS and a fused-silica capillary column (HP-5MS: 30 m × 0.25 mm i.d., film thickness 0.25 μm). The initial column temperature was set at 60°C for 10 min and then increased at 3°C/min till 220°C. The temperature was held at 220°C for 10 min and raised to 240°C by increments of 1°C/min; the injector port temperature was 250°C with the carrier gas of helium at a flow rate of 0.8 ml/min. Ionization voltage of MS in the EI-mode was 70 eV and ionization source temperature at 250°C with a mass range of 35–465 amu. The volatile components were identified by comparison of their retention indices relative to *n*-alkanes (C6-C28) and mass spectra with those of authentic compounds by means of NIST and Wiley databases and with the Adams library spectra.

Bacterial Strains

The antibacterial activity of oregano oil was tested against a panel of MDR bacteria isolated from combat casualties, including seven Gram-negative strains *A. baumannii* (AF0004, AF0005, IQ0012, and IQ0013) and *P. aeruginosa* (AF0001, IQ0042, and IQ0046), and four Gram-positive MRSA (AF0003, IQ0064, IQ0103, and IQ0211). All the bacterial isolates were obtained from San Antonio Military Medical Center under a Materials Transfer Agreement and demonstrated MDR according to the microbiology tests performed at the United States Army Institute of Surgical Research (**Table 2**). Amongst the *A. baumannii* and *P. aeruginosa* tested, only strains of IQ0012, IQ0013, and IQ0042 were susceptible to imipenem; the rest of strains were resistant to all antibiotics tested. The five MRSA strains were resistant to amikacin, ampicillin, cefazolin, cefoxitin, and erythromycin, but susceptible to gentamicin, levofloxacin, nitrofurantoin, and tetracycline. In addition, luminescent strains of *P. aeruginosa* (PA01) and MRSA USA300 were used in the *in vivo* study, allowing real-time monitoring of infection in the mouse burn wounds *in vivo* via bioluminescence imaging (Dai et al., 2013; Zhang et al., 2014; Wang et al., 2016).

Determinations of Minimum Inhibitory Concentration (MIC)

In order to determine a MIC, a broth microdilution assay was employed as previously described (Joshi et al., 2010; Gao et al., 2011). Stock solution of oregano oil was prepared at 40 mg/ml in DMSO and twofold dilutions (0.04–1.28 mg/ml) of the stock EO in brain heart infusion (BHI) medium were added into 96-well plates for bactericidal tests. In each well, 20 μL of the suspensions containing 10^8 CFU/ml of bacteria was added to 180 μL of the above medium containing oregano oil at varying concentrations. Medium supplemented with a similar amount of DMSO only severed as controls. The microplates were incubated at 37°C for 24 h and examined for bacterial growth. The first well without turbidity was determined as a MIC value. All assays were performed in triplicate.

Antibiofilm Activity

Bacteria were incubated in trypticase soy broth (TSB) with 0.1% glucose at 37°C for 18 h, after which the cultures were harvested by centrifugation and washed twice with PBS. Bacterial suspensions with an optical density of OD_{600} equal to 0.1 in TSB were added to 96-well plates at 100 μL/well, followed by incubation at 37°C under static condition for 24 h to form biofilms. Oregano oil was added at indicated concentrations and incubated with the biofilms for 1 h, after which biofilms were washed twice with PBS and bacterial viability was determined using an Alamar Blue assay. TSB without bacteria was used as a negative control. All experiments were performed in triplicate.

Assessment of Possible Resistance Development to Oregano Oil

To study any potential development of resistance to oregano oil, three representative strains (*A. baumannii* AF0005, *P. aeruginosa* IQ0042, and MRSA IQ0064) were propagated for 20 generations in the presence of sublethal doses of oregano oil as previously described (Li et al., 2014). Briefly, 200-μL aliquots of the bacterial suspensions (10^7 CFU/ml) were inoculated into 96-well plates and exposed to the sub-MIC (2/3 MIC) of oregano oil at 37°C for 1 h, and the resultant bacteria were labeled as the first generation and tested for a MIC as above. The second generation was obtained by exposing the first generation to its sub-MIC for 1 h and determined for its MIC again. The procedure was repeated for up to 20 times. Oregano-resistance was determined by any significant increases in the MIC of successive generations.

Transmission Electron Microscopy (TEM)

To determine bactericidal mechanism of oregano oil, *A. baumannii* AF0005 and *P. aeruginosa* IQ0042 were investigated as the representative strains for oregano-induced ultrastructural damages using transmission electron microscopy (TEM). Bacterial suspensions were fixed in 2.5% glutaraldehyde plus 2% paraformaldehyde overnight at 4°C. Fixed cells were collected by centrifugation at 4,000 × g for 5 min and rinsed with 0.1 M sodium cacodylate buffer (pH 7.2) for three times. After the final wash, hot agar was added to each pellet and the cell pellets were post-fixed in 2% osmium tetroxide for 1 h, dehydrated with a graded ethanol series, embedded in fresh Epon, and then polymerized at 60°C for 48 h. Ultra-thin sections were cut on ultramicrotome and collected onto 200 mesh bare copper grids. Samples were stained for 30 min with uranyl acetate and lead citrate and examined with a CM-10 TEM (Philips, Eindhoven, Netherlands).

Scanning Electron Microscopy (SEM)

To investigate the ultrastructural changes of bacterial biofilms caused by oregano oil, scanning electron microscopy (SEM) was performed using the representative strains of *P. aeruginosa* IQ0042 and MRSA IQ0064. Briefly, biofilms of IQ0042 and IQ0064 were grown for 24 h on sterilized squares of ACLAR 33C (Electron Microscopy Sciences, Hatfield, PA, United States), and treated for 1 h with oregano oil at 0.75 mg/ml or 0.3 mg/ml, respectively. Untreated and oregano-treated biofilms were fixed at 4°C for 24 h in 0.1 M sodium cacodylate buffer containing 2.5% glutaraldehyde, 0.15% alcian blue, and 0.15% safranin O. The fixed biofilms were washed with 0.1 M sodium cacodylate buffer, infiltrated with 2% osmium tetroxide for 2 h, and dehydrated to 100% ethanol. The biofilms were dried using a critical-point dryer (Tousimis Research Corporation, Rockville, MD, United States), mounted on specimen stubs, sputter-coated with 10 nm Cressington 208 platinum (Cressington Scientific Instruments, Watford, United Kingdom), and examined on a S4800 SEM (Hitachi Ltd., Tokyo, Japan). Micrographs were acquired under high vacuum using an accelerating voltage of 3.0 kV.

Animal

Female BALB/c mice at 8 weeks of age and 17–19 g were purchased from Charles River Laboratories (Wilmington, MA, United States). All animal procedures were approved by the Institutional Animal Care and Used Committees (IACUC) of Massachusetts General Hospital (Protocol 2014N000009) and were in accordance with guidelines of the National Institutes of Health.

Treatment of Burn Infection in Mice by Oregano Oil

Mice were anesthetized with an intraperitoneal injection of ketamine-xylazine cocktail and shaved on the lower dorsal skin. The burn was introduced by a brass block (1 cm^2) heated to thermal equilibration with boiling water prior to application of its extremity onto the shaved skin for 5 s, which generated a third-degree burn wound. Sterile saline was intraperitoneally administered at 0.5 ml/mouse to support fluid balance during recovery. Aliquots of 50 μL bacterial suspensions containing 5×10^6 CFU in PBS were inoculated onto the burn 30 min after the injury and remained in place while the mice recovered from anesthesia. Luminescent strains of *P. aeruginosa* PA01 and MRSA USA300 were used as the causative pathogens in the study. At 24 h after bacterial inoculation when the biofilms were formed in the wounds, oregano oil was diluted with grape seed oil, which is commonly used for EO dilution in aromatherapy, at a final concentration of 5 or 10 mg/ml, and topically applied to the infected wounds.

Bioluminescence emission of the bacteria in the wounds was recorded in real time by a Lumina *in vivo* image system (IVIS) (PerkinElmer, Waltham, MA, United States). Bioluminescence images were acquired (60 s exposure, medium binning) at different time points after infection. During imaging, mice were anesthetized in chambers containing 2.0% isoflurane inhalant mixed with oxygen via an IVIS manifold placed within the imaging chamber. Bioluminescence was quantified with the Living Image software (Xenogen).

For measurement of bacterial burden, the infected burn wounds were collected after sacrifice of the mice on day 7 of bacterial inoculation. The collected tissues were homogenized in 2 ml sterile PBS. The resultant homogenate was serially diluted and spotted onto BHI agar plate containing Skirrow's supplement (10 μg/ml vancomycin, 5 μg/ml trimethoprim lactate, and 2500 IU/L polymyxin B). The plates were then incubated at 37°C for 24 h and bacterial colonies were enumerated in a treatment-blind fashion.

Gram Stain

Gram stain was carried out as previously described, with some modifications, to corroborate formation of PA01 biofilms in the infected wounds (Christensen et al., 2013; Wang et al., 2016). Briefly, at 24 h after bacterial inoculation, the infected wounds were excised, fixed in 10% phosphate-buffered formalin for 2 days, and then embedded in paraffin. Tissue sections were cut at 5 μm, de-paraffined, and rehydrated, followed by staining with 0.8% crystal violet in 1% sodium bicarbonate for 1 min and then in gram's iodine for 2 min. After decolorization with acetone/alcohol = 1:1 (v/v), the tissue sections were counterstained with 0.1% safranin O for 2 min, washed, air dried, and mounted with permount (Fisher Scientific, Waltham, MA, United States). Sections were visualized by Hamamatsu NanoZoomer 2.0 HT and the images were processed using NDP viewer software.

Toxicity of Oregano Oil to Mouse Skin *in vivo*

To evaluate any possible toxicity of oregano oil to the skin *in vivo*, mice were shaved on the low dorsal skin 24 h prior to application of oregano oil. Oregano oil *at* 10 mg/ml was applied topically on the shaved area once a day for three consecutive days. Mice treated with PBS served as negative controls. The mice were sacrificed 24 h after the final oregano oil application, and the skin was cross-sectioned using 8 mm biopsy punch for standard histological examination. The tissue sections stained with hematoxylin and eosin (HE) were visualized by Hamamatsu Nanozommer 2.0 HT and the images were processed using NDP viewer software.

DNA damage in oregano oil-treated skin was assessed using the DeadEnd Fluorometric TUNEL system (Promega, Madison, WI, United States), in which damage DNA undergoes end labeling with fluorophore as per the manufacturer's instruction. Briefly, after deparaffinization and rehydration, the tissue sections were incubated with Proteinase K for 10 min to permeabilize the cells, washed, and stained with the TUNEL reaction mixture for 1 h at 37°C in a humidifies chamber. The sections were counterstained with DAPI to mark cell nuclei. Fluorescence images were captured using a FluoView FV1000-MPE confocal microscopy (Olympus Corporation, Tokyo, Japan). For the positive control, tissue sections were pre-treated with 10 unit/ml of RQ1 RNase-free DNase I for 10 min to induce DNA fragmentation before the sections were assayed by the TUNEL staining kit.

Statistical Analyses

Data are presented as means ± standard deviations (SDs). Statistical significance was assessed with two-tailed Student's *t*-test between two groups or one-way ANOVA for multiple group comparison. *P*-values of < 0.05 were considered statistically significant. All statistical analyses were performed using GraphPad Prism 7.0 (GraphPad Software).

RESULTS

GC/MS Analysis of Constituents in Oregano Oil

Chemical ingredients of commercial oregano oil were identified by GC/MS analysis (**Table 1**). The twenty constituents accounted for 97.45% of the total amount of ingredients in

TABLE 1 | Chemical composition (%) of the oregano EO determined by GC-MS analyses.

No.	Constituents	RI[a]	RI[b]	Peak area (%)[c]
1	α-Thujene	926	924	0.21
2	α-Pinene	939	932	1.21
3	Camphene	953	946	0.13
4	1-Octen-3-ol	982	974	0.23
5	Myrcene	991	988	2.12
6	α-Phellandrene	1002	1002	0.62
7	α-Terpinene	1018	1014	0.10
8	*p*-Cymene	1026	1020	5.21
9	Limonene	1031	1024	0.56
10	γ-Terpinene	1060	1054	4.12
11	Terpinolene	1092	1086	0.10
12	Linalool	1100	1095	1.21
13	Borneol	1165	1165	0.35
14	Terpinen-4-ol	1178	1174	0.56
15	Thymol	1295	1289	6.62
16	Carvacrol	1315	1298	72.25
17	Caryophyllene	1426	1417	0.66
18	α-Humulene	1456	1452	0.12
19	β-Bisabolene	1509	1505	0.35
20	Isocaryophyllene oxide	1585	1582	0.72
	Total			97.45

[a]*Retention index relative to C6-C28 n-alkanes on the HP-5MS capillary column.* [b]*Retention index identification by using the Kovats index.* [c]*Expressed as percentage of the total peak area of the chromatograms without correction.*

TABLE 2 | MIC (mg/ml) of the oregano EO and results of antibiotic susceptibility testing for the pathogens.

Species	Strain no.	Oregano	AMK	AMP	ATM	CFZ	FOX	CRO	CXM	CIP	ERY	GEN	IPM	LVX	MEM	NIT	TET
		MIC	R/S	R/S	R/S	R/S	R/S	R/S	R/S	R/S	R/S	R/S	R/S	R/S	R/S	R/S	R/S
A. baumannii	AF0004	0.16	R	R	R	R	R	R	R	R		R	R	R	R	R	R
	IQ0012	0.08	R	R	R	R	R	R	R	R		R	S	R	R	R	R
	AF0005	0.16	R	R	R	R	R	R	R	R		R	R	R	R	R	R
	IQ0010	0.10	R	R	R	R	R	R	R	R		R	S	R	R	R	R
P. aeruginosa	AF0001	0.64	R	R	R	R	R	R	R	R		R	R	R	R	R	R
	IQ0042	0.56	R	R	R	R	R	R	R	R		R	S	R	R	R	R
	IQ0046	0.64	R	R	R	R	R	R	R	R		R	R	R	R	R	R
	PA01	0.56	R	R	R	R	R	R	R	R		R	R	R	R	R	R
Methicillin-resistant *S. aureus*	AF0003	0.16	R	R		R	R	R			R	S		S		S	S
	IQ0064	0.32	R	R		R	R	R			R	S		S		S	S
	IQ0103	0.32	R	R		R	R	R			R	S		S		S	S
	IQ0211	0.16	R	R		R	R	R			R	S		S		S	S
	USA300	0.32	R	R		R	R	R			R	S		S		S	S

AMK, amikacin; AMP, ampicillin; ATM, aztreonam; CFZ, cefazolin; FOX, cefoxitin; CRO, ceftriaxone; CXM, cefuroxime; CIP, ciprofloxacin; ERY, erythromycin; GEN, gentamicin; IPM, imipenem; LVX, levofloxacin; MEM, meropenem; NIT, nitrofurantoin; TET, tetracycline; R, resistant; S, susceptible.

oregano oil. The phenols carvacrol (72.25%) and thymol (6.62%), as well as the monoterpene hydrocarbons *p*-cymene (5.21%), γ-terpinene (4.12%), and α-pinene (1.21%) were the predominant components of oregano oil.

Oregano Oil Effectively Inactivated Bacteria *in vitro* Irrespective of Antibiotic Sensitivity

The MIC values of oregano oil against the 13 bacterial strains are shown in **Table 2**. Oregano oil showed a significant antibacterial activity over PBS controls against *A. baumannii* strains of AF0004, AF0005, IQ0012, and IQ0013 and MRSA strains of AF0003 and IQ0211, with the MICs ranging from 0.08 to 0.16 mg/ml. The MICs were significantly lower than those MICs ranging from 0.32 to 0.64 mg/ml against strains of *P. aeruginosa* and MRSA strains IQ0064, IQ0103, and USA300 (**Table 1**). Oregano oil also exhibited similar antibacterial activities against established biofilms (24-h-old) formed by the 13 bacterial strains within 1 h, with complete inactivation of the biofilms of *A. baumannii*, *P. aeruginosa*, and MRSA at the concentrations of 0.3, 1.0, and 0.4 mg/ml, respectively, in good agreement with the MIC values for planktonic bacterial cells (**Table 1** and **Figure 1**). The results clearly suggest that oregano oil can overcome the obstacles of biofilms and kill bacteria within as sufficiently as planktonic bacteria, in contrast to antibiotics that kills bacterial biofilms poorly.

TEM and SEM Illustrated Ultrastructural Damages of Bacteria

Transmission electron microscopy showed ultrastructural damages of *A. baumannii* AF0005 (**Figure 2B**) and *P. aeruginosa* IQ0042 cells (**Figure 2D**) after exposure to oregano oil for 1 h at 0.16 mg/ml and 0.56 mg/ml, respectively. The cell wall and membrane damages were apparent in *A. baumannii* AF0005 and *P. aeruginosa* IQ0042 cells with a severe leakage of intracellular substances resulting in cell membrane shrinking and separating from cell wall (**Figures 2B,D**, arrows). Moreover, cytoplasmic vacuoles in *A. baumannii* AF0005 (**Figure 2B**, asterisk) and many stainless-vesicles in *P. aeruginosa* IQ0042 (**Figure 2D**, asterisk) were observed. Intracellular structural discontinuation such as dissociation between cell wall and membrane was also seen in *A. baumannii* AF0005 (**Figure 2B**, oval). In comparison, untreated *A. baumannii* AF0005 (**Figure 2A**) and *P. aeruginosa* IQ0042 cells (**Figure 2C**) had intact, clear cell wall and membrane and dense and homogeneous cytoplasm. However, we did not find any significant differences in the ultrastructure between the control and oregano oil-treated MRSA USA300 by TEM (data not shown), which probably hints at different responses of MRSA from *A. baumannii* or *P. aeruginosa*. As with biofilms, dense and thick bacterial biofilm was observed on the dentin surface, comprised of numerous layers of densely concentrated cocci in 24-h-old *P. aeruginosa* IQ0042 (**Figure 2E**) and MRSA IQ0064 (**Figure 2G**) biofilms. The biofilms of *P. aeruginosa* IQ0042 (**Figure 2E**) and MRSA IQ0064 (**Figure 2G**) were treated with oregano oil at 1 mg/ml and 0.4 mg/ml for 1 h, respectively. The cells decohered in the extracellular polymeric matrix, dead

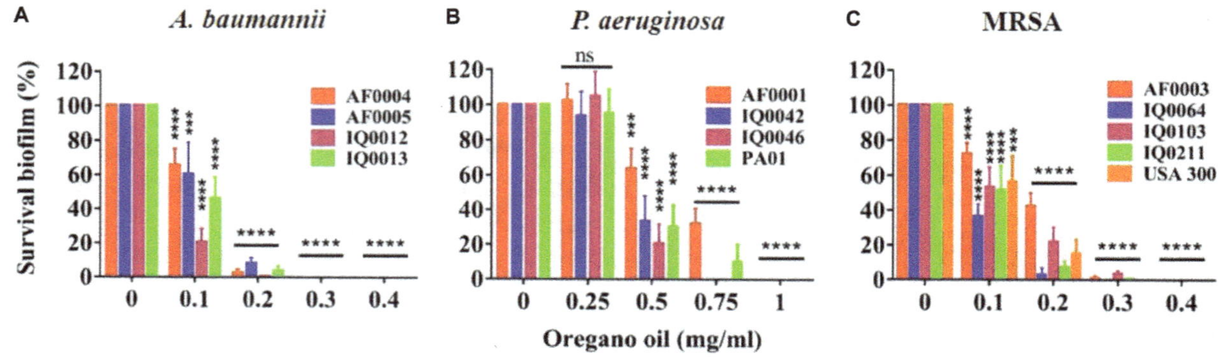

FIGURE 1 | Bacterial viability of 24 h-old-biofilms formed by MDR strains of *A. baumannii* **(A)**, *P. aeruginosa* **(B)**, and MRSA **(C)** after 1 h treatment with oregano oil at indicated concentrations. The viability of bacterial biofilms was determined using an Alamar Blue assay. Data represent means ± SDs. ***$p < 0.001$ and ****$p < 0.0001$ in the presence vs. absence of oregano oil. ns, no significance.

bacteria were readily seen all over, and biofilms were destroyed completely in oregano oil-treated samples (**Figures 2F,H**, arrows). There were only a few bacteria scantly growing on the dentin surface owing to intensive cell death (**Figures 2F,H**).

No Evidence of Resistant Development to Oregano Oil

Risk of resistant development was evaluated with three representative strains: *A. baumannii* AF0005, *P. aeruginosa* IQ0042, and MRSA IQ0064. The bacteria were cultured up to 20 successive passages in the presence of sub-lethal doses of oregano oil for bacterial inactivation. As shown in **Figure 3A**, *A. baumannii* AF0005, *P. aeruginosa* IQ0042, and MRSA IQ0064 retained susceptibility to the original MIC values of 0.16, 0.32, or 0.56 mg/ml, respectively, after 20 cycles of treatment. Moreover, there were no statistically significant differences in the survival rates of all the bacterial strains among the cycles 0, 1, and 20 in the three tested strains, after exposure to oregano oil at the MICs for 24 h (**Figures 3B–D**). The results indicate that resistance to oregano oil of the bacterial strains did not take place under this condition.

Oregano Oil Significantly Reduced Bacterial Burden in Burn Wounds Infected With PA01

Gram stain of histological longitudinal section (**Figure 4A**) and crossing section (**Figure 4B**) of a representative skin specimen demonstrated the presence of PA01 biofilms at 24 h after bacterial inoculation, as evidenced by abundant bacteria densely clustered together (red) in a highly hydrated extracellular matrix on the surface of skin and in the epidermis (**Figure 4A**, outline in red). In addition, highly resilient microbial assemblies were readily found in the dermis suggesting that the PA01 could infect not only the epidermis but also the dermis within 24 h (**Figure 4B**). In successive bacterial luminescence images of representative wounds infected with 5 × 10^6 CFU of PA01, oregano oil treatment at 10 mg/ml almost completely eradicated bacterial luminescence in 60 min, while luminescence remained unchanged during the same period in untreated mice (**Figures 4C,D**). Moreover, there was no recurrence of infection in the following days in oregano oil-treated mice, whereas the mice remained significantly infected in untreated mice in the same experimental period (**Figures 4C,D**). An average reduction in bacterial luminescence of 2.9 $\log_{10}$ and 3.5 $\log_{10}$ were achieved in 60 min at a concentration of 5 or 10 mg/ml of oregano oil, respectively (**Figure 4E**). On the contrary, bacterial luminescence of the wounds in the absence of oregano oil treatment was almost unaltered with only 0.08 $\log_{10}$ reduction during the equivalent period (**Figure 4E**, $P < 0.0001$). A time course study of the mean bacterial luminescence from days 2 to 7 after bacterial inoculation corroborated that the treatment consistently and significantly lowered the luminescence compared to untreated mice during the whole period of the experiment regardless of whether oregano oil was used at 5 or 10 mg/ml (**Figure 4F**). The mean areas under the curve (AUC) of the bioluminescence time course were 6.9 × 10^9 and 2.4 × 10^9 for oregano oil-treated groups at 5 and 10 mg/ml, respectively, but it was 5.9 × 10^{10} for untreated mice ($P < 0.0001$; **Figure 4G**), representing an 8.6-fold or a 24.6-fold reduction of the AUC in infected burns by oregano oil. We next excised the infected wounds on day 7 to determine bacterial CFU remaining in the wounds. There were 6.7 × 10^6 and 2.4 × 10^6 CFU in the wounds treated with oregano oil at a concentration of 5 or 10 mg/ml, respectively, which was significantly lower than the bacterial burden of 6.6 × 10^7 CFU/wound in untreated mice (**Figure 4H**).

Oregano Oil Significantly Reduced Bacterial Burden in Burn Wounds Infected With USA300

As shown in **Figure 5A**, an average reduction in bacterial luminescence of 2.9 $\log_{10}$ was attained when the infected wounds were treated with oregano oil at 5 mg/ml for 40 min, which was highly significant compared to only 0.4 $\log_{10}$ decline of the bioluminescence in the absence of oregano oil during the same period ($P < 0.0001$; **Figure 5A**). The diminished bacterial luminescence was persistent for 7 days after a single oregano

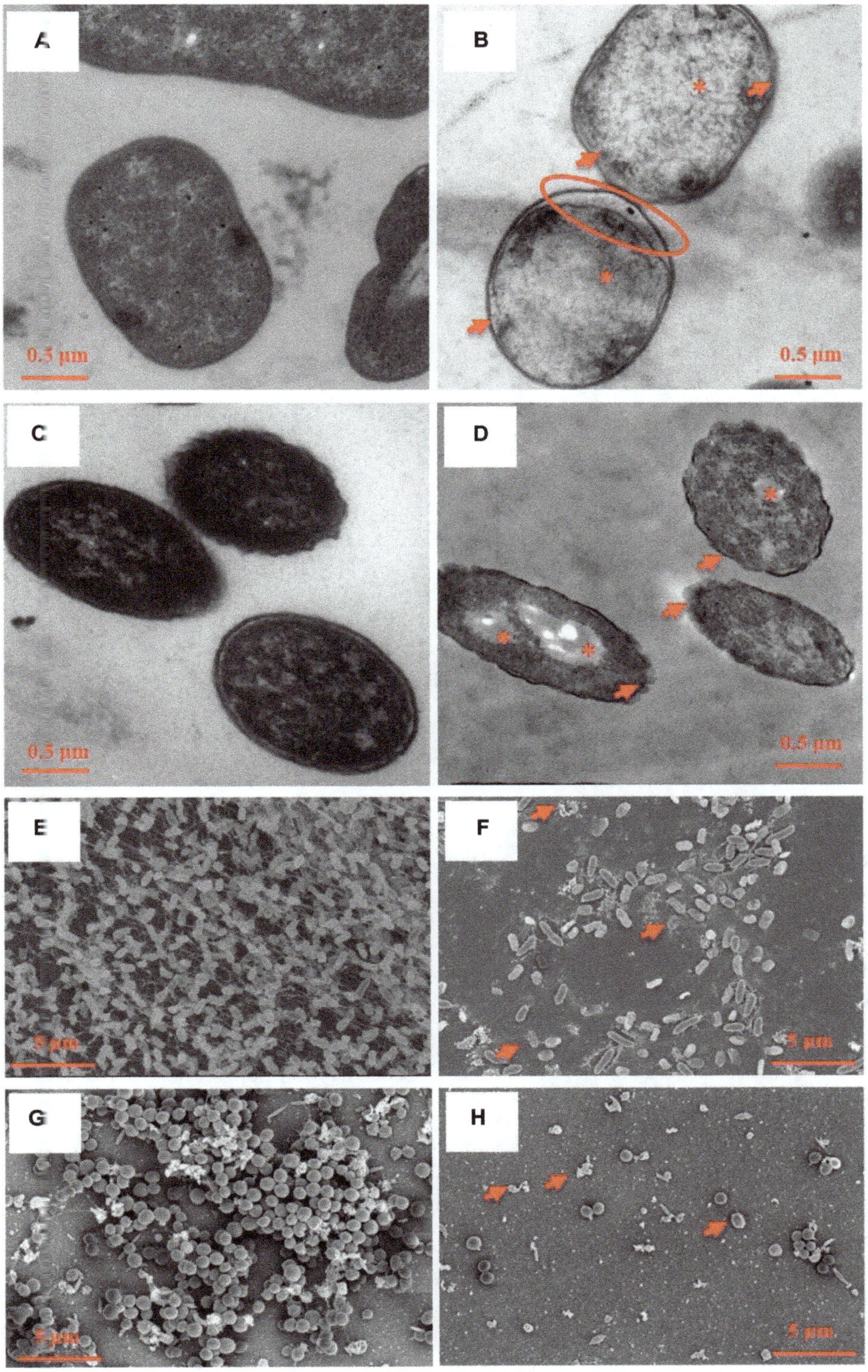

FIGURE 2 | Representative TEM images of planktonic cells **(A–D)** and SEM images of bacterial biofilms **(E–H)** with **(B,D,E,F)** or without **(A,C,E,G)** oregano oil treatment for 1 h. Oregano oil was used at 0.16 mg/ml for *A. baumannii* AF0005 cells, 0.56 mg/ml for *P. aeruginosa* IQ0042 cells, 1.0 mg/ml for *P. aeruginosa* IQ0042 biofilms, and 0.4 mg/ml for MRSA IQ0064 biofilm. **(A,B)** *A. baumannii* AF0005 cells; **(C,D)** *P. aeruginosa* IQ0042 cells; **(E,F)** *P. aeruginosa* IQ0042 biofilms; and **(G,H)** MRSA IQ0064 biofilms. Shown are cell wall and membrane damages **(B,D; arrows)**; dissociation between cell wall and membrane **(B; oval)**, cytoplasmic vacuoles and bubbles **(B,D; asterisk)**, and cell collapse **(F,H, arrows)**. The number of bacteria was drastically reduced after oregano oil treatment in **(F,H)** as compared to untreated controls **(E,G)**.

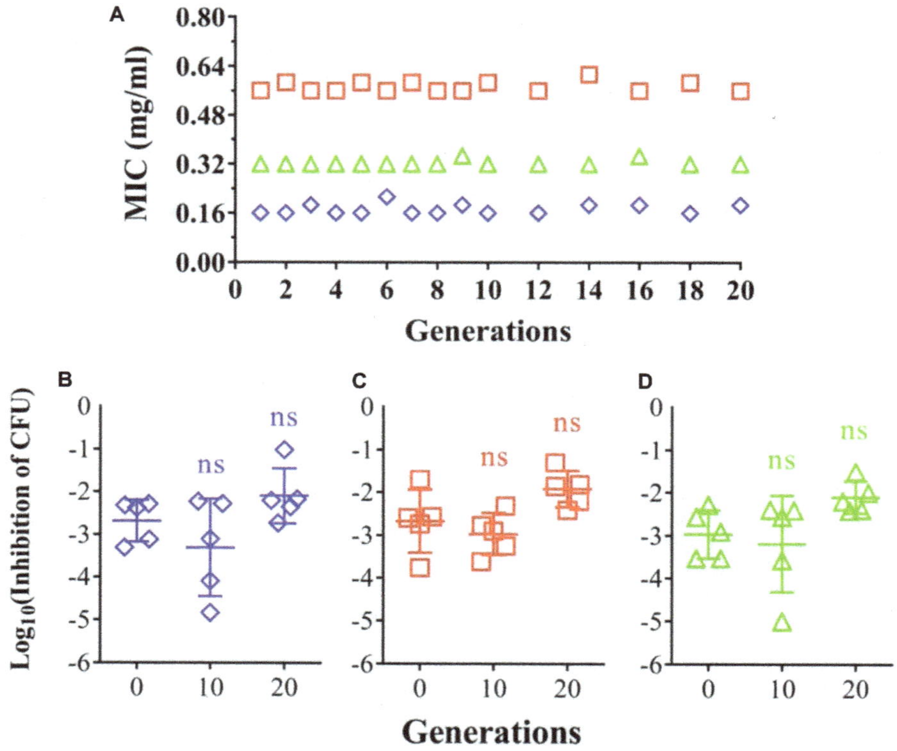

FIGURE 3 | Possible development of bacterial resistance to oregano oil. **(A)** *A. baumannii* AF0005, *P. aeruginosa* IQ0042, and MRSA IQ0064 were passaged for 20 generations each in the presence of indicated MIC doses of oregano oil. The inhibition rate of *A. baumannii* AF0005 **(B)**, *P. aeruginosa* IQ0042 **(C)**, or MRSA IQ0064 **(D)** was unaltered when the bacteria of indicated generations were exposed to oregano oil at an initial MIC concentration. ns, no significance.

oil treatment at 5 mg/ml (**Figure 5B**). The mean AUC of the bioluminescence were 3.7×10^7 in oregano oil-treated group, but it was 1.8×10^9 for untreated mice ($P < 0.0001$; **Figure 5C**), a 48.6-fold reduction of the AUC by oregano oil treatment. In accordance with this, a single dose of oregano oil treatment diminished bacterial load to 2.7×10^7 CFU/mouse that was 18-fold lower than 4.8×10^8 CFU/mouse in the untreated group ($P < 0.0001$; **Figure 5D**).

No Side Effects in Mouse Skin Caused by Oregano Oil

There was no noticeable skin reaction, as visualized with the naked eye, after three consecutive days of oregano oil treatment at 10 mg/ml (**Figure 6B**) when compared to untreated skin (**Figure 6A**). On the histological levels, the skin maintained an undisturbed structure with a clear layer of healthy epidermal cells on the top of the dermis, indistinguishable to mock-treated skins (**Figures 6C,D**). Genotoxicity was next evaluated by a TUNEL assay to examine any DNA damage induced by oregano oil. In comparison with mock-treated controls, there was no any apparent increase of DNA staining in oregano oil-treated skin (**Figures 6E,F**), while the staining was readily seen in the positive control in which skin section was treated with DNase I (**Figure 6G**). The absence of any oregano oil-induced skin reaction and DNA damage after a 3-day treatment suggests that topical application of oregano oil is neither cytotoxic nor genotoxic to the host.

DISCUSSION

In seeking non-antibiotic microbicides, we have screened dozens of EOs from Chinese indigenous aromatic plants/spices because EOs have been long recognized as one of the most promising natural products for safe microbicides in folk medicines (Lu et al., 2013a,b,c). The selection was initially based on their antiseptic applications in the food industry and in agricultures after an extensive database search. Among the dozen EOs tested, about one third showed significant antibacterial activities against clinically and agricultural important microbes (Lu et al., 2013a,b,c). Oregano oil stood out as one of the best ones in terms of safety and efficacy. We thus detailed the bactericidal activity of oregano oil against 11 MDR clinical isolates of *P. aeruginosa, A. baumannii* and MRSA as well as two bioluminescent strains of *P. aeruginosa* PA01 and MRSA USA300 in the current study. Oregano oil effectively killed all the bacterial strains tested, with the MICs ranging from 0.08 to 0.64 mg/ml and at an order of sensitivity of *A. baumannii* > MRSA > *P. aeruginosa* (**Table 1**). The finding is in agreement with previous studies demonstrating that oregano oil and its main component carvacrol had a higher MIC against *P. aeruginosa*

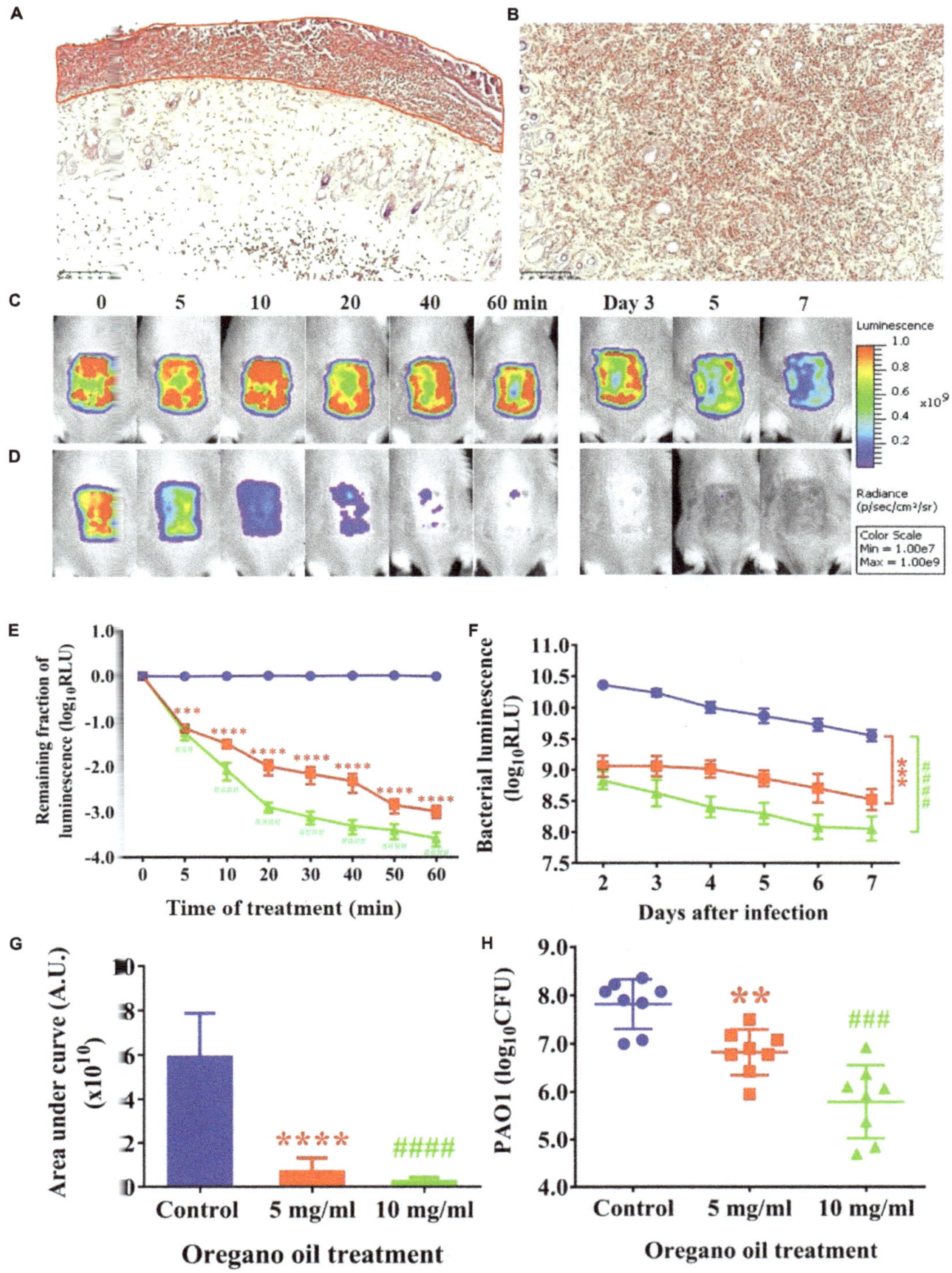

FIGURE 4 | Oregano oil treatment of PA01 infections in the burn wounds. **(A,B)** Gram-stained longitudinal section **(A)** and crossing section **(B)** of a representative wound showing the presence of PA01 biofilms outlined in red. The skin sample was harvested 24 h after bacterial inoculation. **(C,D)** Successive bacterial luminescence images of representative wounds infected with 5×10^6 CFU of luminescent PA01 with **(D)** and without **(C)** oregano oil at 10 mg/ml. The oregano oil was topically applied onto the wounds at 24 h after bacterial inoculation. **(E)** A dose response of mean bacterial luminescence of the wounds infected with 5×10^6 CFU of PA01 in the presence or absence of oregano oil treatment at 5 or 10 mg/ml. **(F)** Time courses of mean bacterial luminescence of the infected wounds in the presence or absence of oregano oil treatment at 5 or 10 mg/ml from days 2 to 7. **(G)** Mean areas under the bacterial luminescence curves **(F)**, representing the overall bacterial burden of infected wounds. **(H)**. The wounds were treated with grape seed oil (control) or oregano oil 24 h after infection and bacterial CFU were quantified on day 7 after bacterial inoculation. RLU, relative luminescence units; A.U., arbitrary units. The data represent means ± SDs (n = 8). $^{**}p < 0.01$, $^{###}$ or $^{***}p < 0.001$ and $^{####}$ or $^{****}p < 0.0001$ in the presence vs. absence of oregano oil. ns, no significance.

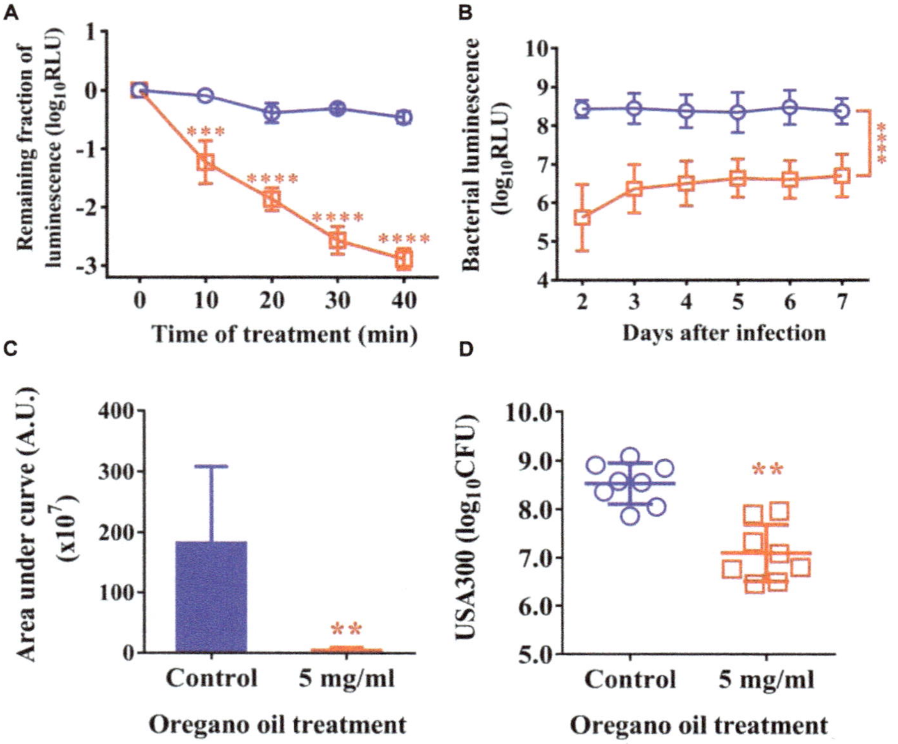

FIGURE 5 | Oregano oil treatment of MRSA USA300 in infected wounds. **(A)** The change in mean bacterial luminescence of the wounds infected with 5×10^6 CFU of USA300 with or without 5 mg/ml oregano oil treatment. **(B)** Time courses of mean bacterial luminescence of the infected wounds with and without oregano oil treatment. **(C)** Mean areas under the bacterial luminescence curves in **(B)**. **(D)** The wounds were treated with grape seed oil (control) or oregano oil once 24 h after infection and bacterial CFU were quantified on day 7 after bacterial inoculation. The data represent means ± SDs ($n = 8$). $^{**}p < 0.01$, $^{***}p < 0.001$, and $^{****}p < 0.0001$ in the presence vs. absence of 5 mg/ml of oregano oil.

compared to other species, such as *S.* spp. (Nostro et al., 2007), *Chromobacterium violaceum, Salmonella typhimurium,* and *S. aureus* (Burt et al., 2014). Similar to the clinical isolates, oregano oil also inactivated standard strains of *A. baumannii* ATCC 19606 (Rosato et al., 2010), *P. aeruginosa* ATCC 27853 and *S. aureus* ATCC 29213 (Bouhdid et al., 2009), with the MICs 0.15 mg/mL, 1 mg/mL, and 0.33 mg/mL, respectively, which are comparable to our investigation. Previous studies suggested that Gram-negative bacteria appeared to be more resistant than Gram-positive bacteria in response to EO (Tepe et al., 2005; Longaray Delamare et al., 2007; Gilles et al., 2010). This relative resistance of Gram-negative over Gram-positive bacteria may be ascribed to their cell wall structure and outer membrane arrangement. The outer membrane of Gram-negative bacteria is rich in lipopolysaccharide molecules, relatively impermeable to lipophilic compounds, thereby presenting a barrier to penetration of EO antimicrobial substances (Gao et al., 2011). It may be also associated with the enzymes in the periplasmic space, which are capable of breaking down the antimicrobial substances upon their entrance of the cells (Nikaido, 1996). However, our studies disagreed with these observations and found Gram-negative *A. baumannii* was more sensitive to oregano oil than Gram-positive MRSA. This different outcome suggests that antibacterial activity of oregano oil may not depend on the type of Gram reaction in contrast to other EOs, a possibility that is supported by the studies of Gao et al. (2011). In their studies, Gram-negative bacteria *Klebsiella pneumoniae* was the most sensitive bacteria whereas the Gram-positive bacteria *Listeria monocytogenes* was the most resistant strain to the *Sphallerocarpus gracilis* seed EO (Gao et al., 2011).

The possibility that the cell wall and membrane were primary targets of oregano oil was supported by TEM imaging of the ultrastructure of the bacteria. We found damages of the cell wall and membranes, occurrent with cytoplasmic vacuoles, stainless-vesicles, and disruption and discontinuation of the intracellular structures in a large number of bacterial cells after oregano oil treatment (**Figures 2B,E**). This finding is consistent with an association of the antibacterial activity of oregano oil/carvacrol with disturbance of membrane embedded proteins and disruption of lipids, RNA synthesis, ATPase activity, and efflux pump previously demonstrated (Simoes et al., 2009; Tapia-Rodriguez et al., 2017). Moreover, oregano oil may cause an imbalance in intracellular osmotic pressure owing to a leakage of cytoplasmic contents following cell wall and membrane damages, and formation of cytoplasmic vacuoles, eventually inducing cell necrosis, although more investigations are required to conclude the mechanism in detail.

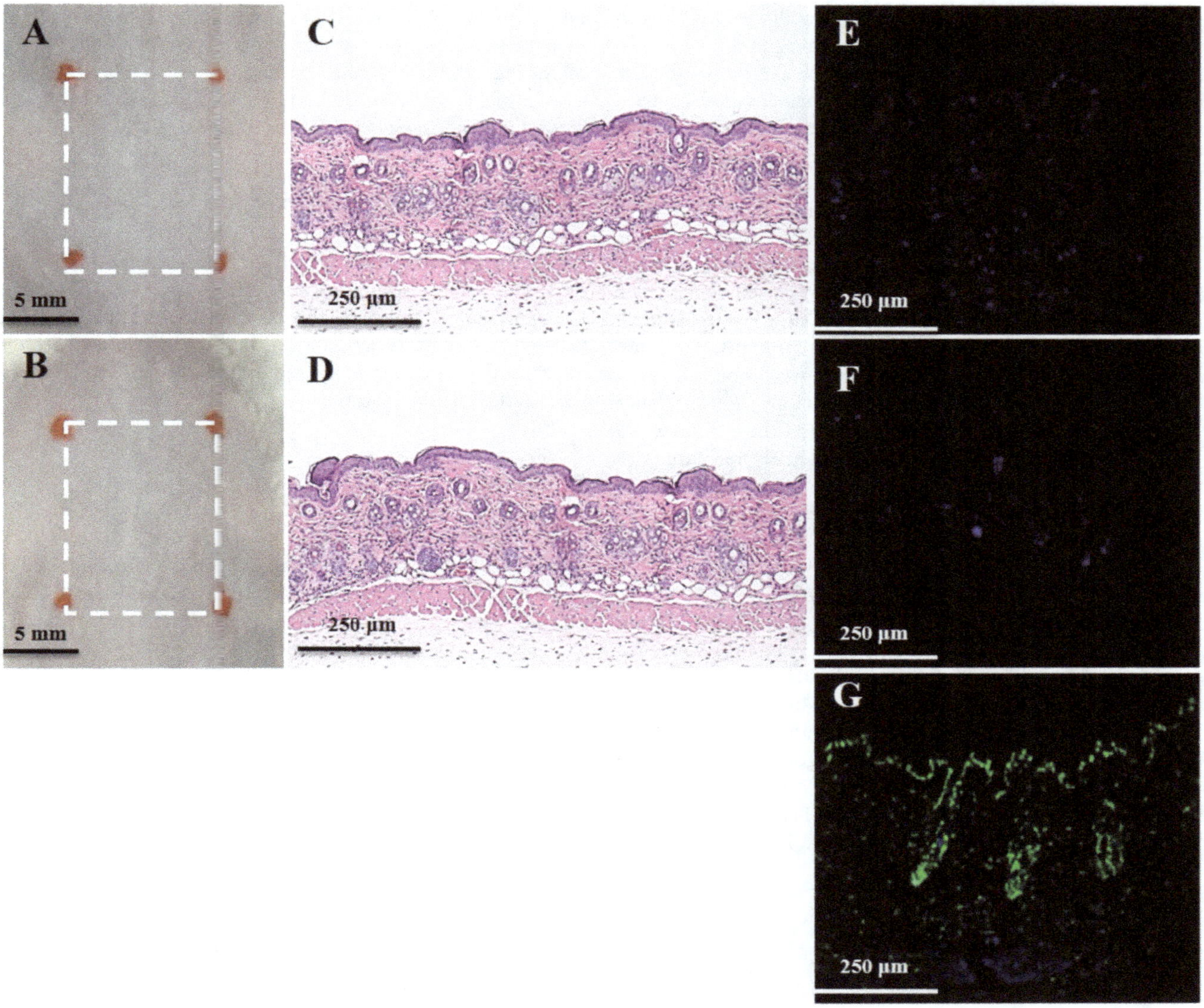

FIGURE 6 | Toxicity evaluation of oregano oil to normal mouse skins. The dorsal skin of mice was topically treated with **(A,C,E)** or without 10 mg/ml oregano oil **(B,D,F)** once a day for three consecutive days. On day 4, the skins were photographed **(A,B)**, followed by histological examination **(C,D)**. The skin sections were also TUNEL stained **(E,F)**. DNase I treated skin samples **(G)** were TUNEL stained in parallel as positive-staining controls.

Biofilms are sessile organizations of bacterial cells with a strong adherence to surfaces. Biofilm-associated microbial cells are well protected by an extracellular matrix that comprises exopolysaccharides, proteins and DNA and is poorly permeable (Donlan, 2002; Husain et al., 2015). Systemic antibiotics administered to treat bacterial infections frequently fails at least in part due to the poor permeability of biofilms. Interestingly, oregano oil was capable of biofilm-killing at least at an early stage (24-h-old biofilms) as efficiently as planktonic cells. Biofilms of *A. baumannii*, *P. aeruginosa*, and MRSA were eliminated by oregano oil at a concentration of 0.3, 1.0, or 0.4 mg/ml, respectively, similar to the corresponding MICs attained in planktonic cells. The similarity can be extended to the order of sensitivity with *P. aeruginosa* biofilms more resistant than MRSA biofilms than *A. baumannii* biofilms (**Figure 1** and **Table 1**). This may be attributed to the superior permeability and lipid solubility of oregano oil to bacterial cell membrane and wall (Magi et al., 2015; Khan et al., 2017). Likewise, the effectiveness of oregano oil to inactivate *S. aureus*, *S. epidermidis*, and *P. aeruginosa* biofilms was also found at similar MICs as those against planktonic cells (Nostro et al., 2007; dos Santos Rodrigues et al., 2017; Tapia-Rodriguez et al., 2017). SEM observations confirmed the physical damage and considerable morphological alteration in the *P. aeruginosa* IQ0042 (**Figures 2E,F**) and MRSA IQ0064 (**Figures 2G,H**) biofilms following oregano oil treatment. These observations raise an intriguing possibility that EO may have advantages over water soluble antibiotics in treatment of biofilms because bacteria living in the biofilms are well known to be more resistant to antibiotics (up to 1,000 times) than their planktonic counterparts, in part owing to poor permeability of biofilms to the antibiotics (Ceri et al., 1999; Caraher et al., 2007).

One concern of using oregano oil as an alternative for the treatment of infections in clinics will be whether MDR bacteria can develop resistance to oregano oil. Although this remains largely unaddressed to date, our results suggest that resistance may not be readily developed because 20 passages in the presence of sublethal concentrations of oregano oil did not alter their susceptibility to the oil (**Figure 3A**). Moreover, oregano oil has been used in food prevention and other antiseptic application for centuries and no resistance has been reported so far. It is commonly believed that EOs act at multiple sites within bacterial cells (cell membrane, cell wall, structural proteins, enzymes, nucleic acids, unsaturated lipids, etc.) and would be less likely to induce the development of resistance (Burt, 2004; Simoes et al., 2009; Tapia-Rodriguez et al., 2017). On the contrary, the MIC of conventional antibiotics could gradually increase with a treatment length due to their single action to inactivate the bacteria (Baym et al., 2016; Levin-Reisman et al., 2017).

The bactericidal activity of oregano oil was corroborated in mouse burn models using model bioluminescent strains of Gram-negative *P. aeruginosa* PA01 and Gram-positive MRSA USA300. When applied at 24 h after bacterial inoculation forming early stage biofilms, oregano oil effectively reduced the bacterial burden by 25-folds for PA01 and 49-folds for USA300, respectively, in comparison to untreated wounds. While efficiently inactivating bacteria, oregano oil exhibited no cytotoxicity or genotoxicity to the skin, in good agreement with its long record of safety. Moreover, oregano oil did not adversely affect human keratinocytes (Babili et al., 2011) and was safe when administered orally in mice (Manohar et al., 2001; Preuss et al., 2005; Feng et al., 2017).

In summary, we reported here the effectiveness of oregano oil against a panel of MDR bacteria isolated from combating casualties and demonstrated for the first time efficacy of oregano oil for the treatment of burn infections in mice. The study serves as an initial effort in the pursuit of a novel therapeutic option for wound infections, especially those caused by MDR bacteria.

AUTHOR CONTRIBUTIONS

ML designed and performed all the experiments, analyzed the data, and wrote the manuscript. TD supervised and designed the experiments, analyzed the data, and wrote the paper. CM isolated and characterized all the clinical bacteria and wrote the paper. and MW designed and supervised the study, analyzed the data, and wrote the manuscript.

FUNDING

This study was supported in part by FA9550-16-1-00173, Department of Defense/Air Force Office of Scientific Research Military Photomedicine Program and Department funds to MW and TD.

ACKNOWLEDGMENTS

We thank Drs. Michael R. Hamblin and Ji Wang for stimulating comments and discussions from Massachusetts General Hospital and the staff at the photopathology core at Wellman Center for Photomedicine for assisting transmission electron microscopy and histopathology.

REFERENCES

Akgul, A., and Kivanc, M. (1988). Inhibitory effects of selected Turkish spices and oregano components on some foodborne fungi. *Int. J. Food Microbiol.* 6, 263–268. doi: 10.1016/0168-1605(88)90019-0

Babili, F. E., Bouajila, J., Souchard, J. P., Bertrand, C., Bellvert, F., Fouraste, I., et al. (2011). Oregano: chemical analysis and evaluation of its antimalarial, antioxidant, and cytotoxic activities. *Food Sci.* 3, 512–518. doi: 10.1111/j.1750-3841.2011.02109.x

Baym, M., Lieberman, T. D., Kelsic, E. D., Chait, R., Gross, R., Yelin, I., et al. (2016). Spatiotemporal microbial evolution on antibiotic landscapes. *Science* 353, 1147–1151. doi: 10.1126/science.aag0822

Benito, M., Jorro, G., Morales, C., Pelaez, A., and Fernandez, A. (1996). Labiatae allergy: systemic reactions due to ingestion of oregano and thyme. *Ann. Allergy Asthma Immunol.* 76, 416–418. doi: 10.1016/S1081-1206(10)63456-4

Bloemsma, G. C., Dokter, J., Boxma, H., and Oen, I. M. (2008). Mortality and causes of death nin a burn centre. *Burns* 34, 1103–1107. doi: 10.1016/j.burns.2008.02.010

Bouhdid, S., Abrini, J., Zhiri, A., Espuny, M. J., and Manresa, A. (2009). Investigation of functional and morphological changes in *Pseudomonas aeruginosa* and *Staphylococcus aureus* cells induced by *Origanum compactum* essential oil. *J. Appl. Microbiol.* 106, 1558–1568. doi: 10.1111/j.1365-2672.2008.04124.x

Burt, S. (2004). Essential oils: their antibacterial properties and potential applications in foods – A review. *Int. J. Food Microbiol.* 94, 223–253. doi: 10.1016/j.ijfoodmicro.2004.03.022

Burt, S. A., Ojo-Fakunle, V. T. A., Woertman, J., and Veldhuizen, E. J. A. (2014). The natural antimicrobial carvacrol inhibits quorum sensing in chromobacterium violaceum and reduces bacterial biofilm formation at sub-lethal concentrations. *PLoS One* 9:e93414. doi: 10.1371/journal.pone.0093414

Calhoun, J. H., Murray, C. K., and Manring, M. M. (2008). Multidrug-resistant organisms in military wounds from iraq and afghanistan. *Clin. Orthop.* 466, 1356–1362. doi: 10.1007/s11999-008-0212-9

Caraher, E., Reynolds, G., Murphy, P., McClean, S., and Callaghan, M. (2007). Comparison of antibiotic susceptibility of *Burkholderia cepacia* complex organisms when grown planktonically or as biofilm in vitro. *Eur. J. Clin. Microbiol. Infect. Dis.* 26, 213–216. doi: 10.1007/s10096-007-0256-x

Ceri, H., Olson, M., Stremick, C., Read, R., Morck, D., and Buret, A. (1999). The calgary biofilm device: new technology for rapid determination of antibiotic susceptibilities of bacterial biofilms. *J. Clin. Microbiol.* 37, 1771–1776.

Christensen, L., Breiting, V., Bjarnsholt, T., Eickhardt, S., Hogdall, E., Janssen, M., et al. (2013). Bacterial infection as a likely cause of adverse reactions to polyacrylamide hydrogel fillers in cosmetic surgery. *Clin. Infect. Dis.* 56, 1438–1444. doi: 10.1093/cid/cit067

Crane, D. P., Gromov, K., Li, D., Soballe, K., Wahnes, C., Buechner, H., et al. (2009). Efficacy of colistin-impregnated beads to prevent multidrug-resistant *A. baumannii* implant-associated osteomyelitis. *J. Orthop. Res.* 27, 1008–1015. doi: 10.1002/jor.20847

Dai, T., Gupta, A., Huang, Y., Yin, R., Murray, C. K., Vrahas, M. S., et al. (2013). Blue light rescues mice from potentially fatal *Pseudomonas aeruginosa* burn infection: efficacy, safety, and mechanism of action. *Antimicrob. Agents Chemother.* 57, 1238–1245. doi: 10.1128/AAC.01652-12

Donlan, R. (2002). Biofilms: microbial life on surfaces. *Emerg. Infect. Dis.* 8, 881–890. doi: 10.3201/eid0809.020063

dos Santos Rodrigues, J. B., de Carvalho, R. J., de Souza, N. T., Oliveira, K. d. S., Franco, O. L., Schaffner, D., et al. (2017). Effects of oregano essential oil and carvacrol on biofilms of *Staphylococcus aureus* from food-contact surfaces. *Food Control* 73, 1237–1246. doi: 10.1016/j.foodcont.2016.10.043

Feng, J., Zhang, S., Shi, W., Zubcevik, N., Miklossy, J., and Zhang, Y. (2017). Selective essential oils from spice or culinary herbs have high activity against stationary phase and biofilm borrelia burgdorferi. *Front. Med.* 4:169. doi: 10.3389/fmed.2017.00169

Fitzwater, J., Purdue, G., Hunt, J., and O'Keefe, G. (2003). The risk factors and time course of sepsis and organ dysfunction after burn trauma. *J. Trauma-Injury Infect. Crit. Care* 54, 959–966. doi: 10.1097/01.TA.0000029382.26295.AB

Gao, C., Tian, C., Lu, Y., Xu, J., Luo, J., and Guo, X. (2011). Essential oil composition and antimicrobial activity of *Sphallerocarpus gracilis* seeds against selected food-related bacteria. *Food Control* 22, 517–522. doi: 10.1016/j.foodcont.2010.09.038

Gilles, M., Zhao, J., An, M., and Agboola, S. (2010). Chemical composition and antimicrobial properties of essential oils of three Australian Eucalyptus species. *Food Chem.* 119, 731–737. doi: 10.1016/j.foodchem.2009.07.021

Gomez, R., Murray, C. K., Hospenthal, D. R., Cancio, L. C., Renz, E. M., Holcomb, J. B., et al. (2009). Causes of mortality by autopsy findings of combat casualties and civilian patients admitted to a burn unit. *J. Am. Coll. Surg.* 208, 348–354. doi: 10.1016/j.jamcollsurg.2008.11.012

Hampton, T. (2013). Report reveals scope of US antibiotic resistance threat. *JAMA* 310, 1661–1663. doi: 10.1001/jama.2013.280695

Husain, F. M., Ahmad, I., Khan, M. S., Ahmad, E., Tahseen, Q., Khan, M. S., et al. (2015). Sub-MICs of *Mentha piperita* essential oil and menthol inhibits AHL mediated quorum sensing and biofilm of ram-negative bacteria. *Front. Microbiol.* 6:420. doi: 10.3389/fmicb.2015.00420

Jiang, B., Yin, S., You, B., Huang, G., Yang, Z., Zhang, Y., et al. (2017). A 5-year survey reveals increased susceptibility to glycopeptides for methicillin-resistant *Staphylococcus aureus* isolates from *Staphylococcus aureus* bacteremia patients in a Chinese burn center. *Front. Microbiol.* 8:2531. doi: 10.3389/fmicb.2017.02531

Joshi, S. C., Verma, A. R., and Mathela, C. S. (2010). Antioxidant and antibacterial activities of the leaf essential oils of Himalayan *Lauraceae* species. *Food Chem. Toxicol.* 48, 37–40. doi: 10.1016/j.fct.2009.09.011

Kavanaugh, N. L., and Ribbeck, K. (2012). Selected antimicrobial essential oils eradicate *Pseudomonas* spp. and *Staphylococcus aureus* biofilms. *Appl. Environ. Microbiol.* 78, 4057–4061. doi: 10.1128/AEM.07499-11

Khan, I., Bahuguna, A., Kumar, P., Bajpai, V. K., and Kang, S. C. (2017). Antimicrobial potential of carvacrol against uropathogenic *Escherichia coli* via membrane disruption, depolarization, and reactive oxygen species generation. *Front. Microbiol.* 8:2421. doi: 10.3389/fmicb.2017.02421

Levin-Reisman, I., Ronin, I., Gefen, O., Braniss, I., Shoresh, N., and Balaban, N. Q. (2017). Antibiotic tolerance facilitates the evolution of resistance. *Science* 355, 826–830. doi: 10.1126/science.aaj2191

Li, X., Robinson, S. M., Gupta, A., Saha, K., Jiang, Z., and Moyano, D. F. (2014). Functional gold nanoparticles as potent antimicrobial agents against multi-drug-resistant bacteria. *ACS Nano* 8, 10682–10686. doi: 10.1021/nn5042625

Longaray Delamare, A. P., Moschen-Pistorello, I. T., Artico, L., Atti-Serafini, L., and Echeverrigaray, S. (2007). Antibacterial activity of the essential oils of *Salvia officinalis* L. and *Salvia triloba* L. cultivated in South Brazil. *Food Chem.* 100, 603–608. doi: 10.1016/j.foodchem.2005.09.078

Lopez-Reyes, J. G., Spadaro, D., Gullino, M. L., and Garibaldi, A. (2010). Efficacy of plant essential oils on postharvest control of rot caused by fungi on four cultivars of apples in vivo. *Flavour Fragrance J.* 25, 171–177. doi: 10.1002/ffj.1989

Lu, M., Han, Z., Xu, Y., and Yao, L. (2013a). In vitro and in vivo anti-tobacco mosaic virus activities of essential oils and individual compounds. *J. Microbiol. Biotechnol.* 23, 771–778. doi: 10.4014/jmb.1210.10078

Lu, M., Han, Z., and Yao, L. (2013b). In vitro and in vivo antimicrobial efficacy of essential oils and individual compounds against *Phytophthora parasitica* var. nicotianae. *J. Appl. Microbiol.* 115, 187–198. doi: 10.1111/jam.12208

Lu, M., Han, Z., Xu, Y., and Yao, L. (2013c). Effects of essential oils from Chinese indigenous aromatic plants on mycelial growth and morphogenesis of three phytopathogens. *Flavour Fragrance J.* 28, 84–92. doi: 10.1002/ffj.3132

Magi, G., Marini, E., and Facinelli, B. (2015). Antimicrobial activity of essential oils and carvacrol, and synergy of carvacrol and erythromycin, against clinical, erythromycin-resistant Group A *Streptococci*. *Front. Microbiol.* 6:165. doi: 10.3389/fmicb.2015.00165

Manohar, V., Ingram, C., Gray, J., Talpur, N., Echard, B., Bagchi, D., et al. (2001). Antifungal activities of origanum oil against *Candida albicans*. *Mol. Cell Biochem.* 228, 111–117. doi: 10.1023/A:1013311632207

Munhuweyi, K., Caleb, O. J., Lennox, C. L., van Reenen, A. J., and Opara, U. L. (2017). In vitro and in vivo antifungal activity of chitosan-essential oils against pomegranate fruit pathogens. *Postharvest. Biol. Technol.* 129, 9–22. doi: 10.1016/j.postharvbio.2017.03.002

Nikaido, H. (1996). Multidrug efflux pumps of gram-negative bacteria. *J. Bacteriol.* 178, 5853–5859. doi: 10.1128/jb.178.20.5853-5859.1996

Nostro, A., Roccaro, A. S., Bisignano, G., Marino, A., Cannatelli, M. A., Pizzimenti, F. C., et al. (2007). Effects of oregano, carvacrol and thymol on *Staphylococcus aureus* and *Staphylococcus epidermidis* biofilms. *J. Med. Microbiol.* 56, 519–523. doi: 10.1099/jmm.0.46804-0

Ocana-Fuentes, A., Arranz-Gutierrez, E., Senorans, F. J., and Reglero, G. (2010). Supercritical fluid extraction of oregano (*Origanum vulgare*) essentials oils: anti-inflammatory properties based on cytokine response on THP-1 macrophages. *Food Chem. Toxicol.* 48, 1568–1575. doi: 10.1016/j.fct.2010.03.026

Pandey, A. K., Kumar, P., Singh, P., Tripathi, N. N., and Bajpai, V. K. (2017). Essential oils: sources of antimicrobials and food preservatives. *Front. Microbiol.* 7:2161. doi: 10.3389/fmicb.2016.02161

Preuss, H., Echard, B., Dadgar, A., Talpur, N., Manohar, V., Enig, M., et al. (2005). Effects of essential oils and monolaurin on *Staphylococcus aureus*: in vitro and in vivo studies. *Toxicol. Mech. Methods* 15, 279–285. doi: 10.1080/15376520590968833

Rosato, A., Piarulli, M., Corbo, F., Muraglia, M., Carone, A., Vitali, M. E., et al. (2010). In vitro synergistic action of certain combinations of gentamicin and essential oils. *Curr. Med. Chem.* 17, 3289–3295. doi: 10.2174/092986710792231996

Sakkas, H., and Papadopoulou, C. (2017). Antimicrobial activity of basil, oregano, and thyme essential oils. *J. Microbiol. Biotechnol.* 28, 429–438. doi: 10.4014/jmb.1608.08024

Scott, P., Deye, G., Srinivasan, A., Murray, C., Moran, K., Hulten, E., et al. (2007). An outbreak of multidrug-resistant *Acinetobacter baumannii*-calcoaceticus complex infection in the US military health care system associated with military operations in Iraq. *Clin. Infect. Dis.* 44, 1577–1584. doi: 10.1086/518170

Shen, D., Pan, M., Wu, Q., Park, C., Juliani, H. R., Ho, C., et al. (2010). LC-MS method for the simultaneous quantitation of the anti-inflammatory constituents in oregano (*Origanum* Species). *J. Agric. Food Chem.* 58, 7119–7125. doi: 10.1021/jf100636h

Simoes, M., Bennett, R. N., and Rosa, E. A. S. (2009). Understanding antimicrobial activities of phytochemicals against multidrug resistant bacteria and biofilms. *Nat. Prod. Rep.* 26, 746–757. doi: 10.1039/b821648g

Soylu, E. M., Kurt, S., and Soylu, S. (2010). In vitro and in vivo antifungal activities of the essential oils of various plants against tomato grey mould disease agent *Botrytis cinerea*. *Int. J. Food Microbiol.* 143, 183–189. doi: 10.1016/j.ijfoodmicro.2010.08.015

Soylu, S., Yigitbas, H., Soylu, E. M., and Kurt, S. (2007). Antifungal effects of essential oils from oregano and fennel on *Sclerotinia sclerotiorum*. *J. Appl. Microbiol.* 103, 1021–1030. doi: 10.1111/j.1365-2672.2007.03310.x

Tapia-Rodriguez, M. R., Hernandez-Mendoza, A., Gonzalez-Aguilar, G. A., Martinez-Tellez, M. A., Martins, C. M., and Ayala-Zavala, J. F. (2017). Carvacrol as potential quorum sensing inhibitor of *Pseudomonas aeruginosa* and biofilm production on stainless steel surfaces. *Food Control* 75, 255–261. doi: 10.1016/j.foodcont.2016.12.014

Tepe, B., Daferera, D., Sokmen, A., Sokmen, M., and Polissiou, M. (2005). Antimicrobial and antioxidant activities of the essential oil and various extracts of *Salvia tomentosa* Miller (Lamiaceae). *Food Chem.* 90, 333–340. doi: 10.1016/j.foodchem.2003.09.013

Vento, T. J., Cole, D. W., Mende, K., Calvano, T. P., Rini, E. A., Tully, C. C., et al. (2013). Multidrug-resistant gram-negative bacteria colonization of healthy US military personnel in the US and Afghanistan. *BMC Infect. Dis.* 13:68. doi: 10.1186/1471-2334-13-68

Wang, Y., Beekman, J., Hew, J., Jackson, S., Issler-Fisher, A. C., Parungao, R., et al. (2018). Burn injury: challenges and advances in burn wound healing, infection, pain and scarring. *Adv. Drug Deliv. Rev.* 123, 3–17. doi: 10.1016/j.addr.2017.09.018

Wang, Y., Wu, X., Chen, J., Amin, R., Lu, M., Bhayana, B., et al. (2016). Antimicrobial blue light inactivation of ram-negative pathogens in biofilms: in vitro and in vivo studies. *J. Infect. Dis.* 213, 1380–1387. doi: 10.1093/infdis/jiw070

Yan, F., Azizi, A., Janke, S., Schwarz, M., Zeller, S., and Honermeier, B. (2016). Antioxidant capacity variation in the oregano (*Origanum vulgare* L.) collection of the German National Genebank. *Ind. Crops Prod.* 92, 19–25. doi: 10.1016/j.indcrop.2016.07.038

Zhang, Y., Zhu, Y., Gupta, A., Huang, Y., Murray, C. K., Vrahas, M. S., et al. (2014). Antimicrobial blue light therapy for multidrug-resistant *Acinetobacter baumannii* infection in a mouse burn model: implications for prophylaxis and treatment of combat-related wound infections. *J. Infect. Dis.* 209, 1963–1971. doi: 10.1093/infdis/jit842

9

Changing Antimicrobial Resistance and Epidemiology of Non-Typhoidal *Salmonella* Infection in Taiwanese Children

*Yi-Jung Chang[1,2], Yi-Ching Chen[1,2], Nai-Wen Chen[1], Ying-Jie Hsu[1], Hsiao-Han Chu[1], Chyi-Liang Chen[2] and Cheng-Hsun Chiu[1,2,3]**

[1] Department of Pediatrics, Chang Gung Memorial Hospital, College of Medicine, Chang Gung University, Taoyuan, Taiwan, [2] Molecular Infectious Disease Research Center, Chang Gung Memorial Hospital, Taoyuan, Taiwan, [3] Graduate Institute of Clinical Medical Sciences, College of Medicine, Chang Gung University, Taoyuan, Taiwan

***Correspondence:**
Cheng-Hsun Chiu
chchiu@adm.cgmh.org.tw

Non-typhoidal *Salmonella* (NTS) typically causes self-limiting diarrheal disease but may occasionally lead to invasive infection. This study investigated the epidemiology and antimicrobial resistance of children with NTS infection between 2012 and 2019. We retrospectively analyzed pediatric patients with NTS infections, confirmed by positive cultures, in a tertiary medical center in Taiwan in 2012 and 2019. Clinical features and laboratory data of the patients were collected. Changes in the serogroup category and antimicrobial resistance were also analyzed. Of the total 797 isolates collected, 55 had NTS bacteremia. Compared with the resistance rates in 2012, the rates of resistances to third-generation cephalosporin and ciprofloxacin were significantly higher in 2019 (4.1% vs 14.3%, $P < 0.001$; 1.9% vs 28.6%, $P < 0.001$), especially in groups B, D, and E. Moreover, we observed significantly higher antimicrobial resistance (25.3%) to third-generation cephalosporin, and approximately half the NTS isolates in the infant group were multidrug resistant – a higher rate than those of other age groups in 2019. Invasive NTS often presented with a longer fever duration, lower hemoglobin level and with no elevated C-reactive protein ($P < 0.05$). Non-invasive NTS isolates in 2019 were significantly more resistant to ceftriaxone ($P < 0.001$) and ciprofloxacin ($P < 0.001$) than those in 2012. The antimicrobial resistance of NTS in children has increased progressively in the past decade, and different serogroups exhibited different resistance patterns. During this period, infants showed the highest risk to get a third-generation cephalosporin-resistant NTS infection. The high rates of antimicrobial resistance among children with NTS in Taiwan merit continual surveillance.

Keywords: antimicrobial resistance, bacteremia, *Salmonella*, antibiotics, children

INTRODUCTION

Non-typhoidal *Salmonella* (NTS) infection is a global public health concern; it results in a considerable disease burden in both industrialized and developing countries (Majowicz et al., 2010; Kyu et al., 2018; Roth et al., 2018; Stanaway et al., 2019). NTS typically causes self-limiting diarrheal disease and may also result in invasive NTS (iNTS) infection (Katiyo et al., 2019).

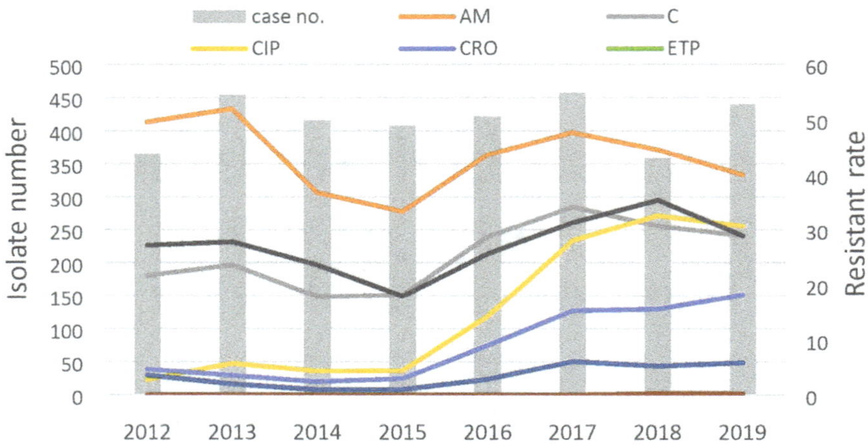

FIGURE 1 | Antibiotic resistant rates of non-typhoidal salmonella from 2012 to 2019.

Approximately 5% of individuals with NTS infection develop invasive diseases, such as bacteremia, meningitis, or septic arthritis, which are especially common in young infants or patients with compromised immune systems (Hohmann, 2001; Feasey et al., 2012). Antimicrobial agents are not recommended for non-severe NTS diarrhea, but they are recommended for people at risk of severe or invasive infection (Ke et al., 2020).

Antimicrobial therapy is the first-line therapy for treating patients with NTS with invasive diseases (Tsai et al., 2011). However, the recognition of NTS bacteremia in children before culture is challenging and rarely reported. Furthermore, resistance to antimicrobial agents has increased worldwide, including in Taiwan (Su et al., 2011; James et al., 2018; Chang et al., 2020). Resistant NTS infection has been reported to be correlated with higher morbidity and mortality (Angelo et al., 2016). Therefore, awareness of changes in antimicrobial resistance and the clinical characteristics of NTS is essential for physicians to arrange effective therapeutic plans to prevent complications.

This study investigated the changing trend of antimicrobial resistance and serogroup distribution in children in northern Taiwan between 2012 and 2019 and the risk factors associated with invasive NTS infection.

MATERIALS AND METHODS

Study Population and Data Collection

The secular trend of antimicrobial resistance of NTS in Chang Gung Memorial Hospital is shown in **Figure 1**. The study enrolled patients aged < 18 years with NTS infection, confirmed by a positive culture, in Chang Gung Memorial Hospital, Linkou, Taiwan, in 2012 and 2019. We retrospectively collected demographic data and clinical characteristics, including patient age, sex, treatment, outcome, serogroup category, and antimicrobial susceptibility from the medical records. In Taiwan, the pediatrician cares patients under 18 of age. In addition, diarrhea is the main cause of morbidity of children under 5 years of age. We stratified participants at different age group, which has been widely validated in many studies. The study was approved by the Research Ethics Committee of Chang Gung Memorial Hospital. (Institutional Review Board Approval No: 201702155B0). All data analyzed were anonymized.

TABLE 1 | Baseline characteristics and clinical features of 797 patients with non-typhoid *Salmonella* infection in 2012 and 2019.

N (%)	2012 (*N* = 363)	2019 (*N* = 434)	*P* value
Males (n, %)	200 (55.1%)	239 (55.1%)	0.994
Age(mean) (y/o)	2.1 (SD = 3.8)	2.4 (SD = 3.8)	0.56
Admission proportion	74.2%	62.7%	<0.001
Admission duration (days)	6.9 ± 16.2	5.4 ± 5.9	0.139
Ampicillin use	27/144(18.8%)	8/195 (4.1%)	<0.001
Ceftriaxone use	82/144(56.9%)	155/195(79.5%)	<0.001
iNTS	23/364 (6.3%)	39/434 (7.9%)	0.123
***Salmonella* serogroups**			
Group B	98/364 (26.9%)	100/434 (23%)	0.206
Group C1	20/364 (5.5%)	29/434 (6.7%)	0.486
Group C2	45/364 (12.4%)	56/434 (12.9%)	0.819
Group D	155/364 (42.6%)	185/434 (42.6%)	0.990
Group E	40/364 (11%)	57/434 (13.1%)	0.356
Antimicrobial resistance			
MDR	44/364 (12.2%)	130/434 (30%)	<0.001
Ampicillin	179/364 (49.3%)	174/434 (40.1%)	0.009
Ceftriaxone	15/364 (4.1%)	62/434 (14.3%)	<0.001
Ciprofloxacin	7/364 (1.9%)	124/433 (28.6%)	<0001
TMP-SMX	99/364 (27.3%)	127/432 (29.4%)	0.508
Ertapenem	0/364 (0%)	3/434 (0.7%)	0.255
Imipenem	0/364 (0%)	5/434 (1.2%)	0.067
Chloramphenicol	79/364 (21.8%)	126/403 (31.3%)	0.003
Flomoxef	12/364 (3.3%)	24/403 (6%)	0.084

iNTS, invasive non-typhoidal Salmonella;
MDR, multi-drug resistance, resistant to ≥3 drug classes;
TMP-SMX: trimethoprim-sulphamethoxazole.

Salmonella Strains and Antimicrobial Susceptibility Testing

We collected stool when the patient had gastrointestinal symptoms. The cerebrospinal fluid was sampled when meningitis is suspected. When a person has symptoms such as urinary irritation or needs to rule out a urinary tract infection, a urine culture would be ordered. At the time of admission in our hospital, each child would have a blood sample taken as usual. The blood samples were sent to microbiology laboratory and incubated in the BACTEC FX automatic blood culture system (Becton Dickinson Diagnostic Instrument Systems, Sparks, MD, United States). The BACTEC FX system monitors the production of carbon dioxide every 10 min and uses a fluorescent signal to indicate positive. The stool samples were planted on HE (Hektoen enteric) and EMB (Eosin Methylene Blue) agar medium, and then incubated at 35°C for 20–24 h. If the same participant had several samples, only 1 sample per patient was collected for downstream analyses. If both blood and stool isolates were available from the same patient, only the blood isolate was analyzed. Our hospital identified each *Salmonella* isolate by using a matrix-assisted laser desorption ionization time-of-flight mass spectrometry automated microbiology system. Serogroups of *Salmonella* isolates were examined with O-antigen antisera (Difco Laboratories, Detroit, MI, United States) by employing the slide agglutination method. We then classified *Salmonella* isolates into five serogroups (group B, C1, C2, D, and E) and other serogroups. The antimicrobial susceptibility of NTS isolates was determined using the Kirby–Bauer disk diffusion method and interpreted according to the Standards for Antimicrobial Susceptibility of the Clinical Laboratory Standards Institute. The CLSI versions M100-S29 in 2019 and M100-S22 in 2012 were used in this study (Clinical and Laboratory Standards Institute [CLSI], 2012, 2019). The following antimicrobial agents were examined: ciprofloxacin, ceftriaxone, ampicillin, chloramphenicol, ertapenem, imipenem, flomoxef, and trimethoprim-sulfamethoxazole (TMP-SMX). In MIC determination, the concentration of ceftriaxone resistant was with MIC 4 μg/mL and intermediate was with MIC 1–4 μg/mL. Meanwhile, the concentration of ciprofloxacin resistant was with MIC 1 μg/ml and intermediate was with MIC 0.5 μg/ml. The MIC range of chloramphenicol was 2.0–8.0 μg/mL. For further statistical analysis, intermediate resistance was regarded as the threshold for resistance. Multi-drug resistance (MDR) was defined as concomitant resistance to ≥three antimicrobial drug classes with the same selection, including ampicillin, ceftriaxone, chloramphenicol, ciprofloxacin, imipenem, TMP-SMX, ertapenem, and flomoxef. To analyze factors associated with invasive NTS in children, patients with *Salmonella* bacteremia, meningitis, or septic arthritis and without invasive salmonellosis were analyzed. For clinical features, only children who had both blood and stool culture performed were analyzed. We further divided the study patients into two groups. Those with diarrhea and negative blood culture were categorized as the non-invasive group. Those had positive results either in blood, CSF, or pus culture would be categorized into the invasive group. Patient eligibility was determined according to factors such as clinical manifestations and laboratory data obtained upon admission.

Statistical Analysis

We completed statistical analysis using SPSS for Windows version 22.0 (SPSS Inc., Chicago, IL, United States). Categorical variables including multiple categories were analyzed using the chi-square test, and continuous variables were examined using

TABLE 2 | Changing antimicrobial resistance in different serogroup between 2012 and 2019.

Antimicrobials	2012	2019	*P* value	OR	95% CI
Serogroup B					
MDR	11.2% (11/98)	32% (32/100)	<0.001	3.72	1.74–7.91
Ceftriaxone	5.1% (5/98)	15% (15/100)	0.021	3.28	1.14–9.41
Ciprofloxacin	1% (1/98)	27.3% (27/99)	<0.001	36.3	4.83–273.95
Ampicillin	53.1% (52/98)	43% (43/100)	0.157	1.49	0.85–2.62
TMP-SMX	26.5% (26/98)	35% (35/100)	0.197	0.671	0.365–1.232
Ertapenem	0% (0/98)	1% (1/100)	1.000	NA	NA
Imipenem	0% (0/98)	2% (2/100)	0.498	NA	NA
Serogroup C1					
MDR	10% (2/20)	34.5% (10/29)	0.089	4.73	0.91–24.64
Ceftriaxone	0% (0/20)	20.7% (6/29)	0.069	NA	NA
Ciprofloxacin	0% (0/20)	44.8% (13/29)	<0.001	NA	NA
TMP-SMX	26.3% (5/19)	32.1% (9/28)	0.668	0.754	0.20–2.74
Ampicillin	47.4% (9/19)	44.8% (13/29)	0.863	1.10	0.34–3.53
Ertapenem	0% (0/19)	3.4% (1/29)	1.000	NA	NA
Imipenem	0% (0/19)	3.4% (1/29)	1.000	NA	NA
Serogroup C2					
MDR	8.9% (4/45)	16.1% (9/56)	0.284	1.96	0.56–6.85
Ceftriaxone	4.4% (2/45)	5.4% (3/56)	1.000	1.21	0.19–7.61
Ciprofloxacin	2.2% (1/45)	19.6% (11/56)	0.007	10.75	1.33–86.85
TMP-SMX	31.1% (14/45)	14.3% (8/56)	0.042	2.70	1.01–7.21
Ampicillin	62.6% (28/45)	23.2% (13/56)	<0.001	5.44	2.29–12.93
Ertapenem	0% (0/45)	0% (0/56)	NA	NA	NA
Imipenem	0% (0/45)	0% (0/56)	NA	NA	NA
Serogroup D					
MDR	14.2% (22/155)	31.4% (58/185)	<0.001	2.76	1.59–4.77
Ceftriaxone	5.2% (8/155)	15.1% (28/185)	0.003	3.27	1.44–7.42
Ciprofloxacin	2.6% (4/155)	27.6% (51/185)	<0.001	14.36	5–40.8
TMP-SMX	27.7% (43/155)	30.4% (56/184)	0.587	0.878	0.548–1.406
Ampicillin	45.8% (71/155)	43.2% (80/185)	0.636	1.10	0.72–1.70
Ertapenem	0% (0/155)	0% (0/185)	NA	NA	NA
Imipenem	0% (0/155)	0.5% (1/185)	1.000	NA	NA
Serogroup E					
MDR	12.5% (5/40)	31.6% (18/57)	0.030	3.23	1.08–9.61
Ceftriaxone	0% (0/40)	14% (8/57)	0.019	NA	NA
Ciprofloxacin	2.5% (1/40)	19.6% (19/57)	<0.001	19.5	2.48–152.98
TMP-SMX	27.5% (11/40)	28.1% (16/57)	0951	0.972	0.394–2.398
Ampicillin	42.5% (17/40)	38.6% (22/57)	0.700	1.17	0.51–2.67
Ertapenem	0% (0/40)	0% (0/57)	NA	NA	NA
Imipenem	0% (0/40)	0% (0/57)	NA	NA	NA

MDR, multi-drug resistance, resistant to ≥3 drug classes; TMP-SMX, trimethoprim/sulfamethoxazole; OR, odds ratio; CI, confidence interval; NA, not applicable.

independent t tests. A p value <0.05 was considered to be statistically significant.

RESULTS

A total of 797 NTS isolates were collected from 781 patients in 2012 and 2019 (363 from 2012 and 434 from 2019), of which 90.7% were isolated from the stool, 6.8% from blood, and 2.5% from other extraintestinal samples (12 isolates from urine, 3 from cerebrospinal fluid, and 2 from pus). The isolates collected from blood and extraintestinal samples were classified as iNTS. The majority (81.5%) of the NTS isolates were obtained from children aged $\leq$ 3 years, and 36.0% of the isolates were from children aged 1–2 years. The most common serogroup was group D (42.6%), followed by group B (24.8%), serogroup C2 (12.6%), and serogroup E (12.1%). The overall resistance rates were 15.1% to ciprofloxacin, 8% to ceftriaxone, 41.4% to ampicillin, 27.8% to chloramphenicol, 2.3% to ertapenem, 3.9% to flomoxef, 0.6% to imipenem, and 28.2% to sulfamethoxazole. **Table 1** presents a comparison of the baseline characteristics of the patients and antimicrobial resistance rates of NTS between 2012 and 2019. The mean age of the two groups was similar (2.1 years vs 2.4 years, P = 0.56). Compared with the resistance rates in 2012, the resistance rates in 2019 to ciprofloxacin (28.6% vs 1.9%, P < 0.001), ceftriaxone (14.3% vs 4.1%, P < 0.001), chloramphenicol (31.3% vs 21.7%, P = 0.003), and sulfamethoxazole (29.4% vs 27.2%, P < 0.001) were significantly higher. Moreover, the ampicillin resistance rate was significantly lower in 2019 than in 2012 (49.2% vs 40.1%, P = 0.01). No significant difference in resistance rate was observed for ertapenem, imipenem, and flomoxef between those 2 years. The incidence of ampicillin as an empirical antibiotic in 2012 was higher than in 2019 (18.8% vs 4.1%, P < 0.001). On the contrary, if directed, most doctors choose ceftriaxone as an empirical antibiotic in 2019 than in 2012 (79.5% vs 56.9%, P < 0.001). The evolution of antimicrobial resistance in different serogroups is presented in **Table 2**. The highest resistance rate to ampicillin was noted in group B (48%), and the highest resistance rate to ciprofloxacin was observed in group C1 (27.1%). We noted significantly increased ciprofloxacin, ceftriaxone, and MDR resistance between 2012 and 2019 in the isolates from group B, group D, and group E. In groups C1 and C2, we also noted an increase in ciprofloxacin resistance in 2019 compared with 2012. **Table 3** presents the differences in antimicrobial resistance by age for 2012 and 2019. In 2019, the patients aged < 1 year had a higher resistance rate to ampicillin (50.6%, P = 0.005), ceftriaxone (25.3%, P = 0.002), TMP-SMX (44.2%, P = 0.001), and chloramphenicol (46.3%, P = 0.003) than did that other age group. The differences in clinical manifestations and laboratory examination results upon admission between the NTS bacteremia group and the non-iNTS group are listed in **Table 4**. Longer fever duration (3.8 ± 2.7, P < 0.001), lower C-reactive protein (CRP) level (39.1 ± 41.8 vs 58.6 ± 55.7, P < 0.001), and lower hemoglobin level (11.6 ± 1.4 vs 12.1 ± 1.2, P = 0.027) were significant factors associated with the NTS bacteremia group. The main outcomes between children with iNTS and those with diarrhea and a negative blood culture was the prolonged hospital stay in iNTS (9.8 ± 9.5 vs 5.8 ± 12.1 p = 0.016). **Table 5** presents the antimicrobial resistance in NTS bacteremia and non-iNTS infections in 2012 and 2019. Non-iNTS isolates in 2019 were significantly more resistant to

TABLE 3 | Changing antimicrobial resistance by different age groups between 2012 and 2019.

AGE	<1 Y	1–2 Y	2–5 Y	>5 Y	P value
2012					
MDR	12.1% (12/99)	11.6% (18/155)	14.9% (14/94)	0% (0/15)	0.426
Ampicillin	48.5% (48/99)	54.2% (84/155)	42.3% (22/52)	43.1% (25/58)	0.279
Ceftriaxone	3% (3/99)	5.2% (8/155)	4.3% (4/94)	0% (0/15)	0.575
Ciprofloxacin	2% (2/99)	1.9% (3/155)	2.1% (2/94)	0% (0/15)	0.895
TMP-SMX	25.3% (25/99)	25.8% (40/155)	34% (32/94)	13.3% (2/15)	0.260
Ertapenem	0% (0/99)	0% (0/155)	0% (0/94)	0% (0/15)	
Imipenem	0% (0/99)	0% (0/155)	0% (0/94)	0% (0/15)	
Chloramphenicol	28.3% (28/99)	22.6% (35/155)	16% (15/94)	6.7% (1/15)	0.094
Flomoxef	4% (4/99)	2.6% (4/155)	4.3% (4/94)	0% (0/15)	0.641
2019					
MDR	42.5% (37/87)	22.2% (40/180)	29.6% (37/125)	38.1% (16/42)	0.005
Ampicillin	50.6% (44/87)	32.8% (59/180)	41.6% (52/125)	19.0% (8/42)	0.036
Ceftriaxone	25.3% (22/87)	8.3% (15/180)	13.6% (17/125)	19.0% (8/42)	0.002
Ciprofloxacin	34.9% (30/86)	23.9% (43/180)	28.8% (36/125)	35.7% (15/42)	0.199
TMP-SMX	44.2% (38/86)	22.3% (40/179)	26.4% (33/125)	38.1% (16/42)	0.001
Ertapenem	2.3% (2/87)	0.6% (1/180)	0% (0/125)	0% (0/42)	0.221
Imipenem	3.4% (3/87)	0.6% (1/180)	0% (0/125)	2.4% (1/42)	0.084
Chloramphenicol	46.3% (37/80)	24.4% (39/160)	27.9 (34/122)	39% (16/41)	0.003
Flomoxef	3.8% (3/80)	4.4% (7/160)	8.2% (10/122)	49.8% (4/41)	0.326

MDR, multi-drug resistance, resistant to ≥3 drug classes.

TABLE 4 | Demographic, clinical manifestations and antimicrobial resistance among iNTS and non-iNTS infections in 2012 and 2019.

	iNTS infections (*n* = 62)	Non-iNTS infections (*n* = 555)	*P* value
Male, *n* (%)	53.2% (33)	56.5% (314)	0.582
Age, y/o, mean ± SD	1.7 ± 2.8	2.3 ± 2.3	0.099
Symptoms at admission			
Fever, *n* (%)	58(93.5%)	512(92.8%)	0.930
Diarrhea, *n* (%)	45(72.6%)	376(68.1%)	0.444
Bloody stools, *n* (%)	19(43.2%)	242(58%)	0.059
Abdominal pain, *n* (%)	9(14.5%)	186(33.7%)	0.001
Vomiting, *n* (%)	18(29%)	208(37.3%)	0.087
Fever duration, days, mean ± SD	3.8 ± 2.4	2.7 ± 2.1	< 0.001
Hospital stay, days, mean ± SD	[illegible].8 ± 9.5	5.8 ± 12.1	0.016
Hb, g/dL, mean ± SD	11.6 ± 1.4	12.1 ± 1.2	0.027
CRP, mg/L, mean ± SD	39.1 ± 58.3	58.6 ± 54.8	0.009
Band form, %, mean ± SD	4.7 ± 6.9	6.9 ± 6.9	0.112
WBC, /μl, mean ± SD	10,803 ± 4,420	10,051 ± 4,168	0.192
Antimicrobial resistance			
2019			
Ampicillin	29.7%	41.6%	0.165
Ceftriaxone	5.4%	14.8%	0.119
Ertapenem	2.7%	0.3%	0.209
Imipenem	2.8%	1.0%	0.353
Ciprofloxacin	30.6%	28.5%	0.790
TMP-SMX	20.6%	30.2%	0.240
Chloramphenicol	66.7%	29.9%	0.073
Flomoxef	40%	5.5%	0.030
2012			
Ampicillin	42.1%	49.7%	0.519
Ceftriaxone	10.5%	3.8%	0.182
Ertapenem	0%	0%	NA
Imipenem	0%	0%	NA
Ciprofloxacin	5.3%	1.7%	0.316
TMP-SMX	15.8%	27.9%	0.248
Chloramphenicol	21.1%	21.8%	1.000
Flomoxef	5.3%	3.2%	0.624

iNTS, invasive non-typhoidal Salmonella;
SD, standard deviation;
TMP-SMX, trimethoprim-sulfamethoxazole.

ceftriaxone (15.1% vs 3.8%, $P < 0.001$) and ciprofloxacin (28.5% vs 1.7%, $P < 0.001$) than those in 2012.

DISCUSSION

Our results indicated that the antimicrobial susceptibility of NTS has changed during the past decade, with several clinically relevant findings. A particularly crucial finding is the significantly higher prevalence of antimicrobial resistance to third-generation cephalosporin in infants. Additionally, the resistance rate to ciprofloxacin and third-generation cephalosporin increased significantly from 2012 to 2019, especially in groups B, D, and E. Furthermore, we observed that most patients with NTS bacteremia presented with fever lasting more than 4 days at admission with a lower systemic inflammatory reaction. This is the first analysis to reveal that *Salmonella* bacteremia is closely associated with longer fever duration and inconsistent lower systemic inflammatory reaction. By contrast, non-blood isolates (mostly local) were generally more resistant than NTS bacteremia isolates.

TABLE 5 | Antimicrobial resistance and serogroups between iNTS and non-iNTS infections in 2012 and 2019.

	iNTS			non-iNTS		
	2012	2019	*P* value	2012	2109	*P* value
Antimicrobial resistance						
Ampicillin	42.1%	27.8%	0.282	49.7%	41.2%	0.020
Ceftriaxone	10.5%	5.6%	0.602	3.8%	15.1%	<0.001
Ertapenem	0%	2.8%	1.000	0%	0.5%	0.502
Imipenem	0%	2.8%	1.000	0%	1.0%	0.128
Ciprofloxacin	5.3%	30.6%	0.041	1.7%	28.5%	<0.001
TMP-SMX	15.8%	20.6%	1.000	27.9%	30.2%	0.518
Chloramphenicol	21.2%	60%	0.126	21.8%	30.9%	0.005
Flomoxef	5.3%	40%	0.099	3.2%	5.5%	0.125
MDR	10.5%	13.9%	1.000	12.2%	31.4%	<0.001
Serogroups						
B	15.8%	22.2%	0.730	27.6%	23.1%	0.159
C1	15.8%	2.8%	0.114	4.7%	7%	0.170
C2	5.3%	16.7%	0.401	12.8%	12.6%	0.926
D	52.6%	41.7%	0.437	42.2%	42.7%	0.891
E	10.5%	13.9%	1.000	11%	13.1%	0.401

iNTS, invasive non-typhoidal Salmonella;
MDR, multi-drug resistance, resistant to ≥3 drug classes;
TMP-SMX, trimethoprim-sulfamethoxazole.

Concern has been growing over the past decades regarding antimicrobial resistance in NTS. Our data demonstrated an increase in overall antimicrobial resistance in *Salmonella* from 20 to 30% in 2012 to as high as 70% in 2019. Previous studies have reported high resistance rates to ampicillin in Taiwan. The increasing rates of resistance have resulted in changes to clinical practice guidelines for treating the disease. Therefore, expensive third-generation cephalosporins are currently the first-choice antibiotics for iNTS infection in children. Our data revealed a significant elevation in ceftriaxone resistance from 2012 to 2019, whereas the resistance rate to ampicillin decreased. These results are in accordance with recent studies indicating the emergence and spread of resistance to third-generation cephalosporin in Taiwan and other Asian countries (Lee et al., 2021). Ampicillin resistance significantly decreased in our study period, possibly because of antibiotic choice.

This study explored various NTS serogroups that are closely associated with antimicrobial resistance. More than half the NTS isolates were classified as MDR, with particularly high resistance in groups B, D, and E. These three groups also had the highest resistance rate to third-generation cephalosporin. In Taiwan, self-transferable bla_{CMY-2}-harboring IncI1 plasmids have been identified in several *Salmonella* serotypes belonging to *Salmonella* groups B and D (Lo et al., 2020). Since 2015, northern Taiwan has experienced an increase in *Salmonella* infections caused by previously rare *Salmonella* Anatum, a serogroup E serotype. Such infections have also been reported in central Taiwan, indicating that this outbreak has already spread throughout the island (Chiou et al., 2019). Coresistance to ceftriaxone and ciprofloxacin is the main feature of the outbreak clone (Feng et al., 2020).

This study highlighted that isolates from infants had significantly higher MDR to ampicillin and third-generation cephalosporin than did isolates from other age groups. This is partly explained by the increase in isolates in infants with serotypes since the early 1990s, which have been associated with MDR (Katiyo et al., 2019). This rather unexpected result may be attributed to human-to-human transmissions. Parents may have more often touched, rinsed, and cooked contaminated meat before feeding other foods to their infants. Moreover, these parents were more willing to purchase meat from traditional markets rather than supermarkets (Feng et al., 2020). One possibility is that parents bought meat from traditional markets, and then, their frequent rinsing spread the *Salmonella* from the surface of the meats to cutting boards, knives, sinks, and finally onto fresh vegetables, fruit, and other ready-to-eat foods that were cross-contaminated and reached the infants through parents or other caregivers. This transmission mode is particularly critical in infants. On the basis of these findings, we recommend that clinicians in Taiwan use third-generation cephalosporins for empirical treatment of NTS bacteremia and determine the exact treatment according to antimicrobial susceptibility results.

Our analyses indicated that ceftriaxone resistance in Taiwan was low in 2012, and our results revealed that the overall resistance rates in the non-iNTS isolates were generally higher than those in the iNTS isolates. We noted significantly lower serum CRP level in patients with NTS bacteremia than in patients without NTS bacteremia. In previous studies, a severity score with CRP served as a guide for prescribing antibiotics for severe NTS infection in children. On the basis of the current findings, we recommend against routinely using antimicrobials to treat uncomplicated NTS gastroenteritis in cases of high CRP level. This finding is consistent with that of Mughini-Gras et al. (2020) who reported that iNTS isolates were generally less resistant than non-iNTS isolates (Mughini-Gras et al., 2020; Ke et al., 2020). NTS bacteremia in this study tended to develop in young children with prolonged fever. The hemoglobin level was also found significantly lower in the invasive group ($P = 0.027$) in our study. Christenson (2013) had reported that patients with hemolytic anemia, malaria, sickle cell anemia, and thalassemia major were more susceptible to invasive *Salmonella* infection (Christenson, 2013). This finding is consistent with previous reports that revealed a longer duration of symptoms, such as fever and diarrhea, before admission in children with bacteremia (Lee et al., 2021). Thus, fever duration can be a suitable rationale for treatment before receiving antimicrobial susceptibility results.

Adopting an 8-year detailed hospitalization dataset from the largest pediatric hospital in Taiwan enabled us to representatively evaluate the trends and characteristics of antimicrobial resistance in pediatric NTS infections. However, this study has some limitations. First, only serogroup data were available in our research, and serotype data were limited. Disease severity and antimicrobial resistance may be associated with different serotypes; therefore, further analysis of serotypes with clinical manifestations or resistance patterns are required to clarify virulence and impact among different serotypes. Second, this was a single-center study; thus, we could not adequately account for the considerable geographic variability in antimicrobial resistance patterns in NTS. Although the data is from a single hospital, Chang Gung Memorial Hospital is the largest in Taiwan. So, the data can reflect the true epidemiology in Taiwan.

This study revealed that the resistance of NTS to fluoroquinolones and third-generation cephalosporins has been increasing in Taiwan. MDR in serogroups B, D, and E remained high. More importantly, cephalosporin resistance was more common in isolates from infants. Prolonged fever was a single factor associated with bacteremia in children with NTS infection.

AUTHOR CONTRIBUTIONS

C-HC and Y-JC: conception and design of the study. N-WC and Y-JH: implementation and data collection. H-HC and Y-CC: analysis and interpretation of the data. Y-JC, C-LC, and C-HC: writing and critical review of the manuscript. All authors contributed to the article and approved the submitted version.

FUNDING

The funders had no role in study design, data collection and analysis, decision to publish, or preparation of the manuscript.

REFERENCES

Angelo, K., Reynolds, J., Karp, B., Hoekstra, R., Scheel, C. M., and Friedman, C. (2016). Antimicrobial resistance among nontyphoidal *Salmonella* Isolated from blood in the United States, 2003–2013. *J. Infect. Dis.* 214, 1565–1570. doi: 10.1093/infdis/jiw415

Chang, Y. J., Chen, M. C., Feng, Y., Su, L. H., Li, H. C., Yang, H. P., et al. (2020). Highly antimicrobial-resistant nontyphoidal *Salmonella* from retail meats and clinical impact in children, Taiwan. *Pediatr. Neonatol.* 61, 432-438. doi: 10.1016/j.pedneo.2020.03.017

Chiou, C. S., Hong, Y. P., Liao, Y. S., Wang, Y. W., Tu, Y. H., Chen, B. H., et al. (2019). New Multidrug-resistant *Salmonella enterica* serovar Anatum clone, Taiwan, 2015-2017. *Emerg Infect Dis.* 25, 144–147. doi: 10.3201/eid2501.181103

Christenson, J. C. (2013). *Salmonella* infections. *Pediatr Rev.* 34, 375–383. doi: 10.1542/pir.34-9-375

Clinical and Laboratory Standards Institute [CLSI] (2012). *Performance Standards for Antimicrobial Susceptibility Testing; Twenty-Two Informational Supplement. CLSI Document M100-22.* Wayne, PA: Clinical and Laboratory Standards Institute.

Clinical and Laboratory Standards Institute [CLSI] (2019). *Performance Standards for Antimicrobial Susceptibility Testing; Twenty-Ninth Informational Supplement. CLSI Document M100-29.* Wayne, PA: Clinical and Laboratory Standards Institute.

Feasey, N. A., Dougan, G., Kingsley, R. A., Heyderman, R. S., and Gordon, M. A. (2012). Invasive non-typhoidal *Salmonella* disease: an emerging and neglected tropical disease in Africa. *Lancet* 379, 2489-2499. doi: 10.1016/S0140-6736(11)61752-2

Feng, Y., Chang, Y. J., Pan, S. C., Su, L. H., Li, H. C., Yang, H. P., et al. (2020). Characterization and source investigation of multidrug-resistant *Salmonella* Anatum from a sustained outbreak, Taiwan. *Emerg. Infect. Dis.* 26, 2951–2955. doi: 10.3201/eid2612.200147

Hohmann, E. L. (2001). Nontyphoidal salmonellosis. *Clin. Infect. Dis.* 32, 263-9. doi: 10.1086/318457

James, S. L., Abate, D., Abate, K. H., Abay, S. M., Abbafati, C., Abbasi, N., et al. (2018). Global, regional, and national incidence, prevalence, and years lived with disability for 354 diseases and injuries for 195 countries and territories, 1990–2017: a systematic analysis for the Global Burden of Disease Study 2017. *Lancet* 392, 1789–1858. doi: 10.1016/S0140-6736(18)32279-7

Katiyo, S., Muller-Pebody, B., Minaji, M., Powell, D., Johnson, A. P., De Pinna, E., et al. (2019). Epidemiology and outcomes of nontyphoidal *Salmonella* Bacteremias from England, 2004 to 2015. *J. Clin. Microbiol.* 57:e01189-18. doi: 10.1128/JCM.01189-18

Ke, Y., Lu, W., Liu, W., Zhu, P., Chen, Q., and Zhu, Z. (2020). Non-typhoidal *Salmonella* infections among children in a tertiary hospital in Ningbo, Zhejiang, China, 2012-2019. *PLoS Negl. Trop. Dis.* 14:e0008732. doi: 10.1371/journal.pntd.0008732

Kyu, H. H., Abate, D., Abate, K. H., Abay, S. M., Abbafati, C., Abbasi, N., et al. (2018). Global, regional, and national disability-adjusted life-years (DALYs) for 359 diseases and injuries and healthy life expectancy (HALE) for 195 countries and territories, 1990–2017: a systematic analysis for the Global Burden of Disease Study 2017. *Lancet* 392, 1859–1922. doi: 10.1016/S0140-6736(18)32335-3

Lee, C. M., Lee, M. S., Yang, T. L., Lee, K. L., Yen, T. Y., Lu, C. Y., et al. (2021). Clinical features and risk factors associated with bacteremia of nontyphoidal salmonellosis in pediatric patients, 2010-2018. *J. Formos. Med. Assoc.* 120, 196–203. doi: 10.1016/j.jfma.2020.04.022

Lo, H. Y., Lai, F. P., and Yang, Y. J. (2020). Changes in epidemiology and antimicrobial susceptibility of nontyphoid *Salmonella* in children in southern Taiwan, 1997-2016. *J. Microbiol. Immunol. Infect.* 53, 585-591. doi: 10.1016/j.jmii.2018.06.004

Majowicz, S. E., Musto, J., Scallan, E., Angulo, F. J., Kirk, M., O'Brien, S. J., et al. (2010). International collaboration on enteric disease 'Burden of Illness' studies. the global burden of nontyphoidal *Salmonella* gastroenteritis. *Clin. Infect. Dis.* 50, 882-889. doi: 10.1086/650733

Mughini-Gras, L., Pijnacker, R., Duijster, J., Heck, M., Wit, B., Veldman, K., et al. (2020). Changing epidemiology of invasive non-typhoid *Salmonella* infection: a nationwide population-based registry study. *Clin. Microbiol. Infect.* 26, 941.e9-941.e14. doi: 10.1016/j.cmi.2019.11.015

Roth, G. A., Abate, D., Abate, K. H., Abay, S. M., Abbafati, C., Abbasi, N., et al. (2018). Global, regional, and national age-sex-specific mortality for 282 causes of death in 195 countries and territories, 1980–2017: a systematic analysis for the Global Burden of Disease Study 2017. *Lancet* 392, 1736–1788. doi: 10.1016/S0140-6736(18)32203-7

Stanaway, J. D., Parisi, A., Sarkar, K., Blacker, B. F., Reiner, R. C., Hay, S. I., et al. (2019). The global burden of non-typhoidal *Salmonella* invasive disease: a systematic analysis for the Global Burden of Disease Study 2017. *Lancet Infect. Dis.* 19, 1312–1324. doi: 10.1016/S1473-3099(19)30418-9

Su, L. H., Teng, W. S., Chen, C. L., Lee, H. Y., Li, H. C., Wu, T. L., et al. (2011). Increasing ceftriaxone resistance in *Salmonellae*, Taiwan. *Emerg. Infect. Dis.* 17, 1086-1890. doi: 10.3201/eid/1706.101949

Tsai, M. H., Huang, Y. C., Lin, T. Y., Huang, Y. L., Kuo, C. C., and Chiu, C. H. (2011). Reappraisal of parenteral antimicrobial therapy for nontyphoidal *Salmonella enteric* infection in children. *Clin. Microbiol. Infect.* 17, 300–305. doi: 10.1111/j.1469-0691.2010.03230.x

10

Nano-Strategies to Fight Multidrug Resistant Bacteria — "A Battle of the Titans"

Pedro V. Baptista[1], Matthew P. McCusker[2†], Andreia Carvalho[1], Daniela A. Ferreira[3], Niamh M. Mohan[3,4], Marta Martins[3]* and Alexandra R. Fernandes[1]**

[1] UCIBIO, Departamento de Ciências da Vida, Faculdade de Ciências e Tecnologia, Universidade Nova de Lisboa, Caparica, Portugal, [2] School of Food Science and Environmental Health, College of Sciences and Health, Dublin Institute of Technology, Dublin, Ireland, [3] Department of Microbiology, Moyne Institute of Preventive Medicine, Schools of Genetics and Microbiology, Trinity College Dublin, University of Dublin, Dublin, Ireland, [4] Nuritas Limited, Dublin, Ireland

***Correspondence:**
Pedro V. Baptista
pmvb@fct.unl.pt
Marta Martins
mmartins@tcd.ie
Alexandra R. Fernandes
ma.fernandes@fct.unl.pt

***†Present Address:**
Matthew P. McCusker,
Kerry Europe, Global Technology & Innovation Centre, Naas, Ireland

Infectious diseases remain one of the leading causes of morbidity and mortality worldwide. The WHO and CDC have expressed serious concern regarding the continued increase in the development of multidrug resistance among bacteria. Therefore, the antibiotic resistance crisis is one of the most pressing issues in global public health. Associated with the rise in antibiotic resistance is the lack of new antimicrobials. This has triggered initiatives worldwide to develop novel and more effective antimicrobial compounds as well as to develop novel delivery and targeting strategies. Bacteria have developed many ways by which they become resistant to antimicrobials. Among those are enzyme inactivation, decreased cell permeability, target protection, target overproduction, altered target site/enzyme, increased efflux due to over-expression of efflux pumps, among others. Other more complex phenotypes, such as biofilm formation and quorum sensing do not appear as a result of the exposure of bacteria to antibiotics although, it is known that biofilm formation can be induced by antibiotics. These phenotypes are related to tolerance to antibiotics in bacteria. Different strategies, such as the use of nanostructured materials, are being developed to overcome these and other types of resistance. Nanostructured materials can be used to convey antimicrobials, to assist in the delivery of novel drugs or ultimately, possess antimicrobial activity by themselves. Additionally, nanoparticles (e.g., metallic, organic, carbon nanotubes, etc.) may circumvent drug resistance mechanisms in bacteria and, associated with their antimicrobial potential, inhibit biofilm formation or other important processes. Other strategies, including the combined use of plant-based antimicrobials and nanoparticles to overcome toxicity issues, are also being investigated. Coupling nanoparticles and natural-based antimicrobials (or other repurposed compounds) to inhibit the activity of bacterial efflux pumps; formation of biofilms; interference of quorum sensing; and possibly plasmid curing, are just some of the strategies to combat multidrug resistant bacteria. However, the use of nanoparticles still presents a challenge to therapy and much more research is needed in order to overcome this. In this review, we will summarize the current research on nanoparticles and other nanomaterials and how these are or can be applied in the future to fight multidrug resistant bacteria.

Keywords: antimicrobial resistance, multidrug resistance, nanomaterials, nanoparticles, plant-based compounds, novel antimicrobial agents, nanotheranostics

INTRODUCTION

Multidrug resistant (MDR) bacteria remain the greatest challenge in public health care. The numbers of infections produced by such resistant strains are increasing globally. This acquired resistance of pathogens presents a key challenge for many antimicrobial drugs. Recent advances in nanotechnology offer new prospects to develop novel formulations based on distinct types of nanoparticles (NPs) with different sizes and shapes and flexible antimicrobial properties.

NPs may offer a promising solution as they can not only combat bacteria themselves but can also act as carriers for antibiotics and natural antimicrobial compounds (Wang et al., 2017a). While various materials have been explored from liposomal to polymer based nano-drug carriers, metallic vectors, such as gold NPs, are attractive as core materials due to their essentially inert and nontoxic nature (Burygin et al., 2009). Arguably the most attractive aspect of NPs drug delivery systems is their ability to introduce a wide range of therapeutics, either bound to their large surface area or contained within the structure, to the site of infection effectively and safely by having a controlled rate of targeted delivery (Pissuwan et al., 2011; Gholipourmalekabadi et al., 2017). By improving the pharmacokinetic profile and therapeutic index of encapsulated drugs compared to free drug equivalents, the dose required to achieve clinical effects can be dramatically decreased (Gao et al., 2018). This in turn, can reduce the toxicity and the adverse side effects associated with high systemic drug concentrations and frequent dosing (Liu et al. 2009).

This review covers the latest approaches in the development of new nanobiotechnology approaches that may challenge the medical practice to fight bacteria and particularly MDR bacteria.

NANOMATERIALS AGAINST BACTERIA

Nanomaterials have at least one dimension in the nanometer scale range (1–100 nm) that convey particular physical and chemical properties considerably different from those of bulk materials (Wang et al., 2017a). Among the wide range of nanomaterials, particular interest has been directed toward NPs. NPs have a number of features, which make them favorable as vectors for drugs to combat disease-causing pathogens. These include their enhancement of drug solubility and stability (Huh and Kwon, 2011); their ease of synthesis (Gholipourmalekabadi et al., 2017); their biocompatibility with target agents; and their modulated release, which can be controlled by stimuli, such as light, pH and heat (Wang Z. et al., 2017). Their distinctive functionality in drug delivery is achieved by their ultra-small size and vast surface to volume ratios. This is a key competitive advantage over conventional therapies in the treatment of infections caused by intracellular pathogens and MDR strains. Their functionalization with different (bio)molecules is another important feature. These comprise NPs containing Ag, Au, Al, Cu, Ce, Cd, Mg, Ni, Se, Pd, Ti, Zn, and super-paramagnetic Fe (Hemeg, 2017; Slavin et al., 2017). AgNPs are considered the most effective nanomaterial against bacteria but other metallic NPs, such as CuONPs, TiONPs, AuNPs, and Fe_3O_2NPs, have also demonstrated bactericidal effects (Dakal et al., 2016; Hemeg, 2017; Slavin et al., 2017).

While poor membrane transport limits the potency of many antibiotics (Andrade et al., 2013), drug loaded NPs vehicles can enter host cells *via* endocytosis, facilitating their intracellular entry (Wang Z. et al., 2017). Membrane penetration can also be achieved through interactions with surface lipids, for example, using gold NPs in the co-administration of protein-based drugs (Huang et al., 2010). The therapeutic appeal of NPs is enhanced by their ability to confer physical protection against bacterial resistance mechanisms (Huh and Kwon, 2011). Furthermore, the potential to load multiple drug combinations into NPs presents a highly complex antimicrobial mechanism of action, to which, bacteria are unlikely to develop resistance (Huh and Kwon, 2011). Although, this is usually believed to be the case, there are some studies reporting development of bacterial resistance against silver NPs (Panáček et al., 2018). There is also evidence that exposure of bacteria to this type of NPs may increase its antibiotic tolerance (Kaweeteerawat et al., 2017).

NPs can exert their antibacterial activity *via* a multitude of mechanisms, such as: (1) direct interaction with the bacterial cell wall; (2) inhibition of biofilm formation; (3) triggering of innate as well as adaptive host immune responses; (4) generation of reactive oxygen species (ROS); and (5) induction of intracellular effects (*e.g.*, interactions with DNA and/or proteins). Because they do not present the same mechanisms of action of standard antibiotics (**Figure 1**), they can be of extreme use against MDR bacteria (Singh K. et al., 2014; Aderibigbe, 2017; AlMatar et al., 2017; Hemeg, 2017; Natan and Banin, 2017; Rai et al., 2017; Slavin et al., 2017; Zaidi et al., 2017; Bassegoda et al., 2018; Katva et al., 2018; Siddiqi et al., 2018).

Besides the broad-spectrum antibacterial properties that NPs have against Gram-positive and -negative bacteria, NPs have been used as vectors for the delivery of antimicrobial moieties that greatly improve their biocidal properties (Beyth et al., 2015; Rai A. et al., 2016; Singh J. et al., 2016; Esmaeillou et al.,

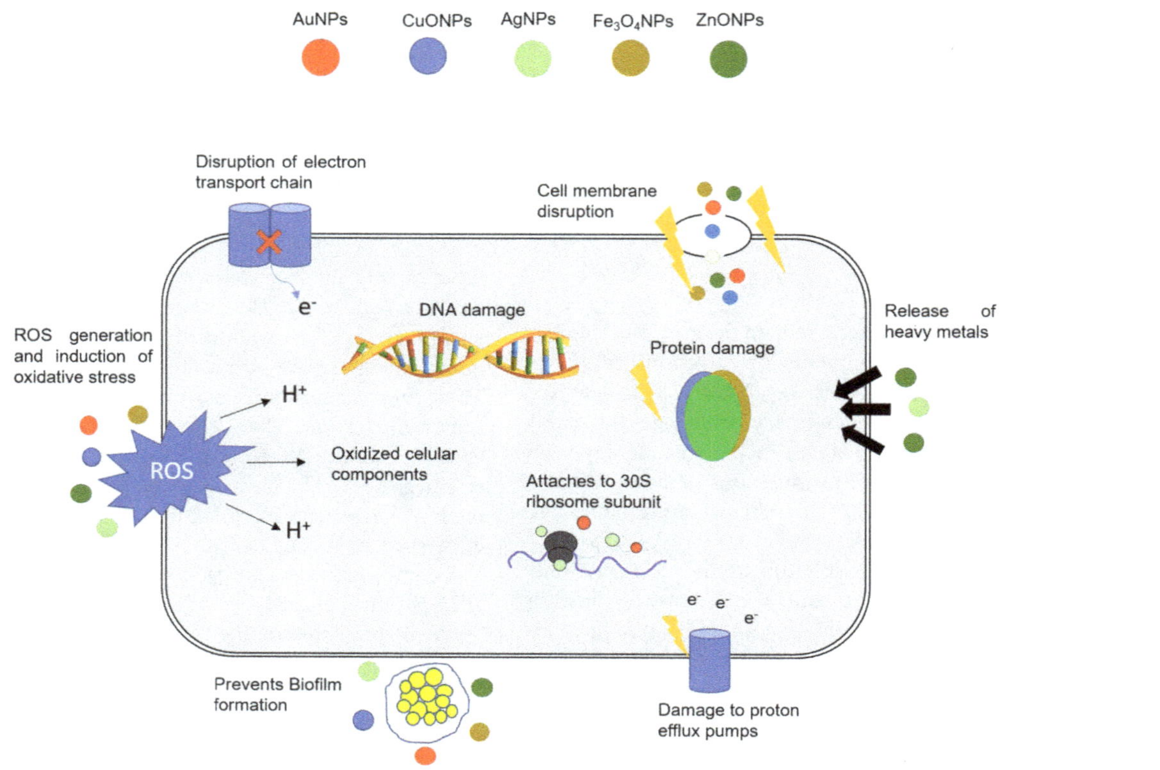

FIGURE 1 | Different mechanisms of action of NPs in bacterial cells. The combination in a single nanomaterial of a multitude of cellular effects may have a tremendous impact in fighting MDR bacteria. DNA, deoxyribonucleic acid; ROS, Reactive oxygen species; AuNPs, gold NPs; CuONPs, Copper oxide NPs; AgNPs, silver NPs; Fe_3O_4NPs, iron oxide NPs; ZnONPs, zinc oxide NPs.

2017; Wang et al., 2017a; Zaidi et al., 2017; Hadiya et al., 2018). Some of the advantages of using NPs as vectors are due to their small and controllable size; their protective action against enzymes that would otherwise destroy antimicrobial compounds; their ability to actively deliver antibiotics; and their capability to combine several therapeutic modalities onto a single nanomaterial (*e.g.*, several antibiotics/compounds onto the same NPs for combined action; combining silencing agents and drugs, etc.) (Turos et al., 2007; Huh and Kwon, 2011; Mohammed Fayaz et al., 2011; Liu et al., 2013; Qi et al., 2013; Li et al., 2014; Ranghar et al., 2014; Thomas et al., 2014; Wang et al., 2014; Payne et al., 2016; Rai A. et al., 2016; Singh J. et al., 2016; Yeom et al., 2016; Esmaeillou et al., 2017; Zaidi et al., 2017; Zong et al., 2017; Hadiya et al., 2018).

NPs carriers can tackle bacterial threats "passively," through prolonged drug retention at the specific infection site, or "actively," through surface conjugation with active molecules that bind a certain target (Wang Z. et al., 2017). The balance between the surface modification interaction strength, the compound release rate and the stability of the conjugate should be carefully considered for the design of an effective "active" delivery strategy (Burygin et al., 2009; Pissuwan et al., 2011). In an attempt to overcome their therapeutic limitations, various research groups have investigated the conjugation of antibiotics to NPs (Tiwari et al., 2011). For example, Saha et al. describe the direct conjugation of ampicillin, streptomycin and kanamycin to gold NPs (Saha et al., 2007). The resulting complexes were shown to have lower minimum inhibitory concentration (MIC) than the free drug counterparts against both Gram -negative and -positive bacteria. While the detailed mechanism of these effects are not explained by the authors in the above case, Fayaz et al. has attempted to uncover how their vancomycin functionalized gold NPs demonstrated activity against strains which are usually vancomycin resistant based either on mutations (vancomycin resistant *Staphylococcus aureus*), or membrane structure (*Escherichia coli*) (Mohammed Fayaz et al., 2011). They propose that only when the antibiotic was complexed with the NPs could this result in nonspecific, multivalent interactions and anchoring of the carrier to the cell wall synthesis proteins. Based on the presence of pits in the cells, which was observed using transmission electron microscopy, the authors concluded that the consequence of the non-specific binding was compromised membrane integrity, and subsequent cell death (Mohammed Fayaz et al., 2011; Gao et al., 2018).

ANTIBACTERIAL MECHANISM OF NPS

The antibacterial activity of NPs against MDR bacteria and biofilms depends on a number of factors, namely, their large surface area in contact with bacteria through electrostatic attraction, van der walls forces or hydrophobic interactions; on the nanoparticle size and stability; together with the drug concentration (Chen et al. 2014; Gao et al., 2014; Li et al., 2015). The interaction of NPs with bacteria generally triggers oxidative stress mechanisms, enzymatic inhibition, protein deactivation and changes in gene expression. Still, the most common antibacterial mechanisms are related to oxidative stress, metal ion release, and non-oxidative mechanisms (Wang et al., 2017a; Zaidi et al., 2017 see **Figure 1**).

Oxidative stress induced by ROS is one of the most important mechanisms assisting the antibacterial activity of NPs (Dwivedi et al., 2014; Rudramurthy et al., 2016). ROS are natural byproducts of cellular oxidative metabolism and have significant important roles in the modulation of cell survival and death, differentiation and cell signaling. In bacteria, ROS are formed from aerobic respiration, and their production is balanced by the cell antioxidant machinery but upon an additional ROS insult, oxidation of biomolecules, and cell components result in severe cellular damage (Li et al., 2012b). The excessive production of ROS leads to a disturbed redox homeostasis resulting in oxidative stress, affecting membrane lipids and altering the structure of DNA and proteins (Dwivedi et al., 2014). It has been shown that while O_2^- and H_2O_2 can be neutralized by endogenous antioxidants, ·OH and singlet oxygen ($^1[O_2]$) lead to acute microbial death (Zaidi et al., 2017). Different NPs may generate distinctive ROS, such as superoxide (O_2^-) or hydroxyl radical (·OH), hydrogen peroxide (H_2O_2), and $^1[O_2]$) (Wang et al., 2017a). In this manner, the level of ROS generated by NPs is dependent on the chemical nature of the NPs themselves. Application of metallic NPs is currently being considered to overcome bacterial infections since they have shown antimicrobial efficacy due to their high surface-to-volume ratio. An increase ratio is usually accompanied by increased production of ROS, including free radicals. Zhang et al. (2013) demonstrated that ROS generation and metal ion release significantly enhanced the antibacterial activity through uncoated AuNPs in aqueous suspension under UV irradiation (365 nm). Umamaheswari (Umamaheswari et al., 2014) demonstrated that the antibacterial activity of AuNPs against *E. coli*, *Salmonella* Typhi, *Pseudomonas aeruginosa* and *Klebsiella pneumoniae* were due to oxidative stress caused by increased intracellular ROS. A recent study (Zhang et al., 2013) evaluated AuNPs and AuNPs -laser combined therapy against *C. pseudotuberculosis* and suggested that the mechanism of action is related with ROS production, that causes an increase of oxidative stress of microbial cells in the form of vacuole formation as an indication of potent activity. This effect was higher with AuNPs-laser causing a rapid loss of bacterial cell membrane integrity due to the fact that laser light enhances at least one fold antimicrobial activity of AuNPs. Several other studies have addressed the role of metal NPs to induce MDR bacteria death *via* oxidative stress (**Table 1**) (Foster et al., 2011; Li et al., 2012b; Rai et al., 2012; Zhang et al., 2013; Reddy L. S. et al., 2014; Singh R. et al., 2014; Pan et al., 2016; Courtney et al., 2017; Ulloa-Ogaz et al., 2017; Zaidi et al., 2017). Indeed, titanium dioxide NPs were shown to adhere to the surface of the bacterial cell and trigger the production of ROS, which in turns lead to damage of the structure of cellular components and consequent cell death (Foster et al., 2011). In another important study using different metal NPs, AgNPs were shown to generate superoxide radicals and hydroxyl radicals, whereas Au, Ni, and Si NPs generated only singlet oxygen, which upon entering the cell produced an antibacterial effect (Zhang et al., 2013). More recently, Reddy and co-workers demonstrated that ZnONPs alone can also act as an effective antibacterial agent *via* the generation of ROS (Reddy L. S. et al., 2014). Exposure to UV irradiation may also potentiate the action of NPs. Li et al. (2012b) reported the augmented antibacterial effects of zinc oxide (ZnO) and titanium oxide (TiO) NPs triggered by UV irradiation as the results of the increased production of superoxide, hydroxyl and singlet oxygen radicals that potentiated bacteria mortality by severe oxidative stress. Graphene oxide–iron oxide NPs have also demonstrated maximum antibacterial activity due to the generation of hydroxyl radicals and diffusion into bacterial cells (Pan et al., 2016). More recently, Ulloa-Ogaz and collaborators demonstrated that copper oxide NPs interact with bacteria, generating an intracellular signaling cascade that trigger oxidative stress and, thus, an antibacterial effect (Ulloa-Ogaz et al., 2017).

Metal oxides slowly release metal ions that are up taken by the cell, reaching the intracellular compartment where they can interact with functional groups of proteins and nucleic acids, such as amino (–NH), mercapto (–SH), and carboxyl (–COOH) groups (Wang et al., 2017a). This interaction alters the cell structure, hampers enzymatic activity and interferes with the normal physiological processes in the bacterial cell. It has been shown that copper oxide (CuO) NPs cause a significant alteration of the expression of key proteins and may inhibit denitrification. Proteomic analysis showed that CuONPs cause an alteration of proteins involved in nitrogen metabolism, electron transfer and transport (Su et al., 2015). Also, the interaction of gold–superparamagnetic iron oxide NPs with bacterial proteins *via* disulfide bonds affects the metabolism and redox system of bacterial cells (Niemirowicz et al., 2014). NPs may also enter bacteria through absorption, releasing metal ions to the surrounding medium and/or binding to the negatively charged functional groups of the bacterial cell membrane. For example, silver ions (from silver NPs) are adsorbed on the cell membrane, leading to protein coagulation (Jung et al., 2008). Jankauskaitl and collaborators described the bactericidal effect of graphene oxide/Cu/Ag NPs against *E. coli*, *P. aeruginosa*, *K. pneumoniae*, *S. aureus*, and Methicillin-resistant *S. aureus* (MRSA) through a possible synergy between multiple toxic mechanisms (Jankauskaite et al., 2016).

Non-oxidative mechanisms involve interaction of the NPs with the cell wall. In bacteria, the cell wall and membrane behave as defensive barriers that protect against environmental insults. Cell membrane components provide different adsorption pathways for the NPs (Lesniak et al., 2013). The cell wall of Gram-negative bacteria is composed of lipoproteins, phospholipids and lipid polysaccharides (LPS), which form a barrier only allowing the entry of certain macromolecules (Zaidi et al., 2017). In Gram-positive bacteria, the cell wall is composed of a thin layer of

TABLE 1 | Nanoparticles against MDR pathogens and their mechanisms of action.

Type of nanoparticles	Targeted bacteria	Antibiotic resistance type	Mechanisms of antibacterial action	References
AgNPs	*Enterococcus faecalis, S. aureus*	Vancomycin-resistant	Combination with vancomycin. Bacterial cell death.	Saeb et al., 2014; Esmaeillou et al., 2017
	Enterococcus		On-going investigations.	Percival et al., 2007
	S. aureus	Methicillin-resistant	Combination with antibiotics.	Brown et al., 2012; Saeb et al., 2014; Esmaeillou et al., 2017
			Physical adhesion to the bacterial cell.	Su et al., 2011
			On-going investigations.	Percival et al., 2007
	E. coli, P. aeruginosa	Ampicillin- resistant	Combination with ampicillin leads to entry into the bacterial cell. Inhibition of cell wall synthesis, protein synthesis and nucleic acid synthesis.	Lara et al., 2010; Brown et al., 2012
	S. aureus, E. coli, P. aeruginosa, K. pneumoniae, E. faecalis, Salmonella Typhimurium, *Bacillus cereus*	Erythromycin-resistant	Cell surface damage and loss of the chain integrity.	Otari et al., 2013
	S. pneumoniae	Teicoplanin-resistant	ROS generation, cellular uptake of silver ions, cascade of intracellular reaction.	Thapa et al., 2017
	E. coli, S. aureus	Ampicillin- resistant		
	E. coli, S. aureus	Tetracycline-resistant	Combination with tetracycline.	Djafari et al., 2016
	P. aeruginosa	Ofloxacin-resistant	Evade multidrug efflux pumps.	Ding et al., 2018
	P. aeruginosa, MRSA, VRE, *Serratia marcescens*	Biofilm formation	Ongoing investigations.	Percival et al., 2007
	Enterobacter cloacae, S. mutans		ROS production and membrane disruption.	Kulshrestha et al., 2017
	S. epidermidis, S. aureus		Penetration in the bacterial biofilm using an external magnetic field.	Mahmoudi and Serpooshan, 2012
	E. coli	MDR	ROS generation.	Zhang et al., 2013; Siddiqi et al., 2018
	E. coli, P. aeruginosa			Ramalingam et al., 2016
	S. aureus, Enterococcus spp., *P. aeruginosa, A. baumannii, Enterobacteriaceae*		Interaction with components of the cells where chemical and physical properties are modified.	Cavassin et al., 2015
	E. coli			Lok et al., 2007
	S. aureus, E. coli, P. aeruginosa, K. pneumoniae, B. subtilis		Penetration in the bacterial cell wall.	Acharya et al., 2018
	P. aeruginosa		Combined therapy, using blue light.	El Din et al., 2016
	E. coli, Pseudomonas fluorescens, Pseudomonas putida, P. aeruginosa, B. subtilis, S. aureus		Disruption of the bacterial cell wall.	Bondarenko et al., 2013

(Continued)

TABLE 1 | Continued

Type of nanoparticles	Targeted bacteria	Antibiotic resistance type	Mechanisms of antibacterial action	References
	A. baumannii		Attach to the cell wall leading to structural changes in the permeability of the cell membrane.	Chang et al., 2017
	P. aeruginosa			Singh K. et al., 2014; Salomoni et al., 2017
	S. aureus, E. coli			Jung et al., 2008; Muniyan et al., 2017
	P. aeruginosa, E. coli		Combination with antibiotics.	Esmaeillou et al., 2017
	E. coli			Karimi et al., 2016
	E. faecalis			Katva et al., 2018
	Salmonella Typhimurium			McShan et al., 2015
	Enterobacteriaceae			Panáček et al., 2016b
	S. aureus, P. aeruginosa, E. coli			Panáček et al., 2016a
	S. aureus, E. coli		Upregulation of the expression of antioxidant genes and ATP pumps.	Nagy et al., 2011
	S. epidermidis	MDR/Biofilm formation	Conjugation with AMP.	Jaiswal et al., 2015
	Mycobacterium smegmatis			Mohanty et al., 2013
	Vibrio fluvialis, P. aeruginosa			Lambadi et al., 2015
	B. subtilis, E. coli			Liu et al., 2013
	E. coli			Pal et al., 2016
	E. coli, Acinetobacter calcoaceticus, Aeromonas bestiarum, B. Subtili, P. fluorescens, Kocuria rhizophila, Micrococcus luteus			Ruden et al., 2009
AuNPs	*S. aureus*	Vancomycin-resistant	Combination with vancomycin.	Mohammed Fayaz et al., 2011
	E. faecalis			Lai et al., 2015
	S. aureus	Methicillin-resistant	Photothermal therapy with ROS generation.	Kuo et al., 2009; Millenbaugh et al., 2015; Mocan et al., 2016; Hu et al., 2017; Ocsoy et al., 2017
			Combination with vancomycin.	Lai et al., 2015
	E. coli, K. pneumoniae	Cefotaxime-resistant	Disruption of the bacterial cell wall, DNA damage.	Shaikh et al., 2017
	S. aureus, E. coli, P. aeruginosa, Enterobacter aerogenes	Ampicillin-resistant	Combination with ampicillin. Lead to entry into the bacterial cell.	Brown et al., 2012
	Streptococcus bovis, S. epidermidis, E. Aerogenes	Kanamycin-resistant	Disruption of the bacterial cell wall.	Payne et al., 2016
	K. 45ellular45, Proteus mirabilis, A. baumannii	Carbapenems-resistant	Disturb of osmotic balance and disrupt the integrity of cell bacterial cell wall.	Shaker and Shaaban, 2017
	P. aeruginosa	Biofilm formation	Interaction with cell surface.	Yu et al., 2016
	S. aureus		Laser excitation of the near IR LSPR lead to an efficient photothermal response with efficient killing of bacteria biofilms.	Pallavicini et al., 2014

(Continued)

TABLE 1 | Continued

Type of nanoparticles	Targeted bacteria	Antibiotic resistance type	Mechanisms of antibacterial action	References
	E. coli, P. aeruginosa, S. aureus		Penetration through biofilm layers and interaction with cellular components.	Ramasamy et al., 2017a,b
	S. epidermidis, S. haemolyticus		Combination with antibiotics.	Roshmi et al., 2015
	Proteus species		Interaction between proteins and NPs.	Vinoj et al., 2015
	E. coli, P. aeruginosa, S. aureus, B. Subtilis		ROS generation.	Wang Z. et al., 2017
	Gram-negative bacteria	MDR	Automated microarray-based system that identifies Gram-negative pathogens from positive blood cultures and resistance mechanism.	Walker et al., 2016
	S. aureus		Photoacoustic detection and photothermal therapy	Galanzha et al., 2012
	E. coli		ROS generation	Zhang et al., 2013
	E. coli		Change of membrane potential and inhibition of ATP synthase; inhibition of the subunit of the ribosome for tRNA binding.	Cui et al., 2012
	E. coli, K. pneumoniae, S. aureus, B. subtilis			Shamaila et al., 2016
	E. coli, K. pneumoniae, E. cloacae		Photodynamic Therapy/ Photothermal therapy.	Khan et al., 2017
	S. aureus, E. coli, E. cloacae, P. aeruginosa			Mocan et al., 2017
	Salmonella Typhimurium			Lin and Hamme, 2015
	S. aureus			Gil-Tomás et al., 2007
	E. coli, S. aureus		Interaction with biomolecules.	Kim D. et al., 2017
	E. coli, K. pneumoniae		Not revealed.	Bresee et al., 2014
	S. aureus, E. coli, P. aeruginosa		Disruption of bacterial cell wall.	Li et al., 2014; Yang et al., 2017
	E. coli		Interaction between lysozyme microbubbles and cell wall.	Mahalingam et al., 2015
	E. coli, S. aureus, Salmonella Typhimurium		Depend of co-existing chemicals that were not removed from AuNPs.	Shareena Dasari et al., 2015; Zhang et al., 2015a
	E. coli, S. aureus, K. pneumoniae		Combination with antibiotics.	Pradeepa et al., 2016
	P. aeruginosa	MDR/Biofilm formation	Conjugation with AMP.	Casciaro et al., 2017
	Staphylococci, Enterococci and other bacterial strain			Kuo et al., 2016
	E. coli, S. aureus, K. pneumoniae, P. aeruginosa			Rai A. et al., 2016
	Salmonella Typhimurium			Yeom et al., 2016
ZnONPs	*K. pneumoniae*	Ampicillin-carbenicillin-resistant	ROS generation and disruption of bacterial cell wall.	Reddy L. S. et al., 2014

(Continued)

TABLE 1 | Continued

Type of nanoparticles	Targeted bacteria	Antibiotic resistance type	Mechanisms of antibacterial action	References
	S. aureus	Methicillin-resistant	Enzyme inhibition.	Cha et al., 2015
	E. coli	*MDR*	ROS generation and disruption of bacterial cell wall.	Li et al., 2012b; Tong et al., 2013; Chakraborti et al., 2014; Gelabert et al., 2016; Nagvenkar et al., 2016
	B. subtilis			Hsueh et al., 2015
	S. aureus			Lakshmi Prasanna and Vijayaraghavan, 2015; Nagvenkar et al., 2016
	Vibrio cholerae			Sarwar et al., 2016
	S. aureus, E. coli, Proteus, Acinetobacter, P. aeruginosa		Combination with antibiotics.	Ehsan and Sajjad, 2017
	S. aureus, E. coli, S. mutants		Depend on components and structure of the bacteria cell wall.	Yu et al., 2014
	S. aureus, P. aeruginosa	Biofilms formation	ROS generation.	Aswathanarayan and Vittal, 2017
	Streptococcus sobrinus			Aydin Sevinç and Hanley, 2010
CuONPs	*E. coli, S. aureus*	MDR	ROS generation.	Singh R. et al., 2014; Chakraborty et al., 2015
	S. aureus, P. aeruginosa			Ulloa-Ogaz et al., 2017
	Paracoccus denitrificans		Modulation of nitrogen metabolism.	Su et al., 2015
	S. aureus	Biofilm formation	Ongoing investigations.	Chen et al., 2014
CuNPs	*S. aureus*	Methicillin-resistant	Copper ions release and subsequently bind with DNA leading to disorder of helical structure.	Kruk et al., 2015
	P. aeruginosa	Biofilm formation	Penetrate the cell wall and damage the nucleic acid.	LewisOscar et al., 2015
	P. aeruginosa	MDR	Generation of Cu hydrosols.	Zhang et al., 2015b
Fe_3O_4NPs	*E. coli*	MDR	Radiofrequency (RF) coupled with magnetic core shell nanoparticles lead to RF-mediated physical perturbation of cell membranes and bacterial membrane dysfunction.	Chaurasia et al., 2016
	S. aureus, P. aeruginosa, E. coli		Penetrate the membrane and interference in the electron transfer.	El-Zowalaty et al., 2015
	Gram-positive and -negative bacteria		ROS generation.	Behera et al., 2012
	Gram-positive and -negative bacteria		Nanotechnology to capture Gram- positive and -negative bacteria.	Reddy P. M. et al., 2014
	S. aureus	Biofilm formation	ROS generation.	Leuba et al., 2013
Al_2O_3NPs	*S. aureus*	Methicillin-resistant	Disruption of bacterial cell wall and ROS generation.	Ansari et al., 2013
	E. coli	MDR	Penetration and accumulation inside bacterial cell wall.	Ansari et al., 2014

(Continued)

TABLE 1 | Continued

Type of nanoparticles	Targeted bacteria	Antibiotic resistance type	Mechanisms of antibacterial action	References
TiO_2NPs	*S. aureus*	Methicillin-resistant	Release ions and react with thiol group of proteins present on bacteria surface.	Roy et al., 2010
	E. coli	MDR	ROS generation and disruption of bacterial cell wall.	Li et al., 2012b
	E. coli and Gram-positive bacteria		Photocatalytic disinfection.	Foster et al., 2011
	E. coli		Peroxidation and decomposition of membrane fatty acids.	Joost et al., 2015
Cu/Zn bimetal NPs	*S. aureus*	Methicillin-resistant	Membrane disruption, DNA damage, inhibition of protein synthesis.	Ashfaq et al., 2016
Au/Ag bimetallic NPs	*Enterococcus*	Vancomycin-resistant	Theranostic system for SERS and aPDT.	Zhou et al., 2018
	E. coli, S. aureus, E. faecalis, P. aeruginosa	Biofilm formation	Disruption of bacterial cell wall and inactivate the proteins and enzymes for ATP production.	Ramasamy et al., 2016
	B. subtilis E. coli, K. pneumoniae, S. aureus	MDR	Combination with antibiotics.	Baker et al., 2017
	P. aeruginosa, E. coli, S. aureus, Micrococcus luteus			Fakhri et al., 2017
	E. coli, S. aureus			dos Santos et al., 2012
Au/Pt bimetallic NPS	*E. coli*	MDR	Damage of the inner membrane, increase intracellular ATP level.	Zhao et al., 2014
Au/ Fe_3O_4NPs	*P. aeruginosa*	MDR	Disruption of bacterial cell wall.	Niemirowicz et al., 2014
Cu/Ni bimetallic NPs	*S. aureus, E. coli, S. mutans*	MDR	Adsorption of ions to the bacteria cells.	Argueta-Figueroa et al., 2014
MgF_2NPs	*S. aureus*	Biofilm formation	Attach and penetrate cell surface leading to disruption in membrane potential, promotes the lipid peroxidation and DNA binding.	Lellouche et al., 2009; Chen et al., 2014
Graphene Oxide NPs	*S. aureus*	Methicillin-resistant	Combine antibiotics with exposure to NIR.	Pan et al., 2016
	E. coli, E. faecalis	MDR	UV irradiation lead to generation of ROS.	Govindaraju et al., 2016
	E. coli, P. aeruginosa, K. pneumoniae, S. aureus		Multiple toxic mechanisms.	Jankauskaite et al., 2016
	E. cloacae, S. mutans	Biofilm formation	ROS generation, release of ions.	Kulshrestha et al., 2017
SeNPs	*S. aureus, E. coli*	MDR	Theranostic nanoplatform for selective imaging and targeted therapy: Disruption of the bacteria cell wall.	Huang et al., 2017
SiNPs	*S. aureus*	Methicillin-resistant	Theranostics nanoprobe for near-infrared fluorescence imaging and photothermal therapy: Disruption of the bacteria cell wall.	Zhao et al., 2017

peptidoglycans and abundant pores that allow the penetration of foreign molecules, leading to covalent binding with proteins and cellular components interrupting the proper functioning of the bacterial cell (Sarwar et al., 2015). In addition, Gram-positive bacteria have a highly negative charge on the surface of the cell wall. For example, LPS provides negatively charged regions on the cell wall of Gram-negative bacteria that attracts NPs; and, since teichoic acid is only expressed in Gram-positive bacteria, the NPs are distributed along the phosphate chain. As such, the antimicrobial effect is more foreshadowed in Gram-positive than -negative bacteria (Wang et al., 2017a). Indeed, Yu and colleagues synthesized a novel hydroxyapatite whisker (HAPw)/zinc oxide (ZnO) NPs and evaluated the antimicrobial effect against *S. aureus*, *E. coli*, and *Streptococcus mutans*. The authors demonstrate that the antibacterial effect depends on the components and structure of the bacterial cell wall. The antibacterial action of these NPs could be improved for Gram-positive bacteria and certain components could prevent the adhesion of ZnO NPs to the bacterial cell barrier (Yu et al., 2014). Ansari et al. reported that the accumulation on NPs in the bacterial cell wall causes irregularly shaped pit, perforation and disturbs metabolic processes (Ansari et al., 2014). In a study carried out by Joost and co-workers, it was demonstrated that a treatment with TiO_2 NPs increased the bacterial cell volume, resulting in membrane leakage (Joost et al., 2015).

BIOFILM FORMATION AND QUORUM-SENSING

Biofilm formation plays an important role in bacterial resistance protecting bacteria and allowing then to evade the action of antibiotics (Lebeaux et al., 2014; Khameneh et al., 2016). The most active fractions of bacteria are now recognized to occur as biofilms, where cells are adhered to each other on surfaces within a self-produced matrix of extracellular polymeric substance (EPS). EPS provide a barrier allowing to inhibit the penetration of antibiotics and further promote antibiotic resistance leading to a serious health threat worldwide since biofilms are resistant to antibiotics penetration and escape innate immune system by phagocytes (Hall-Stoodley et al., 2004; Bjarnsholt, 2013). Numerous experimental evidence show that NPs are capable of disrupting the bacterial membranes and can hinder biofilm formation thus reducing the survival of the microorganism (Peulen and Wilkinson, 2011; Leuba et al., 2013; Pelgrift and Friedman, 2013; Slomberg et al., 2013; Chen et al., 2014; Miao et al., 2016; Yu et al., 2016; Kulshrestha et al., 2017). This way, NPs provide an alternative strategy to target bacterial biofilms with potential to use both antibiotic-free and antibiotic-coated approaches (Gu et al., 2003; Li et al., 2012a; Sathyanarayanan et al., 2013). Earlier reports demonstrated that NPs are able to interfere with biofilm integrity by interacting with EPS and with the bacterial communication - quorum sensing (QS). The properties of NPs must be designed to be able to inhibit biofilm formation namely through size and surface chemistry. The size of NPs is important to it since they must be able to penetrate the EPS matrix and surface chemistry will command the amount of interactions with the EPS (Lundqvist et al., 2008). The majority of the strategies to achieve inhibition of biofilm formation are to target and interfere with QS molecules (Singh et al., 2017).

QS systems in bacterial populations act as major regulatory mechanisms of pathogenesis, namely in the formation of biofilm structures. These systems help bacteria to "communicate" with each other, through the production and detection of signal molecules (Rutherford and Bassler, 2012; Papenfort and Bassler, 2016). Using this cell-to-cell communication, bacterial populations are able to synchronize the expression of their genes, acquiring competitive advantage to respond to changes in the environment (Rutherford and Bassler, 2012). Therefore, QS systems are known to promote the formation of antibiotic tolerant biofilm communities. It is known that biofilm structures are a recalcitrant mode of bacterial growth that increases bacterial resistance to conventional antibiotics (Reen et al., 2018). This way, bacterial biofilms pose a significant challenge to the efficacy of conventional antibiotics being considered an essential platform for antibiotic resistance (Høiby et al., 2011). Taking this into account, it isn't surprising that the targeting and disruption of QS signaling systems and consequently, of the biofilm production, set the pillar for future next-generation anti-virulence therapies to be developed (LaSarre and Federle, 2013; Venkatesan et al., 2015; Jakobsen et al., 2017).

Surface-functionalized NPs with β-cyclodextrin (β-CD) or N-acylated homoserine lactonase proteins (AiiA) are able to interfere with signaling molecules preventing these molecules from reaching its cognate receptor, therefore inhibiting the signal/receptor interaction. This process will "turn off" QS and obstructing the bacterial communication (Kato et al., 2006; Ortíz-Castro et al., 2008). Several papers reported inhibition of biofilm formation namely by gold NPs (AuNPs). Acyl homoserine lactones (AHL) are signaling molecules with a role in bacterial QS and bind directly to transcription factors to regulate gene expression Recently, Gopalakrishnan and colleges synthesized (Vinoj et al., 2015) AuNPs coated AiiA purified from *Bacillus licheniformis*. These AiiA AuNPs inhibited EPs production and demonstrated potent antibiofilm activity against Proteus species at 2–8 μM concentrations without being harmful for the host cells at the 2μM concentration. Sathyanarayanan et al. (2013) demonstrated that using AuNPs there is a significant reduction of *S. aureus* and *P. aeruginosa* biofilms applied in high concentration (exceeding 50 mg/L). A recent study by Yu et al. (2016) demonstrated that AuNPs were able to strongly attenuate biofilm formation of *P. aeruginosa*. The inhibition observed in this study was related with interruption of adhesin- mediated interaction between the bacteria and the substrate surface due to electrostatic attractions between the AuNPs and cell wall surface of *P. aeruginosa*, instead of QS-related molecules. Positive charge AuNPs inhibited significantly *S. aureus* and *P. aeruginosa* biofilm formation (while minimizing mammalian cytotoxicity) (Ramasamy et al., 2016). The use of NPs demonstrates an exclusive approach to penetrate infectious biofilms and target bacterial communication, overcoming this major health issue related with biofilm infections.

Because most of these NPs-based platforms exert their action *via* distinct mechanisms/structures/pathways of those used by traditional antibiotics, combined therapeutic regimens are promising strategies to tackle the surge of multidrug resistant (MDR) bacteria bypassing their defense mechanisms (Pelgrift and Friedman, 2013; Singh K. et al., 2014; Hemeg, 2017; Zaidi et al., 2017). Additionally, NPs have been shown to activate macrophages in a dose dependent manner (Patel and Janjic, 2015) which promotes the host defenses (Hemeg, 2017; Jagtap et al., 2017).

This multi-target action of NPs may overcome multidrug resistance by circumventing several obstacles encountered by traditional antibiotics (Pelgrift and Friedman, 2013; Chen et al., 2014; Singh K. et al., 2014; Hemeg, 2017; Jagtap et al., 2017; Rai et al., 2017; Zaidi et al., 2017). **Table 1** highlights several types of NPs that have shown effective bactericidal activity when administered isolated; combined with standard antibiotics; and/or radiation or as vectors for biocidal delivery allowing killing of MDR bacteria, and in some cases also inhibiting biofilm production.

We will now focus on the different types of metal NPs highlighting their most relevant mechanism/effects against MDR bacteria and/or biofilms structures.

SILVER NANOPARTICLES (AGNPS)

Since the ancient times, silver has been recognized as having antimicrobial effects (Rai et al., 2009; Reidy et al., 2013). Based on all the evidence to date, AgNPs are probably one of the most promising inorganic NPs that can be used for the treatment of bacterial infections (Natan and Banin, 2017). These NPs may be synthesized by traditional chemical reduction or *via* "green" chemistry approaches using plant and/or microbial extracts (Iravani et al., 2014; Ribeiro et al., 2018).

Several mechanisms have been proposed to understand how AgNPs mediate cell death, including cell wall disruption (Lok et al., 2007; Bondarenko et al., 2013), oxidation of cellular components, inactivation of the respiratory chain enzymes, production of ROS, and decomposition of the cellular components (Chen et al., 2014; Rizzello and Pompa, 2014; Dakal et al., 2016). The permeability of the membrane increases after incorporation of AgNPs into the cell membrane. The adsorption of the NPs leads to the depolarization of the cell wall, altering the negative charge of the cell wall to become more permeable. It was demonstrated disruption of the cell wall with subsequent penetration of the NPs. The entry of AgNPs induces ROS that will inhibit ATP production and DNA replication (Zhang et al., 2013; Dakal et al., 2016; Durán et al., 2016; Ramalingam et al., 2016). However, there is evidence that AgNPs can release Ag^{+}, known to exhibit antimicrobial activity, when interacting with thiol-containing proteins, which weaken their functions (Durán et al., 2010). The precise method of the antibacterial mechanism of AgNPs is still not completely understood (Franci et al., 2015; Durán et al., 2016). All the existing data indicates that AgNPs exert several bactericidal mechanisms in parallel, which may explain why bacterial resistance to silver is rare (Karimi et al., 2016). Concerns regarding the cytotoxicity and genotoxicity of AgNPs have been raised (Chopra, 2007) but various authors have conducted clinical trials based on AgNPs and no important clinical alterations have been detected (Munger et al., 2014a,b; Smock et al., 2014). Interestingly, AgNPs have been found to exhibit higher antimicrobial activity than antibiotics like gentamicin or vancomycin against *P. aeruginosa* and MRSA (Saeb et al., 2014). Lara *et al.* showed the potential bactericidal effect of AgNPs against MDR *P. aeruginosa*, ampicillin-resistant *E. coli* O157:H7 and erythromycin-resistant *Streptococcus pyogenes* (Lara et al., 2010). Nagy *et al.*, reported that AgNPs were capable of inhibiting the growth of *S. aureus* and *E. coli via* the up-regulation of the expression of several antioxidant genes and ATPase pumps (Nagy et al., 2011). Dolman *et al.* also showed that the Ag-containing Hydrofiber® dressing and nanocrystalline Ag-containing dressing are effective agents against antibiotic sensitive Gram-negative and -positive bacteria as well as antibiotic resistant bacteria, such as MRSA, Vancomycin-resistant *Enterococci* (VRE) and *Serratia marcescens*, avoiding the formation of biofilms on biomaterials (Percival et al., 2007). Su and collaborators showed that AgNPs immobilized on the surface of nanoscale silicate platelets (AgNP/NSPs) have strong antibacterial activity against MRSA and silver-resistant *E. coli via* generation of ROS (Su et al., 2011). Singh and collaborators showed that AgNPs from *P. amarus* extract exhibited excellent antibacterial potential against MDR strains of *P. aeruginosa* (Singh K. et al., 2014). Recently, two different shaped AgNPs (spheres and rods) were used against Gram-positive and -negative bacteria, both showing promising antibacterial activity against different strains (Acharya et al., 2018).

An emerging practice is to combine AgNPs with antibiotics to enhance antimicrobial potency. Recently, Katya and collaborators showed that the combination of gentamicin and chloramphenicol with AgNPs has a better antibacterial effect in MDR *E. faecalis* than both antibiotics alone (Katva et al., 2018). McShan *et al.* described that AgNPs combined with either one of two-different class of antibiotics (tetracycline and neomycin) can exhibit a synergistic effect, showing an enhanced antibacterial activity at concentrations below the MIC of either the NPs or the antibiotic (McShan et al., 2015). Other authors also reported similar results (Thomas et al., 2014; Panáček et al., 2016a,b; Salomoni et al., 2017). Djafari and collaborators described the synthesis of water-soluble AgNPs using the antibiotic tetracycline as co-reducing and stabilizing agent (AgNPs@TC) and demonstrated their effectiveness against tetracycline-resistant bacteria (Djafari et al., 2016).

Antimicrobial peptides (AMPs) represent one of the forms of defense strategy against infections in living organisms and are emerging as essential tools to kill pathogenic bacteria, since they exhibit broad-spectrum activity and low resistance development (Yeaman, 2003). Lytic peptides are AMPs produced by all organisms. In mammals, they are an innate host defense mechanism against pathogens (Bahar and Ren, 2013). The mechanism of action of AMPs relies on the ability to interact with bacterial membranes or the cell wall, thus inhibiting cellular biochemical pathways and ultimately killing the bacteria (Zhang and Gallo, 2016). Defensins and cathelicidin are two of the larger families of lytic peptides that kill bacteria by disrupting the membrane. Unfortunately, AMPs have poor enzymatic stability, low permeability across biological barriers and may be rapidly degraded in the human body by proteases, which greatly limits their application (Wang, 2014). Immobilization of the peptides onto NPs can increase their stability, enhancing the antimicrobial properties of the NPs and therefore, has the potential to be used as a new tool to tackle antibiotic resistant bacteria (Brandelli, 2012; Rai A. et al., 2016). Indeed, the first author to demonstrate that functionalized AgNPs with peptides increased their antibacterial activity was Ruden and co-workers (Ruden et al., 2009). Based on this strategy several researchers functionalized AgNPs with AMPs (AgNP@AMP) with increases in the antimicrobial activity compared with free AMPs (Ruden et al., 2009; Liu et al., 2013; Mohanty et al., 2013). Polymyxin B is the most used AMP and exhibits antibacterial activity *via* interaction with the endotoxin LPS in the outer membrane of Gram-negative bacteria (Morrison and Jacobs, 1976; Lambadi et al., 2015). It was proved that AgNPs functionalized with polymyxin-B removed almost completely endotoxins from solutions and hindered the formation of biofilm onto surgical blades (Jaiswal et al., 2015; Lambadi et al., 2015). Liu *et al.,* demonstrated that the immobilization of peptides with AgNPs enhanced their antimicrobial activity compared to an unbound peptide and also minimized toxicity of AgNPs compared to using the AgNPs alone (Liu et al., 2013). A recent study by Pal *et al.* describes a system consisting of a cysteine containing AMP conjugated with AgNPs, which demonstrated that the Ag-S bonds increased stability and enhanced antimicrobial activity than conjugation using electrostatic interactions (Pal et al., 2016).

Other methods have been used to improve the antibacterial activity of AgNPs. One of these methods relies on the use of visible blue light, which was previously shown to exhibit strong antibacterial activity (Dai T. et al., 2013; Maclean et al., 2014). El Din and collaborators demonstrated that blue light combined with AgNPs exhibits therapeutic potential to treat MDR infections and can represent an alternative to conventional antibiotic therapy, since the antimicrobial activity of the combination was greater than the components alone. Moreover, this approach proved to be synergistic in the treatment of an unresponsive antibiotic-resistant bacteria responsible for a wound in a horse (El Din et al., 2016). Spherical shaped thioglycolic acid-stabilized AgNPs (TGA-AgNPs) conjugated with vancomycin were used as drug delivery systems and demonstrated to possess increased antimicrobial activity against MDR bacteria such as MRSA and VRE (Esmaeillou et al., 2017).

GOLD NANOPARTICLES (AuNPs)

Metallic gold is considered inert and non-toxic, which may vary when it shifts form metallic bulk to oxidation states (I and II) (Merchant, 1998). Gold NPs (AuNPs) may be synthesized by traditional chemical reduction of a gold salt or *via* "green" chemistry approaches using plant and/or microbial extracts (Shah et al., 2014). The most used and described method is the chemical synthesis based on the reduction of chloroauric acid by citrate (Lee and Meisel, 1982; Fernandes and Baptista, 2017). Some studies have addressed the potential of using AuNPs as antibacterial agents, but some controversy still exists (Cui et al., 2012; Bresee et al., 2014; Shah et al., 2014; Shareena Dasari et al., 2015; Zhang et al., 2015a; Shamaila et al., 2016).

According to Yu H and collaborators, AuNPs are usually not bactericidal at low concentrations and weakly bactericidal at high concentrations (Shareena Dasari et al., 2015; Zhang et al., 2015a). This is possibly due to the effect of co-existing chemicals, such as gold ions, surface coating agents, and chemicals involved in the synthesis that were not completely removed (Shareena Dasari et al., 2015; Zhang et al., 2015a). However, other authors describe that the antibacterial mechanism of AuNPs is associated to (i) the collapse in the membrane potential, hindering ATPase activity causing a deterioration of the cell metabolism; (ii) hindering of the binding subunit of the ribosome to tRNA (Cui et al., 2012); and (iii) Shamaila and co-workers showed that AuNPs may affect the bacterial respiratory chain by attacking nicotinamide (Shamaila et al., 2016). Since AuNPs are non-toxic to the host (Conde et al., 2014; Li et al., 2014; Rajchakit and Sarojini, 2017), the possibility of fine tuning their conjugation chemistry to act as carriers or delivery vehicles of antibiotics or other antibacterial moieties may enhance their bactericidal effect and potentiate the effect of antibiotics (Zhao and Jiang, 2013; Conde et al., 2014; Li et al., 2014; Uma Suganya et al., 2015; Zhang et al., 2015a; Fernandes et al., 2017).

Cationic and hydrophobic functionalized AuNPs were shown to be effective against both Gram-negative and -positive uropathogens, including MRSA. These AuNPs exhibited low toxicity to mammalian cells (biocompatibility) and the development of resistance to these NPs was very low (Li et al., 2014). Vinoj *et al.* demonstrated that coating AuNPs with N-acylated homoserine lactonase proteins (AiiA AuNPs) resulted in a nanocomposite with activity against MDR species compared with AiiA proteins alone (Vinoj et al., 2015). Other approaches were also studied, as adsorbing AuNPs to PVA-lysozyme micro bubbles potentiate the antibacterial activity due to the interaction of AuNPs with cells membranes causing bacterial lysis (Mahalingam et al., 2015). Galic acid capped AuNPs have also been found to be active against Gram-negative and -positive bacteria (Kim D. et al., 2017). Recently, Ramasamy and collaborators described the direct one-pot synthesis of cinnamaldehyde immobilized on gold nanoparticles (CGNPs) with effective biofilm inhibition of more than 80% against Gram-positive bacteria (methicillin-sensitive and -resistant strains of *S. aureus*, MSSA and MRSA, respectively) and Gram-negative (*E. coli* and *P. aeruginosa*) *in vitro* and *in vivo* (Ramasamy et al., 2017a,b). Also, the integration of AuNPs with ultrathin graphitic carbon nitride was described as having high bactericidal performance against both MDR Gram-negative and -positive bacteria, and a high effectiveness in eliminating existing MDR-biofilms and preventing the formation of new biofilms *in vitro* (Wang Z. et al., 2017). Also, conjugation of antibiotics to AuNPs, such as vancomycin, methicillin, etc., increases their intrinsic activity against MDR strains (Mohammed Fayaz et al., 2011; Lai et al., 2015; Roshmi et al., 2015; Payne et al., 2016). Recently Payne and collaborators develop a single-step synthesis of kanamycin-capped AuNPs (Kan-AuNPs) with high antibacterial activity against both Gram-positive and -negative bacteria, including kanamycin resistant bacteria. The authors observed a significant reduction in the MIC against all the bacterial strains tested for Kan-AuNPs when compared to the free drug. This higher efficacy was due to the disruption of the bacterial envelope, resulting in leakage of the cytoplasmic content and consequent cell death (Payne et al., 2016). Pradeepa and collaborators synthesized AuNPs with bacterial exopolysaccharide (EPS) and functionalized them with antibiotics (levofloxacin, cefotaxime, ceftriaxone and ciprofloxacin). They observed that these AuNPs exhibited excellent bactericidal activity against MDR Gram-positive and -negative bacteria compared to free drugs. *E. coli* was the most susceptible MDR bacteria followed by *K. pneumoniae* and *S. aureus* (Pradeepa et al., 2016). Recently, Yang and collaborators described the effect of small molecule (6-aminopenicillanic acid, APA)-coated AuNPs to inhibit MDR bacteria (Yang et al., 2017). They doped AuNPs into electrospun fibers of poly(ε-caprolactone) (PCL)/gelatin to produce materials that avoid wound infection by MDR bacteria and demonstrated *in vitro* and *in vivo* that APA-AuNPs reduced MDR bacterial infections (Yang et al., 2017). Shaker and Shaaban evaluated the surface functionalization of AuNPs with carbapenems [imipenem (Ipm) and meropenem (Mem)] as a delivering strategy against carbapenem resistant Gram-negative bacteria isolated from an infected human. Both Ipm-AuNPs and Mem-AuNPs, with 35 nm diameter showed a significant increase in antibacterial activity against all the tested isolates (Shaker and Shaaban, 2017). Also, Shaikh and collaborators described recently the synthesis and characterization of cefotaxime conjugated AuNPs to target drug-resistant CTX-M-producing bacteria. The authors could invert resistance in cefotaxime resistant bacterial strains (i.e., *E. coli* and *K. pneumoniae*) by using cefotaxime-AuNPs. Their results reinforce the efficacy of conjugating an unresponsive antibiotic with AuNPs to restore its efficacy against otherwise resistant bacterial pathogens (Shaikh et al., 2017).

Combination of AuNPs with other approaches has also been demonstrated. Indeed, one of the most extraordinary properties of AuNPs is the capability to transform light into heat under laser irradiation (Mendes et al., 2017; Mocan et al., 2017). This property is extremely important because it can be exploited to develop photothermal nanovectors to destroy MDR bacteria at a molecular level (for a complete review see Mocan et al., 2017). For example, Khan and collaborators showed that the combination of Concanavalin-A (ConA) directed dextran capped AuNPs (GNPDEX-ConA) conjugated with methylene blue (MB) (MB@GNPDEX-ConA) and photodynamic therapy (PDT) enhanced the efficacy and selectivity of MB induced killing of MDR clinical isolates, including *E. coli*, *K. pneumoniae*, and *E. cloacae* (Khan et al., 2017). Gil-Tomas and collaborators described that the functionalization of AuNPs covalently with toluidine blue O–tiopronin forms an enhanced, exceptionally potent antimicrobial agent when activated by white light or 632 nm laser light (Gil-Tomás et al., 2007). Hu and collaborators prepared a mixed charged zwitterion-modified AuNPs consisting of a weak electrolytic 11-mercaptoundecanoic acid (HS-C10-COOH) and a strong electrolytic (10-mercaptodecyl)trimethylammonium bromide (HS-C10-N4) that exhibited *in vivo* and under near-infrared (NIR) light irradiation an enhanced photothermal ablation of MRSA biofilm with no damage to the healthy tissues around the biofilm (Hu et al., 2017). Also, the antibacterial activity of glucosamine-gold nanoparticle-graphene oxide (GlcN-AuNP-GO) and UV-irradiated GlcN-AuNP-GO was evaluated against *E. coli* and *E. faecalis*. Results show that UV irradiation of GlcN-AuNP-GO results in higher antibacterial activity than the standard drug kanamycin (Govindaraju et al., 2016). Ocsoy *et al.* reported the development of DNA aptamer-functionalized AuNPs (Apt@AuNPs) and gold nanorods (Apt@AuNRs) for inactivation of MRSA with targeted PTT (Ocsoy et al., 2017). The authors showed that although both NPs could specifically bind to MRSA cells, Apt@AuNPs and Apt@AuNRs increased resistant cell death for 5% and for more than 95%, respectively through PTT. This difference in induction of cell death was based on the relatively high longitudinal absorption of NIR radiation and strong photothermal conversion capability for the Apt@AuNRs compared to the Apt@AuNPs. However, with the new developments of using AuNPs for hyperthermia in the visible light (Mendes et al., 2017) might additionally potentiate the Apt@AuNPs results observed for these authors (Ocsoy et al., 2017). Recently, Mocan *et al.* also described the synthesis of AuNPs by wet chemistry, their functionalization with IgG molecules following laser irradiation. Their results indicate that administration of IgG-AuNPs following laser irradiation provided an extended and selective bacterial death in a dose dependent manner (Mocan et al., 2016).

In recent years, a new approach relying on the conjugation of AuNPs with AMPs has shown interesting results (Rajchakit and Sarojini, 2017). Indeed, Kuo and collaborators mixed synthetic-peptides containing arginine, tryptophan and cysteine termini [(DVFLG)2REEW4C and (DVFLG)2REEW2C], with aqueous tetrachloroauric acid to generate peptide-immobilized AuNPs [i.e., (DVFLG)2REEW4C-AuNPs and (DVFLG)2REEW2C-AuNPs] that were effective antibacterial agents against *Staphylococci*, *Enterococci*, and antibiotic-resistant bacterial strains (Kuo et al., 2016). Rai and co-workers demonstrated that the use of cecropin-melittin (CM-SH) a known peptide with antibacterial properties (Boman et al., 1989), functionalized in the surface of AuNPs through Au-S bond, showed higher antimicrobial activity and higher stability in media compared with an *in vitro* and *in vivo* infection animal model with the MIC of CM-SH AuNPs four times lower than free CM-SH (Rai A. et al., 2016). Conjugation of AMP with AuNPs usually involves the formation of the Au-S coordinate covalent bond, relying on the amine or thiol groups in peptides or conjugating specific linkers to AMPs with a terminal (N- or C-terminal) cysteine which helps conjugation with gold (Tielens and Santos, 2010; Xue et al., 2014). However, there is one example where covalent conjugation of an AMP to AuNPs has been achieved *via* Au-O bond (Lai et al., 2015). Other approaches use a linker for the conjugation to AuNPs, Poly(ethylene glycol) carboxylic acid (PEGCOOH) covalently bound to AMP showed a significantly increase of the antibacterial and anti-biofilm activity for resistant Gram-negative bacteria (Casciaro et al., 2017). Yeom and co-workers demonstrated the most advanced *in vivo* clinical application for AuNPs@AMP using infected mice and resulting in the inhibition of *Salmonella* Typhimurium colonization in the organs of the animals (Yeom et al., 2016). The reason behind the increased antimicrobial activity of AuNPs@AMP over the free components is that AuNPs can get a higher concentration of the antibiotic at the site of action. These NPs can interact with LPS, proteins in the membrane of the bacteria and in some cases, penetrate the bacterial membrane through the porin channel. This way they can interact with the inner membrane making the AuNPs@AMP conjugate more efficient than the non-conjugated form (Katz and Willner, 2004; Wangoo et al., 2008; Chen J. et al., 2009).

BIMETALLIC NPS

Ag and Au may be used in a single NP to enhance the effects of a drug and reduce the required dose. Alternatively, they can be used alone since they possess antimicrobial properties that are enhanced when combined in the form of bimetallic NPs (Arvizo et al., 2010; Singh R. et al., 2016). The role of Ag against MDR pathogens has been previously described. However, AgNPs are difficult to functionalize with biomolecules and drugs. Such limitation may be circumvented by means of alloy/bimetallic NPs that excel their monometallic counterparts providing improved electronic, optical and catalytic properties (Cho et al., 2005; Shah et al., 2012). As reported above, AuNPs constitute good vectors to the delivery of pharmacologic compounds. Gold(Au)-silver(Ag) alloys are an optimal solution since they combine the antimicrobial effect of silver with the ease of functionalization and improved stability in complex biological media provided by gold (Doria et al., 2010; dos Santos et al., 2012). Fakhri and co-workers synthetized and functionalized AgAuNPs with a tetracycline and concluded that there exists a synergetic effect of the antibiotic with the bimetallic nanoparticle, with greater bactericidal activity of this form in detriment of its free forms. The mechanism of action was established as being the generation of ROS (Fakhri et al., 2017). Also recently, Baker and collaborators described the synthesis and antimicrobial activity of bimetallic AgAuNPs from the cell free supernatant of *Pseudomonas veronii* strain AS41G inhabiting *Annona squamosa L.* The authors showed their synergistic effect with standard antibiotics with 87.5, 18.5, 11.15, 10, 9.7, and 9.4% fold increased activity with bacitracin, kanamycin, gentamicin, streptomycin, erythromycin and chloramphenicol, respectively, against bacitracin resistant strains of *Bacillus subtilis, E. coli,* and *K. pneumoniae* (Baker et al., 2017). Zhao and collaborators have demonstrated the antibacterial activity of AuPtNPs bimetallic NPs against sensitive and drug-resistant bacteria *via* the dissipation of the bacterial membrane potential and the elevation of adenosine triphosphate (ATP) levels (Zhao et al., 2014).

Other types of bimetallic NPs have been studied and their antibacterial activity explored, but in most cases as coating agents and not as a delivery approach and antibacterial activity (Argueta-Figueroa et al., 2014).

METAL OXIDES

Metal oxides NPs are among one of the most explored and studied family of NPs and are known to effectively inhibit the growth of a wide range of sensitive and resistant Gram-positive and -negative bacteria, emerging as hopeful candidates to challenge antimicrobial resistance (Raghunath and Perumal, 2017; Reshma et al., 2017; Kadiyala et al., 2018). Iron oxide (Fe_3O_4), Zinc oxide (ZnO), and Copper oxide (CuO) possess antimicrobial properties and can be applied in clinical care (Sinha et al., 2011). Due to the intrinsic photocatalytic activity of the metal oxides they generate ROS and become powerful agents against bacteria (Tong et al., 2013; Singh R. et al., 2014). These will be described in more detail on the following sections.

IRON OXIDE (FE_3O_4)

The synthesis of iron oxide NPs may be achieved *via* different routes (Babes et al., 1999; Berry and Curtis, 2003). The antibacterial mechanism of these NPs is mainly attributed to dissolved metal ions and the generation of ROS (Wang et al., 2017a). It was shown that superparamagnetic iron oxide NPs interact with microbial cells by penetrating the membrane and interfering with the electron transfer (Behera et al., 2012; El-Zowalaty et al., 2015). Additionally, it has been described that iron oxide NPs can damage macromolecules, including DNA and proteins, through the formation of ROS (Leuba et al., 2013). Pan *et al.* developed a system of reduced graphene oxide (rGO)-iron oxide nanoparticles (rGO-IONP) by the chemical deposition of Fe^{2+}/Fe^{3+} ions on nanosheets of rGO in aqueous ammonia. The *in vivo* results showed maximum antibacterial activity due to the generation of hydroxyl radicals that can cause physical and chemical damage, which inactivated MRSA (Pan et al., 2016).

ZINC OXIDE (ZnO)

ZnO NPs are often used to restrict microorganism growth, being effective against planktonic bacteria, and also inhibiting the formation of biofilms (Hsueh et al., 2015; Sarwar et al., 2016) (Espitia et al., 2012). These NPs can be synthesized by various methods, from green chemistry to sonochemistry (Salem et al., 2015; Ali et al., 2016; Nagvenkar et al., 2016). The antibacterial mechanism of the NPs is partially attributed to two principal factors, the dissolution of metal ion and the generation of ROS (Gelabert et al., 2016; Nagvenkar et al., 2016; Sarwar et al., 2016). ZnO releases Zn^{2+} in liquid medium and is adsorbed on the surface of bacteria or may entry the cell, where it interacts with functional groups in proteins and nucleic acids, hindering enzyme activity and the normal physiological processes (Yu et al., 2014). However, some authors demonstrated that Zn ions have little antimicrobial activity, implying that dissolution of Zn^{2+} might not be the main mechanism of action (Aydin Sevinç and Hanley, 2010). Sarwar and co-workers demonstrated that nanosized ZnO caused significant oxidative stress to *Vibrio cholera*, the damage inflicted was DNA degradation, protein leakage, membrane depolarization and fluidity (Sarwar et al., 2016). Ehsan and Sajjad, described that ZnO NPs impregnated with antibiotics showed good antibacterial activities against *S. aureus*, *Proteus*, *Acinetobacter*, *P. aeruginosa*, and *E. coli*, being that these were resistant to antibiotics but became sensitive in the presence of these NPs with antibiotics (Ehsan and Sajjad, 2017). It was also discovered that these NPs induce the production of ROS even in the dark, and this happens due to the surface defects on the NPs. The different shapes function as enzyme inhibitors, where nanopyramids are the most effective (Cha et al., 2015; Lakshmi Prasanna and Vijayaraghavan, 2015). Recently, Aswathanarayan and Vittal described the antimicrobial effect of ZnO NPs against MDR Gram-positive and -negative pathogens in comparison to gold and iron NPs and these could be used at concentrations less toxic to mammalian cells (Aswathanarayan and Vittal, 2017). ZnO NPs are also known for inhibiting biofilm formation and production of quorum-sensing-dependent virulence factors in *P. aeruginosa* (Lee et al., 2014; García-Lara et al., 2015).

COPPER OXIDE (CuO)

Copper containing NPs have been shown effective against animal and plant pathogens (LewisOscar et al., 2015), impeding formation of MDR biofilms, and showing the potential to serve as antimicrobial coating agents (LewisOscar et al., 2015). Kruk *et al.* and Zhang *et al.* showed that copper NPs are capable of inhibiting the growth of MDR bacteria, namely, *P. aeruginosa* and MRSA (Zhang et al., 2014, 2015b; Kruk et al., 2015). The antimicrobial activity of these NPs is comparable to that of AgNPs but at a lower cost (Kruk et al., 2015). Copper oxide NPs generate ROS that often leads to chromosomal DNA degradation, which seems to highlight a "particle-specific" action rather than resulting from the release of metallic ions (Chakraborty et al., 2015). Su and collaborators investigated the effects of CuONPs on bacterial denitrification and explored the effect on the expression of intracellular proteins. When CuONPs entry into bacteria metabolic functions are affected, such as active transport, electron transfer, and nitrogen metabolism (Su et al., 2015).

NPs can also be complexed with other metals, like gallium. Gallium NPs have been described to facilitate phagosome maturation of macrophages infected with virulent *M. tuberculosis* and therefore being able to inhibit growth of this pathogen (Choi et al., 2017).

THE POTENTIAL FOR NANOTHERANOSTICS

NPs applications in biodetection is huge and more insights on pathogen detection using NPs platforms can be seen in Veigas et al. (2013, 2014, 2015); Costa et al. (2014); Weng et al. (2015); Kim J. et al. (2017); Wang et al. (2017b); Galvan and Yu (2018), and Yang et al. (2018).

Theranostics is a combination of diagnosis and therapy onto a single platform, which allow for timely biodetection and/or real-time monitoring of therapy. By using NPs, this can be translated to the nanoscale—Nanotheranostics. NPs have been applied for multiplex high-throughput diagnostics to assist precision therapy. For example, Verigene® is an AuNPs test commercialized for diagnosis. It is an automated microarray-based system that identifies Gram-negative pathogens from positive blood cultures. Verigene® BC-GN also detects key resistance mechanisms (Walker et al., 2016; Claeys et al., 2018). Others have used, magnetic and functionalized magnetic iron oxide NPs as affinity probes to capture Gram-positive and -negative bacteria. The analyses of captured bacteria using matrix-assisted laser desorption/ionization mass spectrometry was <1 h (Reddy P. M. et al., 2014). One pioneer work on nanotheranostics against bacterial infection was the development of a method for *in vivo* photoacoustic detection and photothermal eradication of *S. aureus*. Two-color gold and multilayer magnetic nanoparticles were functionalized with an antibody cocktail for the targeting of *S. aureus*. These platform demonstrated ultrasensitive detections for circulating bacterial cells (CBCs), *in vivo* magnetic enrichment and PT eradication of CBCs (Galanzha et al., 2012). Recently, Zhou and collaborators developed a silicon 2,3-naphthalocyanine dihydroxide (Nc) and Vancomycin functionalized silica-encapsulated, silver-coated gold NPs (Au@AgNP@SiO2@Nc-Van) as a novel theranostic system for surface-enhanced Raman scattering (SERS) detection and antimicrobial photodynamic therapy (aPDT) of vancomycin (Van)-resistant enterococci (VRE) strains (Zhou et al., 2018). These authors observed a 4–5 logs reduction of bacteria upon *in vitro* aPDT of VRE treated with a nanomolar concentration of the Au@AgNP@SiO2@Nc-Van and an infection regression and even complete eradication of VRE *in vivo* using infected mice (Zhou et al., 2018).

A selenium nanoplatform (Se@PEP-Ru) was designed with excellent fluorescent properties for imaging bacteria and with high antimicrobial properties (Huang et al., 2017). Zhao and co-workers developed an activated theranostics nanoprobe for near-infrared fluorescence imaging and photothermal therapy of MRSA infections, based on SiO2/PAH-cypate nanosystems modified with PEG and Vancomycin-conjugated poly(acrylic acid) molecules (PAAPEG-Van). This probe is activated by bacteria-responsive polyelectrolyte dissociation from silica NPs. The authors believe that this concept can be used as an approach to design and for production of bacteria responsive multifunctional nanomaterials and constitute their ultimate functions in the treatment of drug-resistant bacterial infections (Zhao et al., 2017). Kuo and collaborators developed a nanotheranostics system using Au nanorods conjugated with a hydrophilic photosensitizer, toluidine blue O, that acted as dual-function agents in photodynamic inactivation and hyperthermia against MRSA (Kuo et al., 2009).

CLINICAL TRANSLATION

At present, there are a few metal NPs-based strategies against bacterial infections undergoing clinical trials. The costs associated to the use of nanotechnology platforms are very high, and therefore conventional treatments are preferred. However, these platforms might be preferable in specific situations, with direct impact on the quality of patients life (Caster et al., 2017).

Bio-kil® [3-(Trimethoxysilyl) propyloctadecyldimethyl ammonium chloride] (Cargico Group, Taiwan) is a patented technology that is based on affixing nano-sized antimicrobials onto a large surface area through covalent chemical bonding to form a durable polymer. Bio-kil® eliminates microorganism through a physical biocide process. This type of nanomaterial consists in inorganic metal components and organic quaternary ammonium components. Recently, Bio-Kil® has been shown to reduce the environmental bacterial burden and MDR organisms (Lee et al., 2017).

AgTive (NCT00337714) is a silver-impregnated central venous catheter and has been marketed with the claim to improved bactericidal activity. AgTive catheters are made of polyurethanes impregnated with silver NPs, and their interaction with body fluids and intravenous solutions results in the release of significantly larger amounts of silver ions from the catheter reducing bloodstream infection (Antonelli et al., 2012).

Acticoat is a nanocrystalline silver dressing that acts as an antimicrobial topical, releasing silver into the wound. This nanoformulation has been shown to inhibit *in vitro* biofilms formation in *P. aeruginosa* and *Acinetobacter baumannii* by more than 90% (Potgieter and Meidany, 2017). Madigan Army Medical Center is studying the efficacy of a silver NPs gel SilvaSorb (NCT00659204) and currently is in phase III of the clinical trials. The aim of this study is to compare the antimicrobial efficacy of a one-time application of SilverSorb (AcryMed, Inc., Portland) against the standard antibacterial hand gel Purell (GoJo Industries, Akron), in reducing transient bacterial counts isolated from the hands of 40 patients seeded with *S. marcescens*.

Nano Silver Fluoride is a new formulation that combines silver NPs, chitosan and fluoride and was developed with antimicrobial properties. This nanoformulation has excellent results as antibacterial agent *against S. mutans* and *Lactobacilli*. Currently, is used to prevent dental caries in children (Dos Santos et al., 2014).

Despite this review do not concern liposomal formulations since it refers to clinical translation other formulations involving NPs, such as liposomal formulations, have been also identified as antimicrobial agents. Most of these formulations rely on the incorporation of traditional antibiotics into nanoliposomes to improve distribution and circulation times (Caster et al., 2017). **Table 2** summarizes antimicrobial liposomes, which are undergoing clinical trials. For example, Amikacin (NCT01315691) is a potent aminoglycoside antibiotic that is useful for the treatment of MDR Gram-negative bacteria. Arikace is an inhaled liposomal formulation that encapsulates amikacin composed of dipalmitoyl-phosphatidylcholine (DPPC) and cholesterol (Meers et al., 2008). These formulation have high drug loading and stability when administrated and in phase II trial, there was no notable difference in toxicity between liposomal drug treatment and placebo (Clancy et al., 2013). Another two-inhaled liposomal formulation are currently in clinical trials. Linhaliq (NCT02104245) is a combination of liposomal and aqueous phase ciprofloxacin, whereas Lipoquin (NCT00889967) is a liposomal ciprofloxacin that allows prolonged drug release. Both of these nanoformulation were developed for the treatment of non-cystic fibrosis bronchiectasis (NCFBE) patients with chronic lung infections with *P. aeruginosa*. Phase II in patients with both CF and non-CF bronchiectasis have been completed. After analysis of clinical data from the two different formulations, Linhaliq showed better performance. The Food and Drug Administration (FDA) has designated Linhaliq as a qualified infection disease product and made it eligible for Fast track designation. In 2016, Pulmanic completed two phases III clinical trials, but has not yet been approved by the FDA. The Hadassah Medical Organization (Jerusalem, Israel) has incorporated quaternary ammonium polyethyleneimine (QA-PEI) based polymers into dental composites. The bacterial membrane may be disturbed by the charged quaternary moiety, it also has potent activity against a series of Gram-positive and -negative pathogens (Ortega et al., 2015). In 2013, these nanoformulation completed phase II trials but no data on outcome have been released to date.

MAT2501 is designed to targeted delivery of the antibiotic amikacin while providing an improved safety and tolerability profile. Currently, Matinas Biopharma has reported positive data from the Phase I study in healthy volunteers for the treatment of MDR Gram-negative bacterial infections and is in preparation for a phase II in patients.

OTHER POTENTIAL APPLICATIONS OF NPS

In the case of non-antibiotic therapy, combinations of NPs with essential oils, peptides and other natural compounds have featured as promising antimicrobial strategies. The therapeutic applications of these substances are often limited by their toxicity and volatility (Chen F. et al., 2009; Allahverdiyev et al., 2011). A recent study has shown that chitosan NPs vectors, modified with eugenol and carvacrol essential oils on their surface, were active against *E. coli* and *S. aureus* at concentrations better or equal to unmodified NPs versions (Chen F. et al., 2009). Furthermore, the toxicity of the conjugates toward mouse fibroblasts was significantly less than the pure oils alone. With regards to peptides, the active sequences can be vulnerable to denaturation, aggregation or hydrolysis within end products or in the human body. Colloidal systems containing NPs are at the forefront of peptide research, as they can be designed to encapsulate and protect peptides during biological transit. Water in oil micelles have been successfully used to increase the potency of antimicrobial peptides against *E. coli* (Gontsarik et al., 2016). In another example, liposomes have been used to improve the stability of encapsulated nisin against pH and temperature extremes thereby increasing its potential in food processing (Taylor et al., 2007). Popular NPs vehicle materials

TABLE 2 | Antimicrobial liposomal nanoformulation in clinical development.

Name	Antimicrobial	Clinical trial phase	Target pathogens	ClinicalTrials.gov Identifier
Arikace	Amikacin	III	Gram-negative bacteria	NCT01315691
Lipoquin	Ciprofloxacin	II	Gram-negative bacteria	NCT00889967
Pulmaquin	Ciprofloxacin	III	Gram-negative bacteria	NCT02104245
Silvasorb	Silver	III	Gram-negative bacteria	NCT00659204
MAT2501	Amikacin	–	Gram-negative bacteria	–
QA-PEI	Ammonium Polyehtyleneimine	I-II	Gram-negative and -positive bacteria	NCT01167985

for peptides include phytoglycogen NPs (Bi et al., 2011), chitosan (Wu et al., 2017), pectin (Krivorotova et al., 2017), and alginate (Khaksar et al., 2014).

NPs have also been applied with tremendous success in biodetection systems, namely as sensors and diagnostics platforms with increased sensitivity and selectivity. Due to the decrease in size of the transduction mechanisms provided by NPs, most of these platforms have found applications at point-of-need and/or point-of-care (Costa et al., 2014; Veigas et al., 2014; Weng et al., 2015; Kim J. et al., 2017; Wang et al., 2017b; Galvan and Yu, 2018; Yang et al., 2018). In some cases, diagnostics/sensing and therapeutic properties have been combined onto single NPs, providing for innovative tools – Nanotheranostics. Recently, several nanotheranostics strategies against bacteria have been described (Kuo et al., 2009; DeGrasse, 2012; Dai X. et al., 2013; Khlebtsov et al., 2013; Kim et al., 2013; Gamella et al., 2014; Pei et al., 2014; Setyawati et al., 2014; Patel and Janjic, 2015; Thompson et al., 2015; Jagtap et al., 2017; Mocan et al., 2017; Zhao et al., 2017).

BOTTLENECKS AND FUTURE CHALLENGES OF NPS

Despite the foreseen potential of NPs for medical applications, there are still several bottlenecks related with their acute and long-term exposure in humans. Several routes of exposure must be considered when evaluating NPs exposure, such as oral and gastrointestinal tract, dermal, respiratory system, and endovenous administration directly to the bloodstream (De Matteis, 2017). It is well known also that the physicochemical properties of NPs (e.g., size, shape and surface chemistry) affect their interaction with biological systems, influencing cellular uptake, pharmacokinetics, biodistribution, all of them with direct impact on final biological effects (for recent reviews see Bakand and Hayes, 2016; Xia et al., 2016; De Matteis, 2017; Warheit, 2018). These aspects have been addressed over the past years *via* the evaluation of the *in vitro* and *in vivo* toxicity of metal and metal oxide NPs (Dobrovolskaia et al., 2007; Asharani et al., 2010; Li et al., 2010; Baek and An, 2011; Hackenberg et al., 2011; Conde et al., 2012, 2014; Bondarenko et al., 2013; Ivask et al., 2014; Larsen et al., 2016; Sukwong et al., 2016; Rai et al., 2017), whose conclusions concerning their nanosafety differ depending on the type of assessment. This poses a major concern to effectively draw critical conclusions on NPs safety due to the vast number of different types/shapes/surface modified nanoparticles, the different methods used to evaluate their safety and environmental effects, and also by the fact most of these *in vitro*/*in vivo* studies present acute studies rather than long-term exposure (Bakand and Hayes, 2016; Xia et al., 2016; De Matteis, 2017; Warheit, 2018). Nevertheless, these *in vivo* and *in vitro* studies have been providing clues to the specific mechanisms by which NPs trigger an adverse effect enabling future surface modification of NPs to make them safer and less toxic (De Matteis, 2017). These concerns relating to nanosafety have been addressed and implemented *via* European Commission FP7 and H2020-sponsored programs followed by some relevant conclusions issued by the US National Academy of Science Committee on Research Progress of Environmental Health and Safety Aspects of Engineered Nanomaterials (Warheit, 2018).

Due to the 3Rs (Replacement, Reduction and Refinement) policies of *in vivo* studies, the future challenge of Regulatory Agencies is the standardization of the *in vitro* methodologies to establish the toxicology profile of NPs based on good laboratory practice (GLP) and the construction of flexible and reliable databases in which NPs are classified according to the data derived from these toxicological investigations. Together, these efforts might provide information on the dosage at which a particular NP can be considered safe and thus appropriate for medical use.

CHALLENGES OF CURRENT RESEARCH

As mentioned above, nanomaterials have great potential to prevent and treat bacterial infection, but several challenges remain for the translation to the clinics. Some of these include assessing the interactions of nanoantibiotics with cells, tissues and organs, for dose recalibration and identification of appropriate routes of administration (Sandhiya et al., 2009). The biocompatibility of NPs is generally evaluated through *in vitro* assays, using cell culture. Because NPs, used as antimicrobial agents can enter through skin contact, ingestion, inhalation, oral and intravenous injection, *in vivo* models must also be applied to better understand their effects, including potential toxicity, clearance and metabolism (Beyth et al., 2015). Several studies have shown that intravenously injected NPs accumulate in the colon, lung, bone marrow, liver, spleen and lymphatics (Hagens et al., 2007). Inhalation has also been shown to cause cytotoxicity at the lung, and in the liver, heart and spleen through systemic circulation (Poma and Di Giorgio, 2008; Leucuta, 2013). This is of particular relevance for small NPs because of efficient cellular uptake and transcytosis across epithelial and endothelial cells into the blood and lymphatic circulation. Several NPs systems have demonstrated toxicity in multiple organs, such as free radical-mediated oxidative stress generated by the interaction of antimicrobial NPs with cell components that can result in hepatotoxicity and nephrotoxicity (De Jong and Borm, 2008; Lei et al., 2008).

The effective translation to the clinics will require appropriate guidelines for production and scale-up of manufacturing these nanomaterials, for characterization of the physico-chemical properties and their impact on biocompatibility, for standardization of nanotoxicology assays and protocols to assist easy comparison of data originating from *in vitro* and *in vivo* studies, for the evaluation of their metabolism and mode of action (Duncan and Gaspar, 2011; Bertrand and Leroux, 2012; Beyth et al., 2015; Cordeiro et al., 2016; Rai M. et al., 2016; Zazo et al., 2016). Finally, the community still needs to address the economic impact of translation of these nanomaterials to the clinics.

CONCLUSIONS

Given their vast therapeutic potential, it is becoming increasingly important to understand the mechanisms by which NPs complexes can impact bacterial viability. While one of the beneficial aspects of NPs drug carriers involves "macro-targeting," *i.e.*, specific delivery to the site of infection, understanding the "micro-targeting" of bacterial mechanisms is imperative for the widespread future use of these vectors. Their impact of cell functions such as cell wall permeability, efflux activity, formation of reactive species, and inhibition of essential cellular metabolism and reproduction is of utmost importance.

AUTHOR CONTRIBUTIONS

PB supervision and correction of Nanoparticles part of the manuscript; MPM supervision and correction of MDR bacteria part of the manuscript; AC draft Nanoparticles part of the manuscript, figure draw, tables design; DF draft MDR bacteria part of the manuscript; NM draft MDR bacteria part of the manuscript; MM coordination of MDR bacteria part of the manuscript and final correction and integration; AF coordination of Nanoparticles part of the manuscript and final correction and integration.

ACKNOWLEDGMENTS

This work was supported by the Unidade de Ciências Biomoleculares Aplicadas-UCIBIO, which is financed by National Funds from FCT/MEC (PTDC_CVT-EPI_6685_2014; UID/Multi/04378/2013) and co-financed by the ERDF under the PT2020 Partnership Agreement (POCI-01-0145-FEDER-007728). DF is funded by the Trinity College Dublin Postgraduate Research (1252) Studentship. NM is funded by the Irish Research Council under the employment-based programme EBPPG/2015/233 in conjunction with Nuritas limited. We would like to acknowledge Ana Sofia Santos for preliminary revision of the manuscript.

REFERENCES

Acharya, D., Singha, K. M., Pandey, P., Mohanta, B., Rajkumari, J., and Singha, L. P. (2018). Shape dependent physical mutilation and lethal effects of silver nanoparticles on bacteria. *Sci. Rep.* 8:201. doi: 10.1038/s41598-017-18590-6

Aderibigbe, B. A. (2017). Metal-based nanoparticles for the treatment of infectious diseases. *Molecules* 22:E1370. doi: 10.3390/molecules22081370

Ali, K., Dwivedi, S., Azam, A., Saquib, Q., Al-Said, M. S., Alkhedhairy, A. A., et al. (2016). Aloe vera extract functionalized zinc oxide nanoparticles as nanoantibiotics against multi-drug resistant clinical bacterial isolates. *J. Colloid Interface Sci.* 472, 145–156. doi: 10.1016/j.jcis.2016.03.021

Allahverdiyev, A. M., Kon, K. V., Abamor, E. S., Bagirova, M., and Rafailovich, M. (2011). Coping with antibiotic resistance: combining nanoparticles with antibiotics and other antimicrobial agents. *Expert Rev. AntiInfect. Ther.* 9, 1035–1052. doi: 10.1586/eri.11.121

AlMatar, M., Makky, E. A., Var, I., and Koksal, F. (2017). The role of nanoparticles in the inhibition of multidrug-resistant bacteria and biofilms. *Curr. Drug Deliv.* 15, 470–484. doi: 10.2174/1567201815666171207163504

Andrade, F., Rafael, D., Videira, M., Ferreira, D., Sosnik, A., and Sarmento, B. (2013). Nanotechnology and pulmonary delivery to overcome resistance in infectious diseases. *Adv. Drug Deliv. Rev.* 65, 1816–1827. doi: 10.1016/j.addr.2013.07.020

Ansari, M. A., Khan, H. M., Khan, A. A., Cameotra, S. S., Saquib, Q., and Musarrat, J. (2014). Interaction of Al(2)O(3) nanoparticles with *Escherichia coli* and their cell envelope biomolecules. *J. Appl. Microbiol.* 116, 772–783. doi: 10.1111/jam.12423

Ansari, M. A., Khan, H. M., Khan, A. A., Pal, R., and Cameotra, S. S. (2013). Antibacterial potential of Al2O3 nanoparticles against multidrug resistance strains of *Staphylococcus aureus* isolated from skin exudates. *J. Nanoparticle Res.* 15:1970. doi: 10.1007/s11051-013-1970-1

Antonelli, M., De Pascale, G., Ranieri, V. M., Pelaia, P., Tufano, R., Piazza, O., et al. (2012). Comparison of triple-lumen central venous catheters impregnated with silver nanoparticles (AgTive®) vs conventional catheters in intensive care unit patients. *J. Hosp. Infect.* 82, 101–107. doi: 10.1016/j.jhin.2012.07.010

Argueta-Figueroa, L., Morales-Luckie, R. A., Scougall-Vilchis, R. J., and Olea-Mejía, O. F. (2014). Synthesis, characterization and antibacterial activity of copper, nickel and bimetallic Cu-Ni nanoparticles for potential use in dental materials. *Prog. Nat. Sci. Mater. Int.* 24, 321–328. doi: 10.1016/j.pnsc.2014.07.002

Arvizo, R., Bhattacharya, R., and Mukherjee, P. (2010). Gold nanoparticles: opportunities and challenges in nanomedicine. *Expert Opin. Drug Deliv.* 7, 753–763. doi: 10.1517/17425241003777010

Asharani, P. V., Xinyi, N., Hande, M. P., and Valiyaveettil, S. (2010). DNA damage and p53-mediated growth arrest in human cells treated with platinum nanoparticles. *Nanomedicine* 5, 51–64. doi: 10.2217/nnm.09.85

Ashfaq, M., Verma, N., and Khan, S. (2016). Copper/zinc bimetal nanoparticles-dispersed carbon nanofibers: a novel potential antibiotic material. *Mater. Sci. Eng. C* 59, 938–947. doi: 10.1016/j.msec.2015.10.079

Aswathanarayan, J. B., and Vittal, R. R. (2017). Antimicrobial, biofilm inhibitory and anti-infective activity of metallic nanoparticles against pathogens *MRSA* and *Pseudomonas aeruginosa* PA01. *Pharm. Nanotechnol.* 5, 148–153. doi: 10.2174/2211738505666170424121944

Aydin Sevinç, B., and Hanley, L. (2010). Antibacterial activity of dental composites containing zinc oxide nanoparticles. *J. Biomed. Mater. Res. B Appl. Biomater.* 94, 22–31. doi: 10.1002/jbm.b.31620

Babes, L., Denizot, B., Tanguy, G., Le Jeune, J. J., and Jallet, P. (1999). Synthesis of iron oxide nanoparticles used as MRI contrast agents: a parametric study. *J. Colloid Interface Sci.* 212, 474–482. doi: 10.1006/jcis.1998.6053

Baek, Y.-W., and An, Y.-J. (2011). Microbial toxicity of metal oxide nanoparticles (CuO, NiO, ZnO, and Sb2O3) to *Escherichia coli, Bacillus subtilis*, and *Streptococcus aureus*. *Sci. Total Environ.* 409, 1603–1608. doi: 10.1016/j.scitotenv.2011.01.014

Bahar, A., and Ren, D. (2013). Antimicrobial peptides. *Pharmaceuticals* 6, 1543–1575. doi: 10.3390/ph6121543

Bakand, S., and Hayes, A. (2016). Toxicological considerations, toxicity assessment, and risk management of inhaled nanoparticles. *Int. J. Mol. Sci.* 17:E929. doi: 10.3390/ijms17060929

Baker, S., Pasha, A., and Satish, S. (2017). Biogenic nanoparticles bearing antibacterial activity and their synergistic effect with broad spectrum antibiotics:emerging strategy to combat drug resistant pathogens. *Saudi Pharm. J.* 25, 44–51. doi: 10.1016/j.jsps.2015.06.011

Bassegoda, A., Ivanova, K., Ramon, E., and Tzanov, T. (2018). Strategies to prevent the occurrence of resistance against antibiotics by using advanced materials. *Appl. Microbiol. Biotechnol.* 102, 2075–2089. doi: 10.1007/s00253-018-8776-0

Behera, S. S., Patra, J. K., Pramanik, K., Panda, N., and Thatoi, H. (2012). Characterization and evaluation of antibacterial activities of chemically synthesized iron oxide nanoparticles. *World J. Nano Sci. Eng.* 2, 196–200. doi: 10.4236/wjnse.2012.24026

Berry, C. C., and Curtis, A. S. G. (2003). Functionalisation of magnetic nanoparticles for applications in biomedicine. *J. Phys. D. Appl. Phys.* 36, R198–R206. doi: 10.1088/0022-3727/36/13/203

Bertrand, N., and Leroux, J. C. (2012). The journey of a drug-carrier in the body: an anatomo-physiological perspective. *J. Control. Release* 161, 152–163. doi: 10.1016/j.jconrel.2011.09.098

Beyth, N., Houri-Haddad, Y., Domb, A., Khan, W., and Hazan, R. (2015). Alternative antimicrobial approach: nano-antimicrobial materials. *Evid. Based Complement. Altern. Med.* 2015, 1–16. doi: 10.1155/2015/246012

Bi, L., Yang, L., Narsimhan, G., Bhunia, A., and Yao, Y. (2011). Designing carbohydrate nanoparticles for prolonged efficacy of antimicrobial peptide. *J. Control Release* 150, 150–156. doi: 10.1016/j.jconrel.2010.11.024

Bjarnsholt, T., (2013). The role of bacterial biofilms in chronic infections. *APMIS* 121, 1–58. doi: 10.1111/apm.12099

Boman, H. G., Wade, D., Boman, I. A., Wåhlin, B., and Merrifield, R. B. (1989). Antibacterial and antimalarial properties of peptides that are cecropin-melittin hybrids. *FEBS Lett.* 259, 103–106. doi: 10.1016/0014-5793(89)81505-4

Bondarenko, O., Ivask, A., Käkinen, A., Kurvet, I., and Kahru, A. (2013). Particle-cell contact enhances antibacterial activity of silver nanoparticles. *PLoS ONE* 8:e64060. doi: 10.1371/journal.pone.0064060

Brandelli, A. (2012). Nanostructures as promising tools for delivery of antimicrobial peptides. *Mini Rev. Med. Chem.* 12, 731–741. doi: 10.2174/138955712801264774

Bresee, J., Bond, C. M., Worthington, R. J., Smith, C. A., Gifford, J. C., Simpson, C. A., et al. (2014). Nanoscale structure–activity relationships, mode of action, and biocompatibility of gold nanoparticle antibiotics. *J. Am. Chem. Soc.* 136, 5295–5300. doi: 10.1021/ja408505n

Brown, A. N., Smith, K., Samuels, T. A., Lu, J., Obare, S. O., and Scott, M. E. (2012). Nanoparticles functionalized with ampicillin destroy multiple-antibiotic-resistant isolates of *Pseudomonas aeruginosa* and *Enterobacter aerogenes* and methicillin-resistant *Staphylococcus aureus*. *Appl. Environ. Microbiol.* 78, 2768–2774. doi: 10.1128/AEM.06513-11

Burygin, G., Khlebtsov, B., Shantrokha, A., Dykman, L., Bogatyrev, V., Khlebtsov, N., et al. (2009). On the enhanced antibacterial activity of antibiotics mixed with gold nanoparticles. *Nanoscale Res. Lett.* 4, 794–801. doi: 10.1007/s11671-009-9316-8

Casciaro, B., Moros, M., Rivera-Fernández, S., Bellelli, A., de la Fuente, J. M., and Mangoni, M. L. (2017). Gold-nanoparticles coated with the antimicrobial peptide esculentin-1a(1-21)NH2 as a reliable strategy for antipseudomonal drugs. *Acta Biomater.* 47, 170–181. doi: 10.1016/j.actbio.2016.09.041

Caster, J. M., Patel, A. N., Zhang, T., and Wang, A. (2017). Investigational nanomedicines in 2016: a review of nanotherapeutics currently undergoing clinical trials. *Wiley Interdiscip. Rev. Nanomed. Nanobiotechnol.* 9:e1416. doi: 10.1002/wnan.1416

Cavassin, E. D., de Figueiredo, L. F. P., Otoch, J. P., Seckler, M. M., de Oliveira, R. A., Franco, F. F., et al. (2015). Comparison of methods to detect the *in vitro* activity of silver nanoparticles (AgNP) against multidrug resistant bacteria. *J. Nanobiotechnol.* 13, 1–16. doi: 10.1186/s12951-015-0120-6

Cha, S. H., Hong, J., McGuffie, M., Yeom, B., Vanepps, J. S., and Kotov, N. A. (2015). Shape-dependent biomimetic inhibition of enzyme by nanoparticles and their antibacterial activity. *ACS Nano* 9, 9097–9105. doi: 10.1021/acsnano.5b03247

Chakraborti, S., Mandal, A. K., Sarwar, S., Singh, P., Chakraborty, R., and Chakrabarti, P. (2014). Bactericidal effect of polyethyleneimine capped ZnO nanoparticles on multiple antibiotic resistant bacteria harboring genes of high-pathogenicity island. *Colloids Surf. B. Biointerfaces* 121, 44–53. doi: 10.1016/j.colsurfb.2014.03.044

Chakraborty, R., Sarkar, R. K., Chatterjee, A. K., Manju, U., Chattopadhyay, A. P., and Basu, T. (2015). A simple, fast and cost-effective method of synthesis of cupric oxide nanoparticle with promising antibacterial potency: unraveling the biological and chemical modes of action. *Biochim. Biophys. Acta Gen. Subj.* 1850, 845–856. doi: 10.1016/j.bbagen.2015.01.015

Chang, T. Y., Chen, C. C., Cheng, K. M., Chin, C. Y., Chen, Y. H., Chen, X. A., et al. (2017). Trimethyl chitosan-capped silver nanoparticles with positive surface charge: their catalytic activity and antibacterial spectrum including multidrug-resistant strains of *Acinetobacter baumannii*. *Colloids Surf. B. Biointerfaces* 155, 61–70. doi: 10.1016/j.colsurfb.2017.03.054

Chaurasia, A. K., Thorat, N. D., Tandon, A., Kim, J. H., Park, S. H., and Kim, K. K. (2016). Coupling of radiofrequency with magnetic nanoparticles treatment as an alternative physical antibacterial strategy against multiple drug resistant bacteria. *Sci. Rep.* 6, 1–13. doi: 10.1038/srep33662

Chen, C. W., Hsu, C. Y., Lai, S. M., Syu, W. J., Wang, T. Y., and Lai, P. S. (2014). Metal nanobullets for multidrug resistant bacteria and biofilms. *Adv. Drug Deliv. Rev.* 78, 88–104. doi: 10.1016/j.addr.2014.08.004

Chen, F., Shi, Z., Neoh, K., and Kang, E. (2009). Antioxidant and antibacterial activities of eugenol and carvacrol-grafted chitosan nanoparticles. *Biotechnol Bioeng.* 104, 30–39. doi: 10.1002/bit.22363

Chen, J., Hessler, J. A., Putchakayala, K., Panama, B. K., Khan, D. P., Hong, S., et al. (2009). Cationic nanoparticles induce nanoscale disruption in living cell plasma membranes. *J. Phys. Chem. B* 113, 11179–11185. doi: 10.1021/jp9033936

Cho, K. H., Park, J. E., Osaka, T., and Park, S. G. (2005). The study of antimicrobial activity and preservative effects of nanosilver ingredient. *Electrochim. Acta* 51, 956–960. doi: 10.1016/j.electacta.2005.04.071

Choi, S. R., Britigan, B. E., Moran, D. M., and Narayanasamy, P. (2017). Gallium nanoparticles facilitate phagosome maturation and inhibit growth of virulent *Mycobacterium tuberculosis* in macrophages. *PLoS ONE* 12:e0177987. doi: 10.1371/journal.pone.0177987

Chopra, I. (2007). The increasing use of silver-based products as antimicrobial agents: a useful development or a cause for concern? *J. Antimicrob. Chemother.* 59, 587–590. doi: 10.1093/jac/dkm006

Claeys, K. C., Heil, E. L., Pogue, J. M., Lephart, P. R., and Johnson, J. K. (2018). The Verigene dilemma: gram-negative polymicrobial bloodstream infections and clinical decision making. *Diagn. Microbiol. Infect. Dis.* 91, 144–146. doi: 10.1016/j.diagmicrobio.2018.01.012

Clancy, J. P., Dupont, L., Konstan, M. W., Billings, J., Fustik, S., Goss, C. H., et al. (2013). Phase II studies of nebulised Arikace in CF patients with *Pseudomonas aeruginosa* infection. *Thorax* 68, 818–825. doi: 10.1136/thoraxjnl-2012-202230

Conde, J., Doria, G., and Baptista, P. V. (2012). Noble metal nanoparticles applications in cancer. *J. Drug Deliv.* 2012:751075. doi: 10.1155/2012/751075

Conde, J., Larguinho, M., Cordeiro, A., Raposo, L. R., Costa, M., Santos, S., et al. (2014). Gold-Nanobeacons for gene therapy : evaluation of genotoxicity, cell toxicity and proteome profiling analysis. *Nanotocicology* 8, 521–532. doi: 10.3109/17435390.2013.802821

Cordeiro, M., Ferreira Carlos, F., Pedrosa, P., Lopez, A., and Baptista, P. V. (2016). Gold nanoparticles for diagnostics: advances towards points of care. *Diagnostics* 6:43. doi: 10.3390/diagnostics6040043

Costa, M. N., Veigas, B., Jacob, J. M., Santos, D. S., Gomes, J., Baptista, P. V., et al. (2014). A low cost, safe, disposable, rapid and self-sustainable paper-based platform for diagnostic testing: lab-on-paper. *Nanotechnology* 25:94006. doi: 10.1088/0957-4484/25/9/094006

Courtney, C. M., Goodman, S. M., Nagy, T. A., Levy, M., Bhusal, P., Madinger, N. E., et al. (2017). Potentiating antibiotics in drug-resistant clinical isolates via stimuli-activated superoxide generation. *Sci. Adv.* 3:e1701776. doi: 10.1126/sciadv.1701776

Cui, Y., Zhao, Y., Tian, Y., Zhang, W., Lu, X., and Jiang, X. (2012). The molecular mechanism of action of bactericidal gold nanoparticles on *Escherichia coli*. *Biomaterials* 33, 2327–2333. doi: 10.1016/j.biomaterials.2011.11.057

Dai, T., Gupta, A., Murray, C. K., Vrahas, M. S., Tegos, G. P., and Hamblin, M. R. (2013). Blue Light for infectious diseases: *Propionibacterium acnes*, *Helicobacter pylori*, and beyond? *Drug Resist.* 15, 223–236. doi: 10.1016/j.drup.2012.07.001.Blue

Dai, X., Fan, Z., Lu, Y., and Ray, P. C. (2013). Multifunctional nanoplatforms for targeted multidrug-resistant-bacteria theranostic applications. *ACS Appl. Mater. Interfaces* 5, 11348–11354. doi: 10.1021/am403567k

Dakal, T. C., Kumar, A., Majumdar, R. S., and Yadav, V. (2016). Mechanistic basis of antimicrobial actions of silver nanoparticles. *Front. Microbiol.* 7:1831. doi: 10.3389/fmicb.2016.01831

De Jong, W. H., and Borm, P. J., a (2008). Drug delivery and nanoparticles:applications and hazards. *Int. J. Nanomedicine* 3, 133–149. doi: 10.2147/IJN.S596

De Matteis, V. (2017). Exposure to inorganic nanoparticles: routes of entry, immune response, biodistribution and *in vitro/in vivo* toxicity evaluation. *Toxics* 5:E29. doi: 10.3390/toxics5040029

DeGrasse, J. A. (2012). A single-stranded DNA aptamer that selectively binds to *Staphylococcus aureus* enterotoxin B. *PLoS ONE* 7:e33410. doi: 10.1371/journal.pone.0033410

Ding, F., Songkiatisak, P., Cherukuri, P. K., Huang, T., and Xu, X.-H. N. (2018). Size-dependent inhibitory effects of antibiotic drug nanocarriers against *Pseudomonas aeruginosa*. *ACS Omega* 3, 1231–1243. doi: 10.1021/acsomega.7b01956

Djafari, J., Marinho, C., Santos, T., Igrejas, G., Torres, C., Capelo, J. L., et al. (2016). New synthesis of gold- and silver-based nano-tetracycline composites. *ChemistryOpen* 5, 206–212. doi: 10.1002/open.201600016

Dobrovolskaia, M. A., McNeil, S. E., and Neil, S. E. M. (2007). Immunological properties of engineered nanomaterials. *Nat. Nanotechnol.* 2, 469–478. doi: 10.1038/nnano.2007.223

Doria, G., Larguinho, M., Dias, J. T., Pereira, E., Franco, R., and Baptista, P., V (2010). Gold-silver-alloy nanoprobes for one-pot multiplex DNA detection. *Nanotechnology* 21:255101. doi: 10.1088/0957-4484/21/25/255101

dos Santos, M. M., Queiroz, M. J., and Baptista, P. V. (2012). Enhancement of antibiotic effect via gold:silver-alloy nanoparticles. *J. Nanoparticle Res.* 14:859. doi: 10.1007/s11051-012-0859-8

Dos Santos, V. E., Filho, A. V., Ribeiro Targino, A. G., Pelagio Flores, M. A., Galembeck, A., Caldas, A. F., et al. (2014). A new "silver-Bullet" to treat caries in children - Nano Silver Fluoride: a randomised clinical trial. *J. Dent.* 42, 945–951. doi: 10.1016/j.jdent.2014.05.017

Duncan, R., and Gaspar, R. (2011). Nanomedicine(s) under the microscope. *Mol. Pharm.* 8, 2101–2141. doi: 10.1021/mp200394t

Durán, N., Durán, M., de Jesus, M. B., Seabra, A. B., Fávaro, W. J., and Nakazato, G. (2016). Silver nanoparticles: a new view on mechanistic aspects on antimicrobial activity. *Nanomed. Nanotechnol. Biol. Med.* 12, 789–799. doi: 10.1016/j.nano.2015.11.016

Durán, N., Marcato, P. D., De Conti, R., Alves, O. L., Costa, F. T. M., and Brocchi, M. (2010). Potential use of silver nanoparticles on pathogenic bacteria, their toxicity and possible mechanisms of action. *J. Braz. Chem. Soc.* 21, 949–959. doi: 10.1590/s0103-50532010000600002

Dwivedi, S., Wahab, R., Khan, F., Mishra, Y. K., Musarrat, J., and Al-Khedhairy, A. A. (2014). Reactive oxygen species mediated bacterial biofilm inhibition via zinc oxide nanoparticles and their statistical determination. *PLoS ONE* 9:e111289. doi: 10.1371/journal.pone.0111289

Ehsan, S., and Sajjad, M. (2017). Bioinspired synthesis of zinc oxide nanoparticle and its combined efficacy with different antibiotics against multidrug resistant bacteria. *J. Biomater. Nanobiotechnol.* 8, 159–175. doi: 10.4236/jbnb.2017.82011

El Din, S. N., El-Tayeb, T. A., Abou-Aisha, K., and El-Azizi, M. (2016). *In vitro* and *in vivo* antimicrobial activity of combined therapy of silver nanoparticles and visible blue light against *Pseudomonas aeruginosa*. *Int. J. Nanomedicine* 11, 1749–1758. doi: 10.2147/IJN.S102398

El-Zowalaty, M. E., Al-Ali, S. H. H., Husseiny, M. I., Geilich, B. M., Webster, T. J., and Hussein, M. Z. (2015). The ability of streptomycin-loaded chitosan-coated magnetic nanocomposites to possess antimicrobial and antituberculosis activities. *Int. J. Nanomed.* 10, 3269–3274. doi: 10.2147/IJN.S74469

Esmaeillou, M., Zarrini, G., Rezaee, M. A., Mojarrad, J. S., and Bahadori, A. (2017). Vancomycin capped with silver nanoparticles as an antibacterial agent against multi-drug resistance bacteria. *Adv. Pharm. Bull.* 7, 479–483. doi: 10.15171/apb.2017.058

Espitia, P. J. P., Soares, N., de, F. F., Coimbra, J. S. dos, R., de Andrade, N. J., Cruz, R. S., and Medeiros, E. A. A. (2012). Zinc oxide nanoparticles: synthesis, antimicrobial activity and food packaging applications. *Food Bioprocess Technol.* 5, 1447–1464. doi: 10.1007/s11947-012-0797-6

Fakhri, A., Tahami, S., and Naji, M. (2017). Synthesis and characterization of core-shell bimetallic nanoparticles for synergistic antimicrobial effect studies in combination with doxycycline on burn specific pathogens. *J. Photochem. Photobiol. B Biol.* 169, 21–26. doi: 10.1016/j.jphotobiol.2017.02.014

Fernandes, A. R., and Baptista, P. V. (2017). Gene silencing using multifunctionalized gold nanoparticles for cancer therapy. *Methods Mol. Biol.* 1530, 319–336. doi: 10.1007/978-1-4939-6646-2_19

Fernandes, A. R., Jesus, J., Martins, P., Figueiredo, S., Rosa, D., Martins, L. M., et al. (2017). Multifunctional gold-nanoparticles: a nanovectorization tool for the targeted delivery of novel chemotherapeutic agents. *J. Control. Release* 245, 52–61. doi: 10.1016/j.jconrel.2016.11.021

Foster, H. A., Ditta, I. B., Varghese, S., and Steele, A. (2011). Photocatalytic disinfection using titanium dioxide: spectrum and mechanism of antimicrobial activity. *Appl. Microbiol. Biotechnol.* 90, 1847–1868. doi: 10.1007/s00253-011-3213-7

Franci, G., Falanga, A., Galdiero, S., Palomba, L., Rai, M., Morelli, G., et al. (2015). Silver nanoparticles as potential antibacterial agents. *Molecules* 20, 8856–8874. doi: 10.3390/molecules20058856

Galanzha, E. I., Shashkov, E., Sarimollaoglu, M., Beenken, K. E., Basnakian, A. G., Shirtliff, M. E., et al. (2012). *In vivo* magnetic enrichment, photoacoustic diagnosis, and photothermal purging of infected blood using multifunctional gold and magnetic nanoparticles. *PLoS ONE* 7:e45557. doi: 10.1371/journal.pone.0045557

Galvan, D. D., and Yu, Q. (2018). Surface-enhanced raman scattering for rapid detection and characterization of antibiotic-resistant bacteria. *Adv. Healthc. Mater.* doi: 10.1002/adhm.201701335. [Epub ahead of print].

Gamella, M., Guz, N., Mailloux, S., Pingarrón, J. M., and Katz, E. (2014). Antibacterial drug release electrochemically stimulated by the presence of bacterial cells - theranostic approach. *Electroanalysis* 26, 2552–2557. doi: 10.1002/elan.201400473

Gao, W., Chen, Y., Chang, Y., Zhang, Y., Chang, Q., and Zhang, L. (2018). Nanoparticle-based local antimicrobial drug delivery. *Adv Drug Deliv Rev.* 127, 46–57. doi: 10.1016/j.addr.2017.09.015

Gao, W., Thamphiwatana, S., Angsantikul, P., and Zhang, L. (2014). Nanoparticle approaches against bacterial infections. *Wiley Interdiscip. Rev. Nanomed. Nanobiotechnol.* 6, 532–547. doi: 10.1002/wnan.1282

García-Lara, B., Saucedo-Mora, M. Á., Roldán-Sánchez, J. A., Pérez-Eretza, B., Ramasamy, M., Lee, J., et al. (2015). Inhibition of quorum-sensing-dependent virulence factors and biofilm formation of clinical and environmental *Pseudomonas aeruginosa* strains by ZnO nanoparticles. *Lett Appl Microbiol.* 61, 299–305. doi: 10.1111/lam.12456

Gelabert, A., Sivry, Y., Gobbi, P., Mansouri-Guilani, N., Menguy, N., Brayner, R., et al. (2016). Testing nanoeffect onto model bacteria: impact of speciation and genotypes. *Nanotoxicology* 10, 216–225. doi: 10.3109/17435390.2015.1048323

Gholipourmalekabadi, M., Mobaraki, M., Ghaffari, M., Zarebkohan, A., Omrani, V., Urbanska, A., et al. (2017). Targeted drug delivery based on gold nanoparticle derivatives. *Curr. Pharm. Des.* 23, 2918–2929. doi: 10.2174/1381612823666170419105413

Gil-Tomás, J., Tubby, S., Parkin, I. P., Narband, N., Dekker, L., Nair, S. P., et al. (2007). Lethal photosensitisation of *Staphylococcus aureus* using a toluidine blue O–tiopronin–gold nanoparticle conjugate. *J. Mater. Chem.* 17:3739. doi: 10.1039/b706615e

Gontsarik, M., Buhmann, M., Yaghmur, A., Ren, Q., Maniura-Weber, K., and Salentinig, S. (2016). Antimicrobial peptide - driven colloidal transformations in liquid crystalline nanocarriers. *J. Phys. Chem. Lett.* 7, 3482–3486. doi: 10.1021/acs.jpclett.6b01622

Govindaraju, S., Samal, M., and Yun, K. (2016). Superior antibacterial activity of GlcN-AuNP-GO by ultraviolet irradiation. *Mater. Sci. Eng. C* 69, 366–372. doi: 10.1016/j.msec.2016.06.052

Gu, H., Ho, P. L., Tong, E., Wang, L., and Xu, B. (2003). Presenting vancomycin on nanoparticles to enhance antimicrobial activities. *Nano Lett.* 3, 1261–1263. doi: 10.1021/nl034396z

Hackenberg, S., Scherzed, A., Kessler, M., Hummel, S., Technau, A., Froelich, K., et al. (2011). Silver nanoparticles: evaluation of DNA damage, toxicity and functional impairment in human mesenchymal stem cells. *Toxicol. Lett.* 201, 27–33. doi: 10.1016/j.toxlet.2010.12.001

Hadiya, S., Liu, X., Abd El-Hammed, W., Elsabahy, M., and Aly, S. A. (2018). Levofloxacin-loaded nanoparticles decrease emergence of fluoroquinolone resistance in *Escherichia coli*. *Microb. Drug Resist.* doi: 10.1089/mdr.2017.0304. [Epub ahead of print].

Hagens, W. I., Oomen, A. G., de Jong, W. H., Cassee, F. R., and Sips, A. J. A. M. (2007). What do we (need to) know about the kinetic properties of nanoparticles in the body? *Regul. Toxicol. Pharmacol.* 49, 217–229. doi: 10.1016/j.yrtph.2007.07.006

Hall-Stoodley, L., Costerton, J. W., and Stoodley, P. (2004). Bacterial biofilms: from the Natural environment to infectious diseases. *Nat. Rev. Microbiol.* 2, 95–108. doi: 10.1038/nrmicro821

Hemeg, H. A. (2017). Nanomaterials for alternative antibacterial therapy. *Int. J. Nanomed.* 12, 8211–8225. doi: 10.2147/IJN.S132163

Høiby, N., Ciofu, O., Johansen, H. K., Song, Z.-J., Moser, C., Jensen, P. Ø., et al. (2011). The clinical impact of bacterial biofilms. *Int J Oral Sci.* 3, 55–65. doi: 10.4248/IJOS11026

Hsueh, Y. H., Ke, W. J., Hsieh, C., Te, L.in, K. S., Tzou, D. Y., and Chiang, C. L. (2015). ZnO nanoparticles affect bacillus subtilis cell growth and biofilm formation. *PLoS ONE* 10:e0128457. doi: 10.1371/journal.pone.0128457

Hu, D., Li, H., Wang, B., Ye, Z., Lei, W., Jia, F., et al. (2017). Surface-adaptive gold nanoparticles with effective adherence and enhanced photothermal ablation of methicillin-resistant *Staphylococcus aureus* biofilm. *ACS Nano* 11, 9330–9339. doi: 10.1021/acsnano.7b04731

Huang, N., Chen, X., Zhu, X., Xu, M., and Liu, J. (2017). Ruthenium complexes/polypeptide self-assembled nanoparticles for identification of bacterial infection and targeted antibacterial research. *Biomaterials* 141, 296–313. doi: 10.1016/j.biomaterials.2017.07.005

Huang, Y., Yu, F., Park, Y., Wang, J., Shin, M., Chung, H., et al. (2010). Co-administration of protein drugs with gold nanoparticles to enable percutaneous delivery. *Biomaterials* 31, 9086–9091. doi: 10.1016/j.biomaterials.2010.08.046

Huh, A. J., and Kwon, Y. J. (2011). "Nanoantibiotics": a new paradigm for treating infectious diseases using nanomaterials in the antibiotics resistant era. *J. Control. Release* 156, 128–145. doi: 10.1016/j.jconrel.2011.07.002

Iravani, S., Korbekandi, H., Mirmohammadi, S. V., and Zolfaghari, B. (2014). Synthesis of silver nanoparticles: chemical, physical and biological methods. *Res. Pharm. Sci.* 9, 385–406.

Ivask, A., Juganson, K., Bondarenko, O., Mortimer, M., Aruoja, V., Kasemets, K., et al. (2014). Mechanisms of toxic action of Ag, ZnO and CuO nanoparticles to selected ecotoxicological test organisms and mammalian cells *in vitro*: a comparative review. *Nanotoxicology* 8, 57–71. doi: 10.3109/17435390.2013.855831

Jagtap, P., Sritharan, V., and Gupta, S. (2017). Nanotheranostic approaches for management of bloodstream bacterial infections. *Nanomedicine* 13, 329–341. doi: 10.1016/j.nano.2016.09.005

Jaiswal, S., Bhattacharya, K., McHale, P., and Duffy, B. (2015). Dual effects of β-cyclodextrin-stabilised silver nanoparticles: enhanced biofilm inhibition and reduced cytotoxicity. *J. Mater. Sci. Mater. Med.* 26, 1–10. doi: 10.1007/s10856-014-5367-1

Jakobsen, T. H., Tolker-Nielsen, T., and Givskov, M. (2017). Bacterial biofilm control by perturbation of bacterial signaling processes. *Int. J. Mol. Sci.* 18:E1970. doi: 10.3390/ijms18091970

Jankauskaite, V., Vitkauskiene, A., Lazauskas, A., Baltrusaitis, J., Prosyčevas, I., and Andrulevičius, M. (2016). Bactericidal effect of graphene oxide/Cu/Ag nanoderivatives against *Escherichia coli, Pseudomonas aeruginosa, Klebsiella pneumoniae, Staphylococcus aureus* and Methicillin-resistant *Staphylococcus aureus*. *Int. J. Pharm.* 511, 90–97. doi: 10.1016/j.ijpharm.2016.06.121

Joost, U., Juganson, K., Visnapuu, M., Mortimer, M., Kahru, A., Nommiste, E., et al. (2015). Photocatalytic antibacterial activity of nano-TiO2 (anatase)-based thin films: effects on *Escherichia coli* cells and fatty acids. *J. Photochem. Photobiol. B* 142, 178–185. doi: 10.1016/j.jphotobiol.2014.12.010

Jung, W. K., Koo, H. C., Kim, K. W., Kim, S. H., Park, Y. H., Jung, W. K., et al. (2008). Antibacterial activity and mechanism of action of the silver ion in *Staphylococcus aureus* and *Escherichia coli*. *Appl. Environ. Microbiol.* 74, 2171–2178. doi: 10.1128/AEM.02001-07

Kadiyala, U., Kotov, N. A., and VanEpps, J. S. (2018). Antibacterial metal oxide nanoparticles: challenges in interpreting the literature. *Curr. Pharm. Des.* 24, 896–903. doi: 10.2174/1381612824666180219130659

Karimi, F., Dabbagh, S., Alizadeh, S., and Rostamnia, S. (2016). Evaluation of AgClNPs@SBA-15/IL nanoparticle-induced oxidative stress and DNA mutation in *Escherichia coli*. *Appl. Microbiol. Biotechnol.* 100, 7161–7170. doi: 10.1007/s00253-016-7593-6

Kato, N., Morohoshi, T., Nozawa, T., Matsumoto, H., and Ikeda, T. (2006). Control of gram- negative bacterial quorum sensing with cyclodextrin immobilized cellulose ether gel. *J. Incl. Phenom. Macrocycl. Chem.* 56, 55–59. doi: 10.1007/s10847-006-9060-y

Katva, S., Das, S., Moti, H. S., Jyoti, A., and Kaushik, S. (2018). Antibacterial synergy of silver nanoparticles with gentamicin and chloramphenicol against *Enterococcus faecalis*. *Pharmacogn. Mag.* 13, S828–S833. doi: 10.4103/pm.pm_120_17

Katz, E., and Willner, I. (2004). Integrated nanoparticle-biomolecule hybrid systems: synthesis, properties, and applications. *Angew. Chem. Int. Ed.* 43, 6042–6108. doi: 10.1002/anie.200400651

Kaweeteerawat, C., Na Ubol, P., Sangmuang, S., Aueviriyavit, S., and Maniratanachote, R. (2017). Mechanisms of antibiotic resistance in bacteria mediated by silver nanoparticles. *J. Toxicol. Environ. Health A.* 80, 1276–1289. doi: 10.1080/15287394.2017.1376727

Khaksar, R., Hosseini, S., Hosseini, H., Shijaee-Aliabadi, S., Mohammadifa, M., Mortazavian, A. M., et al. (2014). Nisin-loaded alginate-high methoxy pectin microparticles: preparation and physicochemical characterisation. *Int. J. Food Sci. Technol.* 49, 2076–2082. doi: 10.1111/ijfs.12516

Khameneh, B., Diab, R., Ghazvini, K., and Fazly Bazzaz, B. S. (2016). Breakthroughs in bacterial resistance mechanisms and the potential ways to combat them. *Microb. Pathog.* 95, 32–42. doi: 10.1016/j.micpath.2016.02.009

Khan, S., Khan, S. N., Meena, R., Dar, A. M., Pal, R., and Khan, A. U. (2017). Photoinactivation of multidrug resistant bacteria by monomeric methylene blue conjugated gold nanoparticles. *J. Photochem. Photobiol. B* 174, 150–161. doi: 10.1016/j.jphotobiol.2017.07.011

Khlebtsov, B. N., Tuchina, E. S., Khanadeev, V. A., Panfilova, E. V., Petrov, P. O., Tuchin, V. V., et al. (2013). Enhanced photoinactivation of *Staphylococcus aureus* with nanocomposites containing plasmonic particles and hematoporphyrin. *J. Biophotonics* 6, 338–351. doi: 10.1002/jbio.201200079

Kim, D., Kim, M., Shinde, S., Sung, J., and Ghodake, G. (2017). Cytotoxicity and antibacterial assessment of gallic acid capped gold nanoparticles synthesized at ambient temperature. *Coll. Surfaces B Biointerfaces* 149, 162–167. doi: 10.1016/j.colsurfb.2016.10.017

Kim, J., Kim, H., Park, J. H., and Jon, S. (2017). Gold nanorod-based photo-PCR system for one-step, rapid detection of bacteria. *Nanotheranostics* 1, 178–185. doi: 10.7150/ntno.18720

Kim, J.-W., Galanzha, E. I., Zaharoff, D. A., Griffin, R. J., and Zharov, V. P. (2013). Nanotheranostics of circulating tumor cells, infections and other pathological features *in vivo*. *Mol. Pharm.* 10, 813–830. doi: 10.1021/mp300577s

Krivorotova, T., Staneviciene, R., Luksa, J., Serviene, E., and Sereikaite, J. (2017). Impact of pectin esterification on the antimicrobial activity of nisin-loaded pectin particles. *Biotechnol. Prog.* 33, 245–251. doi: 10.1002/btpr.2391

Kruk, T., Szczepanowicz, K., Stefanska, J., Socha, R. P., and Warszynski, P. (2015). Synthesis and antimicrobial activity of monodisperse copper nanoparticles. *Coll. Surfaces B Biointerfaces* 128, 17–22. doi: 10.1016/j.colsurfb.2015.02.009

Kulshrestha, S., Qayyum, S., and Khan, A. U. (2017). Antibiofilm efficacy of green synthesized graphene oxide-silver nanocomposite using Lagerstroemia speciosa floral extract: a comparative study on inhibition of gram-positive and gram-negative biofilms. *Microb. Pathog.* 103, 167–177. doi: 10.1016/j.micpath.2016.12.022

Kuo, W.-S., Chang, C.-N., Chang, Y.-T., and Yeh, C.-S. (2009). Antimicrobial gold nanorods with dual-modality photodynamic inactivation and hyperthermia. *Chem. Commun.* 28, 4853–4855. doi: 10.1039/b907274h

Kuo, Y.-L., Wang, S.-G., Wu, C.-Y., Lee, K.-C., Jao, C.-J., Chou, S.-H., et al. (2016). Functional gold nanoparticle-based antibacterial agents for nosocomial and antibiotic-resistant bacteria. *Nanomedicine* 11, 2497–2510. doi: 10.2217/nnm-2016-0232

Lai, H. Z., Chen, W. Y., Wu, C. Y., and Chen, Y. C. (2015). Potent antibacterial nanoparticles for pathogenic bacteria. *ACS Appl. Mater. Interfaces* 7, 2046–2054. doi: 10.1021/am507919m

Lakshmi Prasanna, V., and Vijayaraghavan, R. (2015). Insight into the mechanism of antibacterial activity of ZnO: surface defects mediated reactive oxygen species even in the dark. *Langmuir* 31, 9155–9162. doi: 10.1021/acs.langmuir.5b02266

Lambadi, P. R., Sharma, T. K., Kumar, P., Vasnani, P., Thalluri, S. M., Bisht, N., et al. (2015). Facile biofunctionalization of silver nanoparticles for enhanced antibacterial properties, endotoxin removal, and biofilm control. *Int. J. Nanomed.* 10, 2155–2171. doi: 10.2147/IJN.S72923

Lara, H. H., Ayala-Núñez, N. V., Ixtepan Turrent, L., del, C., and Rodríguez Padilla, C. (2010). Bactericidal effect of silver nanoparticles against multidrug-resistant bacteria. *World J. Microbiol. Biotechnol.* 26, 615–621. doi: 10.1007/s11274-009-0211-3

Larsen, S. T., Jackson, P., Poulsen, S. S., Levin, M., Jensen, K. A., Wallin, H., et al. (2016). Airway irritation, inflammation, and toxicity in mice following inhalation of metal oxide nanoparticles. *Nanotoxicology* 10, 1254–1262. doi: 10.1080/17435390.2016.1202350

LaSarre, B., and Federle, M. J. (2013). Exploiting quorum sensing to confuse bacterial pathogens. *Microbiol. Mol. Biol. Rev.* 77, 73–111. doi: 10.1128/MMBR.00046-12

Lebeaux, D., Ghigo, J.-M., and Beloin, C. (2014). Biofilm-related infections: bridging the gap between clinical management and fundamental aspects of recalcitrance toward antibiotics. *Microbiol. Mol. Biol. Rev.* 78, 510–543. doi: 10.1128/MMBR.00013-14

Lee, J. H., Kim, Y. G., Cho, M. H., and Lee, J. (2014). ZnO nanoparticles inhibit *Pseudomonas aeruginosa* biofilm formation and virulence factor production. *Microbiol Res.* 169, 888–896. doi: 10.1016/j.micres.2014.05.005

Lee, P. C., and Meisel, D. (1982). Adsorption and surface-enhanced Raman of dyes on silver and gold sols. *J. Phys. Chem.* 86, 3391–3395. doi: 10.1021/j100214a025

Lee, W. S., Hsieh, T. C., Shiau, J. C., Ou, T. Y., Chen, F. L., Liu, Y. H., et al. (2017). Bio-Kil, a nano-based disinfectant, reduces environmental bacterial burden and multidrug-resistant organisms in intensive care units. *J. Microbiol. Immunol. Infect.* 50, 737–746. doi: 10.1016/j.jmii.2016.04.008

Lei, R., Wu, C., Yang, B., Ma, H., Shi, C., Wang, Q., et al. (2008). Integrated metabolomic analysis of the nano-sized copper particle-induced hepatotoxicity and nephrotoxicity in rats: a rapid *in vivo* screening method for nanotoxicity. *Toxicol. Appl. Pharmacol.* 232, 292–301. doi: 10.1016/j.taap.2008.06.026

Lellouche, J., Kahana, E., Elias, S., Gedanken, A., and Banin, E. (2009). Antibiofilm activity of nanosized magnesium fluoride. *Biomaterials* 30, 5969–5978. doi: 10.1016/j.biomaterials.2009.07.037

Lesniak, A., Salvati, A., Santos-Martinez, M. J., Radomski, M. W., Dawson, K. A., and Åberg, C. (2013). Nanoparticle adhesion to the cell membrane and its effect on nanoparticle uptake efficiency. *J. Am. Chem. Soc.* 135, 1438–1444. doi: 10.1021/ja309812z

Leuba, K. D., Durmus, N. G., Taylor, E. N., and Webster, T. J. (2013). Short communication: carboxylate functionalized superparamagnetic iron oxide nanoparticles (SPION) for the reduction of *S. aureus* growth post biofilm formation. *Int. J. Nanomedicine* 8, 731–736. doi: 10.2147/IJN.S38256

Leucuta, S. E. (2013). Systemic and biophase bioavailability and pharmacokinetics of nanoparticulate drug delivery systems. *Curr. Drug Deliv.* 10, 208–240. doi: 10.2174/1567201811310020007

LewisOscar, F., MubarakAli, D., Nithya, C., Priyanka, R., Gopinath, V., Alharbi, N. S., et al. (2015). One pot synthesis and anti-biofilm potential of copper nanoparticles (CuNPs) against clinical strains of *Pseudomonas aeruginosa*. *Biofouling* 31, 379–391. doi: 10.1080/08927014.2015.1048686

Li, H., Chen, Q., Zhao, J., and Urmila, K. (2015). Enhancing the antimicrobial activity of natural extraction using the synthetic ultrasmall metal nanoparticles. *Sci. Rep.* 5:11033. doi: 10.1038/srep11033

Li, J. J., Hartono, D., Ong, C. N., Bay, B. H., and Yung, L. Y. L. (2010). Autophagy and oxidative stress associated with gold nanoparticles. *Biomaterials* 31, 5996–6003. doi: 10.1016/j.biomaterials.2010.04.014

Li, X., Robinson, S. M., Gupta, A., Saha, K., Jiang, Z., Moyano, D. F., et al. (2014). Functional gold nanoparticles as potent antimicrobial agents against multi-drug-resistant bacteria. *ACS Nano* 8, 10682–10686. doi: 10.1021/nn5042625

Li, Y., Yu, S., Wu, Q., Tang, M., Pu, Y., and Wang, D. (2012a). Chronic Al2O3-nanoparticle exposure causes neurotoxic effects on locomotion behaviors by inducing severe ROS production and disruption of ROS defense mechanisms in nematode *Caenorhabditis elegans*. *J. Hazard Mater.* 219–220, 221–230. doi: 10.1016/j.jhazmat.2012.03.083

Li, Y., Zhang, W., Niu, J., and Chen, Y. (2012b). Mechanism of photogenerated reactive oxygen species and correlation with the antibacterial properties of engineered metal oxide nanoparticles. *ACS Nano* 6, 1–22. doi: 10.1021/nn300934k

Lin, Y., and Hamme, I. I., A. T. (2015). Gold nanoparticle labeling based ICP-MS detection/measurement of bacteria, and their quantitative photothermal destruction. *J. Mater. Chem. B* 3, 3573–3582. doi: 10.1039/C5TB00223K

Liu, L., Yang, J., Xie, J., Luo, Z., Jiang, J., Yang, Y. Y., et al. (2013). The potent antimicrobial properties of cell penetrating peptide-conjugated silver nanoparticles with excellent selectivity for Gram-positive bacteria over erythrocytes. *Nanoscale* 5:3834. doi: 10.1039/c3nr34254a

Liu, P. F., Lo, C. W., Chen, C. H., Hsieh, M. F., and Huang, C. M. (2009). Use of nanoparticles as therapy for methicillin-resistant *Staphylococcus aureus* infections. *Curr. Drug Metab.* 10, 875–884. doi: 10.2174/138920009790274522

Lok, C.-N., Ho, C.-M., Chen, R., He, Q.-Y., Yu, W.-Y., Sun, H., et al. (2007). Silver nanoparticles: partial oxidation and antibacterial activities. *J. Biol. Inorg. Chem.* 12, 527–534. doi: 10.1007/s00775-007-0208-z

Lundqvist, M., Stigler, J., Elia, G., Lynch, I., Cedervall, T., and Dawson, K. A. (2008). Nanoparticle size and surface properties determine the protein corona with possible implications for biological impacts. *Proc. Natl. Acad. Sci. U.S.A.* 105, 14265–14270. doi: 10.1073/pnas.0805135105

Maclean, M., McKenzie, K., Anderson, J. G., Gettinby, G., and MacGregor, S. J. (2014). 405 Nm light technology for the inactivation of pathogens and its potential role for environmental disinfection and infection control. *J. Hosp. Infect.* 88, 1–11. doi: 10.1016/j.jhin.2014.06.004

Mahalingam, S., Xu, Z., and Edirisinghe, M. (2015). Antibacterial activity and biosensing of PVA-lysozyme microbubbles formed by pressurized gyration. *Langmuir* 31, 9771–9780. doi: 10.1021/acs.langmuir.5b02005

Mahmoudi, M., and Serpooshan, V. (2012). Silver-coated engineered magnetic nanoparticles are promising for the success in the fight against antibacterial resistance threat. *ACS Nano* 6, 2656–2664. doi: 10.1021/nn300042m

McShan, D., Zhang, Y., Deng, H., Ray, P. C., and Yu, H. (2015). Synergistic antibacterial effect of silver nanoparticles combined with ineffective antibiotics on drug resistant *Salmonella typhimurium* DT104. *J. Environ. Sci. Heal. Part C* 33, 369–384. doi: 10.1080/10590501.2015.1055165

Meers, P., Neville, M., Malinin, V., Scotto, A. W., Sardaryan, G., Kurumunda, R., et al. (2008). Biofilm penetration, triggered release and *in vivo* activity of inhaled liposomal amikacin in chronic *Pseudomonas aeruginosa* lung infections. *J. Antimicrob. Chemother.* 61, 859–868. doi: 10.1093/jac/dkn059

Mendes, R., Pedrosa, P., Lima, J. C., Fernandes, A. R., and Baptista, P., V (2017). Photothermal enhancement of chemotherapy in breast cancer by visible irradiation of gold nanoparticles. *Sci. Rep.* 7, 1–9. doi: 10.1038/s41598-017-11491-8

Merchant, B. (1998). Gold, the noble metal and the paradoxes of its toxicology. *Biologicals* 26, 49–59. doi: 10.1006/biol.1997.0123

Miao, L., Wang, C., Hou, J., Wang, P., Ao, Y., Li, Y., et al. (2016). Aggregation and removal of copper oxide (CuO) nanoparticles in wastewater environment and their effects on the microbial activities of wastewater biofilms. *Bioresour. Technol.* 216, 537–544. doi: 10.1016/j.biortech.2016.05.082

Millenbaugh, N. J., Baskin, J. B., DeSilva, M. N., Elliott, W. R., and Glickman, R. D. (2015). Photothermal killing of *Staphylococcus aureus* using antibody-targeted gold nanoparticles. *Int. J. Nanomed.* 10, 1953–1960. doi: 10.2147/IJN.S76150

Mocan, L., Matea, C., Tabaran, F. A., Mosteanu, O., Pop, T., Puia, C., et al. (2016). Selective *in vitro* photothermal nano-therapy of MRSA infections mediated by IgG conjugated gold nanoparticles. *Sci. Rep.* 6:39466. doi: 10.1038/srep39466

Mocan, L., Tabaran, F. A., Mocan, T., Pop, T., Mosteanu, O., Agoston-Coldea, L., et al. (2017). Laser thermal ablation of multidrug-resistant bacteria using functionalized gold nanoparticles. *Int. J. Nanomed.* 12, 2255–2263. doi: 10.2147/IJN.S124778

Mohammed Fayaz, A., Girilal, M., Mahdy, S. A., Somsundar, S. S., Venkatesan, R., and Kalaichelvan, P. T. (2011). Vancomycin bound biogenic gold nanoparticles: a different perspective for development of anti VRSA agents. *Process Biochem.* 46, 636–641. doi: 10.1016/j.procbio.2010.11.001

Mohanty, S., Jena, P., Mehta, R., Pati, R., Banerjee, B., Patil, S., et al. (2013). Cationic antimicrobial peptides and biogenic silver nanoparticles kill mycobacteria without eliciting dna damage and cytotoxicity in mouse macrophages. *Antimicrob. Agents Chemother.* 57, 3688–3698. doi: 10.1128/AAC.02475-12

Morrison, D. C., and Jacobs, D. M. (1976). Binding of polymyxin B to the lipid A portion of bacterial lipopolysaccharides. *Immunochemistry* 13, 813–818. doi: 10.1016/0019-2791(76)90181-6

Munger, M. A., Hadlock, G., Stoddard, G., Slawson, M. H., Wilkins, D. G., Cox, N., et al. (2014a). Assessing orally bioavailable commercial silver nanoparticle product on human cytochrome P450 enzyme activity. *Nanotoxicology* 5390, 1–8. doi: 10.3109/17435390.2014.948092

Munger, M. A., Radwanski, P., Hadlock, G. C., Stoddard, G., Shaaban, A., Falconer, J., et al. (2014b). *In vivo* human time-exposure study of orally dosed commercial silver nanoparticles. *Nanomedicine Nanotechnology, Biol. Med.* 10, 1–9. doi: 10.1016/j.nano.2013.06.010

Muniyan, A., Ravi, K., Mohan, U., and Panchamoorthy, R. (2017). Characterization and *in vitro* antibacterial activity of saponin-conjugated silver nanoparticles against bacteria that cause burn wound infection. *World J. Microbiol. Biotechnol.* 33:147. doi: 10.1007/s11274-017-2309-3

Nagvenkar, A. P., Deokar, A., Perelshtein, I., and Gedanken, A. (2016). A one-step sonochemical synthesis of stable ZnO–PVA nanocolloid as a potential biocidal agent. *J. Mater. Chem. B* 4, 2124–2132. doi: 10.1039/C6TB00033A

Nagy, A., Harrison, A., and Dutta, P. K. (2011). Silver nanoparticles embedded in zeolite membranes : release of silver ions and mechanism of antibacterial action. *Int. J. Nanomed.* 6, 1833–1852. doi: 10.2147/IJN.S24019

Natan, M., and Banin, E. (2017). From nano to micro: using nanotechnology to combat microorganisms and their multidrug resistance. *FEMS Microbiol. Rev.* 41, 302–322. doi: 10.1093/femsre/fux003

Niemirowicz, K., Swiecicka, I., Wilczewska, A. Z., Misztalewska, I., Kalska-Szostko, B., Bienias, K., et al. (2014). Gold-functionalized magnetic nanoparticles restrict growth of *Pseudomonas aeruginosa*. *Int. J. Nanomed.* 9, 2217–2224. doi: 10.2147/IJN.S56588

Ocsoy, I., Yusufbeyoglu, S., Yilmaz, V., McLamore, E. S., Ildiz, N., and Ulgen, A. (2017). DNA aptamer functionalized gold nanostructures for molecular recognition and photothermal inactivation of methicillin-Resistant *Staphylococcus aureus*. *Coll. Surf. B. Biointerfaces* 159, 16–22. doi: 10.1016/j.colsurfb.2017.07.056

Ortega, A., Farah, S., Tranque, P., Ocana, A. V., Nam-Cha, S. H., Beyth, N., et al. (2015). Antimicrobial evaluation of quaternary ammonium polyethyleneimine nanoparticles against clinical isolates of pathogenic bacteria. *IET Nanobiotechnol.* 9, 342–348. doi: 10.1049/iet-nbt.2014.0078

Ortíz-Castro, R., Martínez-Trujillo, M., and López-Bucio, J. (2008). N -acyl-L-homoserine lactones: a class of bacterial quorum-sensing signals alter post-embryonic root development in *Arabidopsis thaliana*. *Plant Cell Environ.* 31, 1497–1509. doi: 10.1111/j.1365-3040.2008.01863.x

Otari, S. V., Patil, R. M., Waghmare, S. R., Ghosh, S. J., and Pawar, S. H. (2013). A novel microbial synthesis of catalytically active Ag–alginate biohydrogel and its antimicrobial activity. *Dalt. Trans.* 42, 9966–9975. doi: 10.1039/c3dt51093j

Pal, I., Brahmkhatri, V. P., Bera, S., Bhattacharyya, D., Quirishi, Y., Bhunia, A., et al. (2016). Enhanced stability and activity of an antimicrobial peptide in conjugation with silver nanoparticle. *J. Colloid Interface Sci.* 483, 385–393. doi: 10.1016/j.jcis.2016.08.043

Pallavicini, P., Don,à, A., Taglietti, A., Minzioni, P., Patrini, M., Dacarro, G., et al. (2014). Self-assembled monolayers of gold nanostars: a convenient tool for near-IR photothermal biofilm eradication. *Chem. Commun.* 50, 1969–1971. doi: 10.1039/C3CC48667B

Pan, W. Y., Huang, C. C., Lin, T. T., Hu, H. Y., Lin, W. C., Li, M. J., et al. (2016). Synergistic antibacterial effects of localized heat and oxidative stress caused by hydroxyl radicals mediated by graphene/iron oxide-based nanocomposites. *Nanomed. Nanotechnol. Biol. Med.* 12, 431–438. doi: 10.1016/j.nano.2015.11.014

Panáček, A., Kvítek, L., Smékalová, M., Večerová, R., Kolár, M., Röderová, M., et al. (2018). Bacterial resistance to silver nanoparticles and how to overcome it. *Nat Nanotechnol.* 13, 65–71. doi: 10.1038/s41565-017-0013-y

Panáček, A., Smékalová, M., Kilianová, M., Prucek, R., Bogdanová, K., Věčerová, R., et al. (2016a). Strong and nonspecific synergistic antibacterial efficiency of antibiotics combined with silver nanoparticles at very low concentrations showing no cytotoxic effect. *Molecules* 21, 1–17. doi: 10.3390/molecules21010026

Panáček, A., Smékalová, M., Večerová, R., Bogdanová, K., Röderová, M., Kolár, M., et al. (2016b). Silver nanoparticles strongly enhance and restore bactericidal activity of inactive antibiotics against multiresistant *Enterobacteriaceae*. *Colloids Surfaces B Biointerfaces* 142, 392–399. doi: 10.1016/j.colsurfb.2016.03.007

Papenfort, K., and Bassler, B. (2016). Quorum-sensing signal-response systems in gram-negative bacteria. *Nat Rev Microbiol.* 14, 576–588. doi: 10.1038/nrmicro.2016.89

Patel, S. K., and Janjic, J. M. (2015). Macrophage targeted theranostics as personalized nanomedicine strategies for inflammatory diseases. *Theranostics* 5, 150–172. doi: 10.7150/thno.9476

Payne, J. N., Waghwani, H. K., Connor, M. G., Hamilton, W., Tockstein, S., Moolani, H., et al. (2016). Novel synthesis of kanamycin conjugated gold nanoparticles with potent antibacterial activity. *Front. Microbiol.* 7:607. doi: 10.3389/fmicb.2016.00607

Pei, H., Zuo, X., Zhu, D., Huang, Q., and Fan, C. (2014). Functional DNA nanostructures for theranostic applications. *Acc. Chem. Res.* 47, 550–559. doi: 10.1021/ar400195t

Pelgrift, R. Y., and Friedman, A. J. (2013). Nanotechnology as a therapeutic tool to combat microbial resistance. *Adv. Drug Deliv. Rev.* 65, 1803–1815. doi: 10.1016/j.addr.2013.07.011

Percival, S. L., Bowler, P. G., and Dolman, J. (2007). Antimicrobial activity of silver-containing dressings on wound microorganisms using an *in vitro* biofilm model. *Int. Wound J.* 4, 186–191. doi: 10.1111/j.1742-481X.2007.00296.x

Peulen, T.-O., and Wilkinson, K. J. (2011). Diffusion of nanoparticles in a biofilm. *Environ. Sci. Technol.* 45, 3367–3373. doi: 10.1021/es103450g

Pissuwan, D., Niidome, T., and Cortie, M. (2011). The forthcoming applications of gold nanoparticles in drug and gene delivery systems. *J. Control Release* 149, 65–71. doi: 10.1016/j.jconrel.2009.12.006

Poma, A., and Di Giorgio, M. (2008). Toxicogenomics to improve comprehension of the mechanisms underlying responses of *in vitro* and *in vivo* systems to nanomaterials: a review. *Curr. Genomics* 9, 571–585. doi: 10.2174/138920208786847962

Potgieter, M. D., and Meidany, P. (2017). Evaluation of the penetration of nanocrystalline silver through various wound dressing mediums: an *in vitro* study. *Burns* 44, 596–602. doi: 10.1016/j.burns.2017.10.011

Pradeepa, Vidya, S. M., Mutalik, S., Udaya Bhat, K., Huilgol, P., and Avadhani, K. (2016). Preparation of gold nanoparticles by novel bacterial exopolysaccharide for antibiotic delivery. *Life Sci.* 153, 171–179. doi: 10.1016/j.lfs.2016.04.022

Qi, G., Li, L., Yu, F., and Wang, H. (2013). Vancomycin-modified mesoporous silica nanoparticles for selective recognition and killing of pathogenic gram-positive bacteria over macrophage-like cells. *ACS Appl. Mater. Interfaces* 5, 10874–10881. doi: 10.1021/am403940d

Raghunath, A., and Perumal, E. (2017). Metal oxide nanoparticles as antimicrobial agents: a promise for the future. *Int. J. Antimicrob. Agents* 49, 137–152. doi: 10.1016/j.ijantimicag.2016.11.011

Rai, A., Pinto, S., Velho, T. R., Ferreira, A. F., Moita, C., Trivedi, U., et al. (2016). One-step synthesis of high-density peptide-conjugated gold nanoparticles with antimicrobial efficacy in a systemic infection model. *Biomaterials* 85, 99–110. doi: 10.1016/j.biomaterials.2016.01.051

Rai, M. K., Deshmukh, S. D., Ingle, A. P., and Gade, A. K. (2012). Silver nanoparticles: the powerful nanoweapon against multidrug-resistant bacteria. *J. Appl. Microbiol.* 112, 841–852. doi: 10.1111/j.1365-2672.2012.05253.x

Rai, M., Ingle, A. P., Gaikwad, S., Gupta, I., Gade, A., and Silvério da Silva, S. (2016). Nanotechnology based anti-infectives to fight microbial intrusions. *J. Appl. Microbiol.* 120, 527–542. doi: 10.1111/jam.13010

Rai, M., Ingle, A. P., Pandit, R., Paralikar, P., Gupta, I., Chaud, M. V., et al. (2017). Broadening the spectrum of small-molecule antibacterials by metallic nanoparticles to overcome microbial resistance. *Int. J. Pharm.* 532, 139–148. doi: 10.1016/j.ijpharm.2017.08.127

Rai, M., Yadav, A., and Gade, A. (2009). Silver nanoparticles as a new generation of antimicrobials. *Biotechnol. Adv.* 27, 76–83. doi: 10.1016/j.biotechadv.2008.09.002

Rajchakit, U., and Sarojini, V. (2017). Recent developments in antimicrobial-peptide-conjugated gold nanoparticles. *Bioconjug. Chem.* 28, 2673–2686. doi: 10.1021/acs.bioconjchem.7b00368

Ramalingam, B., Parandhaman, T., and Das, S. K. (2016). Antibacterial effects of biosynthesized silver nanoparticles on surface ultrastructure and nanomechanical properties of gram-negative bacteria viz. *Escherichia coli* and *Pseudomonas aeruginosa*. *ACS Appl. Mater. Interfaces* 8, 4963–4976. doi: 10.1021/acsami.6b00161

Ramasamy, M., Lee, J. H., and Lee, J. (2017a). Direct one-pot synthesis of cinnamaldehyde immobilized on gold nanoparticles and their antibiofilm properties. *Coll. Surfaces B Biointerfaces* 160, 639–648. doi: 10.1016/j.colsurfb.2017.10.018

Ramasamy, M., Lee, J.-H., and Lee, J. (2016). Potent antimicrobial and antibiofilm activities of bacteriogenically synthesized gold-silver nanoparticles against pathogenic bacteria and their physiochemical characterizations. *J. Biomater. Appl.* 31, 366–378. doi: 10.1177/0885328216646910

Ramasamy, M., Lee, J.-H., and Lee, J. (2017b). Development of gold nanoparticles coated with silica containing the antibiofilm drug cinnamaldehyde and their effects on pathogenic bacteria. *Int. J. Nanomed.* 12, 2813–2828. doi: 10.2147/IJN.S132784

Ranghar, S., Sirohi, P., Verma, P., and Agarwal, V. (2014). Nanoparticle-based drug delivery systems : promising approaches against infections. *Braz. Arch. Biol. Technol.* 57, 209–222. doi: 10.1590/S1516-89132013005000011

Reddy, L. S., Nisha, M. M., Joice, M., and Shilpa, P. N. (2014). Antimicrobial activity of zinc oxide (ZnO) nanoparticle against *Klebsiella pneumoniae*. *Pharm. Biol.* 52, 1388–1397. doi: 10.3109/13880209.2014.893001

Reddy, P. M., Chang, K.-C., Liu, Z.-J., Chen, C.-T., and Ho, Y.-P. (2014). Functionalized magnetic iron oxide (Fe3O4) nanoparticles for capturing gram-positive and gram-negative bacteria. *J. Biomed. Nanotechnol.* 10, 1429–1439. doi: 10.1166/jbn.2014.1848

Reen, F. J., Gutiérrez-Barranquero, J. A., Parages, M. L., and O'Gara, F. (2018). Coumarin: a novel player in microbial quorum sensing and biofilm formation inhibition. *Appl Microbiol Biotechnol.* 102, 2063–2073. doi: 10.1007/s00253-018-8787-x

Reidy, B., Haase, A., Luch, A., Dawson, K. A., and Lynch, I. (2013). Mechanisms of silver nanoparticle release, transformation and toxicity: a critical review of current knowledge and recommendations for future studies and applications. *Materials* 6, 2295–2350. doi: 10.3390/ma6062295

Reshma, V. G., Syama, S., Sruthi, S., Reshma, S. C., Remya, N. S., and Mohanan, P. V. (2017). Engineered nanoparticles with antimicrobial property. *Curr. Drug Metab.* 18, 1040–1054. doi: 10.2174/1389200218666170925122201

Ribeiro, A. P. C., Anbu, S., Alegria, E. C. B. A., Fernandes, A. R., Baptista, P. V., Mendes, R., et al. (2018). Evaluation of cell toxicity and DNA and protein binding of green synthesized silver nanoparticles. *Biomed. Pharmacother.* 101, 137–144. doi: 10.1016/j.biopha.2018.02.069

Rizzello, L., and Pompa, P. P. (2014). Nanosilver-based antibacterial drugs and devices: mechanisms, methodological drawbacks, and guidelines. *Chem. Soc. Rev.* 43, 1501–1518. doi: 10.1039/c3cs60218d

Roshmi, T., Soumya, K. R., Jyothis, M., and Radhakrishnan, E. K. (2015). Effect of biofabricated gold nanoparticle-based antibiotic conjugates on minimum inhibitory concentration of bacterial isolates of clinical origin. *Gold Bull.* 48, 63–71. doi: 10.1007/s13404-015-0162-4

Ruden, S., Hilpert, K., Berditsch, M., Wadhwani, P., and Ulrich, A. S. (2009). Synergistic interaction between silver nanoparticles and membrane-permeabilizing antimicrobial peptides. *Antimicrob. Agents Chemother.* 53, 3538–3540. doi: 10.1128/AAC.01106-08

Rudramurthy, G. R., Swamy, M. K., Sinniah, U. R., and Ghasemzadeh, A. (2016). Nanoparticles: alternatives against drug-resistant pathogenic microbes. *Molecules* 21:E836. doi: 10.3390/molecules21070836

Rutherford, S. T., and Bassler, B. L. (2012). Bacterial quorum sensing: its role in virulence and possibilities for its control. *Cold Spring Harb Perspect Med.* 2:a012427. doi: 10.1101/cshperspect.a012427

Roy, A., Parveen, A. R., Koppalkar, A., and Prasad, M. V. N. A. (2010). Effect of nano - titanium dioxide with different antibiotics against methicillin-resistant *Staphylococcus Aureus*. *J. Biomater. Nanobiotechnol.* 1, 37–41. doi: 10.4236/jbnb.2010.11005

Saeb, A. T. M., Alshammari, A. S., Al-brahim, H., and Al-rubeaan, K. A. (2014). Production of silver nanoparticles with strong and stable antimicrobial activity against highly pathogenic and multidrug resistant bacteria. *Sci. World J.* 2:704708. doi: 10.1155/2014/704708

Saha, B., Bhattacharya, J., Mukherjee, A., Ghosh, A., Santra, C., Anjan, K., et al. (2007). *In vitro* structural and functional evaluation of gold nanoparticles conjugated antibiotics. *Nanoscale Res. Lett.* 2, 614–622. doi: 10.1007/s11671-007-9104-2

Salem, W., Leitner, D. R., Zingl, F. G., Schratter, G., Prassl, R., Goessler, W., et al. (2015). Antibacterial activity of silver and zinc nanoparticles against *Vibrio cholerae* and enterotoxic *Escherichia coli*. *Int. J. Med. Microbiol.* 305, 85–95. doi: 10.1016/j.ijmm.2014.11.005

Salomoni, R., Léo, P., Montemor, A. F., Rinaldi, B. G., and Rodrigues, M. (2017). Antibacterial effect of silver nanoparticles in *Pseudomonas aeruginosa*. *Nanotechnol. Sci. Appl.* 10, 115–121. doi: 10.2147/NSA.S133415

Sandhiya, S., Dkhar, S. A., and Surendiran, A. (2009). Emerging trends of nanomedicine - an overview. *Fundam. Clin. Pharmacol.* 23, 263–269. doi: 10.1111/j.1472-8206.2009.00692.x

Sarwar, A., Katas, H., Samsudin, S. N., and Zin, N. M. (2015). Regioselective sequential modification of chitosan via azide-alkyne click reaction: synthesis, characterization, and antimicrobial activity of chitosan derivatives and nanoparticles. *PLoS ONE* 10:e0123084. doi: 10.1371/journal.pone.0123084

Sarwar, S., Chakraborti, S., Bera, S., Sheikh, I. A., Hoque, K. M., and Chakrabarti, P. (2016). The antimicrobial activity of ZnO nanoparticles against *Vibrio cholerae*: variation in response depends on biotype. *Nanomedicine Nanotechnology, Biol. Med.* 12, 1499–1509. doi: 10.1016/j.nano.2016.02.006

Sathyanarayanan, M. B., Balachandranath, R., Genji Srinivasulu, Y., Kannaiyan, S. K., and Subbiahdoss, G. (2013). The effect of gold and iron-oxide nanoparticles on biofilm-forming pathogens. *ISRN Microbiol.* 2013:272086. doi: 10.1155/2013/272086

Setyawati, M. I., Kutty, R. V., Tay, C. Y., Yuan, X., Xie, J., and Leong, D. T. (2014). Novel theranostic DNA nanoscaffolds for the simultaneous detection and killing of *Escherichia coli* and *Staphylococcus aureus*. *ACS Appl. Mater. Interfaces* 6, 21822–21831. doi: 10.1021/am502591c

Shah, A., Latif-Ur-Rahman, Qureshi, R., and Zia-Ur-Rehman (2012). Synthesis, characterization, and application of Au-Ag alloy nanoparticles for the sensing of an environmental toxin, pyrene. *Rev. Adv. Mater. Sci.* 30, 133–149. doi: 10.1007/s10800-015-0807-2

Shah, M., Badwaik, V., Kherde, Y., Waghwani, H. K., Modi, T., Aguilar, Z. P., et al. (2014). Gold nanoparticles: various methods of synthesis and antibacterial applications. *Front. Biosci.* 19, 1320–1344. doi: 10.2741/4284

Shaikh, S., Rizvi, S. M. D., Shakil, S., Hussain, T., Alshammari, T. M., Ahmad, W., et al. (2017). Synthesis and characterization of cefotaxime conjugated gold nanoparticles and their use to target drug-resistant CTX-M-producing bacterial pathogens. *J. Cell. Biochem.* 118, 2802–2808. doi: 10.1002/jcb.25929

Shaker, M. A., and Shaaban, M. I. (2017). Formulation of carbapenems loaded gold nanoparticles to combat multi-antibiotic bacterial resistance: *in vitro* antibacterial study. *Int. J. Pharm.* 525, 71–84. doi: 10.1016/j.ijpharm.2017.04.019

Shamaila, S., Zafar, N., Riaz, S., Sharif, R., Nazir, J., and Naseem, S. (2016). Gold nanoparticles: an efficient antimicrobial agent against enteric bacterial human pathogen. *Nanomaterials* 6:71. doi: 10.3390/nano6040071

Shareena Dasari, T. P., Zhang, Y., and Yu, H. (2015). Antibacterial activity and cytotoxicity of gold (I) and (III) ions and gold nanoparticles. *Biochem. Pharmacol.* 4:199. doi: 10.4172/2167-0501.1000199

Siddiqi, K. S., Husen, A., and Rao, R. A. K. (2018). A review on biosynthesis of silver nanoparticles and their biocidal properties. *J. Nanobiotechnology* 16:14. doi: 10.1186/s12951-018-0334-5

Singh, B. N., Prateeksha, Upreti D. K., Singh, B. R., Defoirdt, T., Gupta, V. K., De Souza, A. O., et al. (2017). Bactericidal, quorum quenching and anti-biofilm nanofactories: a new niche for nanotechnologists. *Crit. Rev. Biotechnol.* 37, 525–540. doi: 10.1080/07388551.2016.1199010

Singh, J., Garg, T., Rath, G., and Goyal, A. K. (2016). Advances in nanotechnology-based carrier systems for targeted delivery of bioactive drug molecules with special emphasis on immunotherapy in drug resistant tuberculosis - a critical review. *Drug Deliv.* 23, 1676–1698. doi: 10.3109/10717544.2015.1074765

Singh, K., Panghal, M., Kadyan, S., Chaudhary, U., and Yadav, J. P., arkas. (2014). Green silver nanoparticles of *Phyllanthus amarus*: as an antibacterial agent against multi drug resistant clinical isolates of *Pseudomonas aeruginosa*. *J. Nanobiotechnology* 12:40. doi: 10.1186/s12951-014-0040-x

Singh, R., Nawale, L., Arkile, M., Wadhwani, S., Shedbalkar, U., Chopade, S., et al. (2016). Phytogenic silver, gold, and bimetallic nanoparticles as novel antitubercular agents. *Int. J. Nanomed.* 11, 1889–1897. doi: 10.2147/IJN.S102488

Singh, R., Smitha, M. S., and Singh, S. P. (2014). The role of nanotechnology in combating multi-drug resistant bacteria. *J. Nanosci. Nanotechnol.* 14, 4745–4756. doi: 10.1166/jnn.2014.9527

Sinha, R., Karan, R., Sinha, A., and Khare, S. K. (2011). Interaction and nanotoxic effect of ZnO and Ag nanoparticles on mesophilic and halophilic bacterial cells. *Bioresour. Technol.* 102, 1516–1520. doi: 10.1016/j.biortech.2010.07.117

Slavin, Y. N., Asnis, J., Hafeli, U. O., and Bach, H. (2017). Metal nanoparticles: understanding the mechanisms behind antibacterial activity. *J. Nanobiotechnology* 15:65. doi: 10.1186/s12951-017-0308-z

Slomberg, D. L., Lu, Y., Broadnax, A. D., Hunter, R. A., Carpenter, A. W., and Schoenfisch, M. H. (2013). Role of size and shape on biofilm eradication for nitric oxide-releasing silica nanoparticles. *ACS Appl. Mater. Interfaces* 5, 9322–9329. doi: 10.1021/am402618w

Smock, K. J., Schmidt, R. L., Hadlock, G., Stoddard, G., Grainger, D. W., and Munger, M. A. (2014). Assessment of orally dosed commercial silver nanoparticles on human *ex vivo* platelet aggregation. *Nanotoxicology* 8, 328–333. doi: 10.3109/17435390.2013.788749

Su, H.-L., Lin, S.-H., Wei, J.-C., Pao, I.-C., Chiao, S.-H., Huang, C.-C., et al. (2011). Novel nanohybrids of silver particles on clay platelets for inhibiting silver-resistant bacteria. *PLoS ONE* 6:e21125. doi: 10.1371/journal.pone.0021125

Su, Y., Zheng, X., Chen, Y., Li, M., and Liu, K. (2015). Alteration of intracellular protein expressions as a key mechanism of the deterioration of bacterial denitrification caused by copper oxide nanoparticles. *Sci. Rep.* 5:15824. doi: 10.1038/srep15824

Sukwong, P., Pissuwan, D., Somkid, K., Kongseng, S., and Yoovathaworn, K. (2016). Respiratory tract toxicity of titanium dioxide nanoparticles and multi-walled carbon nanotubes on mice after intranasal exposure. *Micro Nano Lett.* 11, 183–187. doi: 10.1049/mnl.2015.0523

Taylor, T., Gaysinsky, S., Davidson, P., Bruce, B., and Weiss, J. (2007). Characterization of antimicrobial bearing liposomes by zeta potential, vesicle size, and encapsulation efficiency. *Food Biophys.* 2, 1–9. doi: 10.1007/s11483-007-9023-x

Thapa, R., Bhagat, C., Shrestha, P., Awal, S., and Dudhagara, P. (2017). Enzyme-mediated formulation of stable elliptical silver nanoparticles tested against clinical pathogens and MDR bacteria and development of antimicrobial surgical thread. *Ann. Clin. Microbiol. Antimicrob.* 16, 1–10. doi: 10.1186/s12941-017-0216-y

Thomas, R., Nair, A. P., Kr, S., Mathew, J., and Ek, R. (2014). Antibacterial activity and synergistic effect of biosynthesized AgNPs with antibiotics against multidrug-resistant biofilm-forming coagulase-negative *staphylococci* isolated from clinical samples. *Appl. Biochem. Biotechnol.* 173, 449–460. doi: 10.1007/s12010-014-0852-z

Thompson, M., Blaszykowski, C., Sheikh, S., and Romaschin, A. (2015). A true theranostic approach to medicine: towards tandem sensor detection and removal of endotoxin in blood. *Biosens. Bioelectron.* 67, 3–10. doi: 10.1016/j.bios.2014.07.008

Tielens, F., and Santos, E. (2010). AuS and SH bond formation/breaking during the formation of alkanethiol SAMs on Au(111): a theoretical study. *J. Phys. Chem. C* 114, 9444–9452. doi: 10.1021/jp102036r

Tiwari, P., Vig, K., Dennis, V., and Singh, S. (2011). Functionalised gold nanoparticles and their biomedical applications. *Nanomaterials* 1, 31–63. doi: 10.3390/nano1010031

Tong, G., Du, F., Wu, W., Wu, R., Liu, F., and Liang, Y. (2013). Enhanced reactive oxygen species (ROS) yields and antibacterial activity of spongy ZnO/ZnFe2O4 hybrid micro-hexahedra selectively synthesized through a versatile glucose-engineered co-precipitation/annealing process. *J. Mater. Chem. B* 1, 2647–2657. doi: 10.1039/c3tb20229a

Turos, E., Reddy, G. S. K., Greenhalgh, K., Ramaraju, P., Abeylath, S. C., Jang, S., et al. (2007). Penicillin-bound polyacrylate nanoparticles: restoring the activity of beta-lactam antibiotics against MRSA. *Bioorg. Med. Chem. Lett.* 17, 3468–3472. doi: 10.1016/j.bmcl.2007.03.077

Ulloa-Ogaz, A. L., Piñón-Castillo, H. A., Muñoz-Castellanos, L. N., Athie-García, M. S., Ballinas-Casarrubias, M. D. L., Murillo-Ramirez, J. G., et al. (2017). Oxidative damage to *Pseudomonas aeruginosa* ATCC 27833 and *Staphylococcus aureus* ATCC 24213 induced by CuO-NPs. *Environ. Sci. Pollut. Res.* 24, 22048–22060. doi: 10.1007/s11356-017-9718-6

Uma Suganya, K. S., Govindaraju, K., Ganesh Kumar, V., Stalin Dhas, T., Karthick, V., Singaravelu, G., et al. (2015). Blue green alga mediated synthesis of gold nanoparticles and its antibacterial efficacy against Gram positive organisms. *Mater. Sci. Eng. C* 47, 351–356. doi: 10.1016/j.msec.2014.11.043

Umamaheswari, K., Baskar, R., Chandru, K., Rajendiran, N., and Chandirasekar, S. (2014). Antibacterial activity of gold nanoparticles and their toxicity assessment. *BMC Infect. Dis.* 14:P64. doi: 10.1186/1471-2334-14-S3-P64

Veigas, B., Fernandes, A. R., and Baptista, P. V. (2014). AuNPs for identification of molecular signatures of resistance. *Front. Microbiol.* 5:455. doi: 10.3389/fmicb.2014.00455

Veigas, B., Pedrosa, P., Carlos, F. F., Mancio-Silva, L., Grosso, A. R., Fortunato, E., et al. (2015). One nanoprobe, two pathogens: gold nanoprobes multiplexing for point-of-care. *J. Nanobiotechnology* 13:48. doi: 10.1186/s12951-015-0109-1

Veigas, B., Pedrosa, P., Couto, I., Viveiros, M., and Baptista, P., V (2013). Isothermal DNA amplification coupled to Au-nanoprobes for detection of mutations associated to Rifampicin resistance in *Mycobacterium tuberculosis*. *J. Nanobiotechnology* 11:38. doi: 10.1186/1477-3155-11-38

Venkatesan, N., Perumal, G., and Doble, M. (2015). Bacterial resistance in biofilm-associated bacteria. *Future Microbiol.* 10, 1743–1750. doi: 10.2217/fmb.15.69

Vinoj, G., Pati, R., Sonawane, A., and Vaseeharan, B. (2015). *In vitro* cytotoxic effects of gold nanoparticles coated with functional acyl homoserine lactone lactonase protein from *Bacillus licheniformis* and their antibiofilm activity against proteus species. *Antimicrob. Agents Chemother.* 59, 763–771. doi: 10.1128/AAC.03047-14

Walker, T., Dumadag, S., Lee, C. J., Lee, S. H., Bender, J. M., Abbott, J. C., et al. (2016). Clinical impact of laboratory implementation of verigene BC-GN microarray-based assay for detection of gram-negative bacteria in positive blood cultures. *J. Clin. Microbiol.* 54, 1789–1796. doi: 10.1128/JCM.00376-16

Wang, G. (2014). Human antimicrobial peptides and proteins. *Pharmaceuticals* 7, 545–594. doi: 10.3390/ph7050545

Wang, L., Chen, Y. P., Miller, K. P., Cash, B. M., Jones, S., Glenn, S., et al. (2014). Functionalized nanoparticles complexed with antibiotic efficiently kill MRSA and other bacteria. *Chem. Commun.* 50, 12030–12033. doi: 10.1039/c4cc04936e

Wang, L., Hu, C., and Shao, L. (2017a). The antimicrobial activity of nanoparticles: present situation and prospects for the future. *Int. J. Nanomed.* 12, 1227–1249. doi: 10.2147/IJN.S121956

Wang, L., Huang, F., Cai, G., Yao, L., Zhang, H., and Lin, J. (2017b). An electrochemical aptasensor using coaxial capillary with magnetic nanoparticle, urease catalysis and PCB electrode for rapid and sensitive detection of *Escherichia coli* O157:H7. *Nanotheranostics* 1, 403–414. doi: 10.7150/ntno.22079

Wang, Z., Dong, K., Liu, Z., Zhang, Y., Chen, Z., Sun, H., et al. (2017). Activation of biologically relevant levels of reactive oxygen species by Au/g-C3N4 hybrid nanozyme for bacteria killing and wound disinfection. *Biomaterials* 113, 145–157. doi: 10.1016/j.biomaterials.2016.10.041

Wangoo, N., Suri, C. R., and Shekhawat, G. (2008). Interaction of gold nanoparticles with protein: a spectroscopic study to monitor protein conformational changes. *Appl. Phys. Lett.* 92, 1–4. doi: 10.1063/1.2902302

Warheit, D. B. (2018). Hazard and risk assessment strategies for nanoparticle exposures: how far have we come in the past 10 years? *F1000Res.* 7:376. doi: 10.12688/f1000research.12691.1

Weng, C.-I., Chang, H.-T., Lin, C.-H., Shen, Y.-W., Unnikrishnan, B., Li, Y.-J., et al. (2015). One-step synthesis of biofunctional carbon quantum dots for bacterial labeling. *Biosens. Bioelectron.* 68, 1–6. doi: 10.1016/J.BIOS.2014.12.028

Wu, T., Wu, C., Fang, Z., Ma, X., Chen, S., and Hu, Y. (2017). Effect of chitosan microcapsules loaded with nisin on the preservation of small yellow croaker. *Food Control* 72, 43–52. doi: 10.1016/j.foodcont.2017.04.016

Xia, Q., Li, H., and Xiao, K. (2016). Factors affecting the pharmacokinetics, biodistribution and toxicity of gold nanoparticles in drug delivery. *Curr. Drug Metab.* 17, 849–861. doi: 10.2174/1389200217666160629114941

Xue, Y., Li, X., Li, H., and Zhang, W. (2014). Quantifying thiol-gold interactions towards the efficient strength control. *Nat. Commun.* 5:4348. doi: 10.1038/ncomms5348

Yang, X., Dang, Y., Lou, J., Shao, H., and Jiang, X. (2018). D-alanyl-D-alanine-modified gold nanoparticles form a broad-spectrum sensor for bacteria. *Theranostics* 8, 1449–1457. doi: 10.7150/thno.22540

Yang, X., Yang, J., Wang, L., Ran, B., Jia, Y., Zhang, L., et al. (2017). Pharmaceutical intermediate-modified gold nanoparticles: against multidrug-resistant bacteria and wound-healing application via an electrospun scaffold. *ACS Nano* 11, 5737–5745. doi: 10.1021/acsnano.7b01240

Yeaman, M. R. (2003). Mechanisms of antimicrobial peptide action and resistance. *Pharmacol. Rev.* 55, 27–55. doi: 10.1124/pr.55.1.2

Yeom, J. H., Lee, B., Kim, D., Lee, J., kook, Kim, S., Bae, J., et al. (2016). Gold nanoparticle-DNA aptamer conjugate-assisted delivery of antimicrobial peptide effectively eliminates intracellular *Salmonella enterica serovar Typhimurium*. *Biomaterials* 104, 43–51. doi: 10.1016/j.biomaterials.2016.07.009

Yu, J., Zhang, W., Li, Y., Wang, G., Yang, L., Jin, J., et al. (2014). Synthesis, characterization, antimicrobial activity and mechanism of a novel hydroxyapatite whisker/nano zinc oxide biomaterial. *Biomed. Mater.* 10:015001. doi: 10.1088/1748-6041/10/1/015001

Yu, Q., Li, J., Zhang, Y., Wang, Y., Liu, L., and Li, M. (2016). Inhibition of gold nanoparticles (AuNPs) on pathogenic biofilm formation and invasion to host cells. *Sci. Rep.* 6:26667. doi: 10.1038/srep26667

Zaidi, S., Misba, L., and Khan, A. U. (2017). Nano-therapeutics : a revolution in infection control in post antibiotic era. *Nanomed. Nanotechnol. Biol. Med.* 13, 2281–2301. doi: 10.1016/j.nano.2017.06.015

Zazo, H., Colino, C. I., and Lanao, J. M. (2016). Current applications of nanoparticles in infectious diseases. *J. Control. Release* 224, 86–102. doi: 10.1016/j.jconrel.2016.01.008

Zhang, L., and Gallo, R. L. (2016). Antimicrobial peptides. *Curr. Biol.* 26, R14–R19. doi: 10.1016/j.cub.2015.11.017

Zhang, W., Li, Y., Niu, J., and Chen, Y. (2013). Photogeneration of reactive oxygen species on uncoated silver, gold, nickel, and silicon nanoparticles and their antibacterial effects. *Langmuir* 29, 4647–4651. doi: 10.1021/la400500t

Zhang, Y., Shareena Dasari, T. P., Deng, H., and Yu, H. (2015a). Antimicrobial activity of gold nanoparticles and ionic gold. *J. Environ. Sci. Health. C. Environ. Carcinog. Ecotoxicol. Rev.* 33, 286–327. doi: 10.1080/10590501.2015.1055161

Zhang, Y., Zhu, P., Li, G., Wang, W., Chen, L., Lu, D. D., et al. (2015b). Highly stable and re-dispersible nano Cu hydrosols with sensitively size-dependent catalytic and antibacterial activities. *Nanoscale* 7, 13775–13783. doi: 10.1039/C5NR03414K

Zhang, Y., Zhu, P., Li, G., Zhao, T., Fu, X., Sun, R., et al. (2014). Facile preparation of monodisperse, impurity-free, and antioxidation copper nanoparticles on a large scale for application in conductive ink. *ACS Appl. Mater. Interfaces* 6, 560–567. doi: 10.1021/am404620y

Zhao, Y., and Jiang, X. (2013). Multiple strategies to activate gold nanoparticles as antibiotics. *Nanoscale* 5:8340. doi: 10.1039/c3nr01990j

Zhao, Y., Ye, C., Liu, W., Chen, R., and Jiang, X. (2014). Tuning the composition of AuPt bimetallic nanoparticles for antibacterial application. *Angew Chem Int* 53, 8127–8131. doi: 10.1002/anie.201401035

Zhao, Z., Yan, R., Yi, X., Li, J., Rao, J., Guo, Z., et al. (2017). Bacteria-activated theranostic nanoprobes against methicillin-resistant *Staphylococcus aureus* infection. *ACS Nano* 11, 4428–4438. doi: 10.1021/acsnano.7b00041

Zhou, Z., Peng, S., Sui, M., Chen, S., Huang, L., Xu, H., et al. (2018). Multifunctional nanocomplex for surface-enhanced Raman scattering imaging and near-infrared photodynamic antimicrobial therapy of vancomycin-resistant bacteria. *Coll. Surfaces B Biointerfaces* 161, 394–402. doi: 10.1016/j.colsurfb.2017.11.005

Zong, J., Cobb, S. L., and Cameron, N. R. (2017). Peptide-functionalized gold nanoparticles: versatile biomaterials for diagnostic and therapeutic applications. *Biomater. Sci.* 5, 872–886. doi: 10.1039/C7BM00006E

11

Impact of *mcr-1* on the Development of High Level Colistin Resistance in *Klebsiella pneumoniae* and *Escherichia coli*

*Xiao-Qing Zhu[1,2†], Yi-Yun Liu[1,2†], Renjie Wu[1,2], Haoliang Xun[1,2], Jian Sun[1,2], Jian Li[3], Yaoyu Feng[2,4] and Jian-Hua Liu[1,2]**

[1] College of Veterinary Medicine, Guangdong Provincial Key Laboratory of Veterinary Pharmaceutics Development and Safety Evaluation, Key Laboratory of Zoonosis of Ministry of Agricultural and Rural Affairs, National Risk Assessment Laboratory for Antimicrobial Resistance of Microorganisms in Animals, South China Agricultural University, Guangzhou, China, [2] Guangdong Laboratory for Lingnan Modern Agriculture, Guangzhou, China, [3] Biomedicine Discovery Institute and Department of Microbiology, School of Biomedical Sciences, Monash University, Clayton, VIC, Australia, [4] College of Veterinary Medicine, Center for Emerging and Zoonotic Diseases, South China Agricultural University, Guangzhou, China

***Correspondence:**
Jian-Hua Liu
jhliu@scau.edu.cn

† These authors have contributed equally to this work

Plasmid-mediated colistin resistance gene *mcr-1* generally confers low-level resistance. The purpose of this study was to investigate the impact of *mcr-1* on the development of high-level colistin resistance (HLCR) in *Klebsiella pneumoniae* and *Escherichia coli*. In this study, *mcr-1*-negative *K. pneumoniae* and *E. coli* strains and their corresponding *mcr-1*-positive transformants were used to generate HLCR mutants *via* multiple passages in the presence of increasing concentrations of colistin. We found that for *K. pneumoniae,* HLCR mutants with minimum inhibitory concentrations (MICs) of colistin from 64 to 1,024 mg/L were generated. Colistin MICs increased 256- to 4,096-fold for *mcr-1*-negative *K. pneumoniae* strains but only 16- to 256-fold for the *mcr-1*-harboring transformants. For *E. coli*, colistin MICs increased 4- to 64-folds, but only 2- to 16-fold for their *mcr-1*-harboring transformants. Notably, *mcr-1* improved the survival rates of both *E. coli* and *K. pneumoniae* strains when challenged with relatively high concentrations of colistin. In HLCR *K. pneumoniae* mutants, amino acid alterations predominately occurred in *crrB*, followed by *phoQ*, *crrA*, *pmrB*, *mgrB*, and *phoP*, while in *E. coli* mutants, genetic alterations were mostly occurred in *pmrB* and *phoQ*. Additionally, growth rate analyses showed that the coexistence of *mcr-1* and chromosomal mutations imposed a fitness burden on HLCR mutants of *K. pneumoniae*. In conclusion, HLCR was more likely to occur in *K. pneumoniae* strains than *E. coli* strains when exposed to colistin. The *mcr-1* gene could improve the survival rates of strains of both bacterial species but could not facilitate the evolution of high-level colistin resistance.

Keywords: *mcr-1*, *Enterobacterales*, colistin, resistance, fitness cost

INTRODUCTION

Infections caused by multidrug-resistant pathogens pose significant risks to public health worldwide (Ruhnke et al., 2014; Huang et al., 2018). Owing to a limited number of effective antimicrobial agents, colistin has been reused and is considered to be the last therapeutic agent; however, resistance to colistin has been increasingly reported (Liu et al., 2016; Srinivas and Rivard, 2017). Previously, colistin resistance was mainly caused by mutations in chromosomal genes, including *pmrAB*, *phoPQ*, *crrAB*, and the negative regulator *mgrB* (Wright et al., 2015; Poirel et al., 2017; Srinivas and Rivard, 2017), which resulted in the modification of lipid A with positively charged residues, such as phosphoethanolamine and/or 4-amino-4-deoxy-L-arabinose. However, plasmid-mediated colistin resistance genes have also emerged recently. Since, we reported the first case of plasmid-mediated colistin resistance gene (*mcr-1*) in 2015 (Liu et al., 2016), several variants of *mcr* genes (*mcr-2* to *mcr-10*) have been reported worldwide (Shi et al., 2020; Wang et al., 2020).

Similar to plasmid-mediated quinolone resistance genes, *mcr-1* generally confers low-level colistin resistance (2–8 mg/L) (Jeong et al., 2008; Jacoby et al., 2014; Liu et al., 2016). However, it is unknown whether the presence of *mcr-1* can facilitate the selection of a higher level of colistin resistance, as reported for *qnr* family genes (Jeong et al., 2008; Jacoby et al., 2014). Furthermore, the available data show that the prevalence of *mcr-1* is significantly higher in *Escherichia coli* than that in *Klebsiella pneumoniae* (Quan et al., 2017; Eiamphungporn et al., 2018). Additionally, in clinical *K. pneumoniae* isolates, colistin resistance is mostly mediated by chromosomal mutations, which usually confer higher levels of resistance (16–1,024 mg/L) than that conferred by *mcr* (Cannatelli et al., 2014; Liu et al., 2016; Jayol et al., 2017). It seems that *K. pneumoniae* is more likely to generate chromosomal mutations but is less likely to harbor *mcr-1* compared to the phenomenon observed in *E. coli*. Nevertheless, a previous study showed that after a single overnight exposure to twofold minimum inhibitory concentrations (MICs) of colistin, *mcr-1* facilitated the development of high-level colistin resistance (HLCR; MIC $\geq$ 32 mg/L) mutants in *E. coli* but did not affect the HLCR mutation rates in *K. pneumoniae* (Zhang et al., 2019). However, another study reported that MCR-negative strains could be induced to higher level of colistin resistance than MCR-positive strains after step-wise induction (Luo et al., 2019). Thus, the impact of *mcr-1* on the development of high level colistin resistance in *K. pneumoniae* and *E. coli*, and whether similar probability and frequency of mutations will be observed in *E. coli* and *K. pneumoniae* under selection with increasing concentrations of colistin remain unclear.

In this study, we investigated and compared the development of HLCR and chromosomal mutations among strains of *E. coli* and *K. pneumoniae*, with or without *mcr-1*, *via* multiple passages in the presence of increasing colistin concentrations.

MATERIALS AND METHODS

Bacterial Strains and Plasmids

Klebsiella pneumoniae P11, HZ7H152, and YX6P94K and *E. coli* ATCC 25922, C600, and ZYTF186 were used as *mcr-1*-negative parental strains for this study. The sources and resistance phenotypes of these strains are listed in **Supplementary Table 1**. To construct an *mcr-1*-harboring plasmid, *mcr-1* was cloned from pHNSHP45 (GenBank accession number KP347127.1) to pHSG575 using the primer pair listed in **Supplementary Table 2**, which yielded pHSG575-*mcr-1* (Takeshita et al., 1987). The recombinant plasmid was transformed into *E. coli* ATCC 25922 by electroporation, whereas the original plasmid pHNSHP45 was transformed into *K. pneumoniae* P11, HZ7H152, and YX6P94K and *E. coli* C600 and ZYTF186. Transformants were selected on Luria–Bertani (LB) medium containing 2 mg/L colistin. The presence of *mcr-1* in the transformants was confirmed as per previously described methods (Liu et al., 2016).

Whole-Genome Sequencing and Analysis

The whole genomic DNA of four strains, *K. pneumoniae* P11, HZ7H152, and YX6P94K and *E. coli* ZYTF186, was sequenced using Illumina HiSeq 2000 (Illumina, San Diego, CA, United States). Sequence reads were assembled into contigs using SOAPdenovo version 2.04. Resistance genes were explored using ResFinder[1]. The whole-genome sequences of two laboratory strains, *E. coli* C600 and ATCC 25922 (GenBank accession numbers NZ_CP031214.1 and NZ_CP009072.1, respectively), were obtained from NCBI and used as reference genomes.

Antimicrobial Susceptibility Testing

Minimum inhibitory concentrations of colistin were determined using Mueller–Hinton (MH) broth microdilution following the recommendations of the Clinical and Laboratory Standards Institute (Matuschek et al., 2018). *E. coli* ATCC 25922 was used as a reference strain.

Induction of Colistin Resistance by Conducting Serial Passages

Serial passaging was performed as per previously described methods (San Millan et al., 2016), with minor modifications. As shown in **Supplementary Figure 1**, strains were incubated on MH agar plates at 37°C to obtain single colonies. For each strain, 48 colonies were randomly selected and inoculated in separate wells of 96-well plates containing colistin-free LB broth to obtain overnight cultures. The overnight cultures were inoculated in 0.2 mL of LB broth with colistin (0.5 × MIC) in a new 96-well plate. Following a 24-h incubation at 37°C, the cultures were diluted 1:100 and transferred to a new plate containing a double concentration of colistin relative to that used on the previous day. The serial passages were performed until no surviving populations were observed.

[1] https://cge.cbs.dtu.dk//services/ResFinder/

Surviving populations were defined considering growth indicated by OD_{600} (optical density at 600 nm) > 0.10 ± 0.02. The number of surviving populations was recorded for all treatments over time. For each strain, 5–10 surviving populations were selected along the concentration gradient of colistin from low to high, with priority selection of populations that survived at the highest concentration. Subsequently, the populations were separately plated on fresh LB agar to obtain single colonies, and three colonies were randomly selected from each population to determine their susceptibility to colistin and resistance mechanisms.

Genetic Alterations in Colistin-Resistant Mutants

Chromosomal genes (*mgrB*, *pmrAB*, *phoPQ*, and *crrAB*) associated with colistin resistance were amplified by PCR and sequenced using the primers listed in **Supplementary Table 2**. Genetic alterations that occurred in colistin-resistant mutants were determined by comparing the resulting sequences to their corresponding parental reference genomes.

In vitro Growth Rate Assay

Forty-four HLCR K. pneumoniae mutants with different mutations, including equal numbers of *mcr-1*-negative and *mcr-1*-positive derivatives, were selected incubated in fresh MH broth under shaking (180 rpm) conditions at 37°C. The overnight cultures were inoculated in fresh MH broth, and OD_{600} was measured using the Multiskan Spectrum microplate spectrophotometer (Thermo Labsystems, Franklin, MA, United States). The growth rates were determined by plotting the logarithm of OD_{600} versus time. Data analysis was performed using a non-parametric Mann–Whitney *U*-test, followed by Dunn's multiple comparison test (Zwietering et al., 1990).

Accession Numbers

The whole genome sequencing data of *K. pneumoniae* P11, HZ7H152, *K. variicola* YX6P94K (subtype of *K. pneumoniae*) and *E. coli* ZYTF186 have been deposited in GenBank with accession numbers JAFKAD010000000, JAFKAE010000000, JAFKAG010000000, and JAFKAF010000000, respectively.

RESULTS

Development of Resistance to Colistin via Serial Passages of *Escherichia coli*

Colistin-resistant *E. coli* mutants were obtained under increasing colistin pressure. The final induction concentrations of colistin, which inhibited the growth of all *E. coli* strains, ranged from 32 to 64 mg/L. As shown in **Figures 1A–C**, initially, the surviving populations of the *mcr-1*-negative parental strains (ATCC 25922, C600, and ZYTF186) plummeted in response to a challenge with 2 mg/L colistin, while those of their corresponding *mcr-1*-positive derivatives did not show a marked decline until the colistin concentration reached 16 mg/L. Furthermore, when exposed to relatively high concentrations of colistin (16 and 32 mg/L), *mcr-1*-positive derivatives showed higher survival rates than those of their corresponding *mcr-1*-negative strains, demonstrating that *mcr-1* could enhance the survival rate of *E. coli* at higher colistin concentrations.

After the serial colistin challenge, the highest MICs of colistin for *mcr-1*-positive *E. coli* derivatives reached 32 mg/L, while those for *mcr-1*-negative derivatives only reached 16 mg/L (**Figure 2A**). Colistin MIC values for all mutants ranged from 2 to 32 mg/L (n = 9), suggesting that it was difficult for *E. coli* to generate HLCR mutants. Compared with their basal MICs, those for the *mcr-1*-negative strains (ATCC 25922/pHSG575, C600, and ZYTF186) increased 4- to 64-fold, while the MIC values for their corresponding *mcr-1*-positive derivatives merely showed 2- to 16-fold increases, suggesting that the presence of *mcr-1* did not facilitate the generation of higher colistin resistance in *E. coli*.

Development of Resistance to Colistin via Serial Passages of *Klebsiella pneumoniae*

Compared with *E. coli*, *K. pneumoniae* strains, with or without *mcr-1*, were more likely to generate HLCR mutations. *K. pneumoniae* strains could survive up to extremely high concentrations of colistin (256–1,024 mg/L) (**Figures 1D–F**). Notably, the contribution of *mcr-1* in improving the survival odds of *K. pneumoniae* was initially remarkable, however, it was weakened at higher concentrations of colistin. For example, compared with those of the parent strains of *K. pneumoniae* (YX6P94K and HZ7H152), more populations of their *mcr-1*-harboringtransformants survived when the concentrations of colistin were lower than 32 mg/L (**Figures 1E,F**). However, the contribution of *mcr-1* gradually diminished in the presence of >64 mg/L colistin. Furthermore, the number of P11/pHNSHP45 subsets was initially higher but decreased to fewer than that of the parent strain P11 upon exposure to more than 4 mg/L colistin (**Figure 1D**).

After serial passages, the colistin MIC values for *K. pneumoniae* mutants ranged from 64 to >1,024 mg/L (**Figure 2B**). Particularly, the colistin MICs increased 256- to 4,096-fold for *mcr-1*-negative mutants but only 16- to 256-fold for their respective *mcr-1*-harboring transformants.

Genetic Alterations in *pmrAB* and *phoPQ* in *Escherichia coli*

Although most *E. coli* strains failed to generate HLCR, 36 derivatives that survived at relatively high concentrations of colistin (16–32 mg/L), including 18 *mcr-1*-negative and 18 *mcr-1*-positive derivatives, were selected to determine the presence of mutations in key genes related to colistin resistance (*mgrB*, *pmrAB*, and *phoPQ*). As shown in **Supplementary Table 3**, alterations mainly occurred in *pmrB* (21/36, 58.3%), followed by *phoQ* (15/36, 41.7%), and *pmrA* (9/36, 25.0%), most of which were associated with different amino acid substitutions, except frameshift mutations found in the *pmrB* gene (n = 6). No mutations were observed in *phoP* or *mgrB*.

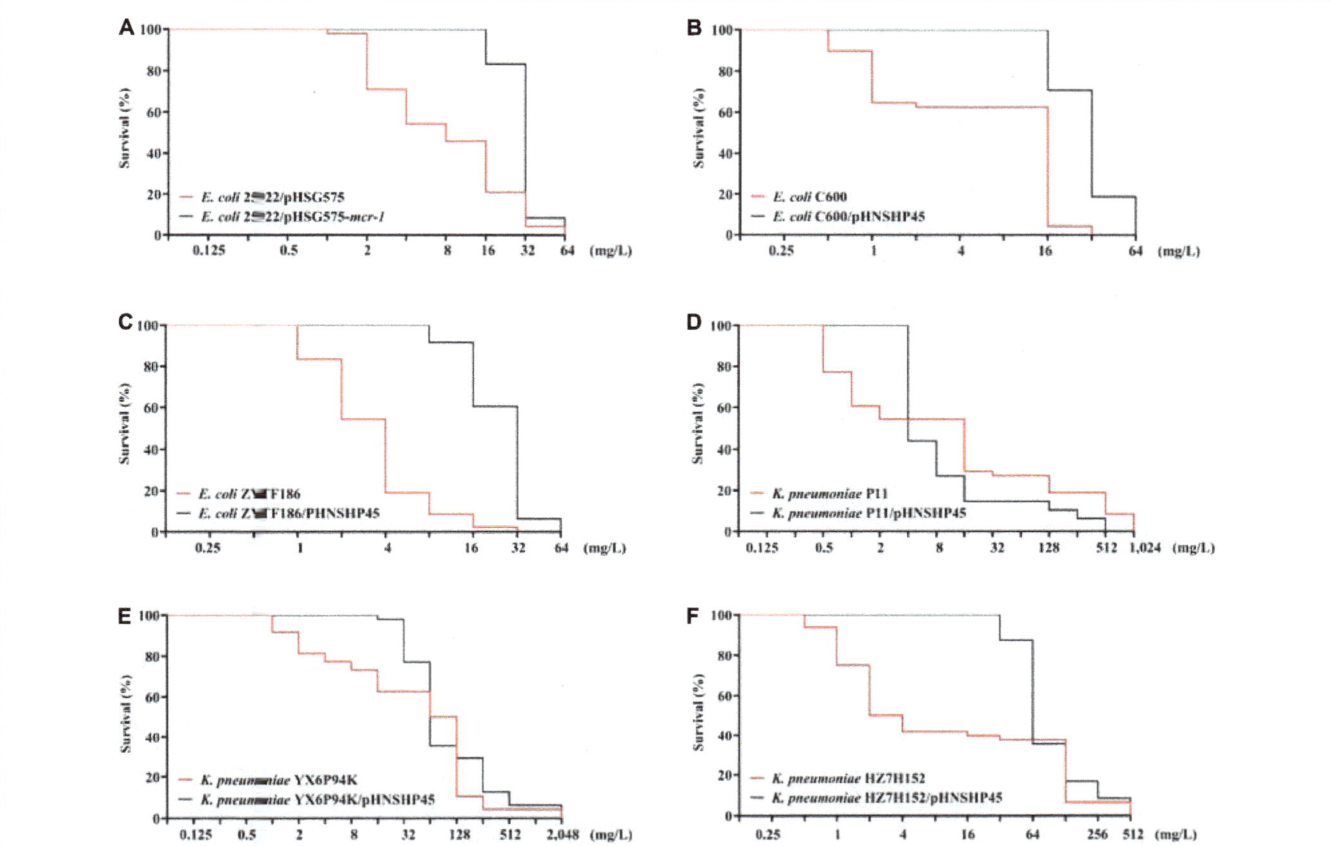

FIGURE 1 | Survival curves of *E. coli* **(A–C)** and *K. pneumoniae* strains **(D–F)** and their *mcr-1*-positive transformants in the presence of increasing concentrations of colistin.

Genetic Alterations in *mgrB*, *pmrAB*, *phoPQ*, and *crrAB* in *Klebsiella pneumoniae*

A total of 156 HLCR *K. pneumoniae* mutants, including 75 *mcr-1*-negative and 81 *mcr-1*-positive derivatives, were examined for the presence of mutations in the *mgrB*, *pmrAB*, *phoPQ*, and *crrAB* genes. The HLCR mutants showed a remarkable multiplicity of mutations in these genes (**Figure 3**, **Table 1**, and **Supplementary Table 4**). Among these mutants, genetic changes predominately occurred in *crrB* (62/156, 39.7%), followed by *phoQ* (41/156, 26.3%), *crrA* (35/156, 22.4%), *pmrB* (28/156, 17.9%), *mgrB* (27/156, 17.3%), and *phoP* (23/156, 14.7%). In 55 mutants, mutations were occurred in two or three genes (**Table 1**). No mutations were observed in *pmrA*.

There were evident differences in mutations between the *mcr-1*-negative and *mcr-1*-positive isolates (**Figure 3A**, **Table 1**, and **Supplementary Table 4**). *phoQ* and *mgrB* alterations were more frequent in the *mcr-1*-negative derivatives (41.3 and 32.0%, respectively) than in the *mcr-1*-positive derivatives (12.3 and 3.7%, respectively). By contrast, the *mcr-1*-positive derivatives predominantly harbored mutations in *crrA* (26/81, 32.1%) and *pmrB* (19/81, 23.5%), both of which only occurred in 12.0% (9/75) of the *mcr-1*-negative derivatives. Moreover, of the 55 mutants with genetic change(s) in two or three genes, 34 (34/75, 45.3%) were *mcr-1*-negative derivatives and 21 (21/81, 25.9%) were *mcr-1*-positive derivatives (**Table 1**).

Regarding mutational patterns, alterations were mainly associated with amino acid substitutions or frameshift mutations (**Table 1** and **Supplementary Table 4**), except for insertion sequences (ISs), which were almost exclusively associated with *mgrB* (**Table 1** and **Supplementary Table 4**). Among 27 derivatives with alterations in *mgrB*, 18 (66.7%) were characterized by insertional inactivation of *mgrB*, which was truncated by one of the ISs, namely IS*Kpn26* (n = 3), IS*903B* (n = 6), IS*Kpn14* (n = 3), IS*Ecp1* (n = 3), or IS*1R* (n = 3) (**Supplementary Figure 2**). Additionally, *crrB* was first observed to be truncated by IS*1R* in three derivatives (**Supplementary Figure 2**).

Impacts of Mutations on the Growth of HLCR *Klebsiella pneumoniae* Strains

To determine whether the genetic changes in *mgrB*, *pmrAB*, *phoPQ*, and *crrAB* could impose a fitness cost on *K. pneumoniae* strains, we determined the growth rates of HLCR mutants harboring different mutations. In the *mcr-1*-negative groups, most of the HLCR mutants showed subtle advantages in the

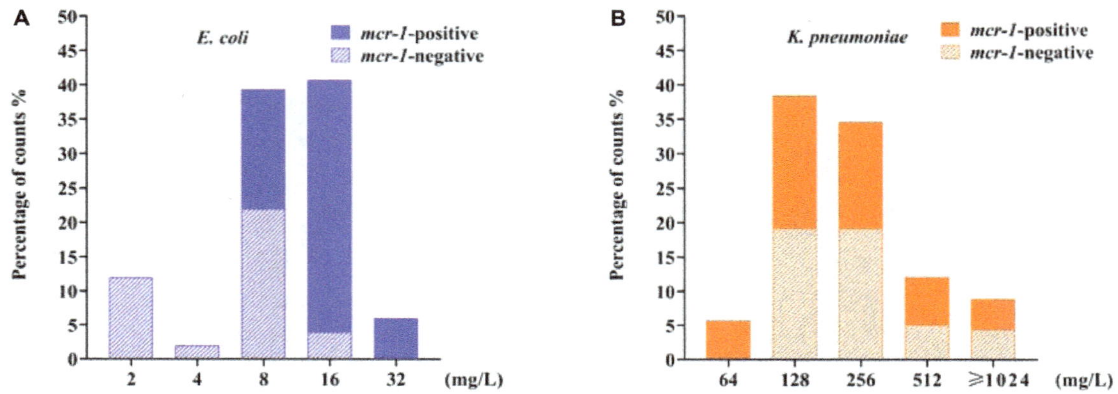

FIGURE 2 | Distributions of colistin minimum inhibitory concentration (MIC) values among *E. coli* and *K. pneumoniae* mutants after induction of colistin resistance *in vitro*. **(A)** Data for 90 *mcr-1*-positive and 60 *mcr-1*-negative *E. coli* derivatives. **(B)** Data for 81 *mcr-1*-positive and 75 *mcr-1*-negative *K. pneumoniae* derivatives. *E. coli* data are indicated in blue, and *K. pneumoniae* data are indicated in orange.

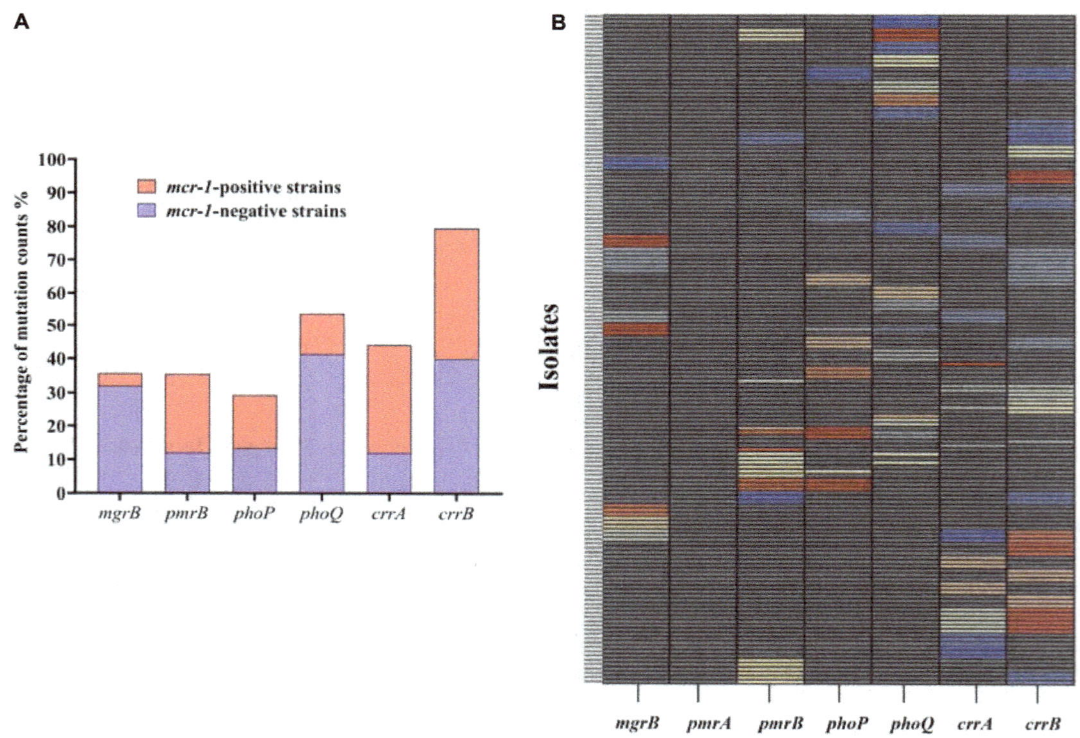

FIGURE 3 | Occurrence of genetic alterations in *mgrB*, *pmrAB*, *phoPQ*, and *crrAB* in *K. pneumoniae*. **(A)** Distribution of mutations in different genes in 81 *mcr-1*-positive and 75 *mcr-1*-negative *K. pneumoniae* derivatives. **(B)** Profiles of genetic alterations in key genes related to colistin resistance, with 53 unique combinations in the 156 colistin-resistant *K. pneumoniae* derivatives. Each unique mutation in each colistin resistance gene is represented by a different color. Specific information on the mutations can be found in **Supplementary Table 4**.

growth rates compared with those of their wild-type parent strains (**Figure 4A**), except for one mutant (*phoQ* V38G), which exhibited a substantial reduction in the growth rate ($p < 0.01$), and three isolates (13.6%) with different mutations, which showed significant advantages in the growth rates ($p < 0.05$). Conversely, among the *mcr-1*-positive HLCR mutants, none exhibited remarkable growth advantages, and most mutants showed slow growth rates compared to their corresponding parent strains (**Figure 4B**). Additionally, 13 individual mutants (59.1%) exhibited significant biological costs for growth ($n = 1$, $p < 0.05$; $n = 9$, $p < 0.01$; $n = 3$, $p < 0.001$). Overall, most chromosomal mutations alone resulted in no burden on growth of HLCR mutants; however, the fitness cost was observed in most *mcr-1*-harboring HLCR mutants.

TABLE 1 | Number of *K. pneumoniae* derivatives with genomic mutation(s) in colistin resistance genes after stepwise induction.

Genome alterations on single gene	Genetic alterations	No. of strains	No. of *mcr-1*-negative strains	No. of *mcr-1*-positive strains
mgrB	Insertional inactivation by ISs	9	6	3
	FMs	2	2	0
pmrB	FMs	5	0	5
	Amino acid substitutions	3	0	3
phoP	Amino acid substitutions	3	0	3
	FMs	3	0	3
phoQ	Amino acid substitutions	33	27	6
crrA	Amino acid substitutions	9	0	9
	FMs	8	0	8
crrB	Amino acid substitutions	21	6	15
	Amino acid substitution, FM	1	0	1
	FM	1	0	1
	Insertional inactivation by ISs, amino acid substitutions	3	0	3
Total strains with mutations in single gene		64.7% (101)	54.7% (41/75)	74.1% (60/81)
Genome alterations on two or three genes	*pmrB* and *phoQ* amino acid substitutions	5	3	2
	phoP and *crrB* amino acid substitutions	9	9	0
	pmrB and *crrB* amino acid substitutions	3	3	0
	mgrB FMs, *crrA* amino acid substitutions	6	6	0
	mgrB FMs, *crrB* amino acid substitutions	6	6	0
	mgrB FM, *phoPQ* amino acid substitution	1	1	0
	crrA FMs, *crrB* amino acid substitutions	3	0	3
	pmrB amino acid substitution and FM, *phoP* amino acid substitution	1	0	1
	pmrB and *phoPQ* amino acid substitution	1	0	1
	phoPQ amino acid substitution	1	0	1
	pmrB amino acid substitution, *phoP* FM	1	0	1
	pmrB and *phoP* amino acid substitutions	3	0	3
	pmrB FMs, *crrB* amino acid substitutions	6	3	3
	mgrB insertional inactivation by ISs, *crrAB* amino acid substitutions	3	3	0
	crrA amino acid substitutions, *crrB* FMs	6	0	6
Total strains associate with mutations in two or more genes		35.3% (55/156)	45.3% (34/75)	25.9% (21/81)

IS, insertion sequence; FM, frameshift mutation.

DISCUSSION

Although the presence of *mcr-1* confers low-level resistance to colistin, there is a concern regarding whether the presence of *mcr-1* can accelerate the development of HLCR. In this study, we found that *mcr-1* did not potentiate the development of HLCR in *E. coli* and *K. pneumoniae,* as the colistin MICs for *mcr-1*-negative derivatives obtained *via* serial colistin challenges were similar to those of their corresponding *mcr-1*-harboring transformants. Moreover, the fold increases in the colistin MICs were higher for *mcr-1*-negative strains than those for their *mcr-1*-harboring transformants. Although the presence of *mcr-1* could not facilitate the evolution of colistin resistance in these two species of bacteria, *mcr-1* could improve their survival rates upon exposure to relatively high concentrations of colistin (16–32 mg/L), which indicated that the presence of *mcr-1* might enhance the survival ability of bacteria under clinical colistin pressure, thereby potentially leading to treatment failure.

Previous reports have shown that the mechanisms of resistance to colistin significantly vary between clinical *K. pneumoniae* and *E. coli* isolates. In *K. pneumoniae*, colistin resistance, including HLCR, is usually caused by chromosomal mutations (Cannatelli et al., 2014; Jayol et al., 2017), whereas in *E. coli*, colistin resistance is mainly associated with the presence of *mcr-1* (Huang et al., 2017). Herein, we demonstrated that compared with *E. coli*, *K. pneumoniae* strains were more likely to develop HLCR by genetic alterations of the two-component systems (TCSs, e.g., PmrAB and PhoPQ) and their regulators (MgrB and CrrAB) when exposed to increasing concentrations of colistin *in vitro*. Previous studies have demonstrated that the TCSs play crucial roles in regulating the expression of genes for lipid A modifications in both *K. pneumoniae* and *E. coli* strains (Poirel et al., 2017; Srinivas and Rivard, 2017). This result partly explains the clinical phenomenon of HLCR being more common in *K. pneumoniae* compared to *E. coli* isolates. However, the mechanism underlying why TCSs and their regulators in

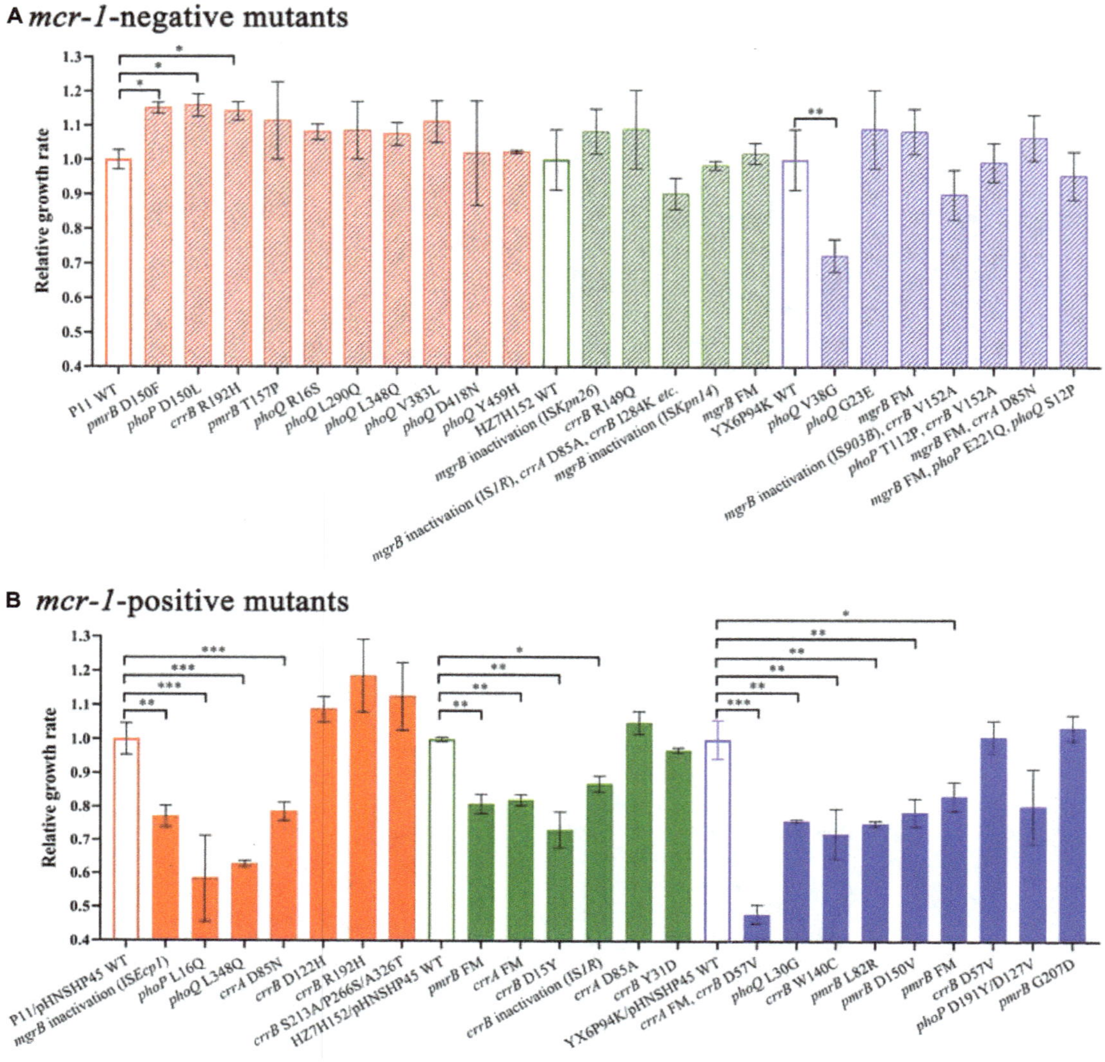

FIGURE 4 | Relative growth rates of *mcr-1*-negative **(A)** and *mcr-1*-positive **(B)** *K. pneumoniae* mutants and their parental strains. The maximal growth rates are presented as relative values compared with the wild-type growth rate (set to 1.0). The relevant mutated genes of each strain are indicated below the chart. $^{*}p < 0.05$; $^{**}p < 0.01$; $^{***}p < 0.001$. Error bars represent standard deviation values. WT, wild-type; FM, frameshift mutation.

K. pneumoniae are more likely to occur genetic alteration under the selective pressure of colistin than those in *E. coli* is unclear and needs further study.

After colistin exposure, alterations were detected in genes (*mgrB*, *pmrAB*, *phoPQ*, and *crrAB*) associated with colistin resistance. In *E. coli*, alterations mainly occurred in *pmrB*, followed by *phoQ*, and no mutations were observed in the *mgrB* or *phoP* gene. However, in HLCR *K. pneumoniae* variants, mutations were more complex and diverse and occurred in all the indicated genes, except *pmrA*. Genetic changes mainly occurred in *crrB* and *phoQ* (**Figure 3A**), in contrast to a previous report which stated that alterations in *mgrB* played a primary role in colistin resistance in *K. pneumoniae* (Cannatelli et al., 2014). However, consistent with previous reports (Kim et al., 2019; Yang et al., 2020), in both *E. coli* and *K. pneumoniae,* the histidine kinase genes *crrB*, *pmrB*, and *phoQ* seemed to be more common sites for mutations compared to the response regulatory genes *crrA*, *pmrA*, and *phoP*. It is possible that the sensor kinases can directly sense environmental stimuli and are therefore more likely to undergo mutations to confer protection against adverse stimuli, such as colistin pressure (Huang et al., 2020). The detected *mgrB*-disrupting ISs, IS*Kpn26*, IS*903B*, IS*Kpn14*, IS*Ecp1*, and IS*1R*, were similar to those found in other studies (Shamina et al., 2020; Yang et al., 2020). Although recent studies have shown that amino acid substitution mutations in *crrB* or IS disruptions are responsible for HLCR (Wright et al., 2015; Jayol et al., 2017; McConville et al., 2020), mutations in *crrAB* in clinical isolates have rarely been reported, possibly due to few tests performed for this newly identified two-component system and the deletion of *crrAB* in some *K. pneumoniae* strains (Wright et al., 2015).

Moreover, most of the mutations observed in this study have not been previously reported; thus, further studies are warranted to elucidate the potential contributions of these novel mutations to colistin resistance.

Remarkably, there were differences in the occurrence of chromosomal mutations in *mcr-1*-positive and *mcr-1*-negative *K. pneumoniae* isolates. In most (74.1%) *mcr-1*-positive derivatives, genetic alteration(s) only occurred in single gene involved in colistin resistance, while half of the *mcr-1*-negative derivatives harbored multiple mutations, thereby implying that the coexistence of chromosomal mutations and *mcr-1* might impose a severe fitness burden on *K. pneumoniae.* To test this hypothesis, we compared the growth rates of *mcr-1*-positive and *mcr-1*-negative strains with those of their relevant HLCR mutants and found that HLCR mutants derived from *mcr-1*-negative strains exhibited almost no fitness cost, while HLCR mutants of *mcr-1*-positive strains showed an evident fitness cost. Previous studies have shown that the fitness cost attributed to chromosomal mutations or the acquisition of wild-type *mcr-1*-harboring plasmids seemed to be insignificant (Cannatelli et al., 2015; Wu et al., 2018); however, increased expression of *mcr-1* could impose a significant fitness burden on host bacteria (Yang et al., 2017; Liu et al., 2020). Our results demonstrated that the coexistence of chromosomal mutations and *mcr-1* was disadvantageous for *K. pneumoniae*, which might partly explain the lack of clinical strains with both chromosomal mutations and *mcr-1* (Nang et al., 2018).

In conclusion, we demonstrated that compared with *E. coli*, *K. pneumoniae* was more likely to develop HLCR by acquiring chromosomal mutations. Although *mcr-1* could not facilitate the selection of HLCR mutants, it could improve the survival rates of bacteria at relatively high concentrations of colistin, which might result in treatment failure.

AUTHOR CONTRIBUTIONS

J-HL designed the study. X-QZ, RW, and HX performed the experiments and collected the data. X-QZ, Y-YL, RW, and HX analyzed and interpreted the data. X-QZ and Y-YL wrote the draft of the manuscript. J-HL, Y-YL, X-QZ, JS, JL, and YF edited and revised the manuscript. All authors have read and approved the manuscript. J-HL coordinated the whole project.

FUNDING

This work was supported in part by the National Natural Science Foundation of China (No. 31830099 and 31625026), the Guangdong Local Innovation Team Program (No. 2019BT02N054), the 111 Project (No. D20008), and the Innovation Team Project of Guangdong University (No. 2019KCXTD001).

REFERENCES

Cannatelli, A., Giani, T., D'Andrea, M. M., Di Pilato, V., Arena, F., Conte, V., et al. (2014). MgrB inactivation is a common mechanism of colistin resistance in *KPC*-producing *Klebsiella pneumoniae* of clinical origin. *Antimicrob. Agents Chemother.* 58, 5696–5703. doi: 10.1128/aac.03110-14

Cannatelli, A., Santos-Lopez, A., Giani, T., Gonzalez-Zorn, B., and Rossolini, G. M. (2015). Polymyxin resistance caused by *mgrB* inactivation is not associated with significant biological cost in *Klebsiella pneumoniae. Antimicrob. Agents Chemother.* 59, 2898–2900. doi: 10.1128/aac.04998-14

Eiamphungporn, W., Yainoy, S., Jumderm, C., Tan-Arsuwongkul, R., Tiengrim, S., and Thamlikitkul, V. (2018). Prevalence of the colistin resistance gene *mcr-1* in colistin-resistant *Escherichia coli* and *Klebsiella pneumoniae* isolated from humans in Thailand. *J. Glob. Antimicrob. Resist.* 15, 32–35. doi: 10.1016/j.jgar.2018.06.007

Huang, J., Li, C., Song, J., Velkov, T., Wang, L., Zhu, Y., et al. (2020). Regulating polymyxin resistance in Gram-negative bacteria: roles of two-component systems PhoPQ and PmrAB. *Future Microbiol.* 15, 445–459. doi: 10.2217/fmb-2019-0322

Huang, X., Yu, L., Chen, X., Zhi, C., Yao, X., Liu, Y., et al. (2017). High prevalence of colistin resistance and *mcr-1*gene in *Escherichia coli* isolated from food animals in China. *Front. Microbiol.* 8:562. doi: 10.3389/fmicb.2017.00562

Huang, Y. H., Chou, S.-H., Liang, S.-W., Ni, C.-E., Lin, Y.-T., Huang, Y. W., et al. (2018). Emergence of an XDR and carbapenemase-producing hypervirulent *Klebsiella pneumoniae* strain in Taiwan. *J. Antimicrob. Chemother.* 73, 2039–2046. doi: 10.1093/jac/dky164

Jacoby, G. A., Strahilevitz, J., and Hooper, D. C. (2014). Plasmid-mediated quinolone resistance. *Microbiol. Spectr.* 2:10.

Jayol, A., Nordmann, P., Brink, A., Villegas, M. V., Dubois, V., and Poirel, L. (2017). High-level resistance to colistin mediated by various mutations in the *crrB* gene among carbapenemase-producing *Klebsiella pneumoniae. Antimicrob. Agents Chemother.* 61:e01423-17.

Jeong, J. Y., Kim, E. S., Choi, S. H., Kwon, H. H., Lee, S. R., Lee, S. O., et al. (2008). Effects of a plasmid-encoded *qnr*A1 determinant in *Escherichia coli* strains carrying chromosomal mutations in the *acrAB* efflux pump genes. *Diagn. Microbiol. Infect. Dis.* 60, 105–107. doi: 10.1016/j.diagmicrobio.2007.07.015

Kim, S., Woo, J. H., Kim, N., Kim, M. H., Kim, S. Y., Son, J. H., et al. (2019). Characterization of chromosome-mediated colistin resistance in *Escherichia coli* isolates from livestock in Korea. *Infect. Drug Resist.* 12, 3291–3299. doi: 10.2147/idr.s225383

Liu, Y. Y., Wang, Y., Walsh, T. R., Yi, L. X., Zhang, R., Spencer, J., et al. (2016). Emergence of plasmid-mediated colistin resistance mechanism MCR-1 in animals and human beings in China: a microbiological and molecular biological study. *Lancet Infect. Dis.* 16, 161–168. doi: 10.1016/s1473-3099(15)00424-7

Liu, Y. Y., Zhu, Y., Wickremasinghe, H., Bergen, P. J., Lu, J., Zhu, X. Q., et al. (2020). Metabolic perturbations caused by the over-expression of *mcr-1* in *Escherichia coli. Front. Microbiol.* 11:588658. doi: 10.3389/fmicb.2020.588658

Luo, Q., Niu, T., Wang, Y., Yin, J., Wan, F., Yao, M., et al. (2019). In vitro reduction of colistin susceptibility and comparative genomics reveals multiple differences between MCR-positive and MCR-negative colistin-resistant *Escherichia coli. Infect. Drug Resist.* 12, 1665–1674. doi: 10.2147/idr.s210245

Matuschek, E., Åhman, J., Webster, C., and Kahlmeter, G. (2018). Antimicrobial susceptibility testing of colistin - evaluation of seven commercial MIC products against standard broth microdilution for *Escherichia coli, Klebsiella pneumoniae, Pseudomonas aeruginosa*, and *Acinetobacter spp. Clin. Microbiol. Infect.* 24, 865–870. doi: 10.1016/j.cmi.2017.11.020

McConville, T. H., Annavajhala, M. K., Giddins, M. J., Macesic, N., Herrera, C. M., Rozenberg, F. D., et al. (2020). CrrB positively regulates high-level polymyxin resistance and virulence in *Klebsiella pneumoniae. Cell Rep.* 33:108313. doi: 10.1016/j.celrep.2020.108313

Nang, S. C., Morris, F. C., Mcdonald, M. J., Han, M. L., Wang, J., Strugnell, R. A., et al. (2018). Fitness cost of *mcr-1*-mediated polymyxin resistance in *Klebsiella pneumoniae. J. Antimicrob. Chemother.* 73, 1604–1610. doi: 10.1093/jac/dky061

Poirel, L., Jayol, A., and Nordmann, P. (2017). Polymyxins: antibacterial activity, susceptibility testing, and resistance mechanisms encoded by plasmids or chromosomes. *Clin. Microbiol. Rev.* 30, 557–596. doi: 10.1128/cmr.00064-16

Quan, J., Li, X., Chen, Y., Jiang, Y., Zhou, Z., Zhang, H., et al. (2017). Prevalence of *mcr-1* in *Escherichia coli* and *Klebsiella pneumoniae* recovered from bloodstream infections in China: a multicentre longitudinal study. *Lancet Infect. Dis.* 17, 400–410. doi: 10.1016/s1473-3099(16)30528-x

Ruhnke, M., Arnold, R., and Gastmeier, P. (2014). Infection control issues in patients with haematological malignancies in the era of multidrug-resistant bacteria. *Lancet Oncol.* 15:e0606-19.

San Millan, A., Escudero, J. A., Gifford, D. R., Mazel, D., and Maclean, R. A. (2016). Multicopy plasmids potentiate the evolution of antibiotic resistance in bacteria. *Nat. Ecol. Evol.* 1:10.

Shamina, O. V., Kryzhanovskaya, O. A., Lazareva, A. V., Alyabieva, N. M., Polikarpova, S. V., Karaseva, O. V., et al. (2020). Emergence of a ST307 clone carrying a novel insertion element MITE *Kpn1* in the *mgrB* gene among carbapenem-resistant *Klebsiella pneumoniae* from Moscow, Russia. *Int. J. Antimicrob. Agents* 55:105850. doi: 10.1016/j.ijantimicag.2019.11.007

Shi, X., Li, Y., Yang, Y., Shen, Z., Wu, Y., and Wang, S. (2020). Global impact of mcr-1-positive *Enterobacteriaceae* bacteria on "one health". *Crit. Rev. Microbiol.* 46, 565–577. doi: 10.1080/1040841x.2020.1812510

Srinivas, P., and Rivard, K. (2017). Polymyxin resistance in gram-negative pathogens. *Curr. Infect. Dis. Rep.* 19:38.

Takeshita, S., Sato, M., Toba, M., Masahashi, W., and Hashimoto-Gotoh, T. (1987). High-copy-number and low-copy-number plasmid vectors for *lacZ* alpha-complementation and chloramphenicol- or kanamycin-resistance selection. *Gene* 61, 63–74. doi: 10.1016/0378-1119(87)90365-9

Wang, C., Feng, Y. A.-O., Liu, L., Wei, L., Kang, M., and Zong, Z. A.-O. X. (2020). Identification of novel mobile colistin resistance gene *mcr-10*. *Emerg. Microb. Infect.* 9, 508–516. doi: 10.1080/22221751.2020.1732231

Wright, M. S., Suzuki, Y., Jones, M. B., Marshall, S. H., Rudin, S. D., Van Duin, D., et al. (2015). Genomic and transcriptomic analyses of colistin-resistant clinical isolates of *Klebsiella pneumoniae* reveal multiple pathways of resistance. *Antimicrob. Agents Chemother.* 59, 536–543. doi: 10.1128/aac.04037-14

Wu, R., Yi, L. X., Yu, L. F., Wang, J., Liu, Y., Chen, X., et al. (2018). Fitness Advantage of *mcr-1*-bearing IncI2 and IncX4 plasmids in vitro. *Front. Microbiol.* 9:331. doi: 10.3389/fmicb.2018.00331

Yang, Q., Li, M., Spiller, O. B., Andrey, D. A.-O., Hinchliffe, P., Li, H., et al. (2017). Balancing *mcr-1* expression and bacterial survival is a delicate equilibrium between essential cellular defence mechanisms. *Nat. Commun.* 8:2054.

Yang, T. Y., Wang, S. F., Lin, J. E., Griffith, B. T. S., Lian, S. H., Hong, Z. D., et al. (2020). Contributions of insertion sequences conferring colistin resistance in *Klebsiella pneumoniae*. *Int. J. Antimicrob. Agents* 55:105894. doi: 10.1016/j.ijantimicag.2020.105894

Zhang, H., Zhao, D., Quan, J., Hua, X., and Yu, Y. (2019). *mcr-1* facilitated selection of high-level colistin-resistant mutants in *Escherichia coli*. *Clin. Microbiol. Infect.* 25:517.e1-e4.

Zwietering, M. H., Jongenburger, I., Rombouts, F. M., and Van 'T Riet, K. (1990). Modeling of the bacterial growth curve. *Appl. Environ. Microbiol.* 56, 1875–1881.

12

Prediction of Cell-Penetrating Potential of Modified Peptides Containing Natural and Chemically Modified Residues

Vinod Kumar[1,2†], *Piyush Agrawal*[1,2†], *Rajesh Kumar*[1,2†], *Sherry Bhalla*[1], *Salman Sadullah Usmani*[1,2], *Grish C. Varshney*[3] *and Gajendra P. S. Raghava*[1,2*]

[1] *Center for Computational Biology, Indraprastha Institute of Information Technology, Okhla, India,* [2] *Bioinformatics Centre, CSIR-Institute of Microbial Technology, Sector-39A, Chandigarh, India,* [3] *Cell Biology and Immunology, CSIR-Institute of Microbial Technology, Sector-39A, Chandigarh, India*

Correspondence:
Gajendra P. S. Raghava
raghava@iiitd.ac.in

† These authors have contributed equally to this work.

Designing drug delivery vehicles using cell-penetrating peptides is a hot area of research in the field of medicine. In the past, number of *in silico* methods have been developed for predicting cell-penetrating property of peptides containing natural residues. In this study, first time attempt has been made to predict cell-penetrating property of peptides containing natural and modified residues. The dataset used to develop prediction models, include structure and sequence of 732 chemically modified cell-penetrating peptides and an equal number of non-cell penetrating peptides. We analyzed the structure of both class of peptides and observed that positive charge groups, atoms, and residues are preferred in cell-penetrating peptides. In this study, models were developed to predict cell-penetrating peptides from its tertiary structure using a wide range of descriptors (2D, 3D descriptors, and fingerprints). Random Forest model developed by using PaDEL descriptors (combination of 2D, 3D, and fingerprints) achieved maximum accuracy of 95.10%, MCC of 0.90 and AUROC of 0.99 on the main dataset. The performance of model was also evaluated on validation/independent dataset which achieved AUROC of 0.98. In order to assist the scientific community, we have developed a web server "CellPPDMod" for predicting the cell-penetrating property of modified peptides (http://webs.iiitd.edu.in/raghava/cellppdmod/).

Keywords: modified cell-penetrating peptides, machine learning, Random Forest, SVM, *in silico* method, chemical descriptors, antimicrobial peptide

INTRODUCTION

Since the existence of human race, therapeutic molecules have been used to cure human illness and to extend lives (Tosato et al., 2007). In past, thousands of molecules have been studied to combat deadly diseases. The ideal molecule must attain the desired therapeutic effect without causing side effects. A large number of promising therapeutic molecules disparage before reaching to its target (Gupta and Jhawat, 2017). In order to overcome this, several delivery vehicles have been discovered in last three decades, such as nanoparticle (Wang et al., 2018) and lipid carrier conjugate (Xu et al., 2017). Cell-penetrating peptide (CPP) is one of the most emergent and widely accepted drug delivery vehicle, having ability to internalize even into eukaryotic cells in non-disruptive way. These are short peptides of 3 to approximately 40 amino acids, mostly cationic followed by amphipathic in nature (Agrawal et al., 2016). CPPs can transport various biologically active molecules inside microbes as well as mammalian cells (Gao et al., 2014; Kurrikoff et al., 2016). CPPs such as TP10 and pVEC had been shown to significantly inhibit growth of few microbes as *Candida albicans*, *Staphylococcus aureus* as well as *Mycobacterium smegmatis* (Nekhotiaeva et al., 2004). CPPs and cationic antibacterial peptides have similar physicochemical properties, so many CPPs have shown antimicrobial activity (Splith and Neundorf, 2011; Bahnsen et al., 2013; Rodriguez Plaza et al., 2014). The poor membrane permeability of drug molecule always remains a concern in drug designing. In the era of drug resistance, where pathogen membrane provides a significant barrier, intracellular delivery of antibiotics/drugs by the virtue of CPP, proved to be a vital step in combating drug resistance to some extent (Sparr et al., 2013). CPP based conjugates (Ganguly et al., 2008; Jain et al., 2015) and combination therapy has been explored against several resistant pathogens (Randhawa et al., 2016). They have been proved effective against intracellular pathogens too (Gomarasca et al., 2017).

A universal mechanism of CPP internalization is always proved to be an exploring question, as the involved pathways are not fully clarified yet. The difficulty arises due to differing size, physicochemical properties, as well as concentration of diverse CPP and CPP-conjugates (Guidotti et al., 2017). Several mechanisms have been shown by various CPPs to translocate in to the cell, as micelle formation (Derossi et al., 1996), pore formation (Matsuzaki et al., 1996), membrane thinning (Pouny et al., 1992), endocytosis (Ferreira and Boucrot, 2018) and micropinocytosis (Jones, 2007). Majority of CPP internalization occurs via endocytosis, but several evidences suggest that at a threshold concentration direct penetration does occur (Palm-Apergi et al., 2012). CPPs can be used for intracellular delivery of small molecule-based drug (Lindgren et al., 2006), oligonucleotide (Margus et al., 2012), peptide and protein (Morris et al., 2001) and trans-epithelial delivery of peptides (Tan et al., 2014).

Despite, numerous properties and potential applications of CPPs, still there use in real life is limited. The primary limitation associated with CPP is endosomal compartment entrapment which reduces the bioavailability of the drug several times. In literature, it has been shown that bioavailability of CPPs can be increased several times by introducing a chemical modification in a CPP (Postlethwaite et al., 1996; Kim et al., 2006; Lundberg et al., 2007; Koppelhus et al., 2008; Aubry et al., 2009). N-terminal stearylation of Arg8 peptide improved the delivery of siRNA (Futaki et al., 2001), C-terminal cysteamidation of MPG peptide improved the delivery of siRNA (Simeoni et al., 2003), cysteine residue modification improved the stability of Tat peptide and thus enhances the plasmid delivery (Lo and Wang, 2008), Poly-L-ornithine modification in PepFect 14 peptide increases transfection efficiency of oligonucleotide in HeLa pLuc 705 (Ezzat et al., 2011). Thus, it is important to understand chemical modification of residues in a peptide and its impact on cell-penetrating property of peptides.

In the last few years, several computational methods have been developed for the prediction of CPPs. These methods have been developed on various features like amino acid composition (Sanders et al., 2011), dipeptide composition (Tang et al., 2016), binary profile, physiochemical properties and motifs (Gautam et al., 2013). They have also applied Z-scale based method (Sandberg et al., 1998), feature selection techniques (Tang et al., 2016), classifiers like Random Forest (RF) (Wei et al., 2017), Support Vector Machine (SVM) (Sanders et al., 2011). Beside this, few more methods have been developed in recent years for predicting CPPs with high accuracy (Chen et al., 2015; Tang et al., 2016; Wei et al., 2017). Best of authors knowledge, all methods developed so far for predicting CPPs are suitable for peptides containing natural residues only, but no method has been developed for predicting cell penetration property of peptides with non-natural and modified residues. In this study, a systematic attempt has been made to develop a machine learning method for predicting cell penetration ability of peptides containing non-natural and modified residues. Machine learning technique derive features/rules from the experimentally validated modified CPPs and Non-CPPs are used to predict cell penetration ability of a modified peptide. We hope this method will be useful for researchers working in the field of drug delivery.

MATERIALS AND METHODS

Creation of Dataset for CPPs and Non-CPPs

Cell-penetrating peptides were extracted from CPPsite2.0 database (Agrawal et al., 2016), which provides comprehensive information on wide-range of CPPs. It consists of 1,850 experimentally validated natural and modified CPPs. We remove CPPs that does not contain any modified residue; we also remove peptides whose tertiary structure is not available in the database. Finally, we got 732 chemically modified CPPs whose structure is available in CPPsite 2.0. We assign this set of 732 CPPs as positive set or set of CPPs. To develop any method, we also need equal number of negative examples. In this study, we extracted non-CPPs from SATPdb (Singh et al., 2016) database which maintains information of 19,192 peptides having several properties. We extracted structures of 732 peptides, which may exhibit any characteristic other than cell penetrating property. This set of peptides were assigned as negative set or set of non-CPPs. Finally, we built the dataset that contains 732 CPPs and 732 non-CPPs whose sequence and tertiary structure is available in CPPsites 2.0 or SATPdb.

Datasets for Internal and External Validation

The dataset was divided into two datasets namely training (main) and validation dataset (Bhalla et al., 2017). The training dataset consists of 80% of peptides, 582 CPPs, and 582 non-CPPs. The validation dataset consists of remaining 20% of peptides, 150 CPPs, and 150 non-CPPs. We used training dataset for developing models and for internal validation.

In internal validation, models were trained and tested using commonly used five-fold cross-validation technique (Nagpal et al., 2017). Performance of best model achieved on training dataset, was evaluated on validation dataset. The evaluation of the performance of model on validation or independent dataset is called external validation.

Model Development

Computation of Features From Peptide Structures

Composition Based Features

Atom composition is computed from CPPs and non-CPPs by converting peptide structures in SMILES format using openbabel (O'Boyle et al., 2011). These SMILES were further used to compute atom composition of following atoms C, H, O, N, S, Cl, Br, and F. The atomic composition provided the fixed length of 8 vectors.

$$\text{Fraction of atom}\,(a) = \frac{\text{Total number of atom}\,(a)}{\text{Total number of all possible diatoms}} \times 100 \quad (1)$$

Where atom (a) is one out of 8 atoms.

Diatom Composition

We computed diatom composition of amino acids just like the atomic composition for CPPs and non-CPPs. The diatomic composition provides the composition of the pair of atoms in each residue (e.g., C-C, C-O, etc.) of the peptide, and used to convert the variable length of modified peptides to fixed length feature vectors. The diatomic composition provided the fixed length of 64 (8 × 8) vectors.

$$\text{Fraction of Diatom}(a) = \frac{\text{Total number of Diatom}\,(a)}{\text{Total number of all possible diatoms}} \times 100 \quad (2)$$

Where diatom (a) is one out of 64 diatoms.

Chemical Descriptors

A biological property of any chemical molecule is determined by its chemical descriptors, which have been used in the past to develop QSAR based molecules (Kumar et al., 2015). PaDEL software, a freely available software was used for the calculation of chemical descriptors (Yap 2011). We calculated 15,537 different types of descriptors, including 2D, 3D, and 10 different types of fingerprints. As all descriptors don't correlate with biological activity, we have done feature selection using "CsfSubsetEval" function present in WEKA software (Smith and Frank, 2016) to remove unnecessary descriptors hence reduced noise from dataset.

Computation of Features From Amino Acid Sequence of Peptide

Amino Acid Composition

We substitute the symbol of the modified residue with its original natural amino acid, for calculating amino acid composition for the positive and negative dataset. This left us with the sequence having 20 natural amino acids which generated the vector of 20.

$$AAC\,(a) = \frac{Ra}{N}x100 \quad (3)$$

Here, $AAC\,(a)$ is the percent composition of amino acid (a); R_a is the numbers of residues of type a, and N represents the total number of peptide's residues.

Dipeptide Composition

We also calculated dipeptide composition of the peptides since it provides global information of the peptide. The dipeptide composition was calculated using the formula 4, and it generated the vector of 400 (20 × 20).

$$\text{Fraction of Dipeptide}\,(a) = \frac{\text{Total number of Dipeptide}\,(a)}{\text{Total number of all possible dipeptides}} \times 100 \quad (4)$$

Where dipeptide (a) is one out of 400 dipeptides.

Terminus Composition-Based Model

We also calculated N and C terminus amino acid composition as well as dipeptide composition for developing prediction models. The composition of 5, 10, and 15 residues from N-terminus as well as C-terminus was taken into account. Also, we joined the terminal residues like N5C5, N10C10, and N15C15 and for developing models.

Residue Preference

In order to observe the residue preference at a particular position in the peptide, web-logos were prepared for first 15 N and 15 C-terminals along with their modifications using online WebLogo software (Crooks et al., 2004). These logos provide the position specific frequency of amino acids in a peptide. Each logo consists of stacks of symbols, one stack for each position in the sequence. The overall height of the stack indicates the sequence conservation at that position while the height of symbols within the stack indicates the relative frequency of each amino acid at that position.

Statistical Analysis

To check whether is there any significance difference between modified CPPs and non-CPPs, we performed Welch t-test on the selected features of 2D, 3D and Fingerprints descriptors using in house R-script. Adjusted p-values were calculated using Boneferroni adjustment.

Performance Measure

Different parameters were used to check the performance of various models developed in this study. These parameters are divided into two groups.

Threshold Dependent Parameters

This category includes Sensitivity (Sen), Specificity (Spc), Accuracy (Acc), and Matthews's correlation coefficient (MCC), where Sensitivity is true positive rate, Specificity is true negative rate, accuracy is ability to differentiate true positive and true negative and MCC is a correlation coefficient between observed and predicted. These can be calculated using the following equations.

$$\text{Sensitivity} = \frac{TP}{PS} \times 100 \quad (5)$$

$$\text{Specificity} = \frac{TN}{NS} \times 100 \quad (6)$$

$$\text{Accuracy} = \frac{TP + TN}{PS + NS} \times 100 \quad (7)$$

$$\text{MCC} = \frac{1 - \left(\frac{FN}{PS} \times \frac{FP}{NS}\right)}{\sqrt{\left(1 + \frac{FP-FN}{PS}\right) \times \left(1 + \frac{FN-FP}{NS}\right)}} \quad (8)$$

Where *TP* represents correctly predicted positive, *TN* represents the correctly predicted negative examples, *PS* represents total sequences in positive set, *NS* represents total sequences in negative set, *FP* represents actual negative examples which have been wrongly predicted as positive and *FN* represents wrongly predicted positive examples. This is a well-established method of measuring performance and has been used earlier in many studies (Porto et al., 2017; Agrawal et al., 2018).

Threshold Independent Parameters

In this study, we also used threshold independent measure to evaluate the performance of models. In case of threshold independent measures, Receiver Operating Characteristics (ROC) curve is drawn between false positive and false negative rates. In order to measure performance, Area Under Curve ROC curve is computed called AUROC.

RESULTS

Analysis

We compute percent average composition of atoms in CPPs and non-CPPs to understand the preference of certain types of atoms present in the CPPs and non-CPPs. Overall, the profile is more or less same in both CPPs and non-CPPs.CPPs are slightly rich in H and N atoms whereas non-CPPs are slightly rich in C, O, and S (**Figure S1**). We analyzed the amino acid composition of both positive (CPPs) and negative (Non-CPPs) dataset. It has been observed that certain type of residues like R, K, and Q are more prominent in CPPs; in contrast residues are like C, L, V, P, and G are not preferred in CPPs (**Figure 1**). In the same manner, we also calculated the average amino acid composition of the first 15 N and 15 C- terminal amino acid residues (**Figure S2**). At the N terminal R, Q, I and M are more prominent in CPP as compared to Non-CPP (**Figure S2A**). Similarly at C terminal, R, K and Q are more prominent (**Figure S2B**).

In addition to compositional preference, we also computed preference of different types of residues in CPPs. It was revealed that some specific type of residues was preferred in the positive dataset contain CPPs as compared to the negative dataset contain non-CPPs. Residues like Rand K are highly preferred at various positions CPPs particularly at N terminal (**Figure 2**). Similarly, K and R are mostly preferred at C terminal also (**Figure 3**).

Machine Learning Based Prediction Model

We used various machine-learning approaches like SVM, Random Forest, Naive Bayes, J48 and SMO for developing the prediction model. These models utilize different features or descriptors to discriminate or classify CPPs and non-CPPs. The results are explained in details in the following sections.

Model Based on Peptide Structure

Tertiary structure of a peptide can present all type of modifications. Thus structure of peptide is used to predict cell penetration ability of modified peptide. In this study,

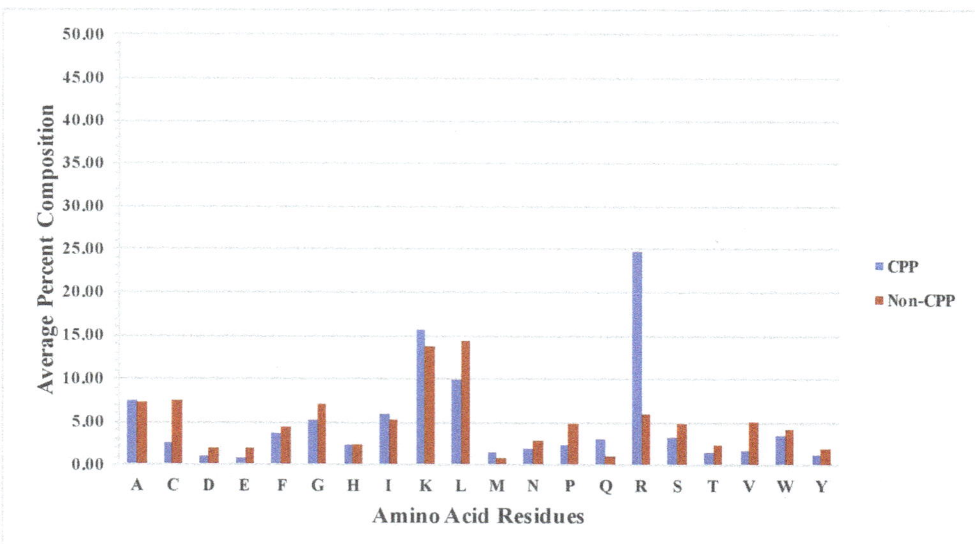

FIGURE 1 | Percentage amino acid composition of CPPs and non-CPPs.

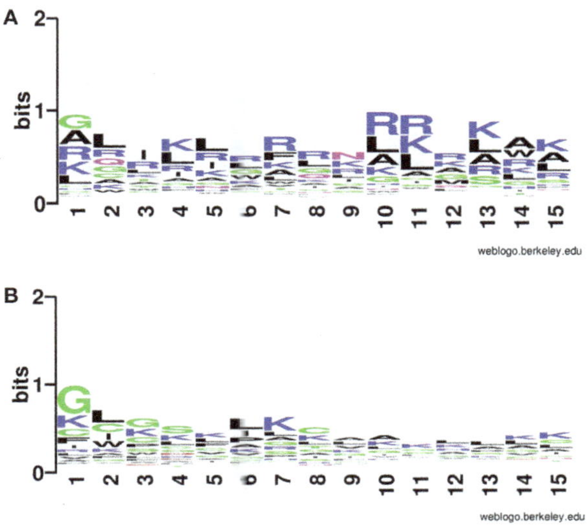

FIGURE 2 | Weblogo illustrating residue preference of first 15 N terminal residues of modified **(A)** CPPs and **(B)** non-CPPs.

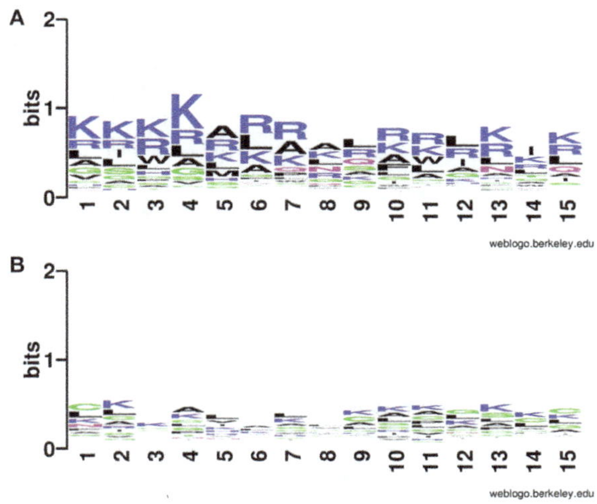

FIGURE 3 | Weblogo illustrating residue preference of first 15 C terminal residues of modified **(A)** CPPs and **(B)** non-CPPs.

we got structure of peptides from databases CPPsite 2.0 and SATPdb. The models were developed using various features of peptide structures. First we developed model using atomic composition of peptides. In order to obtain atomic composition of peptides from its structure, we convert structure from sdf format to SMILES. The atomic composition of peptides was calculated from SMILES of peptide. Prediction models were developed using different classifiers like SVM, RF, Naive Bayes, SMO and J48 using atomic composition as an input feature. Random Forest based classification model provided the highest accuracy of 84.02%, MCC of 0.68 and AUROC of 0.91 on the training dataset. On validation dataset, we achieved maximum accuracy of 78.33%, MCC of 0.57 and AUROC of 0.88. Performance of different classifiers given in **Table 1.** We also developed model using diatom composition of peptides and obtained the highest accuracy of 88.40% with MCC of 0.77. On validation dataset, we achieved maximum accuracy of 91.00% with MCC 0.83. Here SVM based model performed best among all the classifiers used for prediction (**Table 2**).

We developed models individually for 2D descriptors, 3D descriptors, and Fingerprints as well as the single model by combining 2D, 3D descriptors, and Fingerprints. The descriptors were computed using PaDEL software from tertiary structure of peptides (sdf format). The models were developed on the features, selected after performing feature selection, by attribute evaluator named, "CfsSubsetEval" with search method of "BestFirst" at default parameters in the forward direction (amount of backtracking, $N = 5$ and lookup size $D = 1$). In case of 2D descriptors, total 144 descriptors were calculated initially and were reduced to 17 after feature selection. List of the selected features is provided in **Table S1**. We applied different machine learning techniques on these selected features and observed that Random Forest based model achieved the maximum accuracy of 92.34%, MCC of 0.85 and AUROC of 0.97 for the main dataset and 91.67% accuracy, 0.83 MCC and 0.97 AUROC for the validation dataset (**Table 3**).

In case of 3D descriptors, total 47 features were calculated and was reduced to 6 after applying feature selection (**Table S2**). On these features, Random Forest model performed better than other models and achieved maximum accuracy of 76.55%, MCC of 0.53 and AUROC value of 0.85 on the main dataset and 73.49% accuracy, 0.47 MCC and 0.83 AUROC on validation dataset (**Table 4**). The different types of fingerprints generated 14,532 features, which were reduced to 27 after feature selection (**Table S3**). Performance of different classifiers were evaluated on these features (**Table 5**) and once again Random Forest showed the best performance with maximum accuracy of 92.25%, MCC of 0.85 and AUROC of 0.98 on main dataset and accuracy of 92.33%, MCC of 0.85 and AUROC of 0.98 on validation dataset.

Finally, we calculated all the 2D, 3D descriptors and fingerprints at the same time, which generated 15,204 features. Feature selection reduced it down to 48 important features on which different machine learning classifiers were evaluated. Here we observe the maximum accuracy of 95.10%, MCC of 0.90 and AUROC of 0.99 on main dataset and 92.33% accuracy, 0.85 MCC and 0.98 AUROC on validation dataset by Random Forest model (**Table 6**). **Figure 4** shows the AUROC curve as well as AUROC values of different models.

Significance of features

We obtained significant difference between the positive and negative features based on adjusted p-values. P-values were found to be less than 0.05 for most of the features. Therefore, we can say that these features can be used to discriminate modified CPPs and non-CPPs. Mean value of positive and negative features along with their p-value for 2D, 3D, and fingerprint descriptors is provided in **Tables S1–S3**.

TABLE 1 | Performance of different machine learning methods on atom composition.

	Parameter	Main dataset					Validation dataset				
		Sen	**Spc**	**Acc**	**MCC**	**AUROC**	**Sen**	**Spc**	**Acc**	**MCC**	**AUROC**
SVM	$g = 1, c = 9$, j=4	81.10	80.58	80.84	0.62	0.84	79.33	75.33	77.33	0.55	0.81
Random Forest	Ntree = 30	83.33	84.71	84.02	0.68	0.91	79.33	77.33	78.33	0.57	0.88
SMO	$g = 1, c = 2$	77.66	83.51	80.58	0.61	0.80	75.33	82.67	79.00	0.58	0.79
J48	$c = 0.1, m = 1$	75.43	80.58	78.01	0.56	0.82	80.00	76.00	78.00	0.56	0.79
Naive Bayes	Default	74.57	65.46	70.02	0.40	0.80	80.00	69.33	74.67	0.50	0.82

TABLE 2 | Performance of different machine learning methods on diatom composition.

	Parameters	Main dataset					Validation dataset				
		Sen	**Spc**	**Acc**	**MCC**	**AUROC**	**Sen**	**Spc**	**Acc**	**MCC**	**AUROC**
SVM	$g = 0.01, c = 15, j = 2$	90.38	86.43	88.40	0.77	0.93	85.33	96.67	91.00	0.83	0.97
Random Forest	Ntree = 30	88.49	88.49	88.49	0.77	0.94	85.33	82.00	83.67	0.67	0.93
SMO	$g = 0.1, c = 4$	86.25	89.00	87.63	0.75	0.87	86.67	84.00	85.33	0.71	0.85
J48	$c = 0.3, m = 1$	82.47	81.10	81.79	0.64	0.81	85.33	81.33	83.33	0.67	0.82
Naive Bayes	Default	71.65	70.45	71.05	0.42	0.78	72.67	66.67	69.67	0.39	0.77

TABLE 3 | Performance of different machine learning methods on 2D descriptors.

	Parameters	Main dataset					Validation dataset				
		Sen	**Spc**	**Acc**	**MCC**	**AUROC**	**Sen**	**Spc**	**Acc**	**MCC**	**AUROC**
SVM	$g = 0.01, c = 6, j = 2$	89.00	84.48	86.75	0.74	0.92	86.00	82.67	84.33	0.69	0.92
Random Forest	Ntree = 60	92.78	91.90	92.34	0.85	0.97	94.67	88.67	91.67	0.83	0.97
SMO	$g = 0.001, c = 4$	83.16	86.38	84.77	0.70	0.84	81.33	87.33	84.33	0.69	0.84
J48	$c = 0.2, m = 2$	89.52	88.79	89.16	0.78	0.89	90.00	87.33	88.67	0.77	0.89
Naive Bayes	Default	75.09	78.79	76.94	0.54	0.85	74.67	77.33	76.00	0.52	0.84

TABLE 4 | Performance of different machine learning methods on 3D descriptors.

	Parameters	Main dataset					Validation dataset				
		Sen	**Spc**	**Acc**	**MCC**	**AUROC**	**Sen**	**Spc**	**Acc**	**MCC**	**AUROC**
SVM	$g = 1e\text{-}05, c = 15, j = 1$	76.29	74.40	75.34	0.51	0.80	71.14	73.15	72.15	0.44	0.80
Random Forest	Ntree = 700	80.93	72.16	76.55	0.53	0.85	79.87	67.11	73.49	0.47	0.83
SMO	$g = 0.0005, c = 2$	69.42	72.85	71.13	0.42	0.71	63.09	76.51	69.80	040	0.69
J48	$c = 0.1, m = 3$	74.74	76.12	75.43	0.51	0.78	72.48	74.50	73.49	0.47	0.78
Naive Bayes	Default	69.24	74.40	71.82	0.44	0.78	69.80	75.84	72.82	0.46	0.79

TABLE 5 | Performance of different machine learning methods on fingerprints.

	Parameters	Main dataset					Validation dataset				
		Sen	**Spc**	**Acc**	**MCC**	**AUROC**	**Sen**	**Spc**	**Acc**	**MCC**	**AUROC**
SVM	$g = 0.005, c = 15, j = 1$	90.19	88.12	89.16	0.78	0.95	93.33	89.33	91.33	0.83	0.96
Random Forest	Ntree = 600	94.32	90.19	92.25	0.85	0.98	96.67	88.00	92.33	0.85	0.98
SMO	$g = 0.0005, c = 4$	85.54	85.03	85.28	0.71	0.85	88.67	85.33	87.00	0.74	0.87
J48	$c = 0.25, m = 1$	90.02	89.33	89.67	0.79	0.89	88.67	88.67	88.67	0.77	0.90
Naive Bayes	Default	86.40	84.34	85.37	0.71	0.90	82.67	85.33	84.00	0.68	0.90

TABLE 6 | Performance of different machine learning methods on 2D, 3D and fingerprints collectively.

	Parameters	Main dataset					Validation dataset				
		Sen	Spc	Acc	MCC	AUROC	Sen	Spc	Acc	MCC	AUROC
SVM	$g = 1e\text{-}05, c = 15, j = 1$	83.33	79.21	81.27	0.63	0.89	78.67	82.67	80.67	0.61	0.87
Random Forest	Ntree = 60	95.19	95.02	95.10	0.90	0.99	91.33	93.33	92.33	0.85	0.98
SMO	$g = 0.0001, c = 5$	76.80	76.98	76.89	0.54	0.76	75.33	83.33	79.33	0.59	0.79
J48	$c = 0.25, m = 5$	89.69	87.63	88.66	0.77	0.90	84.67	92.00	88.33	0.77	0.92
Naive Bayes	Default	95.19	88.14	91.67	0.84	0.95	92.00	89.33	90.67	0.81	0.96

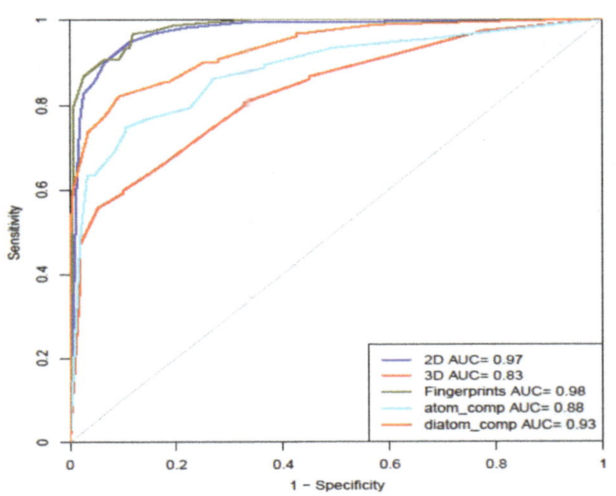

FIGURE 4 | ROC curve showing performance of models on various structural features.

Model Based on Peptide Sequence

It is nearly impossible to present a modified peptide by amino acid sequence. Thus, prediction of modified peptide from there sequence is not possible. Same time generating tertiary structure of a peptide is a tedious job for a biologist. We made an attempt to develop prediction model for cell penetration peptides of modified peptides from their amino acid sequence only by ignoring modifications in peptide. First, we developed simple composition-based models using various machine learning techniques. The SVM based model showed the best performance among all the classifiers used in the study. The accuracy of 91.67%, MCC of 0.83 and AUROC of 0.96 was achieved for the main dataset. On validation dataset, we obtained accuracy of 89.67%, MCC of 0.79 and AUROC of 0.96 (**Table S4**). We also developed SVM based model on first 5, 10, and 15 N and C-terminus residues. Results are given in **Table S5**.

Secondly, we developed models using dipeptide composition, SVM classifier showed the highest accuracy of 91.84%, MCC of 0.84 and AUROC of 0.96 for the main dataset. For independent dataset, the accuracy of 92.33%, MCC of 0.85 and AUROC of 0.97 was achieved (**Table S6**). Results of SVM based models on terminus residues for dipeptide composition is provided in **Table S7**. It is important for users to understand that sequence based model is not alternate to structure based models or alternate to past sequence based models developed for natural peptides. This sequence based is just approximate cell penetration potential of a modified peptide from its amino acid sequence.

Implementation of Webserver

To assist the scientific community, the best models are provided freely at http://webs.iiitd.edu.in/raghava/cellppdmod/. The "PREDICTION" module, consider tertiary structure (PDB format) of the modified peptide as an input and does the prediction. If a user has no structural information, he/she can generate PDB structure of their peptide up to 25 residues in length using server "PEPstrMOD" (Singh et al., 2015) (http://webs.iiitd.edu.in/raghava/pepstrmod/) developed by our group specifically for predicting the structure of the modified peptide. In case of natural peptide user can also use following servers PEP-FOLD (Thevenet et al., 2012) (http://bioserv.rpbs.univ-paris-diderot.fr/services/PEP-FOLD/) and QUARK (Xu and Zhang, 2012) (https://zhanglab.ccmb.med.umich.edu/QUARK/) for predicting structure of peptides. Multiple modification options are provided there, and the user can choose the desired modification. After generating the structure, user can do the prediction on "PREDICTION" module, whether the given modified PDB structure is CPP or non-CPP. Beside the main model, we have also implemented model based on peptide sequence (Subsidiary model). We have also provided a "DOWNLOAD" module from where the user can download the dataset used in this study.

DISCUSSION

CPPs has shown a promising impact in the field of therapeutics or for targeting a specific disease (Bechara and Sagan, 2013). However, the major limitations associated with some of these CPPs is their entrapment of CPP-cargo in endosomal compartments followed by endocytosis and therefore their bioavailability and half-life is severely reduced (Mäe et al., 2009). To overcome this limitation, people have tried to modify the CPP chemically. For example, to increase the delivery of nucleic acid more efficiently, people have introduced chemical modifications like N terminal stearylation (Futaki et al., 2001; Khalil et al., 2004), C-terminal cysteamidation (Simeoni et al., 2003; Morris et al., 2007), residue modifications (Lundberg et al., 2007).Tat is one of the first CPP, discovered from protein of HIV and various studies showed that it enhances the uptake of various drug and protein (Brooks et al., 2005). But DNA delivery by Tat is limited, because of the instability of Tat-DNA complex (Lo and Wang, 2008). Lo and Wang (2008) showed that Cysteine makes the Tat-DNA complex more stable. Incorporation of two cysteine residues results into interpeptide disulphide bond, form by air oxidation once bind to DNA. This enhance the stability of Tat-DNA complex, as well as protect DNA in extracellular environment. Therefore, gene transfection efficiency is more in modified Tat than simple Tat.

Computational algorithms have been proved a wide success in designing therapeutic peptides (Dhanda et al., 2017), therefore a large number of sequence-based model to design CPP has been developed in past. But all of these models have one limitation in common that they can only handle peptides with natural residues. Due to the huge therapeutic importance of modified CPP, prediction and designing of modified CPPs is the need of hour. So, we have developed a computational method, which is based on structural features, can handle the natural as well as modified peptides both. Beside this we have also incorporated a subsidiary model based on the sequence of peptides which consider only natural residues, to handle large number of peptides simultaneously. Here, sequence-based model is not alternate to the methods developed in past to predict natural CPPs.

We have developed various models using machine learning techniques such as SVM, Random Forest, J48, naïve bayes, SMO; individually for atom composition, 2D descriptors, 3D descriptors, and Fingerprints as well as the single model by combining 2D, 3D descriptors, and Fingerprints. We obtain best performance by Random Forest for both combined (2D, 3D, and Fingerprint descriptors) as well as fingerprint with accuracy 92.33% and AUROC 0.98 on validation dataset. As fingerprint alone will be computationally more feasible as compared to the combined method, so we have implemented this model on webserver.

We believe this work will prove a great assist to the researchers aim to design cell penetrating peptide, as well as incorporate different modification and to check their effect on cell penetration ability. In future, we can improve this method, if better art of structure prediction will be developed, as right now PEPstrMOD could tackle only 7–25 amino acid length and other best model I-TASSER only deals with natural residues. So, in conclusion this field must grow simultaneously with the betterment of art-of-structure prediction.

AUTHOR CONTRIBUTIONS

VK and PA generated the dataset. VK, PA, RK, and SB performed the experiments. VK, PA, and RK performed data analysis and prepared the tables and figures. VK, PA, RK, SB, and SU developed the web interface. VK, RK, PA, SU, and GR write the manuscript. GR and GV conceived the idea and coordinated the project.

ACKNOWLEDGMENTS

Authors are thankful to funding agencies J. C. Bose National Fellowship (DST), Council of Scientific and Industrial Research (CSIR), Department of Science and Technology (DST-INSPIRE), Indian Council of Medical Research (ICMR), University Grant Commission (UGC) and Department of Biotechnology (DBT) for fellowships and financial support.

SUPPLEMENTARY MATERIAL

Figure S1 | Percentage atomic composition of modified CPPs and non-CPPs.

Figure S2 | Percentage amino acid composition of CPPs and non-CPPs **(A)** 15 N-terminal residues and **(B)** 15 C-terminal residues.

Table S1 | List of 2D features with their positive mean value, negative mean value and *p*-value.

Table S2 | List of 3D features with their positive mean value, negative mean value and *p*-value.

Table S3 | List of fingerprints with their positive mean value, negative mean value and *p*-value.

Table S4 | Performance of different machine learning methods on amino acid composition.

Table S5 | Performance of SVM method on amino acid composition features of terminus residues.

Table S6 | Performance of different machine learning methods on dipeptide composition.

Table S7 | Performance of SVM method on dipeptide composition features of terminus residues.

REFERENCES

Agrawal, P., Bhalla, S., Chaudhary, K., Kumar, R., Sharma, M., and Raghava, G. P. S. (2018). *In silico* approach for prediction of antifungal peptides. *Front. Microbiol.* 9:323. doi: 10.3389/fmicb.2018.00323

Agrawal, P., Bhalla, S., Usmani, S. S., Singh, S., Chaudhary, K., Raghava, G. P. S., et al. (2016). CPPsite 2.0: a repository of experimentally validated cell-penetrating peptides. *Nucleic Acids Res.* 44, D1098–D1103. doi: 10.1093/nar/gkv1266

Aubry, S., Burlina, F., Dupont, E., Delaroche, D., Joliot, A., Lavielle, S., et al. (2009). Cell-surface thiols affect cell entry of disulfide-conjugated peptides. *FASEB J.* 23, 2956–2967. doi: 10.1096/fj.08-127563

Bahnsen, J. S., Franzyk, H., Sandberg-Schaal, A., and Nielsen, H. M. (2013). Antimicrobial and cell-penetrating properties of penetratin analogs: effect of sequence and secondary structure. *Biochim. Biophys. Acta* 1828, 223–232. doi: 10.1016/j.bbamem.2012.10.010

Bechara, C., and Sagan, S. (2013). Cell-penetrating peptides: 20 years later, where do we stand? *FEBS Lett.* 587, 1693–1702. doi: 10.1016/j.febslet.2013.04.031

Bhalla, S., Chaudhary, K., Kumar, R., Sehgal, M., Kaur, H., Sharma, S., et al. (2017). Gene expression-based biomarkers for discriminating early and late stage of clear cell renal cancer. *Sci. Rep.* 7:44997. doi: 10.1038/srep44997

Brooks, H., Lebleu, B., and Vivès, E. (2005). Tat peptide-mediated cellular delivery: back to basics. *Adv. Drug Deliv. Rev.* 57, 559–577. doi: 10.1016/j.addr.2004.12.001

Chen, L., Chu, C., Huang, T., Kong, X., and Cai, Y.-D. (2015). Prediction and analysis of cell-penetrating peptides using pseudo-amino acid composition and random forest models. *Amino Acids* 47, 1485–1493. doi: 10.1007/s00726-015-1974-5

Crooks, G. E., Hon, G., Chandonia, J.-M., and Brenner, S. E. (2004). WebLogo: a sequence logo generator. *Genome Res.* 14, 1188–1190. doi: 10.1101/gr.849004

Derossi, D., Calvet, S., Trembleau, A., Brunissen, A., Chassaing, G., and Prochiantz, A. (1996). Cell internalization of the third helix of the Antennapedia homeodomain is receptor-independent. *J. Biol. Chem.* 271, 18188–18193. doi: 10.1074/jbc.271.30.18188

Dhanda, S. K., Usmani, S. S., Agrawal, P., Nagpal, G., Gautam, A., and Raghava, G. P. S. (2017). Novel *in silico* tools for designing peptide-based subunit vaccines and immunotherapeutics. *Brief. Bioinform.* 18, 467–478. doi: 10.1093/bib/bbw025

Ezzat, K., Andaloussi, S. E. L., Zaghloul, E. M., Lehto, T., Lindberg, S., Moreno, P. M. D., et al. (2011). PepFect 14, a novel cell-penetrating peptide for oligonucleotide delivery in solution and as solid formulation. *Nucleic Acids Res.* 39, 5284–5298. doi: 10.1093/nar/gkr072

Ferreira, A. P. A., and Boucrot, E. (2018). Mechanisms of carrier formation during clathrin-independent endocytosis. *Trends Cell Biol.* 28, 188–200. doi: 10.1016/j.tcb.2017.11.004

Futaki, S., Ohashi, W., Suzuki, T., Niwa, M., Tanaka, S., Ueda, K., et al. (2001). Stearylated arginine-rich peptides: a new class of transfection systems. *Bioconjug. Chem.* 12, 1005–1011. doi: 10.1021/bc015508l

Ganguly, S., Chaubey, B., Tripathi, S., Upadhyay, A., Neti, P. V. S. V., Howell, R. W., et al. (2008). Pharmacokinetic analysis of polyamide nucleic-acid-cell penetrating peptide conjugates targeted against HIV-1 transactivation response element. *Oligonucleotides* 18, 277–286. doi: 10.1089/oli.2008.0140

Gao, H., Zhang, Q., Yu, Z., and He, Q. (2014). Cell-penetrating peptide-based intelligent liposomal systems for enhanced drug delivery. *Curr. Pharm. Biotechnol.* 15, 210–219. doi: 10.2174/1389201015666140617092552

Gautam, A., Chaudhary, K., Kumar, R., Sharma, A., Kapoor, P., Tyagi, A., et al. (2013). *In silico* approaches for designing highly effective cell penetrating peptides. *J. Transl. Med.* 11:74. doi: 10.1186/1479-5876-11-74

Gomarasca, M., F. C., Martins, T., Greune, L., Hardwidge, P. R., Schmidt, M. A., and Rüter, C. (2017). Bacterium-derived cell-penetrating peptides deliver gentamicin to kill intracellular pathogens. *Antimicrob. Agents Chemother.* 61:e02545-16. doi: 10.1128/AAC.02545-16

Guidotti, G., Brambilla, L., and Rossi, D. (2017). Cell-penetrating peptides: from basic research to clinics. *Trends Pharmacol. Sci.* 38, 406–424. doi: 10.1016/j.tips.2017.01.003

Gupta, S., and Jhawat, V. (2017). Quality by Design (QbD) approach of pharmacogenomics in drug designing and formulation development for optimization of drug delivery systems. *J. Control. Release* 245, 15–26. doi: 10.1016/j.jconrel.2016.11.018

Jain, A., Shah, S. G., and Chugh, A. (2015). Cell penetrating peptides as efficient nanocarriers for delivery of antifungal compound, natamycin for the treatment of fungal keratitis. *Pharm. Res.* 32, 1920–1930. doi: 10.1007/s11095-014-1586-x

Jones, A. T. (2007). Macropinocytosis: searching for an endocytic identity and role in the uptake of cell penetrating peptides. *J. Cell. Mol. Med.* 11, 670–684. doi: 10.1111/j.1582-4934.2007.00062.x

Khalil, I. A., Futaki, S., Niwa, M., Baba, Y., Kaji, N., Kamiya, H., et al. (2004). Mechanism of improved gene transfer by the N-terminal stearylation of octaarginine: enhanced cellular association by hydrophobic core formation. *Gene Ther.* 11, 636–644. doi: 10.1038/sj.gt.3302128

Kim, W. J., Christensen, L. V., Jo, S., Yockman, J. W., Jeong, J. H., Kim, Y.-H., et al. (2006). Cholesteryl oligoarginine delivering vascular endothelial growth factor siRNA effectively inhibits tumor growth in colon adenocarcinoma. *Mol. Ther.* 14, 343–350. doi: 10.1016/j.ymthe.2006.03.022

Koppelhus, U., Shiraishi, T., Zachar, V., Pankratova, S., and Nielsen, P. E. (2008). Improved cellular activity of antisense peptide nucleic acids by conjugation to a cationic peptide-lipid (CatLip) domain. *Bioconjug. Chem.* 19, 1526–1534. doi: 10.1021/bc800068h

Kumar, R., Chaudhary, K., Singh Chauhan, J., Nagpal, G., Kumar, R., Sharma, M., et al. (2015). An *in silico* platform for predicting, screening and designing of antihypertensive peptides. *Sci. Rep.* 5:12512. doi: 10.1038/srep12512

Kurrikoff, K., Gestin, M., and Langel, Ü. (2016). Recent *in vivo* advances in cell-penetrating peptide-assisted drug delivery. *Expert Opin. Drug Deliv.* 13, 373–387. doi: 10.1517/17425247.2016.1125879

Lindgren, M., Rosenthal-Aizman, K., Saar, K., Eiríksdóttir, E., Jiang, Y., Sassian, M., et al. (2006). Overcoming methotrexate resistance in breast cancer tumour cells by the use of a new cell-penetrating peptide. *Biochem. Pharmacol.* 71, 416–425. doi: 10.1016/j.bcp.2005.10.048

Lo, S. L., and Wang, S. (2008). An endosomolytic Tat peptide produced by incorporation of histidine and cysteine residues as a nonviral vector for DNA transfection. *Biomaterials* 29, 2408–2414. doi: 10.1016/j.biomaterials.2008.01.031

Lundberg, P., El-Andaloussi, S., Sütlü, T., Johansson, H., and Langel, U. (2007). Delivery of short interfering RNA using endosomolytic cell-penetrating peptides. *FASEB J.* 21, 2664–2671. doi: 10.1096/fj.06-6502com

Mäe, M. A., El-Andaloussi, S., Lehto, T., and Ulo, L. (2009). Chemically modified cell-penetrating peptides for the delivery of nucleic acids. *Expert Opin. Drug Deliv.* 6, 1195–1205. doi: 10.1517/17425240903213688

Margus, H., Padari, K., and Pooga, M. (2012). Cell-penetrating peptides as versatile vehicles for oligonucleotide delivery. *Mol. Ther.* 20, 525–533. doi: 10.1038/mt.2011.284

Matsuzaki, K., Yoneyama, S., Murase, O., and Miyajima, K. (1996). Transbilayer transport of ions and lipids coupled with mastoparan X translocation. *Biochemistry* 35, 8450–8456. doi: 10.1021/bi960342a

Morris, M. C., Depollier, J., Mery, J., Heitz, F., and Divita, G. (2001). A peptide carrier for the delivery of biologically active proteins into mammalian cells. *Nat. Biotechnol.* 19, 1173–1176. doi: 10.1038/nbt1201-1173

Morris, M. C., Gros, E., Aldrian-Herrada, G., Choob, M., Archdeacon, J., Heitz, F., et al. (2007). A non-covalent peptide-based carrier for *in vivo* delivery of DNA mimics. *Nucleic Acids Res.* 35:e49. doi: 10.1093/nar/gkm053

Nagpal, G., Usmani, S. S., Dhanda, S. K., Kaur, H., Singh, S., Sharma, M., et al. (2017). Computer-aided designing of immunosuppressive peptides based on IL-10 inducing potential. *Sci. Rep.* 7:42851. doi: 10.1038/srep42851

Nekhotiaeva, N., Elmquist, A., Rajarao, G. K., Hällbrink, M., Langel, U., and Good, L. (2004). Cell entry and antimicrobial properties of eukaryotic cell-penetrating peptides. *FASEB J.* 18, 394–396. doi: 10.1096/fj.03-0449fje

O'Boyle, N. M., Banck, M., James, C. A., Morley, C., Vandermeersch, T., and Hutchison, G. R. (2011). Open Babel: an open chemical toolbox. *J. Cheminform.* 3:33. doi: 10.1186/1758-2946-3-33

Palm-Apergi, C., Lönn, P., and Dowdy, S. F. (2012). Do cell-penetrating peptides actually "penetrate" cellular membranes? *Mol. Ther.* 20, 695–697. doi: 10.1038/mt.2012.40

Porto, W. F., Pires, Á. S., and Franco, O. L. (2017). Antimicrobial activity predictors benchmarking analysis using shuffled and designed synthetic peptides. *J. Theor. Biol.* 426, 96–103. doi: 10.1016/j.jtbi.2017.05.011

Postlethwaite, R. J., Garralda, M. E., Eminson, D. M., and Reynolds, J. (1996). Lessons from psychosocial studies of chronic renal failure. *Arch. Dis. Child.* 75, 455–459. doi: 10.1136/adc.75.5.455

Pouny, Y., Rapaport, D., Mor, A., Nicolas, P., and Shai, Y. (1992). Interaction of antimicrobial dermaseptin and its fluorescently labeled analogues with phospholipid membranes. *Biochemistry* 31, 12416–12423. doi: 10.1021/bi00164a017

Randhawa, H. K., Gautam, A., Sharma, M., Bhatia, R., Varshney, G. C., Raghava, G. P. S., et al. (2016). Cell-penetrating peptide and antibiotic combination therapy: a potential alternative to combat drug resistance in methicillin-resistant *Staphylococcus aureus*. *Appl. Microbiol. Biotechnol.* 100, 4073–4083. doi: 10.1007/s00253-016-7329-7

Rodriguez Plaza, J. G., Morales-Nava, R., Diener, C., Schreiber, G., Gonzalez, Z. D., Lara Ortiz, M. T., et al. (2014). Cell penetrating peptides and cationic antibacterial peptides: two sides of the same coin. *J. Biol. Chem.* 289, 14448–14457. doi: 10.1074/jbc.M113.515023

Sandberg, M., Eriksson, L., Jonsson, J., Sjöström, M., and Wold, S. (1998). New chemical descriptors relevant for the design of biologically active peptides. A multivariate characterization of 87 amino acids. *J. Med. Chem.* 41, 2481–2491. doi: 10.1021/jm9700575

Sanders, W. S., Johnston, C. I., Bridges, S. M., Burgess, S. C., and Willeford, K. O. (2011). Prediction of cell penetrating peptides by support vector machines. *PLoS Comput. Biol.* 7:e1002101. doi: 10.1371/journal.pcbi.1002101

Simeoni, F., Morris, M. C., Heitz, F., and Divita, G. (2003). Insight into the mechanism of the peptide-based gene delivery system MPG: implications for delivery of siRNA into mammalian cells. *Nucleic Acids Res.* 31, 2717–2724. doi: 10.1093/nar/gkg385

Singh, S., Chaudhary, K., Dhanda, S. K., Bhalla, S., Usmani, S. S., Gautam, A., et al. (2016). SATPdb: a database of structurally annotated therapeutic peptides. *Nucleic Acids Res.* 44, D1119–D1126. doi: 10.1093/nar/gkv1114

Singh, S., Singh, H., Tuknait, A., Chaudhary, K., Singh, B., Kumaran, S., et al. (2015). PEPstrMOD: structure prediction of peptides containing natural, non-natural and modified residues. *Biol. Direct* 10:73. doi: 10.1186/s13062-015-0103-4

Smith, T. C., and Frank, E. (2016). Introducing machine learning concepts with WEKA. *Methods Mol. Biol.* 1418, 353–378. doi: 10.1007/978-1-4939-3578-9_17

Sparr, C., Purkayastha, N., Kolesinska, B., Gengenbacher, M., Amulic, B., Matuschewski, K., et al. (2013). Improved efficacy of fosmidomycin against Plasmodium and Mycobacterium species by combination with the cell-penetrating peptide octaarginine. *Antimicrob. Agents Chemother.* 57, 4689–4698. doi: 10.1128/AAC.00427-13

Splith, K., and Neundorf, I. (2011). Antimicrobial peptides with cell-penetrating peptide properties and vice versa. *Eur. Biophys. J.* 40, 387–397. doi: 10.1007/s00249-011-0682-7

Tan, J., Cheong, H., Park, Y. S., Kim, H., Zhang, M., Moon, C., et al. (2014). Cell-penetrating peptide-mediated topical delivery of biomacromolecular drugs. *Curr. Pharm. Biotechnol.* 15, 231–239. doi: 10.2174/1389201015666140617094320

Tang, H., Su, Z.-D., Wei, H.-H., Chen, W., and Lin, H. (2016). Prediction of cell-penetrating peptides with feature selection techniques. *Biochem. Biophys. Res. Commun.* 477, 150–154. doi: 10.1016/j.bbrc.2016.06.035

Thevenet, P., Shen, Y., Maupetit, J., Guyon, F., Derreumaux, P., and Tuffery, P. (2012). PEP-FOLD: an updated de novo structure prediction server for both linear and disulfide bonded cyclic peptides. *Nucleic Acids Res.* 40, W288–W293. doi: 10.1093/nar/gks419

Tosato, M., Zamboni, V., Ferrini, A., and Cesari, M. (2007). The aging process and potential interventions to extend life expectancy. *Clin. Interv. Aging* 2, 401–412.

Wang, Y.-R., Chen, G.-X., Yang, S.-Y., and Wei, P. (2018). Barbaloin loaded polydopamine-polylactide-TPGS (PLA-TPGS) nanoparticles against gastric cancer as a targeted drug delivery system: studies *in vitro* and *in vivo*. *Biochem. Biophys. Res. Commun.* 499, 8–16. doi: 10.1016/j.bbrc.2018.03.069

Wei, L., Xing, P., Su, R., Shi, G., Ma, Z. S., and Zou, Q. (2017). CPPred-RF: a sequence-based predictor for identifying cell-penetrating peptides and their uptake efficiency. *J. Proteome Res.* 16, 2044–2053. doi: 10.1021/acs.jproteome.7b00019

Xu, D., and Zhang, Y. (2012). *Ab initio* protein structure assembly using continuous structure fragments and optimized knowledge-based force field. *Proteins* 80, 1715–1735. doi: 10.1002/prot.24065

Xu, J., Zhang, X., Chen, Y., Huang, Y., Wang, P., Wei, Y., et al. (2017). Improved micellar formulation for enhanced delivery for paclitaxel. *Mol. Pharm.* 14, 31–41. doi: 10.1021/acs.molpharmaceut.6b00581

Yap, C. W. (2011). PaDEL-descriptor: an open source software to calculate molecular descriptors and fingerprints. *J. Comput. Chem.* 32, 1466–1474. doi: 10.1002/jcc.21707

13

Advance in Research on *Mycobacterium tuberculosis* FabG4 and Its Inhibitor

Debajyoti Dutta*

Department of Biochemistry, Faculty of Medicine and Dentistry, University of Alberta, Edmonton, AB, Canada

***Correspondence:**
Debajyoti Dutta
ddutta@ualberta.ca;
debajyoti.47@gmail.com

Increasing evidence from recent reports of drug-resistant mycobacterial strains poses a challenge worldwide. Drug-resistant strains often undergo mutations, adopt alternative pathways, and express drug efflux pumps to reduce or eliminate drug doses. Besides these intrinsic resistance mechanisms, bacteria can evade drug doses by forming biofilms. Biofilms are the concerted growth of adherent microorganisms, which can also be formed at the air-water interface. The growth is supported by the extracellular polymer matrix which is self-produced by the microorganisms. Reduced metabolic activity in a nutrient-deficient environment in the biofilm may cause the microorganisms to take alternative pathways that can make the microorganisms recalcitrant to the drug doses. Recent works have shown that *Mycobacterium tuberculosis* expresses several proteins during its growth in biofilm, those when deleted, did not show any effect on mycobacterial growth in normal nutrient-sufficient conditions. Studying these unconventional proteins in mycobacterial biofilms is therefore of utmost importance. In this article, I will discuss one such mycobacterial biofilm-related protein FabG4 that is recently shown to be important for mycobacterial survival in the presence of antibiotic stressors and limited nutrient condition. In an attempt to find more effective FabG4 inhibitors and its importance in biofilm forming *M. tuberculosis*, present knowledge about FabG4 and its known inhibitors are discussed. Based on the existing data, a putative role of FabG4 is also suggested.

Keywords: FabG4, *Mycobacterium tuberculosis*, biofilm, β-oxo acyl-ACP reductase, inhibitor

INTRODUCTION

The ability of *Mycobacterium tuberculosis* to form biofilms was noted almost 120 years ago (Jones, 1896). However, the physiological and molecular basis of biofilm is only beginning to unravel until recently. The first protein that was found to be involved in *M. smegmatis* maturation of biofilm is the chaperone GroEL-1 (Ojha et al., 2005). GroEL-1 deficient mutant of *M. smegmatis* was suggested to lack GroEL-1 interaction with fatty acid synthesis type -II complex thereby reducing the mycolic acid content in biofilms. Mycolic acids are the predominant components of mycobacterial cell envelope that are produced by fatty acid synthesis type-II pathway in mycobacteria. The reason that mycobacterial cell envelope largely contributes to the biofilm attachment endorses mycolic acids may be involved in biofilm formation (Marrakchi et al., 2014). However the physiology of mycobacteria changes as it shifts from planktonic growth to biofilm dependent growth and results in several modifications in the expression level of protein and molecules pertaining to the cell envelope (Ojha et al., 2008; Sambandan et al., 2013; Rastogi et al., 2017). Fatty acid synthesis and its associated pathways for mycobacterial cell envelope synthesis are one of the major areas for developing antitubercular drugs (Zumla et al., 2013). Because of this altered phenotypes and a waxy extra-cellular matrix of biofilm, Mycobacteria become resilient to drug doses (Islam et al., 2012). Therefore the conventional TB drugs may not be as effective for biofilm-forming mycobacteria.

Membrane and cell envelope-associated biofilm-related proteins are particularly of interest as these proteins are likely to be involved in the making of cellular attachment to the biofilms. For example, recent studies have shown that a lipid transporter MmpL11 is specifically required for biofilm formation (Pacheco et al., 2013). Other works have identified a number of proteins specific to mycobacterial growth in the biofilm at air-water interface (Kerns et al., 2014). One of the proteins that are conserved among mycobacterial species is FabG4. The protein was proposed to possess host antigenic property and has a potential to be a biofilm-specific marker (Kerns et al., 2014). In addition to that, FabG4 was recognized as one of the crucial protein for mycobacterial survival in a stressed condition. This article will discuss the known facts about FabG4, its inhibitors, and discuss its possibility to serve as a candidate to study and treat biofilm-related mycobacteria.

IMPORTANCE OF FABG4 IN MYCOBACTERIA

FabG commits the second step of fatty acid synthesis that is to convert β-oxo acyl-ACP to β-hydroxy acyl-ACP. *M. tuberculosis* genome contains multiple FabG homologs. Two of them are conserved among all mycobacterial species, FabG1 and FabG4. FabG1 remain at the focus of attention because it takes part in fatty acid synthesis type-II (Marrakchi et al., 2002). On the other hand, several studies have indicated that FabG4 is not an inactive gene in the *M. tuberculosis* genome. Its expression was first documented in the proteome by using 2-D gel electrophoresis accompanying MALDI-MS analysis (Jungblut et al., 1999) and later verified by others (Rosenkrands et al., 2000; Sinha et al., 2002). Gu et al. (2003), first provide the evidence that the protein is expressed in the mycobacterial membrane fraction. However, it's requirement in mycobacterial physiology was not shown until the comprehensive work done by McFadden and coworkers (Beste et al., 2009). The authors showed that the protein is uniquely required for mycobacterial growth in Roisin's minimal media, which contains limited carbon source (Beste et al., 2009). Proteomics studies have further identified that FabG4 is one of the major proteins which expression is induced by the antibiotic stressor (Sharma et al., 2010). The protein expression was also detected in the drug-resistant strains (Singh et al., 2016; Verma et al., 2017). Most interestingly, FabG4 can functionally complement eukaryotic β-oxoacyl-ACP reductase activity. FabG4, when expressed in the knockout of *ora1* yeast cells can restore the mitochondrial fatty acid synthesis type-II (Gurvitz et al., 2009). Because yeast ORA1 is a mitochondrial FabG1/FabG4 ortholog (Hiltunen et al., 2009), functional complementation of ORA1 with FabG4 is indicative of an active FabG4 protein that can utilize ACP/Coenzyme A tagged β-oxoacyl substrates and is utilized by mycobacteria during limiting resource or antibiotic stressed condition.

UNIQUE FEATURES OF FabG4

Characterization of recombinantly expressed FabG4 has shown that the protein is highly specific for NADH (Dutta et al., 2011). This is intriguingly different from its close relative (33% homology) FabG1 that utilizes NADPH. Crystal structure of the FabG4 complex with NADH reveals that the specificity comes from a single aspartate residue that reduces the volume of the phosphate binding groove of adenosine ribose phosphate moiety of NADPH (Dutta et al., 2013). Crystal structure further shows that FabG4 contains a "flavodoxin-type" structural domain in its N-terminal and a typical ketoreductase domain in its C-terminal (**Figure 1A**). The N-terminal structural domain is also found in modular polyketide synthase ketoreductase domain PlmKR1 (Bonnett et al., 2013). PlmKR1 exists as a monomer but FabG4 is different in the sense that the protein is a dimer, where the N-terminal domain of a protomer makes an extensive interaction with the C-terminal domain of the other protomer. Therefore, FabG4 was designated as "High Molecular weight FabG" (HMwFabG) (Dutta et al., 2011). Typical FabG does not contain this structural domain.

Many of the N-terminal residues (1–19) of FabG4 cannot be traced in crystal structure suggesting that the region has no rigid secondary structure. Most of the N-terminal residues were traced in FabG4 complex with NAD^+ structure (PDB 4FW8) showing a possibility of short helix containing seven residues (21–27) (**Figure 1A**). Long N-terminal sequences in FabGs are also found among eukaryotes, which were suggested to be the signal sequence (Wickramasinghe et al., 2006). Whether it is true for FabG4 is not known, but sequence alignment of HMwFabGs from actinobacteria and many proteobacteria reveals conserved residues Pro30, Leu33, and Arg35 in N-terminal sequence. Truncation of the N-terminal residues does not have any effect on catalytic activity. On the contrary, the C-terminal residues of FabG4 are apparently involved in catalytic activity since its truncation yields with a defective protein (Dutta et al., 2011). This is because the conserved C-terminal residues are engaged in electrostatic interaction with the active site proximal loops (Dutta et al., 2011).

INHIBITORS OF FabG4

Structure of FabG4 and its complex with a substrate mimic hexanoyl-CoA (PDB 3V1U) accelerated the work on structure-based inhibitor design against FabG4 (Dutta et al., 2013) (**Figure 1B**). The particular structure also provides a platform to design FabG specific inhibitors because the structure provided the first evidence of FabG-substrate complex (**Table 1**). The

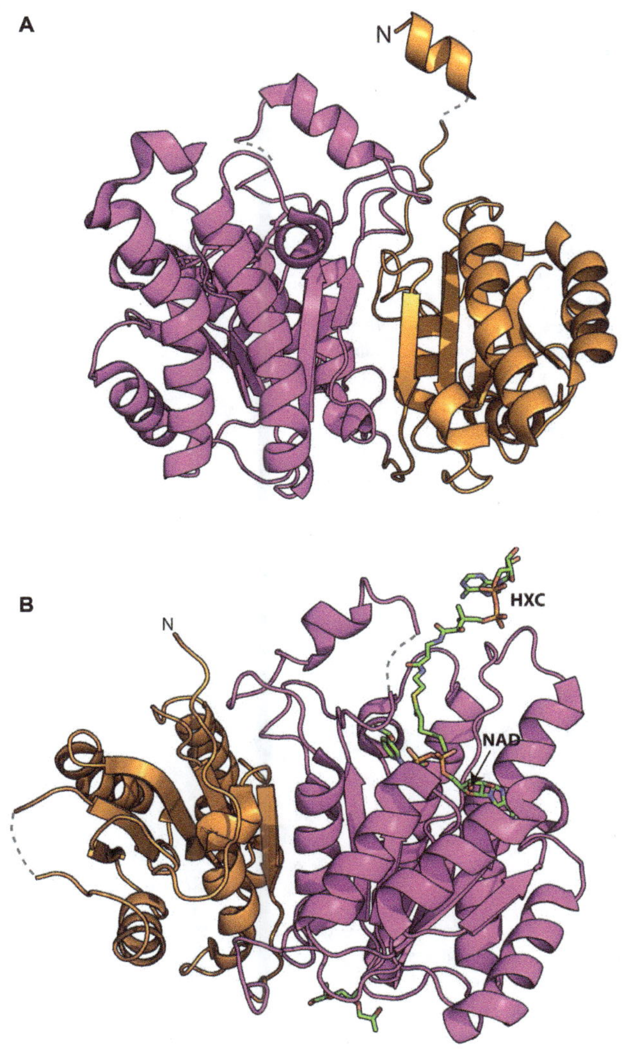

FIGURE 1 | Crystal structures of FabG4: **(A)** N-terminal "flavodoxin type" (orange) and C-terminal ketoreductase (magenta) domains. "N" indicated the N-terminal of the polypeptide chain. The regions those were not be traced in electron density are shown in dotted lines. **(B)** The substrate mimic hexanoyl coenzyme A (HXC) and NAD^+ bound structure shows the putative substrate binding modes.

first reported FabG4 inhibitors are based on the polyphenol compounds (Banerjee et al., 2014, 2015b). Synthesized compounds are also tested against *M. smegmatis* showing the MIC of 5 μg mL^{-1}. Docking studies had revealed that the compounds potentially occupy the NADH binding region with a few hydrogen-bonding interactions with the loop-residues responsible for CoA substrate binding. Another study to design and synthesize the inhibitors based on the common pharmacophores like β-lactam and Isoniazid was also successful inhibiting FabG4 with IC_{50} as low as 15.2 ± 0.5 μM (Banerjee et al., 2015a). Similar to the polyphenol based compounds β-lactam and Isoniazid-based compounds primarily dock on the NADH binding site. Isothermal titration calorimetry indicates two sequential binding sites showing positive cooperativity. Inhibitory effects of β-lactam and Isoniazid-based compounds have shown to be inhibitory toward mycobacterial biofilm formation. Recently, thiophene containing trisubstituted methane compound, *S*-S006-830 was found to have a substantial inhibitory effect on *M. tuberculosis* biofilm formation and possesses antitubercular activity (Singh et al., 2017). FabG4 is one of the three membrane-associated proteins identified to strongly interact with *S*-S006-830. Computational docking study predicts two possible binding sites. One comprises of the region overlapping NADH and CoA substrate binding and the other site is on the N-terminal domain. *S*-S006-830 is special because apart from the NADH-substrate binding site it also targets to the N-terminal structural domain. Two unique FabG inhibitors are worth mentioning in this regard. The first, Pyridomycin analog specifically targets NADH binding proteins and proposed to exhibit inhibitory effects on FabG4 by bridging both NADH and substrate-binding region (Hartkoorn et al., 2014). The second inhibitor was identified using library screening that uniquely binds to the helical dimeric interface of FabG (Cukier et al., 2013). The helical dimeric interface in FabG is responsible of NAD(P)H binding cooperativity (Dutta et al., 2012). All FabG4 and related inhibitors are summarized in **Table 1**.

POSSIBLE ROLE OF THE ENZYME

High Molecular weight FabG are exclusively found among bacteria. Homologous genes of FabG4 are found in actinobacteria and many proteobacteria (Dutta et al., 2011). Genomic analysis of HMwFabG containing bacteria shows another protein coexisting downstream to FabG4 ORF. In *M. tuberculosis* this protein is HtdX (Rv0241c). Both the proteins are conserved among mycobacterial species. Even in *M. leprae* genome where the genomic reduction had happened, retained both *fabG4* and its downstream *htdX* (Cole et al., 2001). However, deletion of *htdX* or *fabG4* does not show any apparent effect on bacterial survival *in vivo* (Sassetti and Rubin, 2003). Nonetheless, the protein is shown to be essential for survival in minimal media (Beste et al., 2009). Presumably, the conditional dependency of *M. tuberculosis* on FabG4 indicates an alternative pathway during limiting resource condition. Another clue is the FabG4 dependency on NADH. The NADH utilizing β-ketoacyl reductase activity of FabG4 is four times higher to the reverse reaction that utilizes NAD^+ for β-hydroxyacyl dehydrogenase activity (Dutta et al., 2013). Compared to NADPH, NADH is the low energy molecule and mostly associates to the catabolic pathways (Cantó et al., 2015). Shifting the coenzyme specificity toward low energy NADH possibly indicates that the bacteria are rewiring its metabolism toward the energy saving mode. Furthermore, FabG4 is isolated from the membrane fraction, which is indicative of its membrane-associated role (Gu et al., 2003; Singh et al., 2017). The role could be either fatty acid synthesis or modification. Notably, the other gene *htdX* was found to be responsive to the inhibitors of cell wall synthesis (Boshoff et al., 2004). Since both *fabG4* and *htdX* are situated in a conserved cluster it is tempting to predict that they are involved in the same

TABLE 1 | Inhibitors of FabG4.

Compound structure	Type of the compounds	General comments	Reference
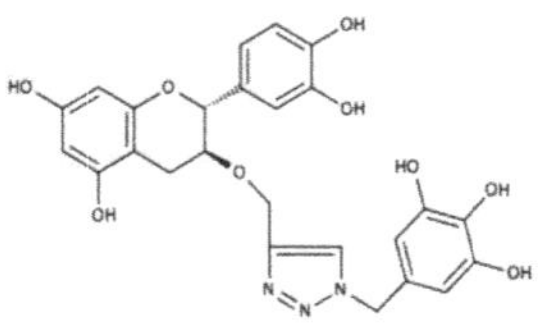	Triazole-polyphenol hybrid compounds	Possibly compete for NADH binding sites; Cooperative sequential binding with two binding sites IC_{50} = 34.9 μM K_i = 0.88 μM MIC = 5 μg ml^{-1}	Banerjee et al., 2014, 2015b
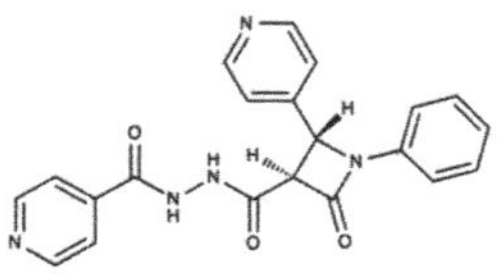	Beta-lactam isoniazid based compounds	Possibly compete for NADH binding sites; Cooperative sequential binding with two binding sites; acts as dual inhibitor of HtdX IC_{50} = 15.2 μM MIC = 15 μg ml^{-1}	Banerjee et al., 2015a
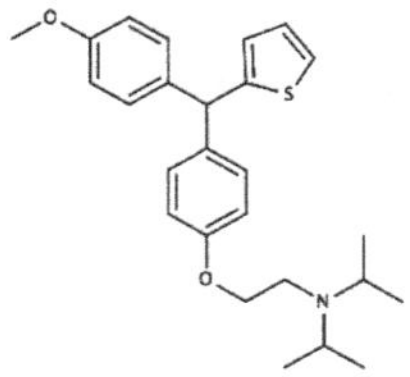	Thiophene containing trisubstituted methane	*S*-Enantiomer has more specificity toward FabG4; combination with rifampicin has a synergistic effect MIC = 3.125 μg ml^{-1}	Singh et al., 2017
Other inhibitors related to FabG4			
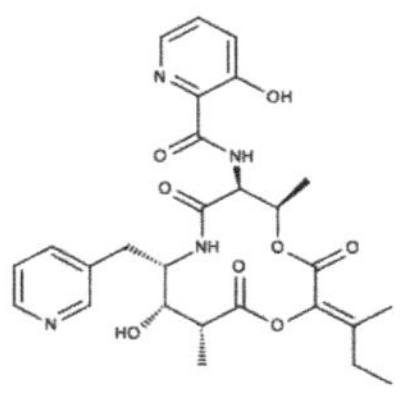	Pyridomycin analogs	An InhA inhibitor that can possibly inhibits FabG4 by binding to the both NADH and substrate binding region	Hartkoorn et al., 2014
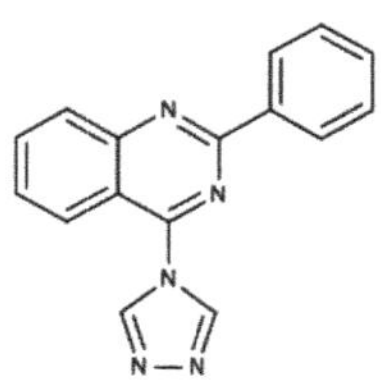	Triazol-quinazoline based compound	Inhibitor identified against *Pseudomonas aeruginosa* FabG from the screening small molecule library, Specifically binds to the helical dimer interface	Cukier et al., 2013

pathway. Both sequence analysis and preliminary enzymatic activities are corroborated that HtdX can commit a dehydratase reaction that is to convert β-hydroxyacyl-CoA to enoylacyl-CoA (Gurvitz, 2009; Sacco et al., 2010; Biswas et al., 2013; Banerjee et al., 2015a). The reaction is theoretically the successive step of FabG4 enzymatic reaction for fatty acid elongation cycle. Altogether the data suggests that during limiting resource condition FabG4 participates into some low-energy requiring pathway that is related to membrane biosynthesis, remodeling or recycling.

FUTURE SCOPE

FabG4 is a host antigenic protein reportedly expressed in mycobacterial biofilms. The protein expression was consistently found in membrane fraction and stressor-induced. As a conserved gene in all mycobacterial species, FabG4 can be a biomarker for biofilm. Although, FabG4 inhibitors are manifested antitubercular activity more experiments are needed to call it a drug target. Role of FabG4 and its connection with the membrane in mycobacteria also require further experimentations. To study FabG4 importance in biofilm forming *M. tuberculosis* it is, therefore, necessary to find out its targeting and interaction with other proteins. Identifying the role of FabG4 in mycobacteria might provide a hint of a new aspect of a survival strategy. The second aspect is the strategy to design more specific inhibitors of FabG4. While the C-terminal domain of FabG4 is common among FabGs, inhibitors against its N-terminal structural domain might be a way to target the protein more specifically. Designing the fluorophore inhibitors against its structural domain could be a way to find out its role *in vivo*.

AUTHOR CONTRIBUTIONS

DD is solely responsible for the conception or design, drafting, and revising the work.

ACKNOWLEDGMENTS

The author thanks Professor Amit Kumar Das, Department of Biotechnology, Indian Institute of Technology Kharagpur for his guidance during Ph.D. The author also thanks Professor Amit Basak, Department of Chemistry, Indian Institute of Technology Kharagpur and Dr. Deb Ranjan Banerjee and Rupam Biswas for their contribution to the FabG4 work from Indian Institute of Technology Kharagpur.

REFERENCES

Banerjee, D. R., Biswas, R., Das, A. K., and Basak, A. (2015a). Design, synthesis and characterization of dual inhibitors against new targets FabG4 and HtdX of *Mycobacterium tuberculosis*. *Eur. J. Med. Chem.* 100, 223–234. doi: 10.1016/j.ejmech.2015.06.007

Banerjee, D. R., Dutta, D., Saha, B., Bhattacharyya, S., Senapati, K., Das, A. K., et al. (2014). Design, synthesis and characterization of novel inhibitors against mycobacterial β-ketoacyl CoA reductase FabG4. *Org. Biomol. Chem.* 12, 73–85. doi: 10.1039/c3ob41676c

Banerjee, D. R., Senapati, K., Biswas, R., Das, A. K., and Basak, A. (2015b). Inhibition of *M. tuberculosis* β-ketoacyl CoA reductase FabG4 (Rv0242c) by triazole linked polyphenol-aminobenzene hybrids: comparison with the corresponding gallate counterparts. *Bioorg. Med. Chem. Lett.* 25, 1343–1347. doi: 10.1016/j.bmcl.2015.01.014

Beste, D. J., Espasa, M., Bonde, B., Kierzek, A. M., Stewart, G. R., and McFadden, J. (2009). The genetic requirements for fast and slow growth in mycobacteria. *PLoS One* 4:e5349. doi: 10.1371/journal.pone.0005349

Biswas, R., Dutta, D., and Das, A. K. (2013). Cloning, overexpression, purification, crystallization and preliminary X-ray diffraction analysis of Rv0241c (HtdX) from *Mycobacterium tuberculosis* H37Rv. *Acta Crystallogr. Sect. F Struct. Biol. Cryst. Commun.* 69, 1110–1113. doi: 10.1107/S1744309113023452

Bonnett, S. A., Whicher, J. R., Papireddy, K., Florova, G., Smith, J. L., and Reynolds, K. A. (2013). Structural and stereochemical analysis of a modular polyketide synthase ketoreductase domain required for the generation of a *cis*-alkene. *Chem. Biol.* 20, 772–783. doi: 10.1016/j.chembiol.2013.04.014

Boshoff, H. I., Myers, T. G., Copp, B. R., McNeil, M. R., Wilson, M. A., and Barry, C. E. III (2004). The transcriptional responses of *Mycobacterium tuberculosis* to inhibitors of metabolism: novel insights into drug mechanisms of action. *J. Biol. Chem.* 279, 40174–40184. doi: 10.1074/jbc.M406796200

Cantó, C., Menzies, K. J., and Auwerx, J. (2015). NAD^+ metabolism and the control of energy homeostasis: a balancing act between mitochondria and the nucleus. *Cell Metab.* 22, 31–53. doi: 10.1016/j.cmet.2015.05.023

Cole, S. T., Eiglmeier, K., Parkhill, J., James, K. D., Thomson, N. R., Wheeler, P. R., et al. (2001). Massive gene decay in the leprosy bacillus. *Nature* 409, 1007–1011. doi: 10.1038/35059006

Cukier, C. D., Hope, A. G., Elamin, A. A., Moynie, L., Schnell, R., Schach, S., et al. (2013). Discovery of an allosteric inhibitor binding site in 3-Oxo-acyl-ACP reductase from *Pseudomonas aeruginosa*. *ACS Chem. Biol.* 8, 2518–2527. doi: 10.1021/cb4005063

Dutta, D., Bhattacharyya, S., and Das, A. K. (2012). Crystal structure and fluorescence studies reveal the role of helical dimeric interface of staphylococcal FabG1 in positive cooperativity for NADPH. *Proteins* 80, 1250–1257. doi: 10.1002/prot.24024

Dutta, D., Bhattacharyya, S., Mukherjee, S., Saha, B., and Das, A. K. (2011). Crystal structure of FabG4 from *Mycobacterium tuberculosis* reveals the importance of C-terminal residues in ketoreductase activity. *J. Struct. Biol.* 174, 147–155. doi: 10.1016/j.jsb.2010.11.012

Dutta, D., Bhattacharyya, S., Roychowdhury, A., Biswas, R., and Das, A. K. (2013). Crystal structure of hexanoyl-CoA bound to β-ketoacyl reductase FabG4 of *Mycobacterium tuberculosis*. *Biochem. J.* 450, 127–139. doi: 10.1042/BJ20121107

Gu, S., Chen, J., Dobos, K. M., Bradbury, E. M., Belisle, J. T., and Chen, X. (2003). Comprehensive proteomic profiling of the membrane constituents of a *Mycobacterium tuberculosis* strain. *Mol. Cell. Proteomics* 2, 1284–1296. doi: 10.1074/mcp.M300060-MCP200

Gurvitz, A. (2009). The essential mycobacterial genes, fabG1 and fabG4, encode 3-oxoacyl-thioester reductases that are functional in yeast mitochondrial fatty acid synthase type 2. *Mol. Genet. Genomics* 282, 407–416. doi: 10.1007/s00438-009-0474-2

Gurvitz, A., Hiltunen, J. K., and Kastaniotis, A. J. (2009). Heterologous expression of mycobacterial proteins in *Saccharomyces cerevisiae* reveals two physiologically functional 3-hydroxyacyl-thioester dehydratases, HtdX and HtdY, in addition to HadABC and HtdZ. *J. Bacteriol.* 191, 2683–2690. doi: 10.1128/JB.01046-08

Hartkoorn, R. C., Pojer, F., Read, J. A., Gingell, H., Neres, J., Horlacher, O. P., et al. (2014). Pyridomycin bridges the NADH- and substrate-binding pockets of the enoyl reductase InhA. *Nat. Chem. Biol.* 10, 96–98. doi: 10.1038/nchembio.1405

Hiltunen, J. K., Schonauer, M. S., Autio, K. J., Mittelmeier, T. M., Kastaniotis, A. J., and Dieckmann, C. L. (2009). Mitochondrial fatty acid synthesis type II: more than just fatty acids. *J. Biol. Chem.* 284, 9011–9015. doi: 10.1074/jbc.R800068200

Islam, M. S., Richards, J. P., and Ojha, A. K. (2012). Targeting drug tolerance in mycobacteria: a perspective from mycobacterial biofilms. *Expert Rev. Anti Infect. Ther.* 10, 1055–1066. doi: 10.1586/eri.12.88

Jones, A. C. (1896). On the so-called tubercle bacilli. *Report of the 66th Meeting of the British Association for the Advancements of Science*. London: John Murray, 1015–1016.

Jungblut, P. R., Schaible, U. E., Mollenkopf, H. J., Zimny-Arndt, U., Raupach, B., Mattow, J., et al. (1999). Comparative proteome analysis of *Mycobacterium tuberculosis* and *Mycobacterium bovis* BCG strains: towards functional genomics of microbial pathogens. *Mol. Microbiol.* 33, 1103–1117. doi: 10.1046/j.1365-2958.1999.01549.x

Kerns, P. W., Ackhart, D. F., Basaraba, R. J., Leid, J. G., and Shirtliff, M. E. (2014). *Mycobacterium tuberculosis* pellicles express unique proteins recognized by the host humoral response. *Pathog. Dis.* 70, 347–358. doi: 10.1111/2049-632X.12142

Marrakchi, H., Ducasse, S., Labesse, G., Montrozier, H., Margeat, E., Emorine, L., et al. (2002). MabA (FabG1), a *Mycobacterium tuberculosis* protein involved in the long-chain fatty acid elongation system FAS-II. *Microbiology* 148, 951–960. doi: 10.1099/00221287-148-4-951

Marrakchi, H., Lanéelle, M. A., and Daffé, M. (2014). Mycolic acids: structures, biosynthesis, and beyond. *Chem. Biol.* 21, 67–85. doi: 10.1016/j.chembiol.2013.11.011

Ojha, A., Anand, M., Bhatt, A., Kremer, L., Jacobs, W. R. Jr., and Hatfull, G. F. (2005). GroEL1: a dedicated chaperone involved in mycolic acid biosynthesis during biofilm formation in mycobacteria. *Cell* 123, 861–873. doi: 10.1016/j.cell.2005.09.012

Ojha, A. K., Baughn, A. D., Sambandan, D., Hsu, T., Trivelli, X., Guerardel, Y., et al. (2008). Growth of *Mycobacterium tuberculosis* biofilms containing free mycolic acids and harbouring drug-tolerant bacteria. *Mol. Microbiol.* 69, 164–174. doi: 10.1111/j.1365-2958.2008.06274.x

Pacheco, S. A., Hsu, F. F., Powers, K. M., and Purdy, G. E. (2013). MmpL11 protein transports mycolic acid-containing lipids to the mycobacterial cell wall and contributes to biofilm formation in *Mycobacterium smegmatis*. *J. Biol. Chem.* 288, 24213–24222. doi: 10.1074/jbc.M113.473371

Rastogi, S., Singh, A. K., Pant, G., Mitra, K., Sashidhara, K. V., and Krishnan, M. Y. (2017). Down-regulation of PE11, a cell wall associated esterase, enhances the biofilm growth of *Mycobacterium tuberculosis* and reduces cell wall virulence lipid levels. *Microbiology* 163, 52–61. doi: 10.1099/mic.0.000417

Rosenkrands, I., King, A., Weldingh, K., Moniatte, M., Moertz, E., and Andersen, P. (2000). Towards the proteome of *Mycobacterium tuberculosis*. *Electrophoresis* 21, 3740–3756. doi: 10.1002/1522-2683(200011)21:17<3740::AID-ELPS3740>3.0.CO;2-3

Sacco, E., Slama, N., Bäckbro, K., Parish, T., Laval, F., Daffé, M., et al. (2010). Revisiting the assignment of Rv0241c to fatty acid synthase type II of *Mycobacterium tuberculosis*. *J. Bacteriol.* 192, 4037–4044. doi: 10.1128/JB.00386-10

Sambandan, D., Dao, D. N., Weinrick, B. C., Vilchèze, C., Gurcha, S. S., Ojha, A., et al. (2013). Keto-mycolic acid-dependent pellicle formation confers tolerance to drug-sensitive *Mycobacterium tuberculosis*. *mBio* 4:e00222-13. doi: 10.1128/mBio.00222-13

Sassetti, C. M., and Rubin, E. J. (2003). Genetic requirements for mycobacterial survival during infection. *Proc. Natl. Acad. Sci. U.S.A.* 100, 12989–12994. doi: 10.1073/pnas.2134250100

Sharma, P., Kumar, B., Singhal, N., Katoch, V. M., Venkatesan, K., Chauhan, D. S., et al. (2010). Streptomycin induced protein expression analysis in *Mycobacterium tuberculosis* by two-dimensional gel electrophoresis & mass spectrometry. *Indian J. Med. Res.* 132, 400–408.

Singh, A., Gupta, A. K., Gopinath, K., Sharma, D., Sharma, P., Bisht, D., et al. (2016). Comparative proteomic analysis of sequential isolates of *Mycobacterium tuberculosis* sensitive and resistant Beijing type from a patient with pulmonary tuberculosis. *Int. J. Mycobacteriol.* 5(Suppl. 1), S123–S124. doi: 10.1016/j.ijmyco.2016.10.028

Singh, P., Kumar, S. K., Maurya, V. K., Mehta, B. K., Ahmad, H., Dwivedi, A. K., et al. (2017). S-Enantiomer of the antitubercular compound S006-830 complements activity of frontline TB drugs and targets biogenesis of *Mycobacterium tuberculosis* cell envelope. *ACS Omega* 2, 8453–8465. doi: 10.1021/acsomega.7b01281

Sinha, S., Arora, S., Kosalai, K., Namane, A., Pym, A. S., and Cole, S. T. (2002). Proteome analysis of the plasma membrane of *Mycobacterium tuberculosis*. *Comp. Funct. Genomics.* 3, 470–483. doi: 10.1002/cfg.211

Verma, R., Pinto, S. M., Patil, A. H., Advani, J., Subba, P., Kumar, M., et al. (2017). Quantitative proteomic and phosphoproteomic analysis of H37Ra and H37Rv strains of *Mycobacterium tuberculosis*. *J. Proteome Res.* 16, 1632–1645. doi: 10.1021/acs.jproteome.6b00983

Wickramasinghe, S. R., Inglis, K. A., Urch, J. E., Müller, S., van Aalten, D. M., and Fairlamb, A. H. (2006). Kinetic, inhibition and structural studies on 3-oxoacyl-ACP reductase from *Plasmodium falciparum*, a key enzyme in fatty acid biosynthesis. *Biochem. J.* 393, 447–457. doi: 10.1042/BJ20050832

Zumla, A., Nahid, P., and Cole, S. T. (2013). Advances in the development of new tuberculosis drugs and treatment regimens. *Nat. Rev. Drug Discov.* 12, 388–404. doi: 10.1038/nrd4001

14

Complete Genome Sequences of Two Novel KPC-2-Producing IncU Multidrug-Resistant Plasmids From International High-Risk Clones of *Escherichia coli* in China

Wenhao Wu[1,2†], Lingling Lu[3†], Wenjia Fan[1], Chun Chen[4], Dazhi Jin[5], Hongying Pan[1*] and Xi Li[5*]

[1] Department of Infectious Diseases, Zhejiang Provincial People's Hospital, People's Hospital of Hangzhou Medical College, Hangzhou, China, [2] Medical College, Qingdao University, Qingdao, China, [3] Adicon Clinical Laboratories, Hangzhou, China, [4] Department of Pneumology, Zhejiang Provincial People's Hospital, People's Hospital of Hangzhou Medical College, Hangzhou, China, [5] Centre of Laboratory Medicine, Zhejiang Provincial People's Hospital, People's Hospital of Hangzhou Medical College, Hangzhou, China

***Correspondence:**
Xi Li
lixi_0611@163.com
Hongying Pan
hypanzjsrmyy@126.com

† These authors have contributed equally to this work and share first authorship

The rapidly increasing prevalence of *Klebsiella pneumoniae* carbapenemase 2 (KPC-2)-producing bacteria has become a serious challenge to public health. Currently, the bla_{KPC-2} gene is mainly disseminated through plasmids of different sizes and replicon types. However, the plasmids carrying the bla_{KPC-2} gene have not been fully characterized. In this study, we report the complete genome sequences of two novel bla_{KPC-2}-harboring incompatibility group U (IncU) plasmids, pEC2341-KPC and pEC2547-KPC, from international high-risk clones of *Escherichia coli* isolated from Zhejiang, China. Two KPC-2-producing *E. coli* isolates (EC2341 and EC2547) were collected from clinical samples. Whole-genome sequencing (WGS) analysis indicated that EC2341 and EC2547 belonged to the ST410 and ST131 clones, respectively. S1-nuclease pulsed-field gel electrophoresis (S1-PFGE), Southern blot and conjugation experiments confirmed the presence of the bla_{KPC-2} gene on the pEC2341-KPC plasmid and that this was a conjugative plasmid, while the bla_{KPC-2} gene on the pEC2547-KPC plasmid was a non-conjugative plasmid. In addition, plasmid analysis further revealed that the two bla_{KPC-2}-harboring plasmids have a close evolutionary relationship. To the best of our knowledge, this is the first report of *E. coli* strains carrying the bla_{KPC-2} gene on IncU plasmids. The emergence of the IncU-type bla_{KPC-2}-positive plasmid highlights further dissemination of bla_{KPC-2} in *Enterobacteriaceae*. Therefore, effective measures should be taken immediately to prevent the spread of these bla_{KPC-2}–positive plasmids.

Keywords: *E. coli*, KPC-2, IncU plasmid, high-risk clones, whole genome sequencing

INTRODUCTION

The rapidly increasing prevalence of KPC-producing bacteria has become a serious challenge to public health (Suay-García and Pérez-Gracia, 2019). At the time of writing (April 2021), 82 variants of KPC enzymes (KPC-1 to KPC-82) have been identified among gram-negative bacteria worldwide[1]. Among these carbapenemases, KPC-2 was first identified from a *Klebsiella pneumoniae* strain in the United States in 2003 (Smith Moland et al., 2003) and attracted extensive attention because of its rapid worldwide dissemination. Currently, the $bla_{KPC\text{-}2}$ gene is prevalent in *K. pneumoniae* strains, and the sequence type 258 (ST258) clone has successfully spread worldwide (Munoz-Price et al., 2013).

Although not as common as in *K. pneumoniae*, the $bla_{KPC\text{-}2}$ gene has also been identified in *Escherichia coli* strains. Some reports, including two from our group, have recently found that the $bla_{KPC\text{-}2}$ gene was present in the ST131-type *E. coli* strains, which are international multidrug-resistant high-risk clones (Du et al., 2020; Wang et al., 2020). KPC-2-producing *E. coli* strains were isolated not only from humans but also from animals, such as cattle (Vikram and Schmidt, 2018), swine (Liu et al., 2018) and cats (Sellera et al., 2018). Unfortunately, $bla_{KPC\text{-}2}$ has also been identified in environmental samples [urban rivers (Xu et al., 2015), drinking water (Mahmoud et al., 2020), and vegetables (Wang et al., 2018)], indicating its presence in the environment. In addition, $bla_{KPC\text{-}2}$ was further disseminated through plasmids of different sizes and replicon types (Mathers et al., 2017), such as the pKpQIL-like plasmid (Chen et al., 2014b), the IncFIA plasmid (Chen et al., 2014a), the IncI2 plasmid (Chen et al., 2013), the IncX3 plasmid (Fuga et al., 2020), the IncP-6 plasmid (Hu et al., 2019) and the IncN plasmid (Schweizer et al., 2019). The movement of bla_{KPC} plasmids into *E. coli* strains that are known pathogens of urinary tract and intra-abdominal infections raises clinical concerns (Bratu et al., 2007). Plasmid transfer will further lead to continued spread of resistance and limit clinical treatment options (Chen et al., 2014). However, plasmids carrying the $bla_{KPC\text{-}2}$ gene have not been fully characterized.

In the present study, we reported the complete sequences of two novel $bla_{KPC\text{-}2}$-harboring IncU plasmids from international high-risk clones of *E. coli* ST131 and ST410 isolates from China. In addition, the whole genome sequence revealed that the two $bla_{KPC\text{-}2}$-positive plasmids have a close evolutionary relationship.

MATERIALS AND METHODS

Bacterial Strains

In a retrospective study, 109 carbapenem-resistant *Enterobacteriaceae* strains were isolated from June 2018 to September 2019. Common carbapenemase genes (bla_{KPC}, bla_{NDM}, bla_{VIM}, and bla_{IMP}) were amplified, and the positive products were sequenced. Two KPC-2-producing *E. coli* strains were included in this study and further identified by the VITEK MS system (bioMérieux, Marcy-l'Etoile, France).

[1]http://www.ncbi.nlm.nih.gov/pathogens/submit_beta_lactamase/

Antimicrobial Susceptibility Testing

Antimicrobial susceptibility testing was carried out using the broth microdilution method according to the protocol of CLSI guidelines (CLSI, 2020). Minimum inhibitory concentrations (MICs) were interpreted according to the guideline document established by Clinical and Laboratory Standards Institute (CLSI, 2020). For tigecycline and polymyxin E, the MIC results were categorized in accordance with the breakpoints defined by the European Committee on Antimicrobial Susceptibility Testing criteria[2]. *E. coli* ATCC 25922 was used as a quality control strain.

S1-PFGE and Southern Blot Hybridization

The plasmid location of the $bla_{KPC\text{-}2}$ gene was determined by Southern blot experiments according to the previous study (Wang et al., 2020). Briefly, whole chromosomal DNA was digested with S1-nuclease (TaKaRa, Japan). The digested fragments were electrophoresed on a CHEF-mapper XA pulsed-field gel electrophoresis (PFGE) system (Bio-Rad, United States) for 18 h at 14°C. The DNA fragments were transferred to a positively charged nylon membrane (Millipore, United States) and then hybridized with a digoxigenin-labeled $bla_{KPC\text{-}2}$-specific probe. The fragments was detected by an NBT/BCIP color detection kit (Roche, Germany). The *Salmonella enterica* serotype *Braenderup* H9812 was used as the size marker.

Conjugation Experiments

A filter-mating experiment was performed with *E. coli* J53 as the recipient strain and $bla_{KPC\text{-}2}$-positive isolates as the donor strains. Transconjugants were selected on Mueller-Hinton agar plates supplemented with 300 mg/L sodium azide and 100 mg/L ampicillin. The transconjugants were confirmed by PCR sequencing and antimicrobial susceptibility testing.

Whole Genome Sequencing and Plasmid Analysis

Total genomic DNA extraction and analysis were carried out according to previously described methods (Wang et al., 2020). Briefly, the QIAamp DNA MiniKit (Qiagen, Valencia, CA, United States) was used to extract the genomic DNA of two strains for genome sequencing. A NextEra XT DNA library preparation kit (Illumina, Inc., Cambridge, United Kingdom) was used to prepare the DNA library. Genomic DNA was sequenced on an Illumina HiSeq^{TM} 4000 instrument with a 150-bp paired-end approach at a depth of approximately 200×. The CLC Genomics Workbench 10.0 was used to assemble the raw reads of the strains into draft genomes using. In addition, a Pacific Biosciences RSII DNA sequencing system (PacBio, Menlo Park, CA, United States) was used to obtain the complete genomes of strains EC2341 and EC2547. The resulting sequences were *de novo* assembled using the Hierarchical Genome Assembly Process (HGAP_Assembly.2) with the default settings of the SMRT Analysis v2.3.0 software package.

[2]http://www.eucast.org/clinical_breakpoints

The Rapid Annotation using Subsystems Technology (RAST) annotation website server[3] was used to annotate the genomes. A schematic map of the linear comparison of the two bla_{KPC-2}-positive plasmids and their related plasmids was generated with EasyFig 2.2.2 (Sullivan et al., 2011). Multi-locus sequence typing (MLST) of the strain and incompatibility typing of the bla_{KPC-2}-positive plasmid were performed with the assistance of the PlasmidFinder-1.3 server and the MLST 2.0 server, which are available at the Center for Genomic Epidemiology[4].

In addition, plasmid stability was determined according to a previous study (Li et al., 2018).

Nucleotide Sequence Accession Number

The complete sequences of the plasmids pEC2341-KPC (accession number CP072979) and pEC2547-KPC (accession number CP072981) were deposited in DDBJ/EMBL/GenBank.

RESULTS AND DISCUSSION

Isolate Characteristics

In the present study, two KPC-2-producing isolates were collected from a teaching hospital in Zhejiang, China. *E. coli* strains EC2341 and EC2547 were isolated from urine and sputum, respectively. The antimicrobial susceptibility testing results showed that the bla_{KPC-2}-positive isolates were resistant to carbapenems, cephalosporins, amoxicillin/clavulanate, ciprofloxacin, and amikacin but were susceptible to colistin, tigecycline and ceftazidime-avibactam (**Table 1**).

The MLST results showed that *E. coli* strains EC2547 and EC2341 belonged to ST131 and ST410, respectively. The ST131 clone-type *E. coli* strain emerged in the mid-2000s and has spread worldwide (Can et al., 2015). Similar to clone lineage of ST131, the *E. coli* ST410 strain has been confirmed as another successful clone in *E. coli* (Schaufler et al., 2016). Furthermore, these two clone-type *E. coli* strains have gained a further selective advantage due to acquisition of carbapenem resistance (Du et al., 2020; Lee and Choi, 2020). In addition, other resistance genes, such as $bla_{CTX-M-3}$, $bla_{CTX-M-27}$, *fosA3*, and *qnrS1*, were also detected in the *E. coli* strains by analysis of the genome sequences. Multiple resistance genes were identified in the ST410 and ST131 strains, indicating that these two clone-type strains might be more capable of acquiring resistance genes.

Notably, these two international high-risk clones have caused a wide variety of clinical infections (Roer et al., 2018; Wang et al., 2020) and are associated with treatment failure because of their high virulence potential (Can et al., 2015). In the present study, multiple potential virulence factors were identified by VirulenceFinder analysis of *E. coli* EC2341 and EC2547 strains, such as *ompA* (outer membrane protein A), *fdeC* (adhesin), and *fepC* (iron-enterobactin transporter). bla_{KPC-2} was present in the ST131 and ST410 strains, further supporting the results that these two clone types may become a successful lineage of KPC-2-producing *E. coli* strains.

IncU-Type Plasmid Carrying the bla_{KPC-2} Gene

To ascertain the plasmid location of the bla_{KPC-2} gene, S1-PFGE was performed followed by Southern blot experiments. The bla_{KPC-2} gene was located on two plasmids of different sizes, ca. 80 Kb and ca. 100 Kb (data not shown). The transferability of the two bla_{KPC-2}-positive plasmids was further determined by filter mating experiments. The EC2341 isolate tested could successfully transfer its carbapenem-resistance to *E. coli* strain J53 (**Table 1**), while the EC2547 isolate could not transfer its carbapenem resistance. Additionally, the bla_{KPC-2}-positive plasmids were both stable in the two isolates by plasmid stability experiments. In the absence of antibiotics, the randomly selected strains all carried the bla_{KPC-2}-positive plasmid that was identical to the parental isolate after 12 rounds of subculture on MH agar.

Incompatibility plasmid classification showed that the two bla_{KPC-2}-positive plasmids were both grouped into IncU replicon types. The IncU plasmid incompatibility group was assigned in 1981 (Sirgel et al., 1981) and is a unique group of mobile elements with highly conserved backbone functions and variable antibiotic resistance gene cassettes (Tschäpe et al., 1981; Rhodes et al., 2000). The IncU incompatibility group has been isolated from a number of *Aeromonas* spp. and *E. coli* strains from natural and clinical environments (Tschäpe et al., 1981; Sandaa and Enger, 1994; Adams et al., 1998; Rhodes et al., 2000). Various resistance genes have also been described for IncU plasmids, such as *qnrS2*, *aac(6′)-Ib-cr*, *aadA1* and *aadA2*, *sulI* and *sulII*, *dfrA16* *dfrIIc* *(dfrB3)* and *catAII* (Sørum et al., 2003). However, carbapenem-resistant IncU plasmids have not been found previously. In this study, the bla_{KPC-2} gene was confirmed to be carried on the IncU plasmids. To the best of our knowledge, this is the first report of *E. coli* strains carrying the bla_{KPC-2} gene on IncU plasmids. Our study further demonstrated that plasmids harboring the bla_{KPC-2} gene were diverse.

Sequence Analysis of bla_{KPC-2} IncU Plasmids

Two entire sequences were obtained to further characterize the IncU plasmids carrying bla_{KPC-2}. Sequence analysis showed that plasmid pEC2341_KPC was 76,952 bp in size, had 51.9% G + C content, and harbored 133 predicted ORFs (**Figure 1A**). The core region of pEC2341_KPC includes a replication module (*repE*), one transfer (*tra*) system, and a stability operon (*stbAB* and *umuCD*). Four antimicrobial resistance genes, *qnrS1*, $bla_{CTX-M-13}$, bla_{TEM-1}, and *drfA14*, were detected in this plasmid except for the bla_{KPC-2} gene. In addition, a class 1 integron-like element was also detected in this plasmid. The element is a *dfrA14* gene with its 3′-conserved sequence truncated by the insertion of an *IS*6100 element. Sequence alignments revealed that the plasmid sequences were almost identical to those previously reported plasmids pECN-580 (KF914891) of *E. coli* ECN580 (97% coverage, 99.97% identity) in China (Chen et al., 2014c) and pCRKP-1-KPC (KX928750) of *K. pneumoniae* CRKP-1-KPC (96% coverage, 99.90% identity) in China (unpublished data) (**Figure 2**).

[3]https://rast.nmpdr.org/

[4]http://www.genomicepidemiology.org/

Plasmid pEC2547 contained bla_{KPC-2} and was 94,462 bp in size, with an average G + C content of 49.3% (**Figure 1B**). Compared with plasmid pEC2341_KPC, two other antimicrobial resistance genes, *aar-3* and *acc(6′)Ib*, were identified in this plasmid. Two class 1 integron-like elements were identified in pEC2547_KPC. The first element is same as that in pEC2341_KPC. The second element is an *IntI1-aac(6′)-Ib-cr-aar-3-Tn3* gene cassette located downstream of the bla_{KPC-2} gene.

TABLE 1 | Antibiotic susceptibility used in this study (mg/L).

Strains	AMC	FEP	CAZ	ETP	IPM	MEM	CZA	AMK	CIP	TGC	CST
EC2341	128	>128	>128	64	8	16	0.25	4	>128	<0.0625	0.125
EC2341-J53	64	>128	32	64	4	8	<0.125	4	1	<0.0625	0.25
EC2547	128	>128	>128	>64	8	32	0.125	8	>128	<0.0625	0.125
E. coli ATCC 25922	4	0.125	0.125	0.125	0.125	0.125	<0.125	0.5	0.125	0.125	0.125

Drug susceptibility was determined with broth microdilution method according to the Clinical Laboratory Standards Institute (CLSI) guidelines. AMC, amoxicillin clavulanate; FEP, cefepime; CAZ, ceftazidime; ETP, ertapenem; IPM, imipenem; MEM, meropenem; CZA, ceftazidime-avibactam; AMK, amikacin; CIP, ciprofloxacin; TGC, tigecycline; CST, colistin.

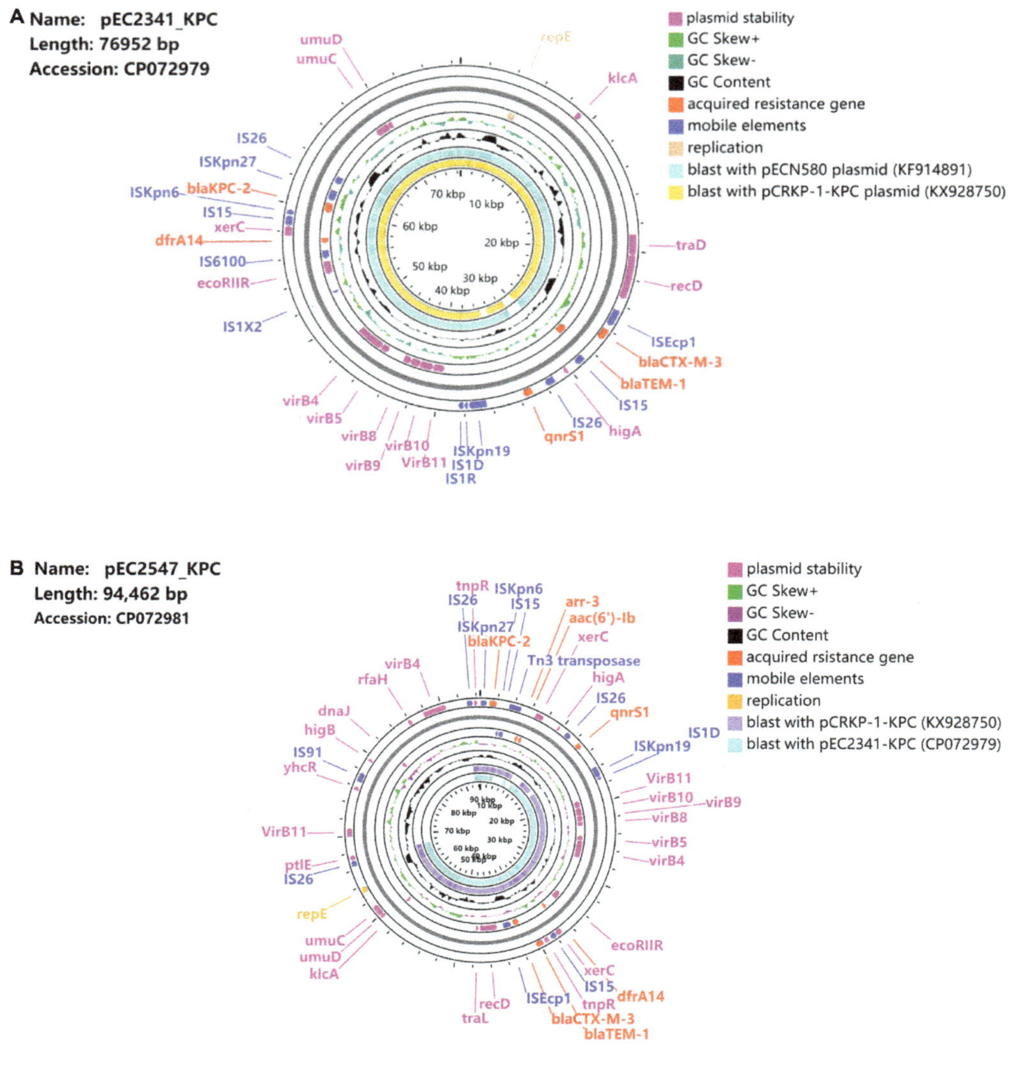

FIGURE 1 | (A) Schematic map of plasmid pEC2341_KPC. Sequence alignment between pECN580 (accession number KF914891) and pCRKP-1-KPC (accession number KX928750) is the outer circle in orange and teal. **(B)** Schematic map of plasmid pEC2547_KPC. Sequence alignment between pEC2341-KPC (accession number CP072979) and pCRKP-1-KPC (accession number KX928750) is the outer circle in teal and blue.

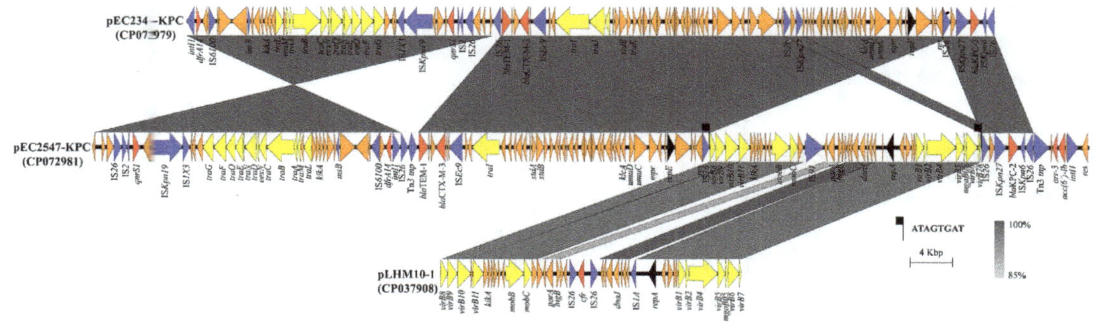

FIGURE 2 | Linear characterization of the plasmids pEC2341-KPC and pEC2547-KPC with closely related plasmid. The gray regions between plasmids indicate nucleotide identity (85–100%) by BLASTn. Arrows indicate predicted ORFs. Primary structural characteristics of plasmids pEC2341-KPC (CP072979), pEC2547-KPC (CP072981), and pLHM10-1 (CP037908). Colored arrows represent open reading frames, with red, yellow, blue, and orange representing antibiotic resistance gene, plasmid transfer related genes, mobile elements and common function genes, respectively.

Notably, sequencing analysis further indicated that pEC2547 might evolve from plasmid pEC2341_KPC of *E. coli* EC2341 (67% coverage, 100% identity) (**Figure 2**). Compared with plasmid pEC2341_KPC, an approximately 24-kb sequence flanked by two *IS26* elements was carried on plasmid pEC2547, which resulted in disruption of the transfer systems of this plasmid. Consistent with our conjugate transfer results, the EC2547 isolate could not transfer its carbapenem resistance to *E. coli* strain J53. The 24-kb sequence was further aligned to an unnamed plasmid of *E. coli* strain LHM10-1 (GenBank accession number CP037908) with 89% coverage and 96.52% identity. This 24-kb composite transposon-like element flanking with two IS26 elements undergoes replicative transposition by the 8-bp target site duplication (TSD) (ATAGTGAT). *IS26* elements have been demonstrated to undergo frequent intramolecular transposition and facilitate recombination between the plasmid or the chromosome (He et al., 2015). These findings suggest that the plasmid pEC2547 was composed of the pEC2341_KPC plasmid and an unnamed plasmid of *E. coli* strain LHM10-1, which was a composite transposon formed by *IS26* (**Figure 2**).

In addition, the bla_{KPC-2} gene carried on the two plasmids was preceded by *IS26*, *IS*Kpn27, and *IS*Kpn6, and followed by *IS26*. In China, bla_{KPC-2} genetic environments can be classified into three main types: Tn4401 with the *IS*Kpn7-bla_{KPC-2}-*IS*Kpn6 core structure, Tn1722-based unit transposons with the *IS*Kpn27-bla_{KPC-2}-*IS*Kpn6 core structure and *IS26*-based composite transposons with the *IS*Kpn27-bla_{KPC-2}-*IS*Kpn6 core structure (Wang et al., 2015). In this study, bla_{KPC-2} genes were both located in an approximately 5-kb composite transposon-like element with the *IS*Kpn27 insertion sequence upstream and the *IS*Kpn6 insertion sequence downstream of the element and flanked by two IS26 elements bracketed by *IS26*, which belonged to the *IS26*-based composite transposon. *IS26*-based composite transposons are mainly carried by IncN-type plasmids. Our plasmids belonged to the IncU type, which led to speculation that the *IS26* elements may promote recombination between the plasmids and explain the movement of the new IncU regions.

CONCLUSION

Overall, we describe here the complete sequences of two novel bla_{KPC-2}-positive IncU plasmids from *E. coli* isolates. The two bla_{KPC-2}-harboring plasmids have a close evolutionary relationship, which highlighted the diversity of these highly promiscuous plasmids. The spread of bla_{KPC-2} harboring multidrug-resistant plasmids, e.g., pEC2341-KPC and pEC2547-KPC, into the international high-risk clones *E. coli* ST131 and ST410, presents tremendous challenges for clinicians. It is important for the IncU-type plasmid to further disseminate bla_{KPC-2} in *Enterobacteriaceae* in order for it to be maintained. Therefore, effective measures should be taken immediately to prevent the spread of these bla_{KPC-2}–positive plasmids.

AUTHOR CONTRIBUTIONS

XL and HP conceived and designed the experiments. WW, LL, and WF performed the experiments. CC and DJ analyzed the data. WW and XL wrote the manuscript. All authors read and approved the final manuscript.

FUNDING

This study was supported by the Public Technology Research Projects of Zhejiang Province, China (LGD21H190001), Natural Science Foundation of Zhejiang Province, China (Q18H010007), and Medical and Health Research Project (2020KY420). The funders had no role in study design, data collection and analysis, decision to publish, or preparation of the manuscript.

REFERENCES

Adams, C. A., Austin, B., Meaden, P. G., and Mcintosh, D. (1998). Molecular characterization of plasmid-mediated oxytetracycline resistance in *Aeromonas salmonicida*. *Appl. Environ. Microbiol.* 64, 4194–4201. doi: 10.1128/aem.64.11.4194-4201.1998

Bratu, S., Brooks, S., Burney, S., Kochar, S., Gupta, J., Landman, D., et al. (2007). Detection and spread of *Escherichia coli* possessing the plasmid-borne carbapenemase KPC-2 in Brooklyn, New York. *Clin. Infect. Dis.* 44, 972–975. doi: 10.1086/512370

Can, F., Azap, O. K., Seref, C., Ispir, P., Arslan, H., and Ergonul, O. (2015). Emerging *Escherichia coli* O25b/ST131 clone predicts treatment failure in urinary tract infections. *Clin. Infect. Dis.* 60, 523–527. doi: 10.1093/cid/ciu864

Chen, L., Chavda, K. D., Al Laham, N., Melano, R. G., Jacobs, M. R., Bonomo, R. A., et al. (2013). Complete nucleotide sequence of a bla_{KPC}-harboring IncI2 plasmid and its dissemination in New Jersey and New York hospitals. *Antimicrob. Agents Chemother.* 57, 5019–5025. doi: 10.1128/aac.01397-13

Chen, L., Chavda, K. D., Melano, R. G., Hong, T., Rojtman, A. D., Jacobs, M. R., et al. (2014a). Molecular survey of the dissemination of two bla_{KPC}-harboring IncFIA plasmids in New Jersey and New York hospitals. *Antimicrob. Agents Chemother.* 58, 2289–2294. doi: 10.1128/aac.02749-13

Chen, L., Chavda, K. D., Melano, R. G., Jacobs, M. R., Koll, B., Hong, T., et al. (2014b). Comparative genomic analysis of KPC-encoding pKpQIL-like plasmids and their distribution in New Jersey and New York Hospitals. *Antimicrob. Agents Chemother.* 58, 2871–2877. doi: 10.1128/aac.00120-14

Chen, L., Hu, H., Chavda, K. D., Zhao, S., Liu, R., Liang, H., et al. (2014c). Complete sequence of a KPC-producing IncN multidrug-resistant plasmid from an epidemic *Escherichia coli* sequence type 131 strain in China. *Antimicrob. Agents Chemother.* 58, 2422–2425. doi: 10.1128/aac.02587-13

Chen, L., Mathema, B., Chavda, K. D., Deleo, F. R., Bonomo, R. A., and Kreiswirth, B. N. (2014). Carbapenemase-producing *Klebsiella pneumoniae*: molecular and genetic decoding. *Trends Microbiol.* 22, 686–696. doi: 10.1016/j.tim.2014.09.003

CLSI (2020). *Performance Standards for Antimicrobial Susceptibility Testing CLSI Supplement M100*, 30th Edn. Wayne, PA: Clinical and Laboratory Standards Institute.

Du, X., Huang, J., Wang, D., Zhu, Y., Lv, H., and Li, X. (2020). Whole genome sequence of an *Escherichia coli* ST131 strain isolated from a patient with bloodstream infection in China co-harbouring bla(KPC-2), bla(CTX-M-3), bla(CTX-M-14), qnrS1, aac(3)-IIa and aac(6′)-Ib-cr genes. *J. Glob. Antimicrob. Resist.* 22, 700–702. doi: 10.1016/j.jgar.2020.06.027

Fuga, B., Ferreira, M. L., Cerdeira, L. T., De Campos, P. A., Dias, V. L., Rossi, I., et al. (2020). Novel small IncX3 plasmid carrying the *bla*(KPC-2) gene in high-risk *Klebsiella pneumoniae* ST11/CG258. *Diagn. Microbiol. Infect. Dis.* 96:114900. doi: 10.1016/j.diagmicrobio.2019.114900

He, S., Hickman, A. B., Varani, A. M., Siguier, P., Chandler, M., Dekker, J. P., et al. (2015). Insertion sequence IS26 reorganizes plasmids in clinically isolated multidrug-resistant bacteria by replicative transposition. *mBio* 6:e00762.

Hu, X., Yu, X., Shang, Y., Xu, H., Guo, L., Liang, Y., et al. (2019). Emergence and characterization of a novel IncP-6 plasmid harboring *bla* (KPC-2) and *qnrS2* genes in *Aeromonas taiwanensis* isolates. *Front. Microbiol.* 10:2132. doi: 10.3389/fmicb.2019.02132

Lee, M., and Choi, T. J. (2020). Species transferability of *Klebsiella pneumoniae* Carbapenemase-2 isolated from a high-risk clone of *Escherichia coli* ST410. *J. Microbiol. Biotechnol.* 30, 974–981. doi: 10.4014/jmb.1912.12049

Li, X., Fu, Y., Shen, M., Huang, D., Du, X., Hu, Q., et al. (2018). Dissemination of *bla*(NDM-5) gene via an IncX3-type plasmid among non-clonal *Escherichia coli* in China. *Antimicrob. Resist. Infect. Control* 7:59.

Liu, X., Liu, H., Wang, L., Peng, Q., Li, Y., Zhou, H., et al. (2018). Molecular characterization of extended-spectrum β-lactamase-producing multidrug resistant *Escherichia coli* from Swine in Northwest China. *Front. Microbiol.* 9:1756. doi: 10.3389/fmicb.2018.01756

Mahmoud, N. E., Altayb, H. N., and Gurashi, R. M. (2020). Detection of carbapenem-resistant genes in *Escherichia coli* isolated from drinking water in khartoum, Sudan. *J. Environ. Public Health* 2020:2571293.

Mathers, A. J., Stoesser, N., Chai, W., Carroll, J., Barry, K., Cherunvanky, A., et al. (2017). Chromosomal integration of the *Klebsiella pneumoniae* carbapenemase gene, *bla*(KPC), in klebsiella species is elusive but not rare. *Antimicrob. Agents Chemother.* 61:e01823-16.

Munoz-Price, L. S., Poirel, L., Bonomo, R. A., Schwaber, M. J., Daikos, G. L., Cormican, M., et al. (2013). Clinical epidemiology of the global expansion of *Klebsiella pneumoniae* carbapenemases. *Lancet Infect. Dis.* 13, 785–796. doi: 10.1016/s1473-3099(13)70190-7

Rhodes, G., Huys, G., Swings, J., Mcgann, P., Hiney, M., Smith, P., et al. (2000). Distribution of oxytetracycline resistance plasmids between aeromonads in hospital and aquaculture environments: implication of Tn1721 in dissemination of the tetracycline resistance determinant *tet A*. *Appl. Environ. Microbiol.* 66, 3883–3890. doi: 10.1128/aem.66.9.3883-3890.2000

Roer, L., Overballe-Petersen, S., Hansen, F., Schønning, K., Wang, M., Røder, B. L., et al. (2018). *Escherichia coli* sequence type 410 is causing new international high-risk clones. *mSphere* 3:e00337-18.

Sandaa, R. A., and Enger, O. (1994). Transfer in marine sediments of the naturally occurring plasmid pRAS1 encoding multiple antibiotic resistance. *Appl. Environ. Microbiol.* 60, 4234–4238. doi: 10.1128/aem.60.12.4234-4238.1994

Schaufler, K., Semmler, T., Wieler, L. H., Wöhrmann, M., Baddam, R., Ahmed, N., et al. (2016). Clonal spread and interspecies transmission of clinically relevant ESBL-producing *Escherichia coli* of ST410–another successful pandemic clone? *FEMS Microbiol. Ecol.* 92:fiv155. doi: 10.1093/femsec/fiv155

Schweizer, C., Bischoff, P., Bender, J., Kola, A., Gastmeier, P., Hummel, M., et al. (2019). Plasmid-mediated transmission of KPC-2 carbapenemase in *Enterobacteriaceae* in critically Ill patients. *Front. Microbiol.* 10:276. doi: 10.3389/fmicb.2019.00276

Sellera, F. P., Fernandes, M. R., Ruiz, R., Falleiros, A. C. M., Rodrigues, F. P., Cerdeira, L., et al. (2018). Identification of KPC-2-producing *Escherichia coli* in a companion animal: a new challenge for veterinary clinicians. *J. Antimicrob. Chemother.* 73, 2259–2261.

Sirgel, F. A., Coetzee, J. N., Hedges, R. W., and Lecatsas, G. (1981). Phage C-1: an IncC group; plasmid-specific phage. *J. Gen. Microbiol.* 122, 155–160. doi: 10.1159/000149385

Smith Moland, E., Hanson, N. D., Herrera, V. L., Black, J. A., Lockhart, T. J., Hossain, A., et al. (2003). Plasmid-mediated, carbapenem-hydrolysing beta-lactamase, KPC-2, in *Klebsiella pneumoniae* isolates. *J. Antimicrob. Chemother.* 51, 711–714. doi: 10.1093/jac/dkg124

Sørum, H., L'abée-Lund, T. M., Solberg, A., and Wold, A. (2003). Integron-containing IncU R plasmids pRAS1 and pAr-32 from the fish pathogen *Aeromonas salmonicida*. *Antimicrob. Agents Chemother.* 47, 1285–1290. doi: 10.1128/aac.47.4.1285-1290.2003

Suay-García, B., and Pérez-Gracia, M. T. (2019). Present and future of carbapenem-resistant *Enterobacteriaceae* (CRE) infections. *Antibiotics* 8:122. doi: 10.3390/antibiotics8030122

Sullivan, M. J., Petty, N. K., and Beatson, S. A. (2011). Easyfig: a genome comparison visualizer. *Bioinformatics* 27, 1009–1010. doi: 10.1093/bioinformatics/btr039

Tschäpe, H., Tietze, E., and Koch, C. (1981). Characterization of conjugative R plasmids belonging to the new incompatibility group IncU. *J. Gen. Microbiol.* 127, 155–160. doi: 10.1099/00221287-127-1-155

Vikram, A., and Schmidt, J. W. (2018). Functional bla(KPC-2) sequences are present in U.S. beef cattle feces regardless of antibiotic use. *Foodborne Pathog. Dis.* 15, 444–448. doi: 10.1089/fpd.2017.2406

Wang, D., Mu, X., Chen, Y., Zhao, D., Fu, Y., Jiang, Y., et al. (2020). Emergence of a clinical *Escherichia coli* sequence type 131 strain carrying a chromosomal bla (KPC-2) gene. *Front. Microbiol.* 11:586764. doi: 10.3389/fmicb.2020.586764

Wang, J., Yao, X., Luo, J., Lv, L., Zeng, Z., and Liu, J. H. (2018). Emergence of *Escherichia coli* co-producing NDM-1 and KPC-2 carbapenemases from a retail vegetable, China. *J. Antimicrob. Chemother.* 73, 252–254. doi: 10.1093/jac/dkx335

Wang, L., Fang, H., Feng, J., Yin, Z., Xie, X., Zhu, X., et al. (2015). Complete sequences of KPC-2-encoding plasmid p628-KPC and CTX-M-55-encoding p628-CTXM coexisted in *Klebsiella pneumoniae*. *Front. Microbiol.* 6:838. doi: 10.3389/fmicb.2015.00838

Xu, G., Jiang, Y., An, W., Wang, H., and Zhang, X. (2015). Emergence of KPC-2-producing *Escherichia coli* isolates in an urban river in Harbin, China. *World J. Microbiol. Biotechnol.* 31, 1443–1450. doi: 10.1007/s11274-015-1897-z

15

Purification and Characterization of an Active Principle, Lawsone, Responsible for the Plasmid Curing Activity of *Plumbago zeylanica* Root Extracts

Rajashree Bhalchandra Patwardhan[1]*, Prashant Kamalakar Dhakephalkar[2]*, Balu Ananda Chopade[3], Dilip D. Dhavale[4] and Ramesh R. Bhonde[5]

[1] Department of Microbiology, Haribhai V. Desai College of Arts, Science and Commerce, Pune University, Pune, India, [2] Bioenergy Group, Agharkar Research Institute, Pune, India, [3] Department of Microbiology, Savitribai Phule Pune University, Aurangabad, India, [4] Department of Chemistry, Savitribai Phule Pune University, Pune, India, [5] School of Regenerative Medicine – Manipal Academy of Higher Education, Bengaluru, India

****Correspondence:***
Rajashree Bhalchandra Patwardhan
dr.rbpatwardhan@gmail.com
Prashant Kamalakar Dhakephalkar
pkdhakephalkar@aripune.org

Plasmid curing is the process of obviating the plasmid encoded functions such as antibiotic resistance, virulence, degradation of aromatic compounds, etc. in bacteria. Several plasmid curing agents have been reported in literature, however, no plasmid curing agent can eliminate all plasmids from different hosts. Hence, there is always a need for novel plasmid curing agents that can be effectively used for reversal of plasmid encoded functions such as virulence, antibiotic resistance, etc. In the present study, an active principle responsible for the plasmid curing activity was purified from roots of *Plumbago zeylanica* by bioassay guided fractionation and identified as 2-hydroxy-1,4-naphthoquinone (lawsone), on the basis of spectral and analytical data such as NMR, GCMS, FTIR. Plasmid curing activity of lawsone was observed against reference as well as wild plasmids (pBR322, pRK2013, R136, pUPI281, and pUPI282) residing in a range of hosts. Curing of plasmid was confirmed by agarose gel electrophoresis. MICs of antibiotics against *A. baumannii* A24 (pUPI281) and *E. coli* (pRK2013) decreased significantly in presence of lawsone suggesting synergy between lawsone and antibiotics. Lawsone also inhibited transfer of plasmid pRK2013 to *E. coli* either by transformation or conjugation. Viability assays (MTT) revealed that lawsone was not toxic to mammalian cells. Thus, the present investigation has revealed lawsone as an effective plasmid curing agent capable of suppressing development and spread of antibiotic resistance. Further, lawsone has important application in basic research to identify phenotypes encoded by the plasmids in plasmid curing experiments. To the best of our knowledge this is the first report of plasmid curing activity of lawsone isolated from roots of *P. zeylanica*.

Keywords: lawsone(2-hydroxy-1, 4 naphthoquinone), *Plumbago zeylanica*, extraction, purification, plasmid curing, antibiotic resistance

INTRODUCTION

Plasmids are independent, circular, self-replicating extra-chromosomal DNA elements with characteristic copy numbers within the host. Various properties encoded by plasmid include resistance to antibiotics and heavy metals, degradation of hydrocarbons, synthesis of bacteriocins and antibiotics, etc. Plasmid mediated antibiotic resistance can be transferred easily from one bacterium to another by transformation, conjugation or mobilization (Opal et al., 2000). Plasmid encoded resistance to multiple antibiotics has been increasingly recognized as a major challenge in the treatment of infections. In addition to the antibiotic resistance, some bacterial plasmids confer pathogenicity as well, to the host cell (Saunders, 1981).

Plasmid curing agents are the chemicals or physical agents that inhibit the replication of plasmid resulting in subsequent elimination of such plasmids from the host population after several replication cycles. Obtaining plasmid cured derivatives is desired in the investigation of bacterial harboring plasmids. Comparison of plasmid harboring strain and its cured derivative allows assigning phenotypic characters to genes located on plasmids. Simultaneous loss of a particular character by curing, gives a strong indication of its plasmid borne genetic character (Trevors, 1986). Further, plasmid curing converts the antibiotic resistant bacterial cells into sensitive ones (Molnar, 1988). Thus, elimination of R-plasmids makes the antibiotic therapy effective. Novel strategies to struggle antimicrobial multidrug resistance are required, and plasmid curing, and anti-plasmid strategies could reduce antimicrobial resistance genes frequency and sensitize bacteria to antibiotics (Michelle et al., 2018).

Plasmid curing agents reported in the scientific literature include sodium lauryl sulfate, ethidium bromide, acridine orange, etc. (Bouanchaud et al., 1969; Chopade et al., 1994). However, it is known from earlier studies that acridine dyes and ethidium bromide cannot be used *in vivo* because of their mutagenicity, carcinogenicity, teratogenicity while SDS, because of its detergent action (Shriram et al., 2010). Hence, these curing agents are not useful in controlling the spread of antibiotic resistance in hospital environment. The curing agents have been effectively used to study plasmid encoded phenotypes in various laboratory studies. Till date no curing agent is known that can universally cure all plasmids from bacterial population. So non-toxic and highly effective plasmid eliminating agents are required to be developed constantly.

Plants are known to produce diverse bioactive substances of chemotherapeutic value (Chopra et al., 1992; Samy and Ignacimuthu, 2000). Ahmad et al. (2000) reported ability of aqueous extracts of *Plumbago zeylanica* to eliminate plasmid encoded antibiotic resistance in *Escherichia coli*. However, active principle responsible was not purified and identified.

In the view of this background, root extracts of *P. zeylanica* were explored for the presence of novel plasmid curing agent that was effective against antibiotic resistant plasmids in *Escherichia coli, Salmonella* Typhi as well as *Acinetobacter baumannii*. In the present investigation, lawsone was purified from the roots of *P. zeylanica* and identified as a plasmid curing agent capable of reversing multiple antibiotic resistance in broad range of clinical isolates as well as reference strains.

MATERIALS AND METHODS

Plant Material

P. zeylanica plants were collected from Western Ghat region of India. The roots were harvested, dried in shade, powdered and used for further extraction procedures. The plant material was authenticated by Botanical Survey of India, Ministry of Environments and forests, Government of India. A voucher specimen (RBPUP1) is deposited at the Herbarium of Botanical Survey of India, Office of Joint Director, Pune, India.

Extraction and Purification of Plasmid Curing Agent From *P. zeylanica* Roots

Active principle responsible for the plasmid curing activity was purified by the bioassay guided fractionation procedure as described previously (Shriram et al., 2008). Air-dried and powdered roots (2.5 kg) of *Plumbago zeylanica* were successively extracted in Soxhlet apparatus with petroleum ether, cyclohexane, benzene, diethyl ether, chloroform, acetone, ethanol, and methanol (according to eluotropic series based on polarity) at boiling temperature for respective solvents (Shriram et al., 2008). Each extract was filtered and concentrated to dryness under vacuum on a rotary evaporator (Heidolph-Germany) and dissolved in 10 ml of dimethyl sulfoxide (DMSO). Isolation and purification of active compounds from *P. zeylanica* roots was performed by column chromatography with silica gel (100–200 mesh) (Sadasivam and Manickam, 1992). Ethanol extract showing antimicrobial and plasmid curing activity was then coarsely fractionated over silica gel using a stepwise gradient solvent system consisting of hexane: ethyl acetate (9:1, 8:2, 7:3, 6:4, 5:5, 4:5, 3:6) to separate the respective fractions (25–40 μm, 3′ 50 cm, eluent hexane-ethyl acetate, flow rate 3 ml/min). TLC analysis was carried out on 0.25 mm precoated silica gel sheets (polygram sil Gluv 254). Chromatographic fractions as well as pure compounds were monitored by TLC, detected by UV light at 250 nm (UV GL-25 Mineralight lamp) and color reaction by spraying with a solution of 2% 2,4-dinitro phenyl hydrazine in methanolic sulphuric acid followed by 5 min heating at 100°C. A total of 83 sub-fractions (10 ml) were collected and monitored by TLC. Sub-fractions 17–23 yielded (64 mg), a single pure compound detected by TLC (hexane-ethyl acetate 7:3, R_f = 0.617). This compound was further purified by preparative TLC (Macherey-Nagel-Germany Precoated TLC plates SIL G-200 UV_{254} 2 mm thickness) using hexane-ethyl acetate solvent system.

Characterization of Purified Plasmid Curing Agent

Melting point was determined in degree Celsius (°C) with Thomas Hoover Capillary Melting point apparatus (New Jersey,

United States). IR spectra were recorded with Perkin Elmer 1600 FTIR and Shimadzu FTIR spectrophotometer as a thin film or in nujol mull or using KBr pellets and were expressed in cm^{-1}. Spectral data on GCMS was acquired with the direct insertion probe on a Shimadzu spectrometer at 70 eV. Isolated compound was analyzed for structure elucidation by techniques such as ^{1}H nuclear magnetic resonance (NMR) and ^{13}C NMR (Choudhary and Atta-ur-Rahman, 1997). The ^{1}H NMR spectra (300 MHz) were recorded in $CDCl_3$ as a solvent on a Varian (mercury) instrument. ^{1}H NMR chemical shifts were expressed in δ (ppm) units, downfield to internal standard TMS (Daniel, 1991). Assignment of signals was confirmed by decoupling experiments.

Microbial Strains and Culture Conditions Used

Bacterial isolates and standard plasmids used in this study are enlisted in **Tables 1, 2**. Clinical isolates of *Acinetobacter* were identified based on their morphological, cultural and biochemical characteristics according to the Bergey's Manual of Systematic Bacteriology (Kloos and Schleifer, 1986) and using API20NE system (Biomeraux, France) as per manufacturer's instructions. All strains were preserved as glycerol stocks at −20°C or as agar slants at 4–8°C. All bacterial cultures were grown on Luria agar at 37°C (Hi Media, Mumbai, India).

Determination of Resistance to Antibiotics

Antibiotic resistance profile was determined by the disk diffusion method (Bauer et al., 1966). Multi-disks containing antibiotics (Don Whitley Scientific Equipments, Mumbai, India) were placed on Muller Hinton agar plates (Hi Media, India) spread with ca. 10^5 cells of actively growing test culture and incubated at 37°C. The inhibition zones measured after 24 h incubation and were interpreted according to the manufacturer's interpretation table. MICs of antibiotics were determined by agar dilution method as described previously (Dhakephalkar and Chopade, 1994). Concentrations of each antibiotic used ranged from 1 μg/ml to 1,024 μg/ml. MIC was interpreted as the lowest concentration of the antibiotic inhibiting bacterial growth.

TABLE 1 | Antibacterial activity of lawsone from *P. zeylanica* ethanol root extract.

Sr. No.	Bacterial strains	Strain designation	MIC (μg/disk)
1	*P. aeruginosa*	PUPU103	800
2	*S. aureus*	PUPU107	400
3	*S.* Typhi	PUST112	200
4	*B. cereus*	PUBL123	200
5	*E. coli*	PUUR119	800
6	*S. dysenteriae*	PUST115	400
7	*B. subtilis*	PUBL126	200
8	*S. marcescens*	PUUR120	>1600
9	*P. mirabilis*	PUUR121	>1600
10	*K. pneumoniae*	PUSP134	800
11	*Enterobacter*	PUST114	800
12	*A. baumannii*	PUBL130	800

MIC (minimum inhibitory concentration) was detected by disk diffusion assay using 10^5 cells as inoculum on NA for bacteria. DMSO without lawsone, used as a solvent control, did not inhibit growth of any of the bacterial cultures tested. All the strains were isolated from clinical specimens like pus, stool, blood, urine, and sputum.

Plasmid Isolation

Plasmid isolation was carried out by alkali lysis method as well as boiling method described by Sambrook et al. (1989). DNA was detected by horizontal agarose gel (0.7%) electrophoresis using Tris-acetate-EDTA buffer (pH 8.0).

Curing of Antibiotic Resistance

The plasmid curing was performed as described earlier by Deshpande et al. (2001). In brief, microbial culture was exposed to different concentrations of curing agent during cultivation in Luria broth at 37°C for 24 h. Subsequently, the culture was serially diluted and plated on Luria agar to obtain isolated colonies. A total of 100 colonies was replica plated on Luria agar with and without antibiotic. Cured derivatives were scored by their failure to grow in presence of antibiotics. Efficiency of curing was calculated as number of colonies showing reversal of antibiotic resistance per 100 colonies tested. Agarose gel electrophoresis was performed to confirm the removal of plasmid DNA from the plasmid cured strain. Effect of pH (range 5.5–8.0), lawsone concentrations (range 64–512 μg/ml) and inoculum densities (range 10^4–10^7 cells/ml) on curing efficiency of lawsone was studied in *E. coli* (pRK2013) and *A. baumannii* (pUPI281). All the experiments were performed at least in duplicate.

Effect of Purified Active Principle (Lawsone) on Transformation of Plasmid

E. coli HB101was used as host for the transformation experiments. Calcium chloride method (Sambrook et al., 1989) was used for the preparation of competent cells. Transformation experiments were performed by "heat shock method" as described previously (Sambrook et al., 1989) using plasmid pRK2013 and competent cells of *E. coli* HB101 as recipient. Transformation efficiency was expressed as number of transformants obtained per μg of plasmid DNA. Purified active principle, at specified concentrations, was added to competent cells along with transforming DNA to evaluate its effect on plasmid transformation.

Effect of Purified Active Principle (Lawsone) on Plasmid Transfer by Conjugation

Conjugation experiments were performed by membrane filter mating method as described by Towner and Chopade (1987). Effect of lawsone on plasmid transfer was studied by incubating both donor *E. coli* (pRK2013) and recipient *E. coli* HB101 (adsorbed on membrane filter) on nutrient agar containing varying concentrations of curing agent. Difference in the percentage efficiency of conjugation in the presence or absence

TABLE 2 | Plasmid curing with purified lawsone.

Strain and plasmid	Size of plasmid	Antibiotic resistance[@]	MIC (μg/ml)	SIC (μg/ml)	Curing efficiency (%)
E. coli K12 (RP4) MTCC 391	56.4 kb	Ap^r, Km^r, Tc^r	512	256	ND
E. coli (pBR 322) MTCC 78	4.3 kb	Ap^r, Tc^r	800	512	11 ± 1.4
E. coli (pRK 2013) MTCC 398	48.0 kb	Ap^r, Km^r	800	512	20 ± 1.4
P. aeruginosa (RIP64) MTCC 1262	95 Mdal	Gm^r, Cm^r	512	256	ND
S. Typhi (R136) MTCC 1264	59 kb	Tc^r	800	512	4.2 ± 0.3
B. subtilis (pUB110) MTCC 1558	4.5 kb	Km^r, Nm^r	800	512	ND
A. baumannii A23 (pUPI280) (present study)	—	Ap^r, Gm^r, Km^r, Cm^r, Am^r	1024	800	ND
A. baumannii A24 (pUPI281) (present study)	—	St^r, Ap^r, Gm^r, Ak^r	800	512	13.5 ± 1.4
A. baumannii A26 (pUPI282) (present study)	—	St^r, Ap^r, Gm^r, Ak^r, Lf^r	512	256	8.5 ± 0.7

MIC, minimum inhibitory concentration; SIC, sub inhibitory concentration. ND, none of the 300 colonies tested showed curing of plasmid. [@]*Am, amoxicillin; Ak, amikacin; Ap, ampicillin; Cm, chloramphenicol; Gm, gentamicin; Km, kanamycin; Lf, lomefloxacin; Nm, neomycin; St, streptomycin; Tc, tetracycline;* ***MTCC (Reference cultures),*** *Microbial Type Culture Collection, Chandigarh, India.*

of curing agent was calculated to evaluate effect of lawsone on transfer of plasmid by conjugation.

Synergistic Action of Lawsone With the Antibiotic: Combination Studies

Synergism between lawsone and antibiotics such as streptomycin and kanamycin was tested against *A. baumannii* (pUPI281) and *E. coli* (pRK2013), respectively. Concentration of lawsone as well as the antibiotic tested was in the range 0–1,000 μg/ml. Actively growing culture was inoculated (10^4 cells/ml) in Luria broth supplemented with varying concentrations of lawsone and streptomycin or kanamycin and incubated at 37°C for 18 h. Culture growth was monitored on spectrophotometer at 600 nm. Interactions of curing agents with antibiotics were assessed by a modified Chequerboard agar dilution method (Charles et al., 1997). Synergistic or otherwise effect of curing agent and antibiotic in combination was evaluated by determining the fractional inhibitory concentration index (minimum FIC index). The FIC was calculated for each combination using the following formula: **FIC A + FIC B = FICI** Where, FICA = MIC of drug A in combination/MIC of drug A alone, and FICB = MIC of drug B in combination/MIC of drug B alone. The FICI was interpreted as follows: synergy = FICI < 0.5; no interaction = FICI > 0.5–4; antagonism = FICI > 4 (Dorsthorst et al., 2002).

Toxicity Testing of Lawsone

Actively growing BHK 21 (baby hamster kidney fibroblast cell line) and AV3 (human amniotic epithelial cell line) cells were obtained from the NCCS repository (Pune, India). These cells were subcultured using TPVG solution (2% trypsin, 0.1% EDTA, and 0.1% glucose in PBS) and seeded on to a 6-well tissue culture plate (Falcon, BD Biosciences, United States) at the concentration of 3×10^5 cells per well with Eagle's minimal essential medium (EMEM) supplemented with 10% fetal calf serum (FCS). Plates were incubated for 24 h for the monolayer formation. The monolayers of both, BHK 21 and AV3 were then exposed to different concentrations of lawsone. Plates were observed under inverted microscope (Olympus IX70) for the cell morphology and floating cell population after 24 h of incubation at 37°C in 5% CO_2 environment. Control cells were grown in absence of lawsone.

MTT Assay for Examination of the Viability of Cells

BHK21 and AV3 cells were seeded in a 96-well tissue culture plate (Falcon, BD Biosciences, United States) and incubated overnight. The cells were then exposed to varying concentrations of lawsone for 24 h. Control cells were not exposed to the lawsone treatment. MTT assay was performed to determine the toxicity of the plasmid curing agent to the cells upon exposure (Bahuguna et al., 2017) In this assay yellow colored 3-(4,5-dimethylazol-2-yl)-2,5-diphenyl-tetrazolium bromide (MTT) is enzymatically converted into purple formazan in the exposed cells. The intensity of purple formazan was measured at 570 nm. using Spectra Max 250 UV-vis microplate reader (Molecular Devices, Sunnyvale, CA, United States). Experiment was performed in duplicate and the average for all wells was shown as cell-viability percentage related to unexposed control cells.

RESULTS

Purification and Identification of Plasmid Curing Agent From *P. zeylanica* Roots

Crude ethanol extract of roots of *P. zeylanica* demonstrated significant antimicrobial as well as plasmid curing activity (Patwardhan, 2007). An active principle responsible for the plasmid curing activity of the ethanol extract of *P. zeylanica* was purified by bioassay guided fractionation. Molecular formula of the purified compound, isolated as yellow crystals, (melting point, 192°C) was established as $C_{10}H_6O_3$ (**Figure 1**) based on GCMS spectral data (molecular ion peak at *m/z* = 174). Further structural characterization was made by UV, FTIR, ^1H NMR and ^{13}C NMR spectroscopic methods. UV λ_{max} at 273 nm for the same compound clearly indicated conjugation in the compound. In the IR spectra, the peak observed at 1,587 cm^{-1} suggested the presence of C=C. The peak at 1,641 cm^{-1} indicated the presence of α, β-unsaturated carbonyl group. The broad band at 3,056–3,350 cm^{-1} was suggestive of hydroxyl group.

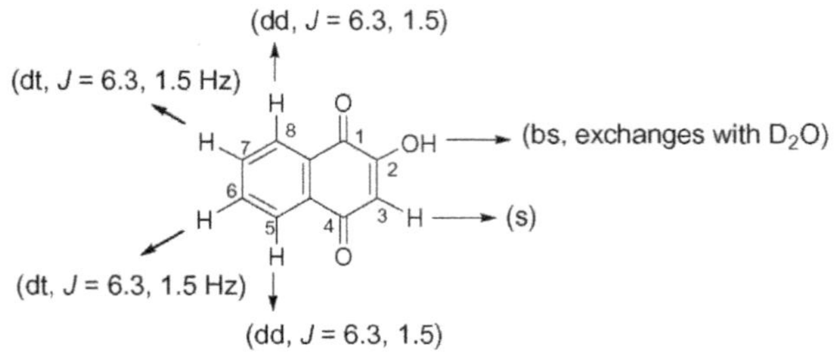

FIGURE 1 | Chemical structure of lawsone demonstrating antimicrobial and plasmid curing activity.

In the ^{1}H-NMR spectrum, the singlet at 6.36 δ was assigned to H-3. The broad singlet 7.33 was due to hydroxyl group which was found to be exchangeable with D_2O. The signal at δ 7.71 appeared as doublet of triplet with J = 6.3 and 1.5 Hz was assigned to either H6 or H7. Similarly, appearance of doublet of triplet at δ 7.79 with J = 6.3 and 1.5 Hz was assigned to either H6 or H7. The signal at δ 8.11, corresponding to two protons, appeared as doublet of doublet with J = 6.3 and 1.5 Hz was assigned to H5 and H8. The compound was identified as lawsone based on spectral data (**Figure 1** and **Table 3**). This data was found to be in good agreement with the spectral and analytical data of lawsone (Sigma, United States) thus confirming our assignment. To the best of our knowledge, this is the first report of lawsone extracted from roots of *Plumbago zeylanica*.

Curing of Antibiotic Resistance by Lawsone

Lawsone inhibited the growth of *A. baumannii, P. aeruginosa, S.* Typhi and *E. coli,* in disk diffusion assay (200–800 μg/disk) (**Table 1**). Plasmid curing activity of lawsone against R-plasmids harbored in reference as well as clinical isolates is illustrated in **Table 2** and **Supplementary Figures S1, S2**. Lawsone cured plasmids pBR322 and pRK2013 at 11% and 20% efficiencies, respectively. Lawsone also cured plasmid R136 in *S.* Typhi at 4.2% curing efficiency. However, it was not able to cure plasmid RP4 in *E. coli.* Lawsone eliminated plasmids pUPI281 and pUPI282

TABLE 3 | ^{1}H NMR and ^{13}C NMR data of lawsone.

Position	^{1}H NMR (δ)	Position	^{13}C NMR (δ)
H-3	6.19 (S)	C-1	184.9
H-5	8.19 (dd, J = 6.3 and 1.4 Hz)	C-2	156.3
H-6	7.72 (dt, J = 6.3 and 1.4 Hz)	C-3	110.7
H-7	7.81 (dt, J = 6.3 and 1.4 Hz)	C-4	181.9
H-8	8.19 (dd, J = 6.3 and 1.4 Hz)	C-4a	132.9
		C-5	133.13
		C-6	126.7
		C-7	126.4
		C-8	135.3
		C-8a	129.4

in *A. baumannii* with 8.5% and 13.5% efficiency, respectively. Curing efficiencies of lawsone observed against plasmids in reference strains as well as clinical isolates of *A. baumannii* were comparable to those observed for conventional curing agents such as DNA-intercalating dyes, acridine orange and ethidium bromide (**Table 4**). Plasmid curing efficiency of lawsone was determined against plasmid pBR322, pRK2013, and pUPI281 at different cell densities of host harboring these plasmids. It was observed that curing efficiencies were higher at lower cell densities (10^4 cells/ml) than at higher cell densities (10^5 cells/ml or 10^6 cells/ml) (**Table 5**). Similarly, increasing concentrations of lawsone (64–512 μg/ml) resulted in higher curing efficiencies when initial inoculum density was maintained constant (**Table 6**). Lawsone could not cure either pUPI281 or pRK2013 at 64 μg/ml or lower concentrations. Plasmid curing activity of lawsone was studied at different pH ranging from 6.0 to 8.0 with plasmids pRK2013 and pUPI281. It was observed that lawsone cured pRK2013 and pUPI281 with curing efficiency of 27% and 17%, respectively at pH 6.0 and 8.0. There exists a possibility of reversal of antibiotic resistance if and when a bacterial culture is grown in absence of antibiotics. Hence, in the present study bacterial culture was grown in absence of antibiotics as well as plasmid curing agent (solvent control). Such culture was plated to obtain isolated colonies in absence of antibiotics. The isolated colonies were replicated on agar media with or without antibiotic to determine the frequency of spontaneous loss of plasmid or reversal of antibiotic resistance. None of the 100 colonies tested were spontaneously cured derivative of plasmid bearing host. However, in this technique only 100 colonies were tested by replica plating. Hence, in another modification, cultures were grown in absence of antibiotics or plasmid curing agents for several generations and then plated on agar media with and without antibiotics. The frequency of spontaneous reversal of antibiotic resistance was found to be less than one in 10^8. This observation was consistent with earlier observation (Inoue, 1997). In comparison, curing efficiencies reported in this study were extremely high (>10^4 times). Both these observations (reversal of antibiotic resistance or plasmid curing observed only upon exposure to plasmid curing agents and not spontaneously) clearly indicated that reversal of antibiotic resistance as a consequence of plasmid curing was not a spontaneous phenomenon but was caused by the exposure of plasmid harboring strains to plasmid curing agent, i.e., lawsone in the present study. In the present investigation, loss of plasmid in the cured derivatives was confirmed by agarose gel electrophoresis analysis (**Figure 2**). Loss of plasmid and not mutation was thus, confirmed as a cause of reversal of antibiotic resistance in the cured derivative. It may be noted here that even mutation could have caused reversal of antibiotic resistance. However, mutagenic activity of the plasmid curing agents is undesired for potential clinical application. Lawsone was able to cure plasmid and inhibit the transfer of plasmid by conjugation as well as by transformation which is significant in containing the spread of antibiotic resistance. Controls did not show loss of plasmids at various pH values, indicating that pH alone did not have any effect on the plasmid curing.

TABLE 4 | Curing of R plasmids with conventional curing agents.

Plasmid	Antibiotic resistance markers	Purified lawsone		Ethidium bromide		Acridine orange	
		Conc. (μg/ml)	Curing efficiency (%)	Conc. (μg/ml)	Curing efficiency (%)	Conc. (μg/ml)	Curing efficiency (%)
RP4	Ap^r, Km^r, Tc^r	256	_	128	13 ± 1.4	64	ND
pBR 322	Ap^r, Tc^r	512	11 ± 1.4	128	21.5 ± 2.1	128	12.5 ± 2.1
pRK 2013	Ap^r, Km^r	512	20 ± 1.4	256	59.5 ± 3.5	128	ND
RIP64	Gm^r, Cm^r	256	_	128	16	256	ND
R136	Tc^r	512	4.2 ± 0.3	256	13.5 ± 0.7	256	ND
pUP110	Km^r, Nm^r	512	_	256	_	128	ND
pUPI 280	Ap^r, Gm^r, Km^r, Cm^r, Am^r	800	_	512	18 ± 2.8	512	6.5 ± 0.7
pUPI 281	St^r, Ap^r, Gm^r, Ak^r	512	13.5 ± 1.4	256	15 ± 1.4	256	17.25 ± 1.06
pUPI 282	St^r, Ap^r, Gm^r, Ak^r, [illegible]f^r	256	8.5 ± 0.7	256	10.25 ± 1.0	256	_

Three hundred clones were tested for each plasmid in the curing experiments. ND, none of the 300 colonies tested showed curing of plasmid.

TABLE 5 | Effect of cell density on plasmid curing efficiency of lawsone.

Plasmid	Curing efficiency (%) at			
	10^4 (cells/ml)	10^5 (cells/ml)	10^6 (cells/ml)	10^7 (cells/ml)
E. coli (pBR 322)	31.3 ± 1.8	16.5 ± 2.1	2 ± 0	ND
E. coli (pRK 2013)	20 ± 1.4	9.3 ± 2.5	4.5 ± 0.7	9 ± 0
A. baumannii (pUPI 281)	12.5 ± 2.1	15.5 ± 2.1	15 ± 0	5.8 ± 1.0

Above desired number of cells were incubated in Luria broth in the presence of 512 μg of lawsone/ml at 37°C for 24 h. Number of clones tested – 300. ND, none of the 300 colonies tested showed curing of plasmid.

Effect of Lawsone on Plasmid Transfer by Conjugation and Transformation

Effect of lawsone on plasmid transfer by conjugation or transformation was investigated with plasmid pRK2013. More than 90% decrease in the frequency of plasmid transfer was observed when conjugation was performed in the presence of lawsone (12.5 μg/ml) by membrane mating method. Plasmid pRK2013 was transferred from *A. baumannii* to *E. coli* with conjugation frequencies of 2.1×10^{-5} and 2×10^{-4} in the presence and absence of lawsone, respectively (**Table 7**). The similar inhibition was observed when the conjugation was performed by broth mating (8.8×10^{-6} and below detection limit). Similarly, lawsone inhibited transfer of plasmid by transformation. Frequency of transformation of *E. coli* HB101 with pRK2013 was observed to be 1.1×10^4 transformants/μg plasmid DNA. However, 63% decrease in the transformation efficiency was observed in the presence of lawsone.

TABLE 6 | Effect of concentration of lawsone on curing efficiency.

Plasmid	Curing efficiency (%) at			
	64 (μg/ml)	128 (μg/ml)	256 (μg/ml)	512 (μg/ml)
E. coli (pBR 322)	ND	ND	13 ± 1.4	31.74 ± 1.06
E. coli (pRK 2013)	ND	ND	20 ± 1.4	22 ± 1.4
A. baumannii (pUPI 281)	ND	7.5 ± 2.1	18 ± 1.4	14.3 ± 0.4

Number of clones tested – 300. 10^4 cells/ml were incubated in the presence of above described concentrations of lawsone at 37°C for 24 h. ND, none of the 300 colonies tested showed curing of plasmid.

TABLE 7 | Effect of lawsone on R plasmid transfer from ampicillin resistant *E. coli* to streptomycin resistant *E. coli* by conjugation.

Conjugation	Frequency of conjugation	
	In absence of curing agent	In presence of curing agent
With membrane filter	2×10^{-4}	2.1×10^{-5}
Without membrane filter	8.8×10^{-6}	Below the detection limit

10^8 cells of donor E. coli (pRK2013) and recipient E. coli (HB101) were mixed and incubated in absence or presence of 12.5 μg of lawsone/ml at 37°C for 24 h. The growth was serially diluted and plated out to score number of transconjugants formed. The data represents average values of two parallel experiments.

Synergistic Action of Lawsone With the Antibiotic: Combination Studies

Synergy between lawsone and antibiotics was investigated against *A. baumannii* (pUPI281) and *E. coli* (pRK2013). The MICs were determined for the curing agent alone and in combination with the different antibiotics by checkerboard assay method. *A. baumannii* (pUPI281) and *E. coli* (pRK2013) were resistant to streptomycin and kanamycin, respectively

(MIC > 1,000 μg/ml). Growth of *A. baumannii* (pUPI281) was inhibited when lawsone and streptomycin were added together at 250 μg/ml concentrations each. Similarly, growth of *E. coli* (pRK2013) was inhibited when lawsone and kanamycin were added together at 100 μg/ml and 250 μg/ml concentrations, respectively. The Fractional Inhibition Concentration (FIC) indices were calculated (**Table 8**). These results clearly indicated that FICI was synergistic (<0.5) for lawsone in combination with antibiotic when used against *A. baumannii*. Additive action of lawsone with antibiotic was observed against *E. coli*. These results suggested that the plasmid curing activity of naphthoquinone directly or indirectly rendered the clinical isolates susceptible to the inhibitory action of antibiotics at significantly lower concentration, and hence, were considered encouraging.

Toxicity Testing and Viability Assay (MTT) of Lawsone

Toxicity testing of lawsone revealed that BHK 21 cells which are fibroblastic in nature are more affected with lawsone than AV3 cells which are epithelial indicating its selective toxicity to fibroblast only. In MTT assay BHK 21 cells showed more drop in % viability with increased concentration of lawsone compared to AV3 Cells (**Table 9** and **Figure 3**).

DISCUSSION

The bioassay guided fractionation of the organic extracts of *P. zeylanica* roots resulted in identification of lawsone as an active principle exhibiting the plasmid curing activity. Lawsone has been reported to be a major constituent of *Lawsonia inermis*. However, to the best of our knowledge, this is the first report of lawsone extracted from roots of *Plumbago zeylanica*. Antimicrobial properties of lawsone have been documented in the literature (Ahmed and Beg, 2001).

Treatment of chronic infections caused by multidrug resistant bacteria is a serious challenge for the physicians. In most of the cases the resistance to multiple antibiotics is mediated by the plasmids. Curing of plasmid-mediated antibiotic resistance in pathogenic strains of bacteria is of great practical importance both in treatment of bacterial infection and in microbial genetics. In the present investigation, curing of plasmids effected by lawsone was confirmed on the basis of reversal of antibiotic resistance phenotype evident from the significant reduction in the MIC of antibiotics; as well as elimination of plasmids in the cured derivatives. Agarose gel electrophoresis revealed presence of plasmid DNA in wild host. However, gel electrophoresis of DNA from cured derivatives revealed loss of the corresponding plasmid band confirming plasmid curing. Plasmid curing was not observed in host exposed to DMSO, a solvent control used for lawsone. Spontaneous loss of plasmid DNA has been reported at low frequency of less than 1 in 10^9 cells· (Inoue, 1997). In comparison curing efficiencies observed in the present study were significantly higher ($>10^4$ times), thus attributing reversal of antibiotic resistance to the exposure of cells to the curing agent (lawsone). Cured strains were tested for the loss of plasmids by agarose gel electrophoresis to confirm that reversal of antibiotic resistance was due to elimination of plasmid carrying genes encoding resistance to antibiotics and not due to mutations. Physical loss of plasmid as evidenced by agarose gel electrophoresis of plasmid DNA preparation of cured strains (**Figure 2**) indicated that genes encoding antibiotic resistance

TABLE 8 | FIC index of individual curing agents and in combination with antibiotics.

Test organism	FIC_c*	FIC_a@	FIC_i#	Interpretation
A. baumannii	0.25	0.133	0.383	Synergistic
E. coli	0.4	0.25	0.65	Additive

**Fractional Inhibition Concentration of curing agent (lawsone).* @*Fractional Inhibition Concentration of antibiotics.* #*Fractional Inhibition Concentration index.*

TABLE 9 | Toxicity testing with MTT assay.

Conc. (μg/ml)	Cell line used			
	BHK 21		AV3	
	Average absorbance	% Viable cells	Average absorbance	% Viable cells
100	0.7715	84.8268	1.1035	98.55
200	0.6625	72.8422	1.1395	97.27
300	0.6650	73.1170	1.064	90.82
400	0.5995	65.9153	0.99	84.50
500	0.6275	68.9939	0.897	76.57
Control blank	0.9095	100	1.1715	100

BHK 21, baby hamster kidney fibroblast cells; AV3, human amnionic epithelial cells. Formula used: % viable cells = (average of test OD/average of control OD) × 100.

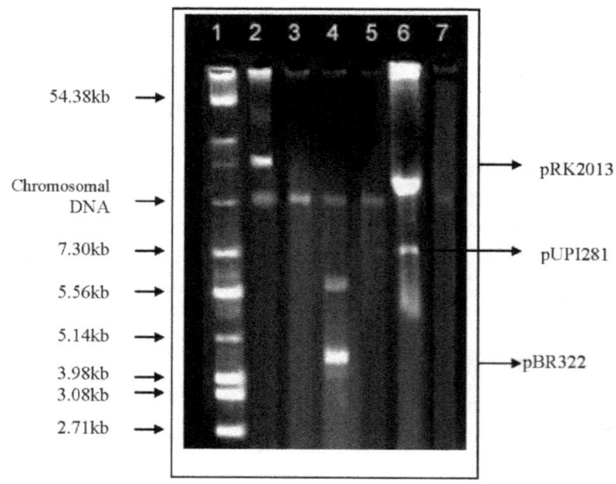

FIGURE 2 | Agarose gel electrophoresis of plasmid DNA in standard strains as well as clinical isolates harboring R-plasmids and their cured derivatives. Lane 1, Reference plasmids from *E. coli* MTCC 131; Lane 2, *E. coli* MTCC398 (pRK2013); Lane 3, Cured derivative of *E. coli* MTCC398; Lane 4, *E. coli* K12 (pBR322); Lane 5, Cured derivative of *E. coli* K12; Lane 6, *Ac. baumannii* A24 (pUPI281); Lane 7, Cured derivative of *Ac. baumannii* A24.

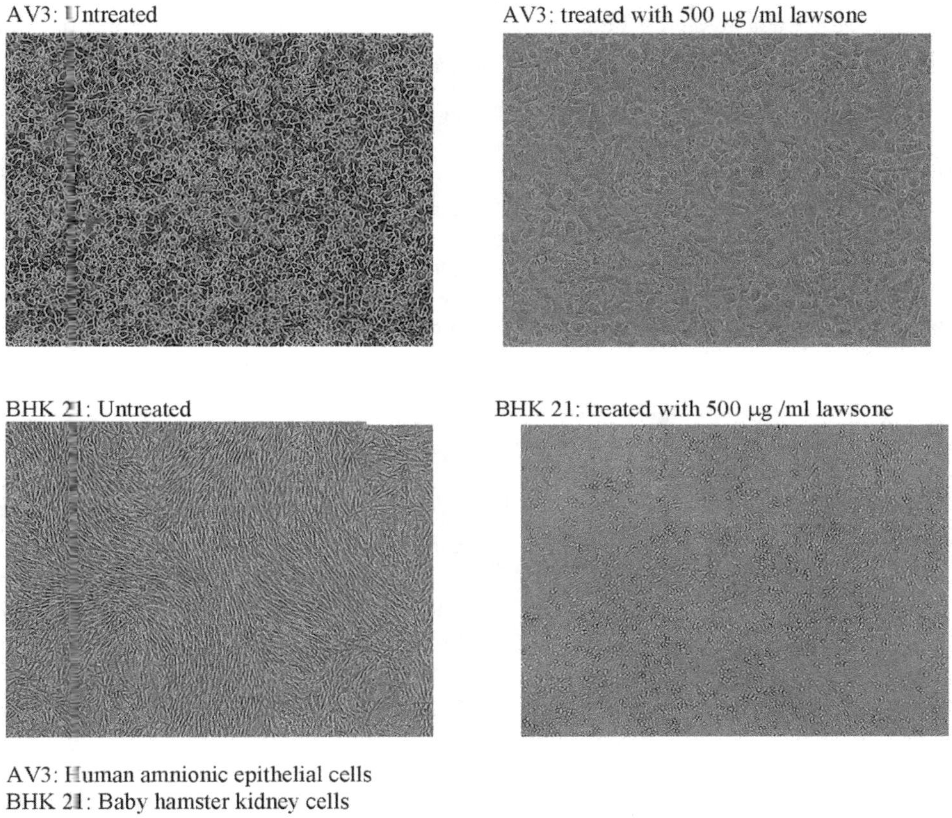

FIGURE 3 | Toxicity testing of lawsone on AV3 and BHK 21 cell lines. AV3, human amnionic epithelial cells; BHK 21, baby hamster kidney cells.

were located on plasmid and that plasmid loss resulted in subsequent loss of antibiotic resistance.

Ability of lawsone to cure plasmid encoded antibiotic resistance in *Acinetobacter* strains is particularly significant since *Acinetobacter* strains are known to act as a reservoir of natural or acquired antibiotic resistance genes in the nosocomial environment facilitating in the spread of antibiotic resistance genes to more pathogenic bacteria (Towner, 1997; Deshpande et al., 2001; Cisneros and Rodriguez-Bano, 2005). Bacteria have tendency to develop resistance against any antimicrobial agent used against them. Concentrations of curing agents used in the plasmid curing experiments were significantly lower than inhibitory concentrations. Hence, it is proposed that chances of bacteria developing any mechanism to inactivate plasmid curing agents or their activity are extremely low. It must be remembered here that plasmids are after all dispensable elements in a bacterial cell.

Plasmids are the extrachromosomal elements that are responsible for development and spread of antibiotic resistance in bacteria. Their role assumes even more significance in the nosocomial environment as plasmid encoded resistance to multiple antibiotics can be transferred from one host to another by inter species transfer modes such as conjugation and/or transformation. Such acquired resistance can make otherwise sensitive pathogens resistant to multiple antibiotics. Thus, making the treatment of infections more difficult and in some cases almost impossible. Ability of lawsone to interfere with interspecies plasmid transfer by conjugation and transformation and thus contain the spread of multi-resistance to antibiotics was investigated in the present study. It was observed that Lawsone not only cured plasmids but also inhibited the transfer of plasmid by both conjugation as well as by transformation. Membrane filter mating technique and broth mating are the two different techniques used to investigate plasmid transfer by conjugation in bacteria. Lawsone was able to inhibit the plasmid transfer by conjugation in both techniques. *Acinetobacter* has been reported as a reservoir of antibiotic resistance genes in nosocomial environment and is frequently reported to be involved in the transfer of multi-resistance to antibiotics. *E. coli* has been the most extensively investigated organism for the inter species gene transfer. Hence, in the present study both organisms were included to investigate the effect of lawsone on inter species plasmid transfer. Ability of lawsone to inhibit plasmid transfer among these organisms may thus assume special significance in nosocomial environment. Ability of lawsone to inhibit plasmid transfer by transformation or conjugation was reported for the first time in the present investigation.

FIC clearly indicated that combination of curing agent and antibiotic was synergistic against *A. baumannii* and additive against *E. coli*. This observation was considered encouraging as it suggested that the plasmid curing activity of naphthoquinone rendered the clinical isolates susceptible to the inhibitory action of antibiotics at significantly lower concentration. Efficacy of extended antibiotic therapy in several microbial infections may be improved with the combination of plasmid curing agent lawsone, as a synergistic drug. Such synergistic combination of antibiotic and lawsone, may serve as a prospective device in selection of appropriate drug therapy that is likely to contribute to the ongoing crusade against microbial drug-resistance.

Plant derived compounds have been previously reported as plasmid curing agents. Such compounds included 8-epidiosbulbin E acetate isolated from the bulbs of *Dioscorea bulbifera* (Shriram et al., 2008); 1'-acetoxychavicol acetate from *Alpinia galanga* (L.) Swartz, (Latha et al., 2009); Plumbagin (5-hydroxy-2-methyl-1,4- naphthoquinone) derived from the root of the tropical/subtropical Plumbago species (Patwardhan et al., 2015), etc. These plasmids curing agents have been proven to be effective at curing plasmids *in vitro*. Unsaturated fatty acids have been shown to be effective conjugation inhibitors in laboratory studies on a variety of plasmids (Lopatkin et al., 2017). Furthermore, they are associated with reduced toxicity on tissue culture cells. Lawsone, a plant derived compound reported in the present investigation has shown dual ability to cure plasmid and also inhibit interspecies plasmid transfer. However, more research is needed to confirm *in vivo* efficacy and to determine potential toxicity of these compounds if administered *in vivo*.

Sauriasari et al. (2007) reported that lawsone was not mutagenic to bacterial strains. However dose dependent cytotoxicity of lawsone was reported in the same study. Cytotoxicity of lawsone was reported to be significantly lower than that of other naphthoquinone derivatives including cisplatin, a widely used anticancer drug (Oliveira et al., 2017). Cytotoxicity of naphthoquinones such as lawsone could be attributed to generation of reactive oxygen species, disruption of mitochondrial functions, inhibition of thymidine incorporation into DNA and DNA intercalation (Aithal et al., 2009; Bonifazi et al., 2010; Klaus et al., 2010; Babula et al., 2012). A series of tests in the published literature have identified lawsone as non-genotoxic agent. Such tests included Ames test, V79 hprt test, Syrian hamster embryo cell transformation assay, bone marrow micronucleus tests in CD1 mice, and bone marrow chromosome aberration test in mice and hamsters (Kirkland and Marzin, 2003). An additional genetic toxicity program performed to clarify *in vivo* genotoxic potential of lawsone revealed that lawsone was devoid of clastogenic potential *in vivo* (Marzin and Kirkland, 2004). Thus, the review of literature illustrating evaluation of genotoxicity of lawsone in a series of *in vivo* and *in vitro* tests has revealed that lawsone is not genotoxic when administered orally up to a dose of 300 mg/kg body weight. Ability of lawsone to intercalate with double stranded DNA has been reported in the published literature (Kirkland and Marzin, 2003). Also, the ability of lawsone to alter the cell membrane by generating free radicle stress has been reported earlier (Sauriasari et al., 2007

). However, the plasmid curing activity reported in the present study was observed at concentration significantly lower than the inhibitory concentrations. Elucidation of exact mechanism by which lawsone effected plasmid curing in bacterial scale is not known at present and requires further extensive investigation.

Thus, in conclusion, this investigation has revealed a compound with an ability to eliminate antibiotic resistance and cure plasmids from pathogenic strains that are resistant to multiple antibiotics without any ill effect on mammalian cells at lower concentrations. The results obtained provide endorsement for investigating the potential value of lawsone in combating clinical drug resistance. The synergistic effect of lawsone with the antibiotic exhibits its tremendous potential in modern day therapeutics. The non-toxic, non-mutagenic, plasmid curing and plasmid transfer inhibiting role of lawsone demands further investigation to make it a potential drug of choice in the treatment of antibiotic resistant bacterial strains; thus, demonstrating a new dimension in antibiotic therapy.

AUTHOR CONTRIBUTIONS

RP, PD, and BC designed and executed the experiments. RP performed the experiments. RP, PD, BC, DD, and RB interpreted the results and analyzed the data. RP, PD, DD, and RB contributed to the writing of the manuscript. RP and PD revised the manuscript.

ACKNOWLEDGMENTS

RP is grateful to University Grants Commission (Teacher Fellowship for the period of two years under FIP according to Xth Plan by UGC; letter No. 34-8/2003 (WRO) dated 25th February, 2004) as well as Principal, Haribhai V. Desai College for teacher fellowship.

REFERENCES

Ahmad, I., Mehmood, Z., Mohammad, F., and Ahmad, S. (2000). Antimicrobial potency and synergistic activity of five traditionally used indian medicinal plants. *J. Med. Arom. Plant Sci.* 2223, 173–176.

Ahmed, I., and Beg, A. Z. (2001). Antimicrobial and phytochemical studies on 45 indian medicinal plants against multidrug resistant human pathogens. *J. Ethnopharmacol.* 74, 113–123. doi: 10.1016/S0378-8741(00)00335-4

Aithal, B. K., Kumar, M. R. S., Rao, B. N., Udupa, N., and Rao, B. S. S. (2009). Juglone, a naphthoquinone from walnut, exerts cytotoxic and genotoxic effects against cultured melanoma tumor cells. *Cell Biol. Int.* 33, 1039–1049. doi: 10.1016/j.cellbi.2009.06.018

Babula, P., Vanco, J., Krejcova, L., Hynek, D., Sochor, J., Adam, V., et al. (2012). Voltammetric characterization of lawsone-copper (II) ternary complexes and their interactions with dsDNA. *Int. J. Electrochem. Sci.* 7, 7349–7366.

Bahuguna, A., Khan, I., Bajpai, V. K., and Kang, S. C. (2017). MTT assay to evaluate the cytotoxic potential of a drug. *Bangladesh J. Pharmacol.* 12, 115–118. doi: 10.3329/bjp.v12i2.30892

Bauer, A. W., Kirby, M. M., Sherris, J. C., and Turck, M. (1966). Antibiotic susceptibility testing by a standardized single disk method. *Am. J. Clin. Pathol.* 36, 493–496. doi: 10.1093/ajcp/45.4_ts.493

Bonifazi, E. L., Rios-Luci, C., Leon, L. G., Burton, G., Padron, J. M., and Misico, R. I. (2010). Antiproliferative activity of synthetic naphthoquinones related to lapachol. First synthesis of 5-hydroxylapachol. *Bioorg. Med. Chem.* 18, 2621–2630. doi: 10.1016/j.bmc.2010.02.032

Bouanchaud, D. D., Scavizzi, M. R., and Chabbert, Y. A. (1969). Elimination by ethidium bromide of antibiotic resistance in enterobacteria and staphylococci. *J. Gen. Microbiol.* 54, 417–425. doi: 10.1099/00221287-54-3-417

Charles, E., Smith, B. E., Foleno, J. F., and Barrett- Frosco, M. B. (1997). Assessment of the synergistic interactions of levofloxacin and ampicillin against *Enterococcus faecium* by the checkerboard agar dilution and time-kill methods. *Diagn. Microbiol. Infect. Dis.* 27, 85–92. doi: 10.1016/S0732-8893(96)00222-2

Chopade, B. A., Patwardhan, R. B., Vaidya, V. C., Khairnar, S., Dhakephalkar, P. K., and Padhye, S. B. (1994). "Curing of antibiotic and metal resistance plasmids in *Acinetobacter baumannii*," in *Tropical Diseases: Molecular Biology and Control Strategies*, eds A. K. Sushil Kumar, G. P. Sen, and R. N. Sharma (New Delhi: CSIR Publications & Information Directorate), 695–703.

Chopra, R. N., Nayer, S. L., and Chopra, I. C. (1992). *In Glossary of Indian Medicinal Plants*, 3rd Edn. New Delhi: Council of Scientific and Industrial Research, 237–246.

Choudhary, M. I., and Atta-ur-Rahman. (1997). "Bioactivity guided isolation of phytochemicals from medicinal plants," in *Photochemical Diversity. A Source of New Industrial Products*, eds S. Wrigley, M. Hayes, R. Thomas, and E. Chrystal (Cambridge: Royal Soc. Chem), 41–52.

Cisneros, J. M., and Rodriguez-Bano, J. (2005). Risk-factors for the acquisition of imipenem-resistant *Acinetobacter baumannii* in spain: a nationwide study. *Clin. Microbiol. Infect.* 11, 874–879. doi: 10.1111/j.1469-0691.2005.01256.x

Daniel, M. (1991). *Methods in Plant Chemistry and Economic Botany*. New Delhi: Kalyani Publishers, 1–4.

Deshpande, N. M., Dhakephalkar, P. K., and Kanekar, P. P. (2001). Plasmid mediated dimethoate degradation in *Pseudomonas aeruginosa* MCMB-427. *Lett. Appl. Microbiol.* 33, 275–279. doi: 10.1046/j.1472-765X.2001.00995.x

Dhakephalkar, P. K., and Chopade, B. A. (1994). High levels of multiple metal resistance and its correlation to antibiotic resistance in environmental isolates of acinetobacter. *Biometals* 7, 67–74. doi: 10.1007/BF00205197

Dorsthorst, T. E., Verweij, D. T., Meis, P. E., Punt, J. F., and Mouton, J. W. (2002). Comparison of fractional inhibitory concentration index with response surface modeling for characterization of in vitro interaction of antifungals against itraconazole-susceptible and resistant *Aspergillus fumigatus* isolates. *Antimicrob. Agents Chemother.* 46, 702–707. doi: 10.1128/AAC.46.3.702-707.2002

Inoue, Y. (1997). Spontaneous loss of antibiotic-resistant plasmids transferred to *Escherichia coli* in experimental chronic bladder infection. *Int. J. Urol.* 4, 285–288. doi: 10.1111/j.1442-2042.1997.tb00191.x

Kirkland, D., and Marzin, D. (2003). An assessment of the genotoxicity of 2-hydroxy-1,4-naphthoquinone, the natural dye ingredient of henna. *Mutat. Res.* 537, 183–199. doi: 10.1016/S1383-5718(03)00077-9

Klaus, V., Hartmann, T., Gambini, J., Graf, P., Stahl, W., Hartwig, A., et al. (2010). 1,4-naphthoquinones as inducers of oxidative damage and stress signaling in HaCaT human keratinocytes. *Arch. Biochem. Biophys.* 496, 93–100. doi: 10.1016/j.abb.2010.02.002

Kloos, W. E., and Schleifer, K. H. (1986). "Genus IV *Staphylococcus*," in *Bergey's Manual of Systematic Bacteriology*, eds P. H. A. Sneath, N. S. Mair, M. E. Sharpe, and J. G. Holt (Baltimore, MD: Williams and Wilkins, Rosenbach), 1013–1035.

Latha, C., Shriram, V. D., Jahagirdar, S. S., Dhakephalkar, P. K., and Rojatkar, S. R. (2009). Antiplasmid activity of 1'-acetoxychavicol acetate from *Alpinia galanga* against multi-drug resistant bacteria. *J. Ethnopharmacol.* 123, 522–525. doi: 10.1016/j.jep.2009.03.028

Lopatkin, A. J., Meredith, H. R., Srimani, J. K., Pfeiffer, C., Durrett, R., and You, L. (2017). Persistence and reversal of plasmid-mediated antibiotic resistance. *Nat. Commun.* 8:1689. doi: 10.1038/s41467-017-01532-1

Marzin, D., and Kirkland, D. (2004). 2-hydroxy-1,4-naphthoquinone, the natural dye of henna, is non-genotoxic in the mouse bone marrow micronucleus test and does not produce oxidative DNA damage in chinese hamster varies cells. *Mutat. Res.* 560, 41–47. doi: 10.1016/j.mrgentox.2004.02.004

Michelle, M. C. B., Maria, L. C., and Laura, J. V. P. (2018). Strategies to combat antimicrobial resistance: anti-plasmid and plasmid curing. *FEMS Microbiol. Rev.* doi: 10.1093/femsre/fuy031 [Epub ahead of print]. doi: 10.1093/femsre/fuy031

Molnar, J. (1988). Antiplasmid activity of tricyclic compounds. Methods and findings. *Exp. Clin. Pharmacol.* 10, 467–474.

Oliveira, K. M., Liany, L. D., Corrêa, R. S., Deflon, V. M., Cominetti, M. R., and Batista, A. A. (2017). Selective Ru (II)/lawsone complexes inhibiting tumor cell growth by apoptosis. *J. Inorg. Biochem.* 176, 66–76. doi: 10.1016/j.jinorgbio.2017.08.019

Opal, S. M., Mayer, K. H., and Medecros, A. A. (2000). "Mechanisms of bacterial resistance," in *Principles and Practice of Infectious Diseases*, 5th Edn, Vol. 2, ed. R. Dolin (New York, NY, Churchill Livingstone), 236–253.

Patwardhan, R. B. (2007). *Herbal Naphthoquinones as Antimicrobial and Plasmid Curing Agents*. Ph.D. thesis, University of Pune, Pune.

Patwardhan, R. B., Shinde, P. S., Chavan, K. R., and Devale, A. (2015). Reversal of plasmid encoded antibiotic resistance from nosocomial pathogens by using plumbago auriculata root extracts. *Int. J. Curr. Microbiol. App. Sci.* 187–198.

Sadasivam, S., and Manickam, A. (1992). *Biochemical Methods for Agricultural Science*. New Delhi: Wiley Eastern Ltd.

Sambrook, J., Fritsch, E. F., and Maniatis, T. (1989). *Plasmid Vectors. In Molecular Cloning: A Laboratory Manual*, 2nd Edn. Cold Spring Harbour, NY: CSH Press.

Samy, R. P., and Ignacimuthu, S. (2000). Antibacterial activity of some folklore medicinal plants used by tribals in Western Ghats of India. *J. Ethnopharmacol.* 69, 63–71. doi: 10.1016/S0378-8741(98)00156-1

Saunders, J. R. (1981). Plasmids and bacterial pathogens. *Nature* 290:362. doi: 10.1038/290362a0

Sauriasari, R., Wang, D. H., Takemura, Y., Tsutsui, K., Masuoka, N., Sano, K., et al. (2007). Cytotoxicity of lawsone and cytoprotective activity of antioxidants in catalase mutant *Escherichia coli*. *Toxicology* 235, 103–111. doi: 10.1016/j.tox.2007.03.019

Shriram, V., Jahagirdar, S., Latha, C., Kumar, V., Puranik, V., Rojatkar, S., et al. (2008). A potential plasmid curing agent, 8- pidiosbulbin E acetate, from *Dioscorea bulbifera* L. against multidrug-resistant bacteria. *Int. J. Antimicrob. Agents* 32, 405–410. doi: 10.1016/j.ijantimicag.2008.05.013

Shriram, V., Jahagirdar, S. C., Latha, C. V., Dhakephalkar, P. K., Rojatkar, S., and Shitole, M. G. (2010). Antibacterial & antiplasmid activities of *Helicteres isora* L. *Indian J. Med. Res.* 132, 94–99.

Towner, K. J. (1997). Clinical importance and antibiotic resistance of *Acinetobacter* spp. Proceedings of a symposium held on 4-5 November 1996 at Eilat, Israel. *J. Med. Microbiol.* 46, 721–746. doi: 10.1099/00222615-46-9-721

Towner, K. J., and Chopade, B. A. (1987). Biotyping of *Acinetobacter calcoaceticus* using the API 2ONE system. *J. Hosp. Infect.* 10, 145–151. doi: 10.1016/0195-6701(87)90140-X

Trevors, J. T. (1986). Plasmid curing in bacteria. *FEMS Microbiol. Rev.* 32, 149–157. doi: 10.1111/j.1574-6968.1986.tb01189.x

16

The Plasmid-Borne *tet*(A) Gene is an Important Factor Causing Tigecycline Resistance in ST11 Carbapenem-Resistant *Klebsiella pneumoniae* Under Selective Pressure

Juan Xu[1], Zhongliang Zhu[2], Yanmin Chen[2], Weizhong Wang[2] and Fang He[2]*

[1] *School of Public Health, Hangzhou Medical College, Hangzhou, China,*

[2] *Department of Clinical Laboratory, Zhejiang Provincial People's Hospital, People's Hospital of Hangzhou Medical College, Hangzhou, China*

***Correspondence:**
Fang He
hetrue@163.com

The emergence and prevalence of tigecycline-resistant *Klebsiella pneumoniae* have seriously compromised the effectiveness of antimicrobial agents in the treatment of infections. To explore the role of the plasmid-borne *tet*(A) gene in tigecycline resistance in carbapenem-resistant *K. pneumoniae* (CRKP), a total of 63 CRKP isolates were collected from a tertiary hospital in Hangzhou, China. The minimum inhibitory concentration (MIC) of tigecycline, mutation rate of *tet*(A) gene, genetic surroundings of *tet*(A)-carrying transmissible plasmid and the contribution of *tet*(A) mutation to tigecycline resistance were analyzed using antimicrobial susceptibility test, whole-genome sequencing, tigecycline resistance evolution experiment, and plasmid conjugation experiment. Our results showed that 52.4% (33 isolates) of the test isolates carried the *tet*(A) gene; among them, 75.8% (25 isolates) exhibited a tigecycline non-susceptible phenotype (MIC = 4 mg/L). Three clonal groups (cluster I, cluster II, and cluster III) were identified in these *tet*(A)-bearing isolates. All 17 isolates belonged to serotype KL21 (cluster I), which differed by only 13 SNPs, suggesting a clonal spread of *tet*(A)-positive ST11 *K. pneumoniae* with serotype KL21 occurred in the sampling hospital. The induction of tigecycline resistance experiments showed that 71.4% of strains evolved *tet*(A) mutations and developed a high-level tigecycline resistance. Eight amino acid substitutions were identified in these mutants. The most common amino acid substitution was A370V, followed by S251A and G300E. Twelve isolates carrying *tet*(A) mutants succeeded in the filter mating experiment with a conjugation efficiency of 10^{-3}–10^{-8}. Tigecycline MICs in *E. coli* EC600 transconjugants with a mutated *tet*(A) were 2 to 8-fold higher than those in *E. coli* EC600 transconjugants with a wild-type *tet*(A). One ColRNAI/IncFII type and two IncFII type *tet*(A)-bearing conjugative plasmids were identified in this study, including a class 1 integron containing multiple antibiotic resistance genes, i.e., *tet*(A), *qnrS1*, bla_{LAP-2}, *catA2*, *sul2*, and *dfrA14*. Our study revealed the wide-spread situation of plasmid-borne *tet*(A) gene in clinical CRKP, and mutation of *tet*(A) is a potential driven force that lead to tigecycline resistance.

Keywords: mutation, plasmid-bearing, tigecycline, *tet*(A), *Klebsiella pneumoniae*

INTRODUCTION

Carbapenem-resistant *Klebsiella pneumoniae* (CRKP) is currently a substantial threat to public health worldwide. CRKP can cause a variety of infections, such as pneumonia, liver abscess, urinary tract infection, and bloodstream infection. CRKP often carry multiple antimicrobial resistance genes in the chromosome and plasmids, enabling the strain to be resistant to almost all antibiotics, except colistin and tigecycline. Tigecycline, the first glycylcycline drug, is an extended-spectrum antibiotic that inhibits protein synthesis by binding to the 30S ribosome and can overcome the mechanisms of tetracycline resistance (Pankey, 2005).

Antibiotics that can treat CRKP infections are limited. Tigecycline remains an important treatment method for CRKP. However, tigecycline resistance has emerged since the approval of this antibiotic and has been reported frequently in Enterobacteriaceae (Hoban et al., 2005). Previous reports have shown that overexpression of resistance-nodulation-cell division (RND)-type efflux pumps is associated with tigecycline resistance in Enterobacteriaceae, such as AcrAB (Ruzin et al., 2005; Keeney et al., 2007; Bratu et al., 2009; He et al., 2015). Ribosomal protein mutation (via the *rpsJ* gene) has also been reported to cause tigecycline resistance in Enterobacteriaceae (Beabout et al., 2015; He et al., 2018; Xu et al., 2020). Recently, the plasmid-mediated mobile tigecycline resistance gene *tet*(X4) and its variants has been reported in Enterobacteriaceae (He et al., 2019; Sun et al., 2019). However, this gene has most often been reported in *Escherichia coli* strains (Zhang et al., 2020), and its role in *K. pneumoniae* is limited.

In 2018, we reported the first case of tigecycline resistance in CRKP mediated by *tet*(A) evolution *in vivo* during tigecycline treatment (Du et al., 2018). Previously, Linkevicius et al. (2016) observed that evolutionary changes in *tet*(A) can cause tigecycline resistance in *E. coli in vitro*. Chiu et al. (2017) considered widespread mutated *tet*(A) gene to be concerning for the possible dissemination of tigecycline resistance in *K. pneumoniae*. To explore the role of *tet*(A) in tigecycline resistance in clinical CRKP isolates, tigecycline minimum inhibitory concentration (MIC) distribution, *tet*(A)-bearing rate, *tet*(A) mutation rate and transmission ability of clinical CRKP isolates were analyzed through antimicrobial susceptibility tests, whole genome sequencing, bioinformatics analysis, and plasmid conjugation experiments.

MATERIALS AND METHODS

CRKP Clinical Isolates

A total of 63 non-repetitive CRKP clinical strains were continuously collected from April 1st to May 30th in 2018 at a tertiary hospital in Hangzhou, China. Strains from different specimens of the same patient or specimens collected from the same patient at different times were considered to be duplicate strains, and only the first strain was selected for subsequent research. **Supplementary Figure 1** outlined the detailed specimen collection information. All of the isolates were identified using the VITEK MS system (bioMérieux, Marcy-l'Étoile, France). The carbapenem resistance genes, bla_{KPC} and bla_{NDM}, as well as the tetracycline resistance gene, *tet*(A), were amplified by PCR and further sent for Sanger sequencing.

Antimicrobial Susceptibility Test

Antimicrobial susceptibility testing was conducted using standard broth microdilution tests and the VITEK 2 system (bioMérieux) with Gram-negative antimicrobial susceptibility testing cards (AST-GN13) following the guidelines of the Clinical and Laboratory Standards Institute (CLSI). Antimicrobial agents: amoxicillin/clavulanate, ceftriaxone, cefepime, cefoxitin, aztreonam, piperacillin/tazobactam, imipenem, meropenem, amikacin, levofloxacin, sulfamethoxazole/trimethoprim, colistin, and tigecycline were used in the test. Antimicrobial susceptibility was determined using breakpoints approved by the CLSI (2019). For tigecycline MIC detection, standard broth microdilution tests were adopted with fresh (<12 h) Mueller-Hinton broth (Cation-adjusted, Oxoid Ltd., Basingstoke, Hampshire, United Kingdom). *E. coli* ATCC 25922 was used for quality control. As there are no CLSI breakpoints for tigecycline, the FDA standard was adopted[1]. The interpretation of colistin MIC was follow by the EUCAST guideline (Breakpoints for 2021)[2].

Quantitative Real-Time PCR

mRNA expression levels of the efflux pump genes, *acrA* and *acrB*, in tigecycline-resistant isolates were examined by quantitative real-time PCR according to our previously published paper (He et al., 2015). The relative expression of each target gene was calibrated against the corresponding expression of *K. pneumoniae* type strain ATCC 13883 (expression = 1), which served as a control with a tigecycline MIC of 0.125 mg/L. Relative expression levels of the two genes were analyzed by the $2^{-\Delta\Delta CT}$ analytical method.

Whole-Genome Sequencing

Isolates confirmed to possess the *tet*(A) gene or resistance to tigecycline were sent for whole-genome sequencing using the Illumina NovaSeq 6000 platform (Illumina Inc., San Diego, CA, United States). In brief, genomic DNA was extracted using a QIAamp DNA Mini Kit (Qiagen, Valencia, CA, United States) and sent for sequencing using the paired-end 2 × 150-bp protocol. The draft genome sequences were assembled using SPAdes 3.13.0. Three strains with *tet*(A) mutants (CRKP52R, CRKP66R, and CRKP78R) were further sent for Nanopore sequencing with a long-read MinION sequencer (Nanopore, Oxford, United Kingdom). Both short Illumina reads and long MinION reads were hybrid assembled using Unicycler (v0.4.7). Complete genome sequences were generated and automatically annotated by the NCBI Prokaryotic Genome Annotation Pipeline (PGAP) server.

[1] https://www.fda.gov/drugs/development-resources/tigecycline-injection-products

[2] https://eucast.org/

Genomic and Phylogenetic Relationship Analysis of *tet*(A)-Positive Isolates

MLST, acquired antibiotic resistance genes (ARGs) and plasmid replicons were analyzed using the BacWGSTdb 2.0 server (Ruan and Feng, 2016; Feng et al., 2020; Ruan et al., 2020). The phylogenetic relationship between *tet*(A)-carrying isolates was analyzed using the (neighbor joining (NJ))/unweighted pair group method with arithmetic mean (UPGMA) phylogeny method (MAFFT version 7) based on a core genome single nucleotide polymorphism strategy (Katoh et al., 2019). A phylogenetic tree was constructed using the resulting SNPs with recombination regions removed using the maximum parsimony algorithm (Jia et al., 2019). The KL type of *K. pneumoniae* was predicted by Kaptive Web (Wick et al., 2018).

Tigecycline Resistance Evolution Experiment *in vitro*

Wild-type *tet*(A)-carrying CRKP clinical isolates were used as parental strains in tigecycline resistance evolution experiments *in vitro*. Tigecycline-resistant mutants were selected by successive passages in MH broth containing increasing concentrations of tigecycline. In brief, one single clone of the parental strain was inoculated in MH broth overnight, and 200 μL of overnight cultures was added to 2 mL of fresh MH broth containing serial concentrations of tigecycline. The selective concentration began at 0.5 mg/L and doubled every 24 h. The protocol was repeated until the mutants grew at a tigecycline concentration of 32 mg/L.

Conjugation Experiment and VITEK MS Identification

Tigecycline-resistant *tet*(A) mutants obtained from tigecycline resistance evolution experiments and their parental strains with wild-type *tet*(A) were used as donors, and rifampicin-resistant *E. coli* EC600 was used as the recipient. Transconjugants were selected on MH agar plates supplemented with tetracycline (16 mg/L) and rifampicin (600 mg/L). *E. coli* EC600 transconjugants were identified using the VITEK MS system, and *tet*(A) gene mutations were further confirmed by PCR and Sanger sequencing. The conjugation efficiency was measured and calculated following the protocol in https://openwetware.org/wiki/conjugation.

Characterization of the *tet*(A)-Bearing Plasmid and Genetic Background of *tet*(A)

Circular comparisons of the *tet*(A)-carrying plasmid were conducted with BLAST Ring Image Generator (BRIG) based on concentric rings (Alikhan et al., 2011). Insertion elements (ISs) located on the plasmids were predicted by application of ISfinder (Siguier et al., 2006). Integrative and conjugative elements (ICEs) were predicted using ICEberg (Liu et al., 2019). The genetic location and background of *tet*(A) were determined by aligning the contigs carrying *tet*(A) with complete genome sequences generated in this study using CLC Genomics Workbench 10.0.1.

Nucleotide Sequence Accession Numbers

We deposited the complete sequences of the CRKP52R, CRKP66R, and CRKP78R *K. pneumoniae* strains and plasmids in GenBank under accession numbers CP066249-CP066253, CP063833-CP063838, and CP066254-CP066259. The draft genome sequences of 33 *tet*(A)-positive strains were deposited in GenBank under accession numbers JAEQKY000000000-JAEQME000000000. The sequence with GenBank accession number AJ517790 was used as the reference for the wild-type *tet*(A) gene with the primary start codon of GTG.

RESULTS

Tigecycline MIC Distribution and Mutations in *rpsJ*, *ramR*, and *tet*(A)

The antimicrobial susceptibility testing results are presented in **Supplementary Table 1**. All isolates were multidrug resistant bacteria with a resistance rate greater than 85% compared to β-lactams, quinolones and aminoglycosides but were still highly sensitive to colistin. The tigecycline MIC distribution of the 63 isolates is presented in **Figure 1A**. All 63 isolates carried bla_{KPC-2} gene, and the *in silico* MLST analysis showed that all strains, except three ST437 strains, one ST751 strain, and one ST15 strain, belonged to ST11. The highest MIC was 16 mg/L for isolate CRKP65, and further WGS results showed that this isolate did not harbor the *tet*(A) gene but had a *rpsJ* mutation (V57L). One isolate, namely, CRKP26, had a tigecycline MIC of 8 mg/L. Further WGS results showed that this strain had a *ramR* mutation (GATCCTG insertion at 222–223 resulted in frameshift mutation) and high expression of the RND efflux pump, AcrAB (**Table 1**), but did not harbor the *tet*(A) gene. Twenty-six isolates had a MIC of 4 mg/L, and among these, 25 isolates harbored wild-type *tet*(A). According to the FDA standard (MIC > 2 mg/L for tigecycline non-susceptible), there were 28 tigecycline non-susceptible isolates, and the non-susceptible rate was 44.4%. The expression levels of the RND efflux pump genes, *acrA* and *acrB*, as well as the mutations in *rpsJ*, *ramR*, and *tet*(A) in tigecycline non-susceptible isolates are presented in **Table 1**. Four isolates (CRKP5, CRKP15, CRKP21, and CRKP26) had a high expression (two-fold increase compare to reference strain) of the AcrAB efflux pump.

Characterizations of *tet*(A)-Positive Isolates and Phylogenetic Analysis

The PCR and Sanger sequencing results showed that 33 of the 63 isolates (52.4%) carried the *tet*(A) gene, all of which were wild-type. The tigecycline MIC distribution of the 33 *tet*(A)-positive isolates is presented in **Figure 1B**, and there were 25 isolates with MIC 4 mg/L (75.8%) and eight isolates (24.2%) with MIC 2 mg/L. Compared with *tet*(A)-negative isolates, the tigecycline MIC is generally increased by two-fold. All 33 isolates belonged to ST11. The antimicrobial resistance genes and serotype based on WGS data of these 33 *tet*(A)-bearing isolates are presented in **Figure 2**. In total, 16 antimicrobial resistance genes were found in these

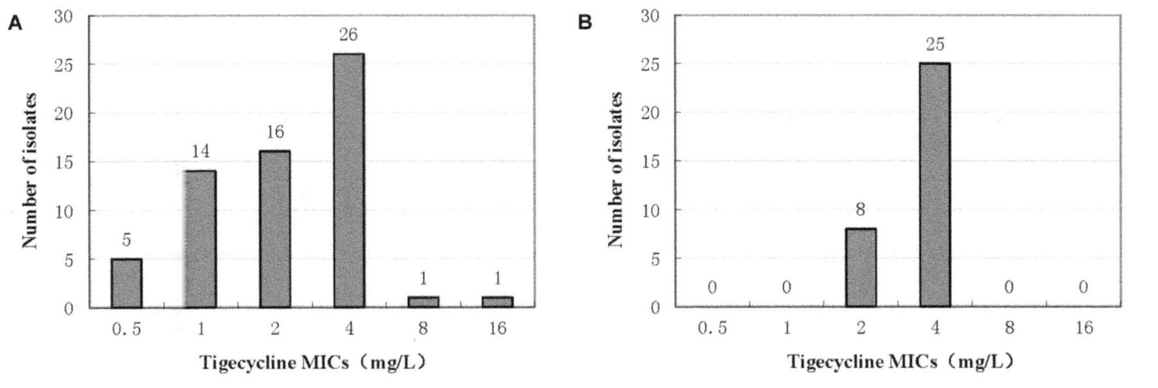

Tigecycline MIC distribution for total 63 CRKP clinical isolates. Tigecycline MIC distribution for 33 *tetA*-bearing isolates.

FIGURE 1 | Tigecycline MIC distributions of 63 CRKP clinical isolates and 33 *tet*(A)-bearing isolates.

TABLE 1 | Expression levels of the *acrA* and *acrB* efflux pump genes and mutation of *rpsJ*, *ramR*, and *tet*(A) in tigecycline non-susceptible isolates.

Isolate	MIC (mg/L)[b]	Relative expression[a]		*Tet*(A)[c]	Mutation	
		acrA	*acrB*		*rpsJ*	*ramR*
ATCC 13883	0.125	1	1	ND	–	–
CRKP5	4	2.16 ± 0.10	1.66 ± 0.31	WT	–	–
CRKP8	4	1.18 ± 0.15	1.27 ± 0.03	WT	–	–
CRKP10	4	1.28 ± 0.11	1.08 ± 0.23	WT	–	–
CRKP15	4	2.38 ± 0.39	2.46 ± 0.40	WT	–	–
CRKP17	4	1.44 ± 0.28	0.99 ± 0.12	WT	–	–
CRKP21	4	2.18 ± 0.15	2.07 ± 0.45	WT	–	–
CRKP22	4	1.03 ± 0.05	0.81 ± 0.17	WT	–	–
CRKP24	4	0.89 ± 0.15	0.75 ± 0.05	WT	–	–
CRKP26	8	3.78 ± 0.29	3.56 ± 0.24	ND	–	GATCCTG insertion at 222–223
CRKP29	4	1.99 ± 0.27	1.83 ± 0.12	WT	–	–
CRKP31	4	0.89 ± 0.20	0.80 ± 0.16	ND		–
CRKP34	4	1.94 ± 0.06	1.81 ± 0.24	WT	–	–
CRKP38	4	1.67 ± 0.30	1.00 ± 0.22	WT	–	–
CRKP39	4	1.42 ± 0.23	0.71 ± 0.06	WT	–	–
CRKP41	4	1.31 ± 0.34	0.78 ± 0.06	WT	–	–
CRKP42	4	0.87 ± 0.12	0.89 ± 0.12	WT	–	–
CRKP43	4	0.78 ± 0.06	0.67 ± 0.02	WT	–	–
CRKP45	4	1.20 ± 0.09	0.98 ± 0.12	WT	–	–
CRKP51	4	1.41 ± 0.28	1.14 ± 0.10	WT	–	–
CRKP52	4	1.35 ± 0.15	1.13 ± 0.14	WT	–	–
CRKP55	4	1.79 ± 0.28	1.25 ± 0.15	WT	–	–
CRKP59	4	1.59 ± 0.60	1.17 ± 0.19	WT	–	–
CRKP61	4	0.81 ± 0.14	0.77 ± 0.15	WT	–	–
CRKP62	4	1.02 ± 0.13	0.73 ± 0.06	WT	–	–
CRKP65	16	1.30 ± 0.25	1.14 ± 0.03	ND	G169C (V57L)	–
CRKP72	4	1.03 ± 0.15	1.28 ± 0.28	WT	–	–
CRKP77	4	1.91 ± 0.54	1.32 ± 0.33	WT	–	–
CRKP80	4	1.17 ± 0.34	0.92 ± 0.12	WT	–	–

[a] *Relative expression compared with K. pneumoniae type strain ATCC 13883 (expression = 1). Results represent the means of three runs ± standard deviation.*
[b] *Tigecycline MIC.*
[c] *ND, tet(A) not detected. WT, wild-type tet(A).*

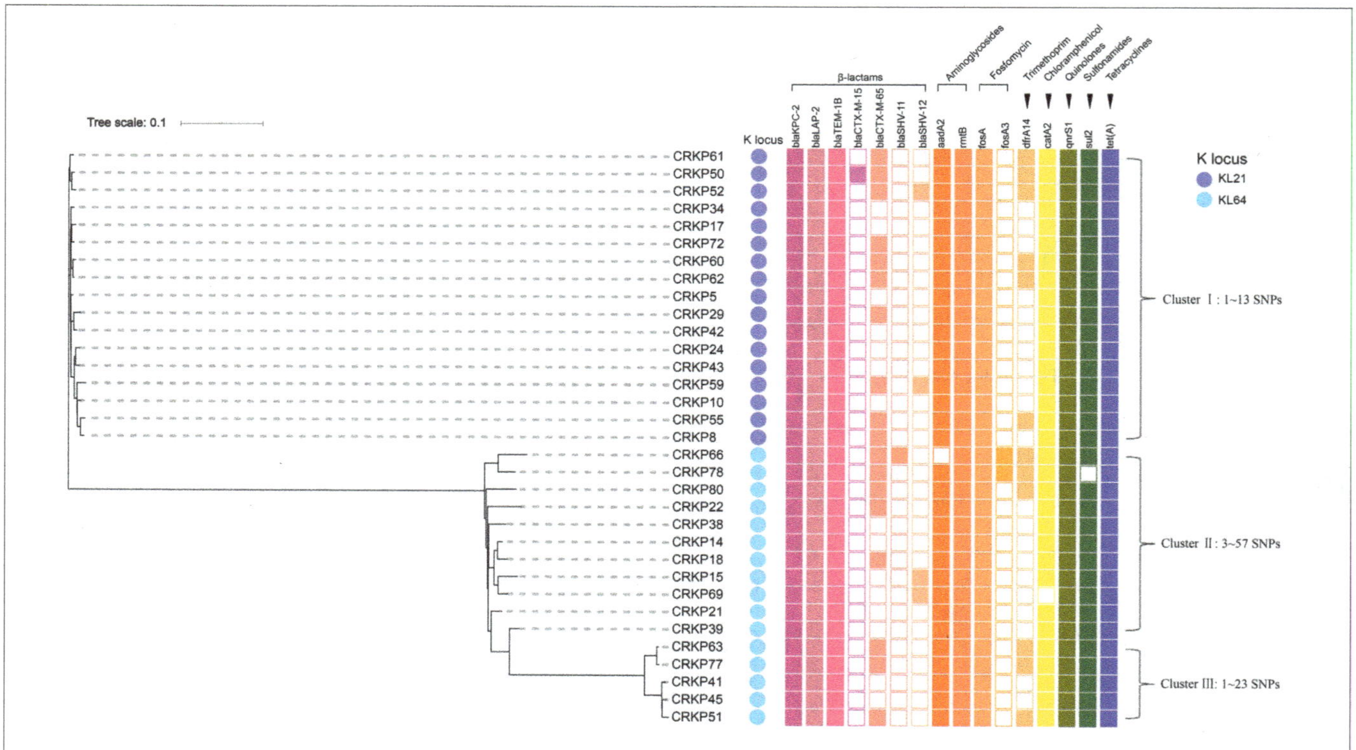

FIGURE 2 | Phylogenetic relationship, antimicrobial resistance genes and serotype analysis based on WGS data of 33 *tet*(A)-bearing CRKP isolates. The cells in different colors indicate the presence of the antimicrobial resistance gene, while the blank cells indicate the absence of the gene. The color of each circle indicates a distinct capsular serotype.

isolates, including bla_{KPC-2}, bla_{LAP-2}, bla_{TEM-1B}, *fosA*, *qnrS1*, *rmtB*, *tet*(A), $bla_{CTX-M-15}$, $bla_{CTX-M-65}$, bla_{SHV-11}, bla_{SHV-12}, *aadA2*, *dfrA14*, *catA2*, *fosA3*, and *sul2*. These isolates were divided into two serotypes (KL21 and KL64). The phylogenetic tree is presented in **Figure 2**, and SNP differences are presented in **Supplementary Figure 2**. Three clonal clusters (cluster I, cluster II, and cluster III) were identified. All 17 isolates belonged to serotype KL21 (cluster I), which differed with 13 SNPs. According to the relatedness criteria recommended for SNP typing schemes of *K. pneumoniae* reported by Schürch et al. (2018), a difference of SNPs ≤18 represents epidemiologically related. Therefore, a clonal spread of *tet*(A)-positive ST11 *K. pneumoniae* with serotype KL21 occurred in the sampling hospital.

Mutations of *tet*(A) in the Tigecycline Resistance Evolution Experiment

All 33 wild-type *tet*(A)-carrying CRKP isolates were subjected to tigecycline resistance evolution experiments *in vitro*. Under successive passages of tigecycline induction in MH broth for approximately 2 weeks, 28 isolates were induced to develop resistance with a tigecycline MIC ≥32 mg/L. PCR and Sanger sequencing detected 20 of the 28 isolates that evolved *tet*(A) mutations (**Table 2**), and the mutation rate was 71.4%. The following eight amino acid substitutions were identified in these mutants: A264V, I248L, A370V, S251A, G300E, G300V, A53G, and G237V. The most common amino acid substitution was A370V, which appeared six times, followed by S251A and G300E (appeared four times each). All 20 *tet*(A) mutants were subjected to conjugation experiments in which they were used as donors, and *E. coli* EC600 was the recipient. Twelve mutants succeeded in the conjugation experiment, and the conjugation efficiency was at a frequency of 10^{-3}–10^{-8} (**Table 2**). The MICs of tigecycline and tetracycline of *E. coli* EC600 transconjugants of *tet*(A) mutants and wild-type *tet*(A) are presented in **Table 2**. In general, tigecycline MICs in *E. coli* EC600 transconjugants of mutated *tet*(A) were 2- to 8-fold higher than *E. coli* EC600 transconjugants of wild-type *tet*(A), and the MICs of tetracycline also increased in eight strains.

Characterization of the *tet*(A)-Bearing Plasmid and Genetic Background of *tet*(A)

The complete genome sequences of three *tet*(A) mutants (CRKP52R, CRKP66R, and CRKP78R) were obtained using Nanopore sequencing. CRKP52R, CRKP66R, and CRKP78R were tigecycline-resistant *tet*(A) mutants collected in the tigecycline resistance evolution experiment. The parental strains of CRKP52R, CRKP66R, and CRKP78R were *K. pneumoniae* strains CRKP52, CRKP66, and CRKP78, respectively. *tet*(A) was located on plasmids in these strains, and three *tet*(A)-bearing plasmids were identified in CRKP52R, CRKP66R, and CRKP78R. The plasmid from CRKP52R was a ColRNAI/IncFII plasmid

TABLE 2 | Tigecycline and tetracycline MICs of *E. coli* EC600 transconjugants of *tet*(A) mutants or wild-type *tet*(A).

Isolates	TGC[c] MICs (mg/L)	*tet*(A)[a]	TGC MICs after tigecycline induction (mg/L)	*tet*(A) mutation after tigecycline induction[b]		Conjugation efficiency	*E. coli* EC600 transconjugant of *tet*(A) mutant[c]		*E. coli* EC600 transconjugant of wild-type *tet*(A)[c]	
				Nucleotide change	Amino acid change		TGC (mg/L)	TC (mg/L)	TGC (mg/L)	TC (mg/L)
CRKP5	4	WT	64	–	–	–	–	–	–	–
CRKP8	4	WT	64	C791T	A264V	$(1.4 \pm 0.6) \times 10$[illegible]	1	64	0.25	64
CRKP10	4	WT	64	–	–	–	–	–	–	–
CRKP14	2	WT	64	A742C	I248L	$(4.8 \pm 1.9) \times 10^{-6}$	2	>256	0.5	128
CRKP15	4	WT	64	–	–	–	–	–	–	–
CRKP17	4	WT	64	–	–	–	–	–	–	–
CRKP18	2	WT	64	–	–	–	–	–	–	–
CRKP21	4	WT	64	–	–	–	–	–	–	–
CRKP22	4	WT	4	–	–	–	–	–	–	–
CRKP24	4	WT	64	C1109T	A370V	Failed	NA	NA	NA	NA
CRKP29	4	WT	64	T751G	S251A	$(6.0 \pm 3.4) \times 10^{-6}$	1	256	0.25	128
CRKP34	4	WT	4	–	–	–	–	–	–	–
CRKP38	4	WT	64	T751G	S251A	$(1.8 \pm 0.9) \times 10^{-3}$	1	64	0.25	64
CRKP39	4	WT	64	G899T	G300V	Failed	NA	NA	NA	NA
CRKP41	4	WT	4	–	–	–	–	–	–	–
CRKP42	4	WT	64	C1109T	A370V	Failed	NA	NA	NA	NA
CRKP43	4	WT	64	G710T T751G	G237V S251A	Failed	NA	NA	NA	NA
CRKP45	4	WT	4	–	–	–	–	–	–	–
CRKP50	2	WT	64	C791T	A264V	$(7.7 \pm 3.3) \times 10^{-7}$	1	128	0.5	64
CRKP51	4	WT	64	G899A	G300E	$(3.7 \pm 1.9) \times 10^{-6}$	2	>256	0.25	128
CRKP52	4	WT	64	G899A	G300E	$(5.2 \pm 2.5) \times 10^{-8}$	1	256	0.25	128
CRKP55	4	WT	64	C1109T	A370V	$(3.2 \pm 1.4) \times 10^{-5}$	1	128	0.5	128
CRKP59	4	WT	64	C1109T	A370V	$(1.1 \pm 0.7) \times 10^{-5}$	1	>256	0.25	128
CRKP60	2	WT	64	G899A	G300E	Failed	NA	NA	NA	NA
CRKP61	4	WT	64	–	–	–	–	–	–	–
CRKP62	4	WT	4	–	–	–	–	–	–	–
CRKP63	2	WT	32	–	–	–	–	–	–	–
CRKP66	2	WT	64	C1109T	A370V	$(1.4 \pm 1.2) \times 10^{-6}$	1	64	0.25	64
CRKP69	2	WT	64	G899A	G300E	$(1.1 \pm 0.5) \times 10^{-4}$	4	>256	0.5	128
CRKP72	4	WT	64	C158G	A53G	Failed	NA	NA	NA	NA
CRKP77	4	WT	64	C1109T	A370V	Failed	NA	NA	NA	NA
CRKP78	2	WT	64	T751G	S251A	$(4.7 \pm 2.8) \times 10^{-6}$	4	>256	0.5	128
CRKP80	4	WT	64	C791T	A264V	Failed	NA	NA	NA	NA

[a]*WT, wild-type tet(A).*

[b]*–, no mutation detected in tet(A).*

[c]*TGC, Tigecycline; TC, Tetracycline. NA, Data not available.*

that was 99,066 bp in size and was designated pCRKP52R-4-tetA. Plasmids from CRKP66R and CRKP78R belonged to the IncFII type with sizes of 87,095 and 86,962 bp, and they were designated pCRKP66R-4-tetA and pCRKP78R-4-tetA, respectively (**Table 3**). Similar *tet*(A)-bearing plasmids in the NCBI GenBank database were searched with the Basic Local Alignment Search Tool (BLAST). We found that IncFII-type and IncFIB-type plasmids with sizes of approximately 90 and 120 kb were common plasmids carrying *tet*(A) in *K. pneumoniae* (**Table 3**). The similarity of the plasmid backbone of these plasmids is presented in **Figure 3**. These IncFII-type plasmids have a plasmid backbone similar to that of ARGs, including *qnrS1*, bla_{LAP-2}, *tet*(A), *catA2*, *sul2*, and *dfrA14*. The *tet*(A) genes in the pCRKP52R-4-tetA plasmid were flanked by the *qnrS1* and bla_{LAP-2} resistance genes on the left and the *catA2*, *sul2*, and *dfrA14* resistance genes on the right, and

TABLE 3 | Detailed information of *tet*(A)-bearing plasmids obtained in this study and the NCBI database.

Plasmid name	Plasmid replicon	Plasmid size	Host bacteria	Antimicrobial resistance genes	Accession number
pCRKP52R-4-tetA	ColRNAI/IncFII	99066bp	*K. pneumoniae*	*qnrS1*, bla_{LAP-2}, *tet*(A), *catA2*, *sul2*, *dfrA14*	CP066252 (this study)
pCRKP66R-4-tetA	IncFII	87095bp	*K. pneumoniae*	*qnrS1*, bla_{LAP-2}, *tet*(A), *catA2*, *sul2*, *dfrA14*	CP063836 (this study)
pCRKP78R-4-tetA	IncFII	86962bp	*K. pneumoniae*	*qnrS1*, bla_{LAP-2}, *tet*(A), *catA2*, *sul2*, *dfrA14*	CP066257 (this study)
pKP18-3-8-IncFII	IncFII	87095bp	*K. pneumoniae*	*qnrS1*, bla_{LAP-2}, *tet*(A), *catA2*, *sul2*, *dfrA14*	MT035876 (NCBI)
pKP18-2079_tetA	IncFII	84699bp	*K. pneumoniae*	*qnrS1*, bla_{LAP-2}, *tet*(A), *sul2*, *dfrA14*	MT090960 (NCBI)
pKP13-53-tet(A)	Col/IncFIB	181383bp	*K. pneumoniae*	*qnrS1*, bla_{LAP-2}, *tet*(A), *sul1*, *dfrA1*, *aac(3)-IId*	MN268580 (NCBI)
p71221-tetA	IncFIB	128170bp	*K. pneumoniae*	*tet*(A), *sul1*, *dfrA1*, *mph(A)*, bla_{SHV-12}, *aph(3')-Ia*	MN310374 (NCBI)
pW08291-tetA	IncFIB	130483bp	*K. pneumoniae*	*tet*(A), *sul1*, *dfrA1*, *mph(A)*, bla_{SHV-12}	MN310376 (NCBI)

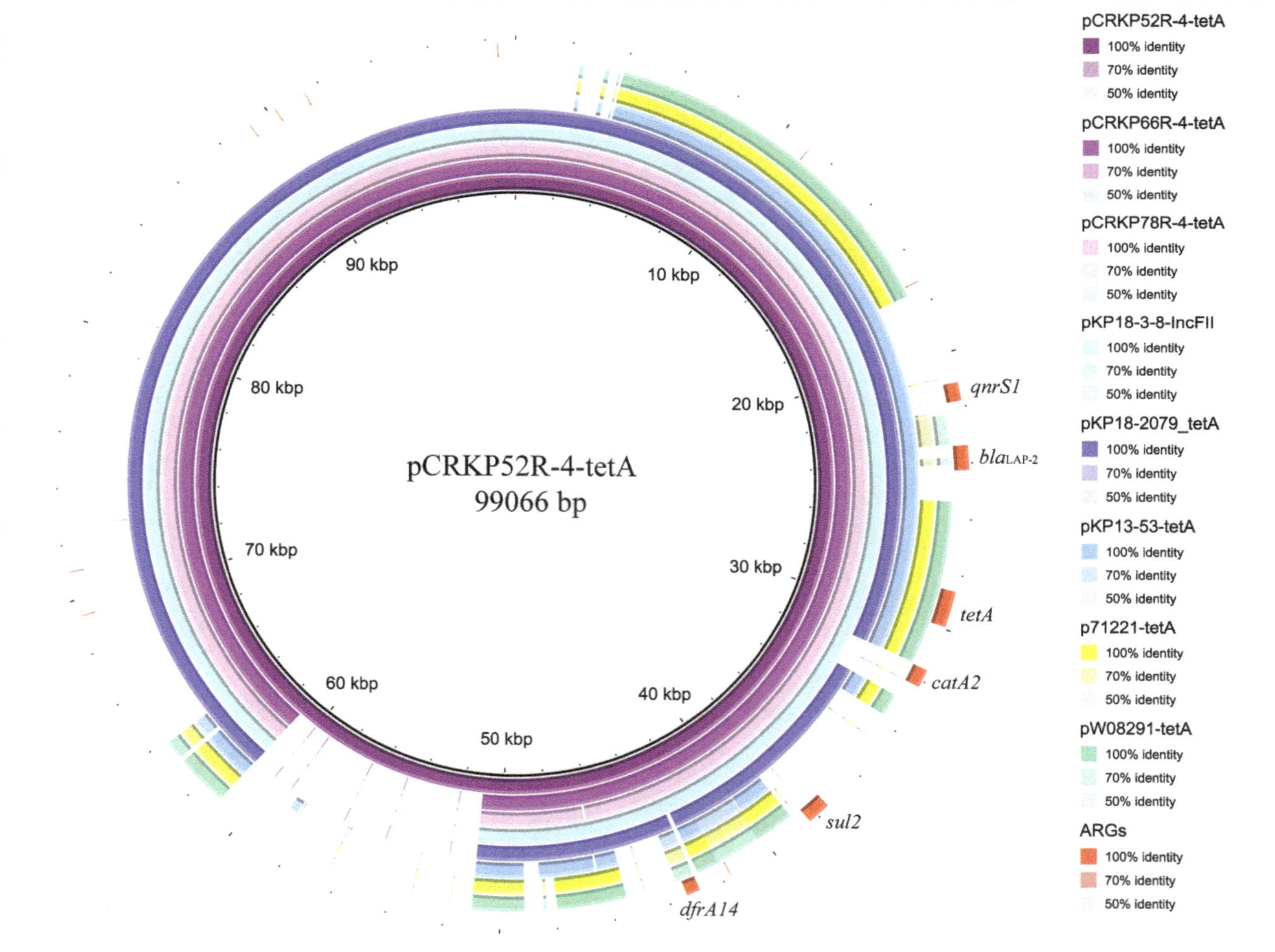

FIGURE 3 | Plasmid backbone comparisons of *tet*(A)-carrying plasmids. Plasmid information is presented in **Table 3**. ARGs are indicated in red.

they were all located in ICEs ranging from 11 to 99 kb in size (**Figure 3**). One class 1 integron (IntI1) was identified in pCRKP52R-4-tetA (from 18944 to 46168 bp), pCRKP66R-4-tetA, and pCRKP78R-4-tetA (**Figure 4**). This integron contains multiple ARGs, including *tet*(A). The *tet*(A) gene was located in the genetic environment, IS*26*-*tetR*-*tet*(A)-*eamA*-*orf*-TnAs1, suggesting that it was acquired by horizontal gene transfer with mobilizable transposons.

DISCUSSION

Carbapenem-resistant *K. pneumoniae* has emerged as an important pathogen worldwide, and the emergence of tigecycline and colistin resistance makes clinical treatment difficult. According to the data obtained in this study, 52.4% of the tested isolates carried the wild-type *tet*(A) gene. Among these isolates, 75.8% of these *tet*(A)-bearing isolates exhibited a tigecycline non-susceptible phenotype. No mutations of *rpsJ* and *ramR* genes were identified in these isolates. We also searched the plasmid-encoded RND efflux pump genes *tmexCD1-toprJ1* in the genome of these strains, but no related genes were found. Compared with *tet*(A)-negative isolates, the tigecycline MIC was generally increased by approximately two-fold in these wild-type *tet*(A)-bearing isolates. Except for three isolates (CRKP5, CRKP15, and CRKP21) had a high expression of the AcrAB efflux pump (**Table 1**), we considered that other undiscovered mechanisms may be utilized in these isolates that work together with wild-type *tet*(A) to mediate tigecycline non-susceptibility. A recent study reported that TetA in synergy with RND-type efflux transporters contribute to tigecycline resistance in *Acinetobacter baumannii* (Foong et al., 2020). This synergy may also exist in *K. pneumoniae*, which warrant further investigation.

tet(A) is a MFS family efflux pump, and mutation in *tet*(A) might result in increased accumulation of tigecycline as a substrate, thus contributing to tigecycline resistance (Linkevicius et al., 2016; Chiu et al., 2017). *tet*(A)-bearing *K. pneumoniae* tended to more easily evolve tigecycline resistance under selective pressure as 71.4% of the strains evolved *tet*(A) mutations and developed high-level tigecycline resistance in our tigecycline resistance evolution experiment *in vitro*. We have previously confirmed the contribution of the S251A Tet(A) variant to tigecycline resistance by transformation experiments (Du et al., 2018). Linkevicius et al. (2016) also confirmed that *tet*(A) mutants of I235F, I248L, S251A, and G300E show increased tigecycline MICs compared to the unmutagenized control. We further conducted transformation experiments on several other mutants (A264V, A370V, G300V, and A53G) identified in this study, and we found these mutants increased the tigecycline MIC in *E. coli* DH5α by 2 to 4-fold compared to the wild-type *tet*(A) control. The degree of tigecycline MIC increase in *E. coli* EC600 transconjugants of *tet*(A) mutants was diverse (**Table 2**), especially for a few transconjugants harboring the same mutation site (e.g., CRKP29, CRKP38, and CRKP78). Linkevicius et al. (2016) confirmed that the magnitude increase of tigecycline MIC depends on the expression level of the *tet*(A) mutant. Thus, we speculated that the difference of the *tet*(A) mutant expression level may be due to the diverse tigecycline MICs in these *E. coli* EC600 transconjugants. *tet*(A) mutants are often located in different types of plasmids, and these plasmids have different promoter and regulatory sequences that may result in different expression levels of *tet*(A).

Multiple types of *tet*(A)-bearing plasmids were retrieved from the NCBI GenBank database, and circular comparison analysis revealed that they have some similar structures, suggesting

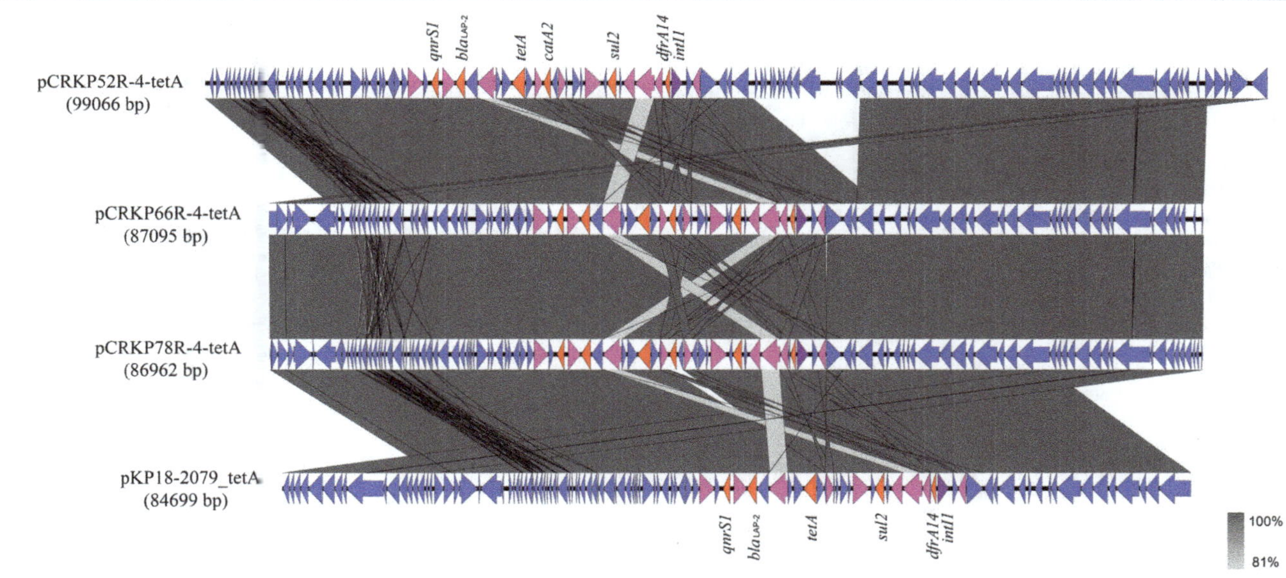

FIGURE 4 | Alignment of integrative elements with *tet*(A) in the pCRKP52R-4-tetA, pCRKP66R-4-tetA, pCRKP78R-4-tetA, and pKP18-2079_tetA plasmids. Resistance genes are indicated in red, and *int1* is indicated in purple. IS elements are indicated in pink, and all other ORFs are indicated in blue.

that genetic exchange and recombination among different types of *tet*(A)-bearing plasmids have occurred (Ribera et al., 2003; Szmolka et al., 2015; Yao et al., 2020). In the three *tet*(A)-bearing plasmids obtained in this study, one class 1 integron containing multiple ARGs, including *tet*(A), was detected. In addition, *tet*(A) mutation occurring under selective pressure may lead to tigecycline treatment failure. Zhang et al. (2019) reported the coexistence of *mcr-1* and the *tet*(A) variant on the same plasmid from a *K. pneumoniae* isolate in human gut, and Yao et al. (2020) also reported an IncFII plasmid co-harboring bla_{IMP-26} and *tet*(A) variant in a clinical *K. pneumoniae* isolate. It seems that *tet*(A) mutants can not only occur in bla_{KPC-2}-carrying plasmids, but also form fusion plasmids with other carbapenem resistance genes and *mcr* gene, which will cause a higher transmission risk of simultaneous resistance to carbapenem, colistin and tigecycline. The emergence and spread of such fusion plasmid needs our attention.

CONCLUSION

In conclusion, our study revealed the wide-spread of plasmid-borne *tet*(A) gene in clinical CRKP, and mutation of *tet*(A) is a potential threat that lead to tigecycline resistance. More attention should be devoted to monitoring the spread of plasmid-borne *tet*(A) in *K. pneumoniae* clinical isolates, especially the emergence of *tet*(A) mutants. Strict administration of tigecycline and classification management of antibiotics must be carried out with precautions.

AUTHOR CONTRIBUTIONS

FH designed the experiments. JX and ZZ performed the experiments and were the major contributors in writing the manuscript. YC and WW analyzed the data. All authors read and approved the final manuscript.

FUNDING

This study was supported by grants from the National Natural Science Foundation of China (81702042), Natural Science Foundation of Zhejiang Province (LQ19H200003), Natural Science Foundation of Zhejiang Provincial Department of Education (Y202044471), and Zhejiang Provincial Medical and Health Science and Technology Plan (2019KY311).

SUPPLEMENTARY MATERIAL

Supplementary Figure 1 | Specimen type and department distribution of 63 non-repetitive CRKP clinical isolates.

Supplementary Figure 2 | Phylogenetic analysis of 33 *tet*(A)-bearing isolates based on the core genome SNP strategy.

REFERENCES

Alikhan, N. F., Petty, N. K., Ben Zakour, N. L., and Beatson, S. A. (2011). BLAST Ring Image Generator (BRIG): simple prokaryote genome comparisons. *BMC Genomics* 12:402. doi: 10.1186/1471-2164-12-402

Beabout, K., Hammerstrom, T. G., Perez, A. M., Magalhaes, B. F., Prater, A. G., Clements, T. P., et al. (2015). The ribosomal S10 protein is a general target for decreased tigecycline susceptibility. *Antimicrob. Agents Chemother.* 59, 5561–5566. doi: 10.1128/aac.00547-15

Bratu, S., Landman, D., George, A., Salvani, J., and Quale, J. (2009). Correlation of the expression of acrB and the regulatory genes marA, soxS and ramA with antimicrobial resistance in clinical isolates of *Klebsiella pneumoniae* endemic to New York City. *J. Antimicrob. Chemother.* 64, 278–283. doi: 10.1093/jac/dkp186

Chiu, S. K., Huang, L. Y., Chen, H., Tsai, Y. K., Liou, C. H., Lin, J. C., et al. (2017). Roles of ramR and tet(A) mutations in conferring tigecycline resistance in carbapenem-resistant *Klebsiella pneumoniae* clinical isolates. *Antimicrob. Agents Chemother.* 61:e00391-17.

CLSI (2019). *Performance Standards for Antimicrobial Susceptibility Testing:* Clinical and Laboratory Standards Institute (CLSI) supplement M100, 29th Edn. Wayne, PA: Clinical and Laboratory Standards Institute.

Du, X., He, F., Shi, Q., Zhao, F., Xu, J., Fu, Y., et al. (2018). The rapid emergence of tigecycline resistance in blaKPC-2 harboring *Klebsiella pneumoniae*, as mediated in vivo by mutation in tetA during tigecycline treatment. *Front. Microbiol.* 9:648. doi: 10.3389/fmicb.2018.00648

Feng, Y., Zou, S., Chen, H., Yu, Y., and Ruan, Z. (2020). BacWGSTdb 2.0: a one-stop repository for bacterial whole-genome sequence typing and source tracking. *Nucleic Acids Res.* 49, D644–D650.

Foong, W. E., Wilhelm, J., Tam, H. K., and Pos, K. M. (2020). Tigecycline efflux in *Acinetobacter baumannii* is mediated by TetA in synergy with RND-type efflux transporters. *J. Antimicrob. Chemother.* 75, 1135–1139. doi: 10.1093/jac/dkaa015

He, F., Fu, Y., Chen, Q., Ruan, Z., Hua, X., Zhou, H., et al. (2015). Tigecycline susceptibility and the role of efflux pumps in tigecycline resistance in KPC-producing *Klebsiella pneumoniae. PLoS One* 10:e0119064. doi: 10.1371/journal.pone.0119064

He, F., Shi, Q., Fu, Y., Xu, J., Yu, Y., and Du, X. (2018). Tigecycline resistance caused by rpsJ evolution in a 59-year-old male patient infected with KPC-producing *Klebsiella pneumoniae* during tigecycline treatment. *Infect. Genet. Evol.* 66, 188–191. doi: 10.1016/j.meegid.2018.09.025

He, T., Wang, R., Liu, D., Walsh, T. r., Zhang, R., Lv, Y., et al. (2019). Emergence of plasmid-mediated high-level tigecycline resistance genes in animals and humans. *Nat. Microbiol.* 4, 1450–1456. doi: 10.1038/s41564-019-0445-2

Hoban, D. J., Bouchillon, S. K., Johnson, B. M., Johnson, J. L., and Dowzicky, M. J. (2005). In vitro activity of tigecycline against 6792 gram-negative and gram-positive clinical isolates from the global tigecycline evaluation and surveillance trial (TEST Program, 2004). *Diagn. Microbiol. Infect. Dis.* 52, 215–227. doi: 10.1016/j.diagmicrobio.2005.06.001

Jia, H., Chen, Y., Wang, J., Xie, X., and Ruan, Z. (2019). Emerging challenges of whole-genome-sequencing-powered epidemiological surveillance of globally distributed clonal groups of bacterial infections, giving *Acinetobacter baumannii* ST195 as an example. *Int. J. Med. Microbiol.* 309:151339. doi: 10.1016/j.ijmm.2019.151339

Katoh, K., Rozewicki, J., and Yamada, K. D. (2019). MAFFT online service: multiple sequence alignment, interactive sequence choice and visualization. *Brief. Bioinform.* 20, 1160–1166. doi: 10.1093/bib/bbx108

Keeney, D., Ruzin, A., and Bradford, P. A. (2007). RamA, a transcriptional regulator, and AcrAB, an RND-type efflux pump, are associated with decreased susceptibility to tigecycline in *Enterobacter cloacae. Microb. Drug Resist.* 13, 1–6. doi: 10.1089/mdr.2006.9990

Linkevicius, M., Sandegren, L., and Andersson, D. I. (2016). Potential of tetracycline resistance proteins to evolve tigecycline resistance. *Antimicrob. Agents Chemother.* 60, 789–796. doi: 10.1128/aac.02465-15

Liu, M., Li, X., Xie, Y., Bi, D., Sun, J., Li, J., et al. (2019). ICEberg 2.0: an updated database of bacterial integrative and conjugative elements. *Nucleic Acids Res.* 47, D660–D665.

Pankey, G. A. (2005). Tigecycline. *J. Antimicrob. Chemother.* 56, 470–480.

Ribera, A., Roca, I., Ruiz, J., Gibert, I., and Vila, J. (2003). Partial characterization of a transposon containing the tet(A) determinant in a clinical isolate of *Acinetobacter baumannii. J. Antimicrob. Chemother.* 52, 477–480. doi: 10.1093/jac/dkg344

Ruan, Z., and Feng, Y. (2016). BacWGSTdb, a database for genotyping and source tracking bacterial pathogens. *Nucleic Acids Res.* 44, D682–D687.

Ruan, Z., Yu, Y., and Feng, Y. (2020). The global dissemination of bacterial infections necessitates the study of reverse genomic epidemiology. *Brief. Bioinform.* 21, 741–750. doi: 10.1093/bib/bbz010

Ruzin, A., Visalli, M. A., Keeney, D., and Bradford, P. A. (2005). Influence of transcriptional activator RamA on expression of multidrug efflux pump AcrAB and tigecycline susceptibility in *Klebsiella pneumoniae. Antimicrob. Agents Chemother.* 49, 1017–1022. doi: 10.1128/aac.49.3.1017-1022.2005

Schürch, A., Arredondo-Alonso, S., Willems, R., and Goering, R. (2018). Whole genome sequencing options for bacterial strain typing and epidemiologic analysis based on single nucleotide polymorphism versus gene-by-gene-based approaches. *Clin. Microbiol. Infect.* 24, 350–354. doi: 10.1016/j.cmi.2017.12.016

Siguier, P., Perochon, J., Lestrade, L., Mahillon, J., and Chandler, M. (2006). ISfinder: the reference centre for bacterial insertion sequences. *Nucleic Acids Res.* 34, D32–D36.

Sun, J., Chen, C., Cui, C. y, Zhang, Y., Liu, X., Cui, Z. h, et al. (2019). Plasmid-encoded tet(X) genes that confer high-level tigecycline resistance in *Escherichia coli. Nat. Microbiol.* 4, 1457–1464. doi: 10.1038/s41564-019-0496-4

Szmolka, A., Lestár, B., Pászti, J., Fekete, P., and Nagy, B. (2015). Conjugative IncF and IncI1 plasmids with tet(A) and class 1 integron conferring multidrug resistance in F18(+) porcine enterotoxigenic *E. coli. Acta Vet. Hung.* 63, 425–443. doi: 10.1556/004.2015.040

Wick, R. R., Heinz, E., Holt, K. E., and Wyres, K. L. (2018). Kaptive web: user-friendly capsule and lipopolysaccharide serotype prediction for *Klebsiella* genomes. *J. Clin. Microbiol.* 56:e00197-18.

Xu, J., Zhao, Z., Ge, Y., and He, F. (2020). Rapid emergence of a pandrug-resistant *Klebsiella pneumoniae* ST11 isolate in an inpatient in a teaching hospital in China after treatment with multiple broad-spectrum antibiotics. *Infect Drug Resist.* 13, 799–804. doi: 10.2147/idr.s243334

Yao, H., Cheng, J., Li, A., Yu, R., Zhao, W., Qin, S., et al. (2020). Molecular characterization of an IncFII(k) plasmid co-harboring bla (IMP-26) and tet(A) variant in a clinical *Klebsiella pneumoniae* isolate. *Front. Microbiol.* 11:1610. doi: 10.3389/fmicb.2020.01610

Zhang, R., Dong, N., Shen, Z., Zeng, Y., Lu, J., Liu, C., et al. (2020). Epidemiological and phylogenetic analysis reveals Flavobacteriaceae as potential ancestral source of tigecycline resistance gene tet(X). *Nat. Commun.* 11:4648.

Zhang, R., Hu, Y. Y., Zhou, H. W., Wang, S. L., Shu, L. B., and Chen, G. X. (2019). Emergence of mcr-1 and the tet(A) variant in a *Klebsiella pneumoniae* isolate from the faeces of a healthy person. *J. Med. Microbiol.* 68, 1267–1268. doi: 10.1099/jmm.0.000932

17

Liposome Entrapment of Bacteriophages Improves Wound Healing in a Diabetic Mouse MRSA Infection

Sanjay Chhibber*, Jasjeet Kaur and Sandeep Kaur

Department of Microbiology, Panjab University, Chandigarh, India

****Correspondence:***
Sanjay Chhibber
sanjaychhibber8@gmail.com

Diabetic populations are more prone to developing wound infections which results in poor and delayed wound healing. Infection with drug resistant organisms further worsen the situation, driving searches for alternative treatment approaches such as phage therapy. Major drawback of phage therapy, however, is low phage persistence *in situ*, suggesting further refinement of the approach. In the present work we address this issue by employing liposomes as delivery vehicles. A liposome entrapped phage cocktail was evaluated for its ability to resolve a *Staphylococcus aureus*-induced diabetic excission wound infection. Two characterized *S. aureus* specific lytic phages, MR-5 and MR-10 alone, in combination (cocktail), or entrapped in liposomes (versus as free phages) were assesed for their therapeutic efficacy in resolving diabetic wound infection. Mice treated with free phage cocktail showed significant reduction in wound bioburden, greater wound contraction and faster tissue healing than with free monophage therapy. However, to further enhance the availability of viable phages the encapsulation of phage cocktail in the liposomes was done. Results of *in vitro* stability studies and *in vivo* phage titer determination, suggests that liposomal entrapment of phage cocktail can lead to better phage persistence at the wound site. A 2 log increase in phage titre, however, was observed at the wound site with liposome entrapped as compared to the free phage cocktail, and this was associaed with increased rates of infection resolution and wound healing. Entrapment of phage cocktails within liposomes thus could represent an attractive approach for treatment of bacterial infections, not responding to antibiotis as increased phage persistence *in vitro* and *in vivo* at the wound site was observed.

Keywords: bacteriophage, diabetes, phage cocktail, liposome, alloxan

INTRODUCTION

Diabetes is a chronic disease that manifests in the form of a chronic hyperglycemia which is associated with a plethora of complications including visual impairment, blindness, kidney disease, nerve damage, amputation, heart disease, and stroke (Loghmani, 2005). WHO has projected diabetes as the 7th leading contributor to death by 2030 (Mathera and Loncar, 2006). In addition, the total number of people with diabetes is projected to rise from 171 million in 2000 to 366 million in 2030 (Wild et al., 2004). Diabetic patients are five times more susceptible to fungal and bacterial infections (Axelrod, 1985). This is due to several factors that include a high glucose level which encourages bacterial growth. Secondly, diabetes decreases a body's blood flow, slowing healing of abrasions, open wounds and other injuries, thus making diabetic individuals more prone to infection (King, 2001). Finally, peripheral neuropathy, a primary complication of diabetes, results in loss of sensation (Pendsey, 2010) and has a central role in the development of foot and wound infections (Bader, 2008; Powlson and Coll, 2010). According to the American Diabetes Association (ADA), 25% of people with diabetes suffer from a wound problem during their lifetime, including infections. *Staphylococcus aureus* is one of the most common pathogens isolated from wounds in diabetic patients. Further, with the spread of methicillin resistant strains of *S. aureus* (MRSA), management of such infections in diabetic population has become challenging. Diabetics who contract MRSA are at a greater risk of harboring more serious, slow-healing wounds (Rogers and Bevilacqua, 2009).

With time, the bacteria in diabetic infections tend to evolve greater resistance to antibiotics (Xavier et al., 2014). Consequently, having a comprehensive treatment plan for MRSA is crucial. Phage therapy seems to be a good option for addressing these problems (Barrow and Soothill, 1997; Bull et al., 2002; Wills et al., 2005; Capparelli et al., 2007; Sunagar et al., 2010; Hsieh et al., 2011; Kumari et al., 2011; Chhibber et al., 2013; Chadha et al., 2016). Fish et al. (2016), on the basis of the success obtained with phage therapy of a diabetic foot infected with *S. aureus*, have suggested that in the future controlled clinical trials can be conducted. The ability of phages to rapidly lyse infected bacteria, their specificity and effectiveness against multidrug-resistant pathogenic bacteria, their ability to self-replicate (auto dosing) (Kumari et al., 2009; Chhibber et al., 2013; Kaur et al., 2014), their natural abundance and their proven clinical safety makes this therapy worth considering in immunocompromised individuals such as diabetic patients (Carlton et al., 2005; Hanlon, 2007). Phage therapy in many cases nevertheless can benefit from approaches that can increase phage retention and persistence at the target sites.

Toward improving phage persistence and retention at diabetic wound sites, we propose here the use of liposome entrapment of phages. Liposomes are composed of natural lipids which are biodegradable, non-immunogenic and non-toxic. Along with these advantages, their structural versatility enables us to design a number of liposome-based formulations (Gregoriadis, 1995). Liposomes also mimic biological membranes in terms of their structure and behavior, which enables them to penetrate the epidermal barrier to a greater extent and thus can be used effectively in treating skin infections (Hua, 2015). Use of drug delivery systems (DDSs) such as liposomes also helps to improve the pharmacological properties of conventional ("free") drugs by altering their pharmacokinetics (PK) and bio-distribution (BD) (Zhang et al., 2013; Zylberberg and Matosevic, 2016). Workers in the past have reported the use of liposomes with entrapped antibiotics or other wound healing agent in treating wound infections (Roesken et al., 2000; Kurilko et al., 2009; Fukui et al., 2012). In recent studies, entrapment of phages in liposomes has also been reported (Colom et al., 2015; Nieth et al., 2015; Singla et al., 2015; Chadha et al., 2017). However, none of these workers have studied the use of liposomes to enhance the stability and persistence of phages for the better therapeutic outcome after treatment of diabetic wound infection caused by MRSA. The present study therefore investigated the therapeutic use of liposome entrapped phage cocktail in treating MRSA mediated skin wound infection in diabetic mice.

MATERIALS AND METHODS

Bacterial Strains and Phage Used

Staphylococcus aureus ATCC 43300 (MRSA) from ATCC, Manassas, VA, United States was used in this study. *S. aureus* specific phages, MR-5 and MR-10, both of which have been isolated and characterized in our laboratory as lytic, dsDNA, tailed phages belonging to Myoviridae family, order Caudovirales were used in the present study (Kaur et al., 2012; Chhibber et al., 2013).

Preparation of Purified High Titer Phage Stocks (MR-5 and MR-10)

High-titer MR-5 and MR-10 suspension was prepared according to the method described by Langley et al. (2003). The inoculated broth was centrifuged and supernatant containing phage collected and passed through a 0.22-μm-pore-size filter. The filtrate was concentrated by using Millipore Labscale TFF system (Pellicon) and 10 K (polyethersulfone) membrane until the sample volume was reduced to 25–30 ml. DNase I (0.25 mg/ml) was added and kept for 1 h at 37°C to digest the free DNA. NaCl (final concentration of 1 M) and polyethylene glycol (PEG) 8000 were added to the concentrated lysate and kept at 4°C overnight. The precipitate was collected, dialyzed against phosphate buffered saline (PBS) overnight at 4°C, passed through an0.22-μm-pore-size filter and stored at 4°C till further use. The phage titer was determined in the final product.

Liposomes

Free phage preparations were entrapped within liposomes to increase their persistence and efficacy. For this a series of optimization experiments were carried to select the exact liposomal formulation for *in vivo* use.

Preparation

The method of Bhatia et al. (2004) was used for the preparation of phage cocktail-loaded liposomes. For preparation of cationic liposomal formulation of phage, phosphatidylcholine:cholesterol: tween 80:stearylamine (7:3:1:0.5) was dissolved in chloroform-methanol mixture (2:1 v/v). Thin film was prepared by a rota-evaporator [Heidolph, Hei-VAP Advantage (ML)] using a hydration temperature of 40°C. Phage suspension (10 ml prepared in PBS [pH 7.2]) was added to the thin film at 40°C and rotated for 10 min to detach the film from the glass wall. The suspension was left overnight at room temperature for swelling. The next day the dispersion is sonicated in a water bath sonicator for 30 min.

Characterization

The morphological characteristics of liposomes were monitored viz. shape, uniformity, and structure by using optical microscope

(Olympus CH20i) at suitable magnification (100X). Morphological analysis of liposomes loaded with phage cocktail was then done using TEM following the procedure of Goodridge et al. (2003). Drops of ultra-centrifuged phage samples (1,00,000 *g* for 2 h, 4°C; L-80, Beckman Instrument, Switzerland) were dropped on nitrocellulose coated grids (diameter, 3 mm; 300 meshes), stained with 2% (w/v) potassium phosphotungstate (pH: 6.8–7.2) for 10 s, and examined under a transmission electron microscope (TEM) (Hitachi H 7500, Tokyo, Japan) at Sophisticated Analytic Instrumentation Facility (SAIF), Panjab University, Chandigarh, India. Particle size and polydispersity index of liposomes was measured by dynamic light scattering (DLS) technique on Beckman coulter instrument (Delsa Nano C) at Department of Chemistry, Panjab University, Chandigarh.

The phage entrapment efficiency of liposomes was determined by modified protamine aggregation method (Gulati et al., 1998). Total phage count was determined by adding Triton × (0.02%) in a ratio of 1:1 v/v so as to disrupt liposomes and release entrapped phage particles. The mixture was then centrifuged (10,000 × *g* for 10 min) and total number of phages in the supernatant was determined using plaque assay. Free phages were separated by protamine aggregation method where protamine sulfate was added at a final concentration of 20 mg/ml. The liposomal phage preparation with added protamine sulfate was allowed to stand overnight. Supernatant was collected and the number of free phage particles was determined using plaque assay. Phage entrapment efficiency was then calculated as total number of non-free phages divided by total number of phages, presented as a percentage.

Animal experiments

Animal experimental protocols were approved by the Institutional Animal Ethics Committee (Approval ID: IAEC/411) of Panjab University, Chandigarh, India and performed in accordance with the guidelines of Committee for the Purpose of Control and Supervision of Experiments on Animals (CPCSEA), Government of India, on animal experimentation. All efforts were made to minimize the suffering of animals.

BALB/c female mice, 4–6 weeks old weighing 20–25 g were used in this study. The animals, obtained from Central Animal House, Panjab University, Chandigarh, India, were kept in polycarbonate cages housed in well-aerated rooms with a 12-h light/12-h dark cycle at 25 ± 2°C, and fed with standard rodent diet and water *ad libitum*. Diabetes as per the protocol of Pan and Liu (2008) was induced by giving two intra-peritoneal injections of alloxan monohydrate (150 mg/kg body weight) at 48-h intervals in mice fasted overnight. One week after the second injection, blood glucose levels (both random as well as fasting) were recorded. The blood sample was obtained by tail clipping method of Oladeinde et al. (2007) and glucose levels were checked using pre-calibrated Glucometer (Optium Xceed).

Wound Model

A diabetic excision wound model was developed following the method of Mendes et al. (2012). *S. aureus* 43300 cultivated overnight in brain heart infusion broth was pelleted and washed twice with PBS. Bacterial suspension was adjusted to achieve a cell density corresponding to a range of bacterial inoculums (10^8, 10^9, and 10^{10} CFU/ml). The number of CFU/ml was confirmed by quantitative plate count. Diabetic BALB/c mice were taken and distributed in four different groups of 14 animals (n = 14) each. The mice were anesthetized by giving 0.1 ml of ketamine-xylazine (50–5 mpk) intraperitoneally. Hair was removed by using commercially available hair removing cream followed by disinfection of the dorsal surface with 70% alcohol. A punch biopsy instrument (diameter 5 mm, accu punch) was used to create a full thickness round wound extending through the panniculus carnosus. The wounds created in all the animals were left open and animals were given ibuprofen suspension (20 mg/ml) in drinking water. Each of the three groups received different doses of inoculum. Animals of the fourth group received same volume of PBS injected into their wound. Two mice from each group were sacrificed on days 1, 3, 5, 7, 10, 15, and 20 post-bacterial challenge by cervical dislocation. Complete epithelial and dermal compartments of wound margins, granulation tissue and adjacent muscle and subcutaneous fat tissue was excised from each individual wound and processed. The tissue was homogenized and dilutions of the homogenates were plated to determine the bacterial burden.

Free Phage Efficacy (Study 1)

In vivo work was divided into two studies. In the first study the therapeutic potential of free phages (monophage therapy as well as cocktail of phages) not involving any delivery system was assessed. For further clarity, phage preparations not entrapped within liposomes have been referred as free monophage (FMP) for, e.g., FMP-MR-5 and FMP-MR-10 and free cocktail of phages (FCP).

For the first study, the therapeutic potential of *S. aureus* 43300-specific phages FMP-MR-5, FMP-MR-10 and their cocktail, FCP, was evaluated in diabetic BALB/c mice. The phages were administered locally at a dose of 10^9 PFU/50 μl, at MOI10 as based on a titer of applied phages of 2×10^{10} PFU/ml, into the wound on its dorsal surface. Diabetic BALB/c mice were randomly divided into five groups (n = 14 per group; as described immediately below) and seven extra animals were put in the infection control group to check the bacterial load on days 1 and 3. In all cases diabetic mice were first infected with *S. aureus* 43300 (10^8 CFU/50 μl) with treatments following 30-min later.

Group 1 (untreated infection control): No phages or clarithromycin applied.
Group 2: Local administration of phage FMP-MR-5 at MOI10.
Group 3: Local administration of phage FMP-MR-10 at MOI10.
Group 4: Local administration of the phage cocktail, FCP (each phage at MOI10 mixed in an equal ratio).
Group 5: Two I/P doses of clarithromycin (10 mpk) given in 12-h intervals.

All of the animals involved in Study 1 were monitored daily for mortality post-bacterial challenge. In addition to mortality, wound bioburden, and phage titer was assessed in surviving animals on different days.

Liposome Entrapped Phage Efficacy (Study 2)

In the second study, liposome entrapped phage cocktail was evaluated for its potential in treatment of diabetic wound infection. Phage cocktail (MR-5 + MR-10, 1:1) entrapped within liposomes shall be referred as liposomes entrapped cocktail of phages (LCP). Results were compared with the groups instead treated with FCP and with clarithromycin. Diabetic BALB/c mice with dermal wounds in this study were randomly divided into a total of four groups (n = 14). As above, in all cases diabetic mice were first infected with *S. aureus* 43300 (10^8 CFU/50 μl) with treatments following 30-min later.

Group 1 (untreated infection control): No phages or clarithromycin applied.
Group 2: Local administration of FCP (each phage at MOI10 mixed in an equal ratio).
Group 3: Local administration of LCP (each phage at MOI10 mixed in an equal ratio).
Group 4: Two I/P doses of clarithromycin (10 mpk) given in 12-h intervals.

All animals in Study 2 were monitored daily for mortality post-bacterial challenge. In addition to mortality, wound bioburden, phage titer, wound contraction rate, MPO, Masson's trichrome staining, histopathological examination, and period of epithelization was also assessed in surviving animals on different days.

Wound microbiology and rate of healing

In both Studies 1 and 2, two mice from each group were sacrificed on days 1, 3, 5, 7, 10, and 15 post-infection by cervical dislocation. Bacterial load (wound bioburden) was assessed as per the method of Park et al. (2009). After disinfection, the wound tissue was carefully excised and homogenized in 1 ml of PBS. This tissue homogenate was then serially diluted and plated for CFUs. Phage titer was determined (in terms of PFU/ml) by centrifuging the homogenate (10,000 g for 10 min at 4°C). The supernatant was filtered through 0.45 μm pore sized filter and the filtrate so obtained was serially diluted and plated on a lawn of *S. aureus* 43300.

Rate of wound contraction, as a percentage, was calculated by measuring the size of the wound (diameter in mm) on each day of all the animals involved in Study 2 using vernier caliper. This data is presented as percentage decrease in wound size. Thus, (initial wound size – wound size on a specific day) × 100. The number of days required for wound healing and eschar to fall off leaving no raw wound behind was taken as period for epithelization.

Myeloperoxidase (MPO) estimation

Two mice from each group (same groups as those described for liposome entrapped phage cocktail protection study, i.e., Study 2 with 14 animals per group) were sacrificed and their wound tissue homogenized. Homogenized samples were processed for MPO determination as per the method of Greenberger et al. (1996). The absorbance was read immediately at 490 nm over a period of 4 min. MPO was calculated as the change in optical density (O.D) × dilution factor (D.F).

Masson's trichrome staining

To assess the wound healing after treatment with LCP, FCP and clarithromycin, collagen formation was checked in each animal group of Study 2. Collagen is used as an essential marker in wound healing studies as it restores the integrity of the skin. Therefore, collagen formation was observed in the skin wound tissue on different days. Samples were fixed on different glass slides, stained as per the protocol[1] and examined under an Olympus microscope (at 100X) to evaluate the amount of collagen formation.

Histopathological examination

Tissue damage and healing following treatment with LCP, FCP, and clarithromycin in Study 2 was assessed on the basis of histopathological examination of infected wound tissue according to the method of Brans et al. (1994). The sections were picked on separate slides, stained with hematoxylin and eosin (Hi-Media, Mumbai) and then examined under a microscope to evaluate the extent of tissue damage and recovery.

Statistical Methods

All the data is expressed as mean ± standard deviation of more than two experimental values for every variable. The statistical significance of difference between groups was determined by Student's t-test (two groups), one-way ANOVA followed by a Tukey test using Sigma Stat, Graph pad prism (GraphPad Software, San Diego, CA, United States). P-value of less than 0.05 was considered statistically significant.

RESULTS

Optimization of Liposomal Formulation and Stability

For phage cocktail entrapment, three different liposomal formulations (7:3:1, 8:2:1, 9:1:1) were made using different ratios of phospholipid phosphatidylcholine (PC), cholesterol (CHOL), and Tween-80. Further, to increase the physical stability of liposomal preparation; positive charge inducer stearylamine (SA) was added in a ratio of 7:3:1:0.5. Liposomal formulation 7:3:1:0.5 showed a minimum liposome size of 230 nm, low PDI of 0.220, uniform liposomes in terms of shape and lamellarity. Both the phages MR-5 and MR-10 (1:1) were entrapped in this liposomal preparation which had an entrapment efficiency of 87% and liposomal size of 212 nm. The photomicrographs (**Figure 1**) obtained after TEM clearly demonstrates presence of phages in the cationic liposomes. LCP was made using 7:3:1:0.5 formulation and tested for stability (drop in phage titer) over a 9 week period. This liposomal preparation had a PDI below 0.3 with minimum size variation and was found to be stable at 4°C in terms of fusion size, aggregation and number of entrapped phages during the entire storage period. Thus, this ratio was selected for further *in vivo* experiments.

[1] http://www.ihcworld.com/_protocols/special_stains/masson_trichrome.htm

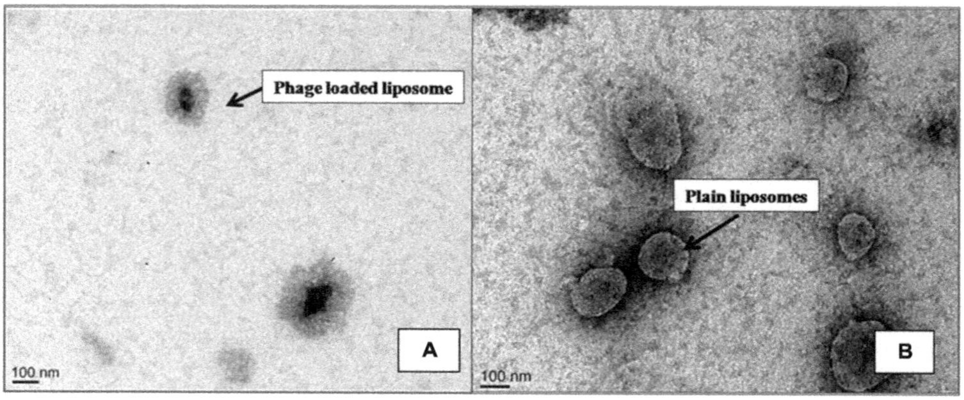

FIGURE 1 | Transmission Electron Micrograph of liposomes. Photomicrograph **(A)** shows phage loaded liposomes. **(B)** Plain liposomes without phage.

Induction of Diabetes in Mice

The average random blood glucose level of normal BALB/c mice was found to be 139 ± 3.8 mg/dl whereas the fasting blood glucose level (after overnight fasting) was 96.2 ± 7.9 mg/dl. Fasting glucose levels were checked daily post-alloxan injection. Mice with fasting blood glucose levels in the range of 150–180 mg/dl, 4–5 days post-injection were termed as moderately diabetic. However, 15 days after alloxan administration, the fasting blood glucose level was found to be 194.6 ± 17.1 mg/dl, whereas the random blood glucose levels were ≥400 mg/dl. Such animals were considered severely diabetic and selected for infection studies.

Excision Wound Infection Model

The excision wound model was developed by inflicting full thickness wound of 5 mm extending through panniculus carnosus with the help of punch biopsy on the dorsal surface of mouse. Since the aim of this study was to assess the efficacy of phages in reducing the mortality and clearing off infection; a high dose of 10^8 CFU/50 μl of *S. aureus* 43300 was chosen as the optimal infectious dose. At this bacterial dose, an acute infection of the inflicted wound was established with 70% of untreated mice exhibiting mortality within 24–48 h post-infection.

Phage Protection Studies

Mortality vs. survival

Animals in all groups were monitored daily for mortality. Untreated mice of Study 1 (group 1) and Study 2 (group 1) exhibited 70% mortality within 24–48 h post-inoculation. However, all treated animals showed no mortality during the experimental period and all infections resolved. This clearly indicated that a single injection of free phages, alone or as cocktail, or liposome-entrapped phages were able to protect the test animals from death.

Wound microbiology

The wound bioburden (bacterial density) and phage titer was also assessed in all the mice groups of Study 1 and Study 2. In Study 1, untreated animals showed an increase in bacterial load that reached ~9 log CFUs/ml by day 3 (peak day). Mice receiving FMP-MR-5, FMP-MR-10, i.e., groups 2 and 3 respectively, showed bacterial loads which instead were 7 log CFUs/ml on day 1 and day 3 followed by a significant decline ($P < 0.05$) to 3 logs on day 10 and sterile wounds by day 15 (**Table 1**). However, mice treated with cocktail, i.e., FCP showed higher reduction in bacterial burden as compared to infection control as well as monophage treated mice on all days. A significant decrease of 3 log ($P < 0.05$) was observed in cocktail treated group on days 3 and 5 as compared to infection control. Clarithromycin treated mice also showed significant reduction on all days with sterile wounds obtained by day 10.

Phage titer for Study 1 is shown in **Figure 2** was also determined on subsequent days post-treatment. Although an initial titer of 10^9 PFU/50 μl (MOI 10) was administered at the wound site, maximum titer of 10^5 PFU/ml was estimated on day 1, which shows a 4 log reduction from the initial phage titer. This phage count was consistent (approximately 10^5 PFU/ml) in all the groups on days 1 and 3, followed by gradual decline on subsequent days with minimum count of 10^2 PFU/ml present on day 10. However, phage titer was higher on all days in the wound of mice receiving FCP as compared to monophage treated animals. No phage particles were detected in the wound of mice receiving either single or cocktail of phages by day 15.

Results in **Table 2** for Study 2 show that the wounds of mice in the infection control (group 1) also had consistently higher bacterial burden (8–9 log CFU/ml) till day 5 followed by decline from day 7 onwards. In FCP treated mice, a significant decrease of 3 log CFU/ml occurred on day 3 and day 5 itself as compared to untreated mice. However, bacterial load (2.21 log CFU/ml) was detected even by day 10. In case of LCP treated mice maximum reduction in bacterial load equivalent to ~4 log CFU/ml ($P < 0.05$) was seen on day 3 (peak day of infection). Negligible counts were obtained on day 7 and this correlated well with visible reduction in wound size by day 7 (**Figure 3**). The wound showed complete healing within 9 days unlike 20 days and less than 15 days required for untreated surviving diabetic mice and FCP treated group, respectively. Animals receiving clarithromycin showed higher reduction in bacterial burden on all days as compared to FCP treated mice

TABLE 1 | Bacterial load (in terms of Log CFU/ml) in skin wound of *S. aureus* 43300 (10^8 CFU/50 μl) infected diabetic BALB/c mice following treatment with FMP (MR-5 and MR-10), FCP and clarithromycin (10 mg/kg/ per i.p.).

Treatment groups (*n* = 14, each group)	Bacterial load (Log CFU/ml) on				
	Day 1	Day 3	Day 5	Day 7	Day 10
Infection control (group 1)	8.37 ± 0.07	9.24 ± 0.26	8.44 ± 0.40	6.84 ± 0.08	NA
FMP-MR-5 (group 2)	7.67 ± 0.8	7.2 ± 0.20	6.29 ± 0.17	5.21 ± 0.38	3.2 ± 0.54
FMP-MR-10 (group 3)	7.69 ± 0.14	7.11 ± 0.20	6.23 ± 0.15	5.14 ± 0.25	3.11 ± 0.31
FCP (group 4)	7.24 ± 0.25	6.83 ± 0.28	5.2 ± 0.40	4.42 ± 0.14	2.10 ± 0.36
Clarithromycin (group 5)	7.16 ± 0.40	6.5 ± 0.36	4.82 ± 0.07	3.18 ± 0.10	(–)

Treatment was given after 30 min of wound inoculation. (–): zero bacterial count; NA: no mice available for determining the wound bio-burden. All values represent mean ± standard error of the mean calculated from three independent values.

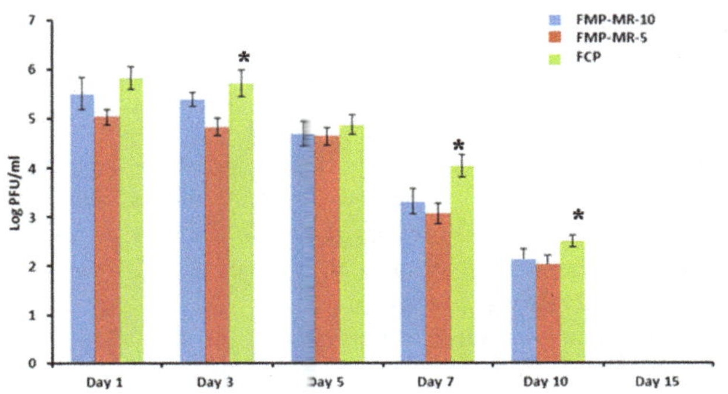

FIGURE 2 | Phage titer (Log PFU/ml) in the wound of *Staphylococcus aureus* 43300 (10^8 CFU/50 μl) infected mice (*n* = 14, each group) following treatment with FMP-MR-10, FMP-MR-5, and FCP on different days post-infection. Error bars represent the standard deviation (SD) from three independent values. $^*P < 0.05$ indicate statistical significant differences (Student's *t*-test) between FMP and FCP treated groups.

and reduction in bacterial load was comparable to that seen in LCP treated animals.

Phage titer in Study 2 in terms of log PFU/ml (**Figure 4**) was maximum on day 1 and thereafter a decrease was noticed on subsequent days in both FCP and LCP treated groups. Maximum titer of 7.45 and 7.12 log PFU/ml on day 1 and day 3 was seen in liposome phage entrapped cocktail (LCP) treated mice as compared to 5.80 and 5.68 log PFU/ml present on day 1 and day 3 in FCP treated group. A decline was seen thereafter due to clearance of its host bacteria as no phage particles were obtained on day 15 and after day 10 with FCP and LCP treated groups, respectively. This shows that entrapment of liposomes led to a significant increase in phage titer by 2 log ($P < 0.05$) at the wound site, which explains the faster wound healing process.

Additional Parameters (Study 2)

Wound contraction

Wound area of all the animal groups was measured with the help of vernier caliper (**Figure 5**). In untreated mice (group 1), an initial wound size of 5 mm persisted until day 3 and it was finally resolved by day 20. In FCP treated animals wound contraction was comparatively slower with wound of 3 mm size evident by day 5 and even by day 12 a wound size of 0.5 mm was observed. However, in case of both LCP treated as well as clarithromycin treated animals, significant decrease in wound size was seen by day 3 onwards as compared to both infection control and FCP treated mice. Minimal wound size of less than 1 mm was observed by day 7 with almost complete closure of wound by day 9 in clarithromycin as well as LCP treated mice. Thus wound closure rates were greater given when phages were encapsulated than when they were not.

Myeloperoxidase (MPO) activity

Neutrophils are the first cells to reach the site of infection or inflammation. MPO is then produced by neutrophils into the extracellular space during degranulation. So as to assess the levels of inflammation or bacterial load MPO levels were measured, and results are presented in **Figure 6**. Highest MPO

TABLE 2 | Bacterial load (in terms of Log CFU/ml) in skin wound of *S. aureus* 43300 (10^8 CFU/50 μl) infected diabetic BALB/c mice following treatment with FCP, LCP, and clarithromycin (10 mg/kg/per i.p.).

Treatment groups (*n* = 14, each group)	Bacterial counts (Log CFU/ml) on				
	Day 1	Day 3	Day 5	Day 7	Day 10
Infection control (group 1)	8.39 ± 0.72	9.08 ± 0.32	8.9.32	6.16 ± 0.27	NA
FCP (group 2)	7.22 ± 0.22	6.78 ± 0.30	5.15.38	4.57 ± 0.44	2.21 ± 0.20
LCP (group 3)	6.22 ± 0.20	5.53 ± 0.41	3.28 ± 0.28	1.84 ± 0.17	(–)
Clarithromycin (group 4)	7.04 ± 0.15	6.28 ± 0.17	4.75 ± 0.45	2.92 ± 0.30	(–)

Treatment was given after 30 min of wound inoculation. (–): zero bacterial count; NA: no mice available for determining the wound bio-burden. All values represent mean ± standard error of the mean calculated from three independent values.

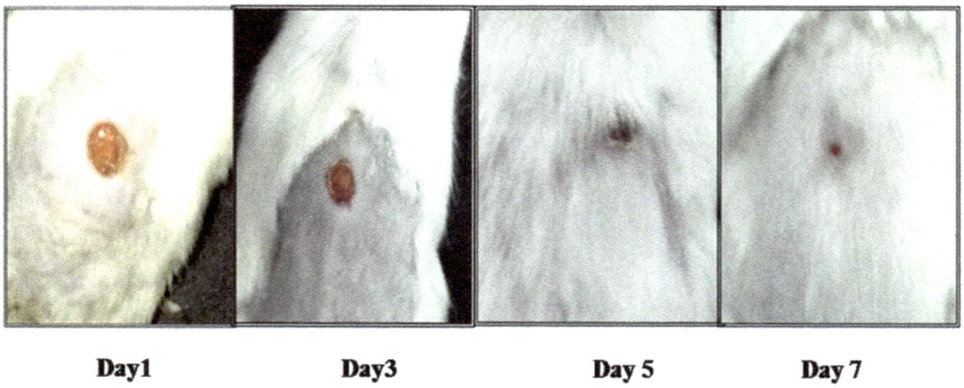

FIGURE 3 | Pictorial representation of wound healing in diabetic BALB/c mice infected with 10^8 CFU/50 μl dose of *S. aureus* 43300 and treated with LCP.

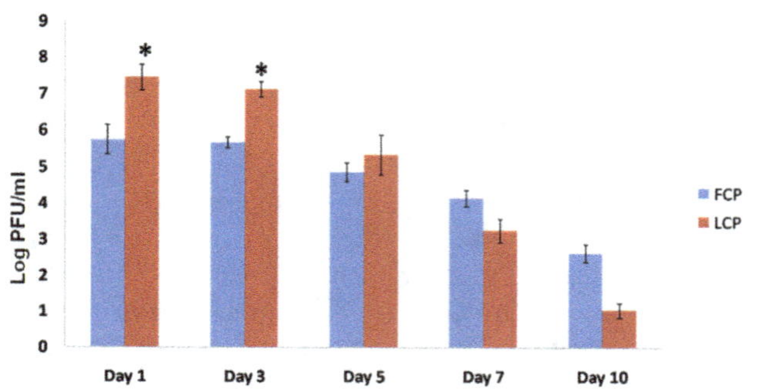

FIGURE 4 | Phage titer (Log PFU/ml) present in the wound of *S. aureus* 43300 (10^8 CFU/50 μl) infected mice (n = 14, each group) following treatment with FCP and LCP on different days post-infection. Error bars represent the standard deviation (SD) from three independent values. $^*P < 0.05$ indicate statistical significant differences (Student's *t*-test) between FCP and LCP treated groups.

levels were present in untreated animals on all days with peak MPO activity of 2.81 units/ml recorded on day 3, that decreased on subsequent days. In case of FCP treated mice, peak MPO activity of 2.41 units/ml was observed on day 1, followed by significant decline thereafter as compared to untreated mice with minimal value of less than 1 unit/ml measured on day 10. However, maximum reduction in MPO levels was seen in mice receiving LCP as it showed peak MPO levels of 1.77 units/ml on day 1 with minimum MPO activity of 0.211 units/ml recorded on day 7 which is significantly less ($P < 0.05$) than activity present in untreated and FCP treated mice Lower levels of MPO activity observed on subsequent days in LCP treated group correlated well with lesser bacterial load seen after treatment. Clarithromycin treated mice also showed significant reduction ($P < 0.05$) in MPO enzyme activity as compared to infection control group and FCP treated group. Thus, these results indicate that neutrophil migration was maximum in untreated animals, while neutrophil migration upon phage and antibiotic treatment decreased due to the decrease in bacterial infection at the site.

Masson's trichrome staining

Wound tissue was taken on day 5 post-infection from all the groups. The tissue of untreated diabetic mice showed little collagen formation as seen in **Figure 7A**. The faint green area seen in the figure depicts early stages of collagen formation. Mostly, growing fibroblast was present in between the majority of blood vessels, capillaries and inflammatory cells, but much less mature collagen fibers were visible with fibroblastic condensation, showing delayed and early stage of wound healing. FCP treated mice (**Figure 7B**) showed growing fibroblasts present between blood vessels and inflammatory cells and thin collagen fibrils, which is an intermediate stage of collagen formation, were common. Mature collagen was also present. The amount of collagen formed was comparatively greater than the untreated mice and less than the cocktail and antibiotic treated groups. LCP treated animals showed maximum formation of mature collagen among all the groups (**Figure 7C**). As is clearly evident that collagen recovered from individual thin fibrils in the dermis into thick bundles or fibers, indicating that mostly mature collagen was present. This correlated well with the less bacterial bioburden on day 5. Together with decreased vascularity and reduced inflammatory cells, the results suggest late stage of wound healing because collagen formation is one of the essential markers of wound healing. Clarithromycin treated animal group also showed presence of mature thick collagen fibers but thin collagen fibrils were comparatively more than LCP treated mice (**Figure 7D**).

Histopathological examination

For histopathological examination, wound tissue was taken on day 5 in order to study tissue damage and extent of wound healing in all the groups. **Figure 8A** depicts wound tissue of untreated animals (group 1). Acute inflammation associated with surface ulceration and breached epidermal layer was seen. A zone of acute inflammatory (AI) reaction with large numbers of infiltrating inflammatory cells and development of vascular granulation tissue (GT) showing large number of capillaries, blood vessels, and inflammatory cells is also visible. But mice receiving FCP (group 2) showed formation of epidermal buds extending toward dermis (**Figure 8B**), growing fibroblasts

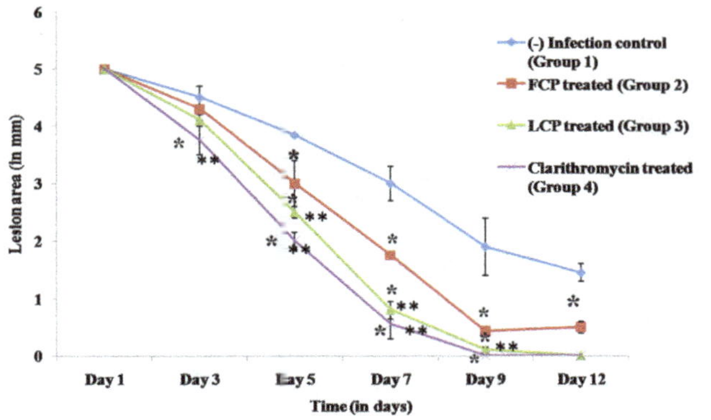

FIGURE 5 | Biometric analysis (mm) of wound area of *S. aureus* 43300 (10^8 CFU/50 μl) infected animals (n = 14, each group) following treatment with FCP, LCP, and clarithromycin. Lesion area was measured on various days post-infection. Error bars represent the standard deviation (SD) from three independent values. *P < 0.05 indicate statistical significant differences (Student's t-test) between infected control and treated groups. **P < 0.05 indicate statistical significant differences between FCP treated and other treated groups (i.e., LCP and clarithromycin treated).

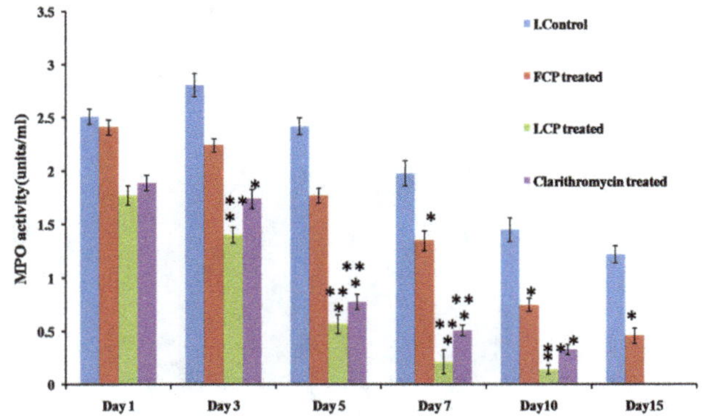

FIGURE 6 | Comparison of MPO levels in the wound tissue of *S. aureus* 43300 (10^8 CFU/50 μl) infected animals (n = 14, each group) following treatment with LCP, FCP, and clarithromycin on different days post-infection. Error bars represent the standard deviation (SD) from three independent values. *P < 0.05 indicate statistical significant differences (Student's t-test) between infected control and treated groups. **P < 0.05 indicate statistical significant differences between FCP treated and other treated groups (i.e., LCP and clarithromycin treated).

in the granulation tissue and collagen formation, indicating healing along with presence of less inflammatory cells. Hair follicles were also visible indicating regeneration of damaged skin. Similarly, clarithromycin treated mice (group 4) showed progressively reduced inflammation with few neutrophils present in the wound tissue (**Figure 8E**). Presence of granulation tissue with fibroblasts, collagen formation, and epidermal buds indicated rapid and significant wound healing in clarithromycin treated group. However, maximum healing with minimum tissue infiltration and damage was clearly visible in the wound tissue of mice treated with LCP as compared to free phage cocktail treated groups (**Figures 8C,D**). In LCP treated group a thick eschar (Ec) over the surface consisting of necrosed cells in dense eosinophillic coagulated protein background was visible. Epidermal healing was accompanied with hyperplasia of epidermis with buds and streaks extending deep into the dermis. Fewer growing fibroblasts and mostly collagen was seen in the granulation tissue with decreased vascularity and reduced inflammatory cells. Presence of hair follicles was also evident. These results indicate significant wound healing by day 5. This effect might be due to the higher number of phages present at the wound site as compared to phage titre in case of FCP treated animals.

DISCUSSION

Bacteriophage therapy represents an attractive treatment option for the eradication of *S. aureus* induced diabetic wound infections. Sunagar et al. (2010) reported significant protection in diabetic mice (90% survival rate) from lethal bacteremia following single injection of *S. aureus* specific phage (phage GRCS). Similarly, Vinodkumar et al. (2011) demonstrated that wounds of diabetic rats which were infected with *S. aureus* were sterilized within 8 days after receiving monophage treatment. Chhibber et al. (2013) focused on the synergistic use of phage and antibiotic in the effective resolution of hindpaw infection in diabetic mice. However, in all of these studies monophage therapy was employed. Monophage based therapies suffer from the drawback of easy emergence of phage resistant bacterial mutants as well as their inability to cover a broad range of possible host targets (Scott et al., 2007; Labrie et al., 2010; Chadha et al., 2016). Thus, use of phage cocktail by incorporating different phages covering the broad host range can provide an effective solution that can be readily delievered without any delay, making it potentialy more effective clinically than monophage therapy (Chan et al., 2013).

In the present study, two already characterized *S. aureus* specific lytic phages, i.e., MR-5 and MR-10 (Kaur et al., 2012; Chhibber et al., 2013) belonging to *Myoviridae* family, were used to study therapeutic efficacy in resolving diabetic wound infection. The main focus of this study was to overcome two major drawbacks of phage therapy. Firstly, therapeutic efficacy of phage cocktail therapy (FCP) was studied and compared with monophage therapy in treatment of MRSA mediated wound infection. The results indicated that when phages were used singly or in cocktail (FCP) there was 100% protection as compared to untreated controls. However, more rapid reduction in bioburden and faster wound healing with FCP treated animals.

Secondly, the problem of potentially low phage retention and persistence *in vivo* was addressed by the use of lipid based carriers, i.e., liposomes. On studying the phage titer post-infection, it was found that phage titer dropped to 10^5 PFU/ml from an initial titer of 10^9 PFU/50 μl within 24 h of phage administration, resulting in presence of low phage number around the wound site. This low titer could be due to phage inactivation by skin's extensive armamentarium of immune-competent cells, that contributed toward delayed phage effect

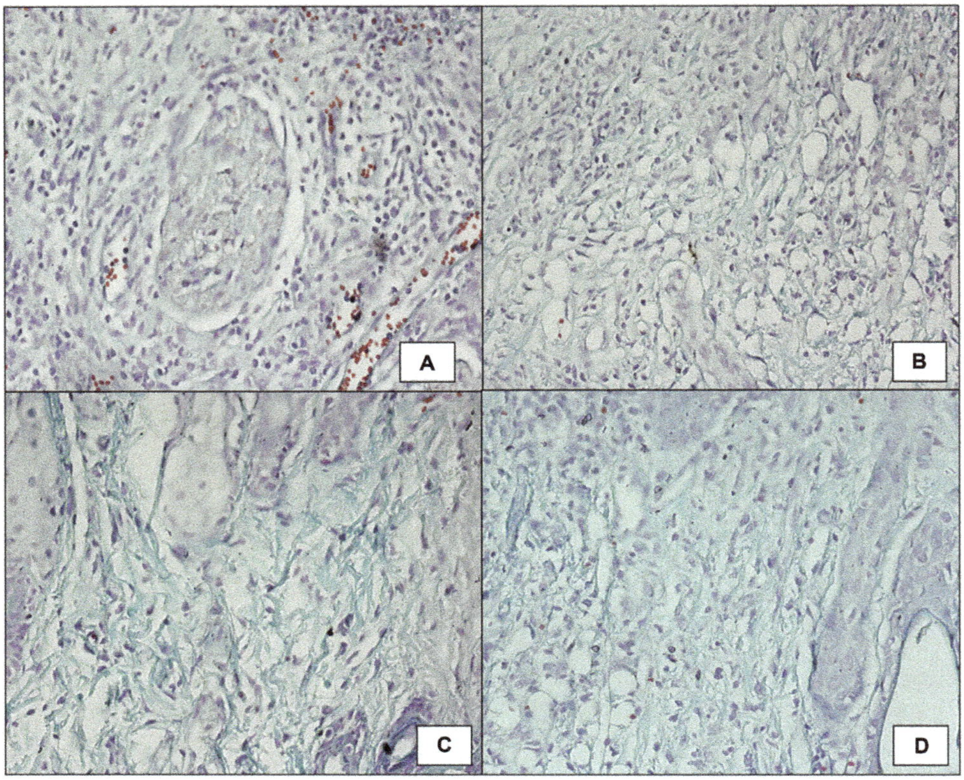

FIGURE 7 | Masson's Trichrome staining (100X) showing collagen formation on day 5 post-infection and treatment in wound tissue of **(A)** infected control mice (diabetic untreated mice) showed fibroblastic condensation along with infiltration of neutrophils. **(B)** Mice treated with FCP showed intermediate stage of collagen formation along with presence of mature collagen fibrils. **(C)** Mice treated with LCP showed thin fibrils of mature collagen present with decreased vascularity and reduced inflammatory cells. **(D)** Mice treated with clarithromycin showed negligible inflamation along with presence of mature collagen fibers, indicating significant wound healing.

(Merril et al., 1996; Keen, 2012; Abedon et al., 2014). The wound bio-burden initially increased as only 10^5 phages were present at the wound site on day 1. The lower number of phage particles probably was unable to tackle the high bacterial load of actively multiplying bacterial population. But as phage growth occurred at the expense of host bacteria, this prevented further increases in bacterial count. This delayed protective response needs to be addressed by preventing rapid phage inactivation and clearance from infection site. Although past workers have made attempts to overcome this problem, however, each approach has its own limitations.

Liposome Entrapment

Our laboratory has for the first time reported successful entrapment of phages within suitable lipid based delivery system, i.e., liposomes that are biocompatible and help to maintain phage titer within *in vivo* system (Singla et al., 2015; Chadha et al., 2017). In another study, encapsulation of *Salmonella* specific phages led to increased stability, prolonged intestinal residence and enhanced therapeutic efficacy (Colom et al., 2015). Liposomes have been regarded as effective DDS due to their GRAS (generally regarded as safe) status, high biocompatibility and high diffusivity in skin as compared to bare drugs (Verma et al., 2003). For drug delivery application liposomes are usually unilamellar and range in diameter from 100 to 300 nm. Large liposomes are rapidly removed from the blood circulation (Barenholz, 1998). Therefore, it is very important to optimize the liposome formulation in terms of size so as to maximize drug loading and minimize leakage and rapid clearance from body. Finally, the cocktail of phages MR-5 and MR-10 (10^9 PFU/50 μl) (1:1) was entrapped within the liposome after optimizing the conditions required for their production and stability. Cocktail entrapped liposomal formulation (LCP) was of unilamellar nature, devoid of any observed aggregation, having a size of 212 nm and exhibited high entrapment efficiency of 87%. Stability studies in terms of size were conducted over a 9 week long period at different temperatures. The liposomal formulation was found to be most stable at 4°C without any physical changes or reduction in number of entrapped phages during storage period. However, at 37°C, an increase in particle size and aggregation was seen in the suspension. Leakage of entrapped drug from the liposomal formulation during storage before administration can lead to poor action of the administered drug (Nallamothu et al., 2006). The results are in consonance with the previous findings of Parmar et al. (2010) who showed that high temperature caused increase in size and aggregation

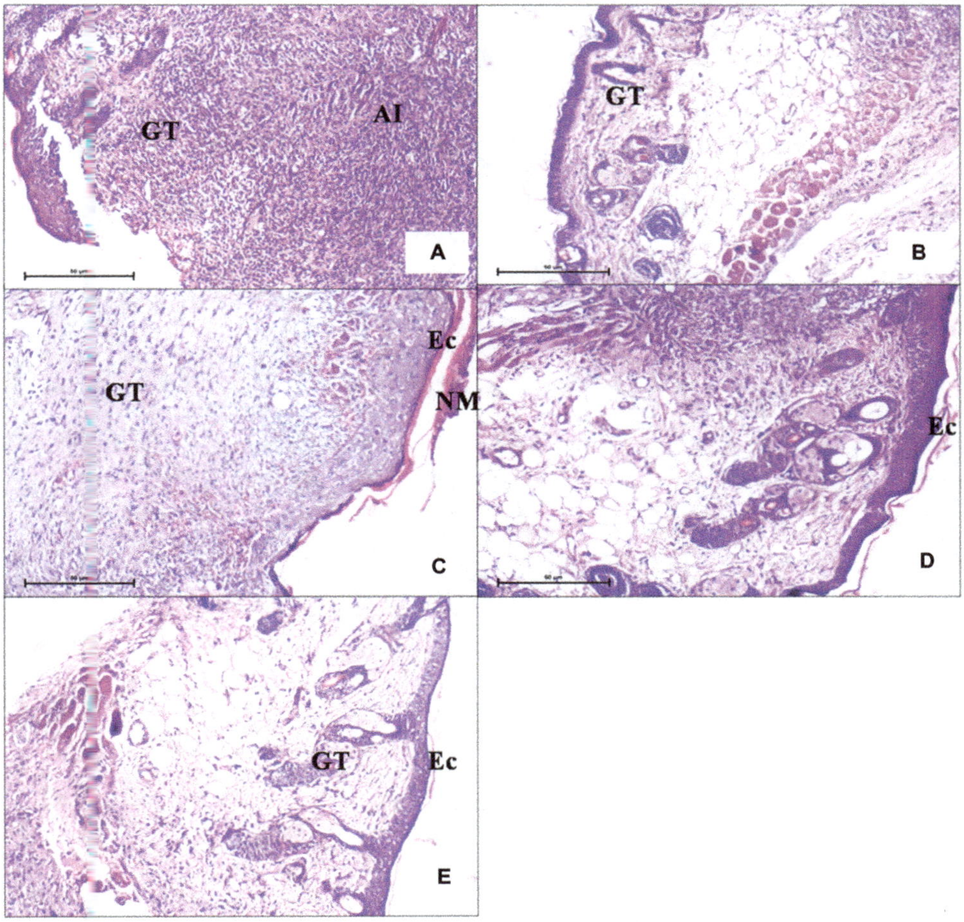

FIGURE 8 | Photomicrographs of wound tissue of **(A)** an infection control mice (diabetic untreated mice) (H and E 100X) showed presence of acute inflammation. **(B)** Mice treated with FCP showed less infiltration of neutrophils and presence of granulation tissue **(C,D)** Mice treated with LCP showed epidermal hyperplasia coupled with reduced inflammation. **(E)** Mice treated with clarithromycin showed nearly normal epidermis with granulation tissue and sweat glands, indicating wound healing (GT, granulation tissue; AI, acute inflammatory; NM, necrotic material; EC, eschar).

as well as leakage of drug from liposomal formulation of budesonide.

The therapeutic efficacy of LCP was evaluated in Study 2. The wound bio-burden correlated well with the visible healing of the wound. No mortality occurred in any of the treatment groups. Maximum reduction was obtained on day 3 in mice treated with liposome entrapped cocktail as compared to infection control group. The entire process of wound healing and re-epithelization was faster and quicker in mice receiving LCP as compared to both untreated diabetic mice as well as animals that received FCP. No phage was present after day 10 in the wound tissue. However, phage titer was higher on all subsequent days in mice treated with liposome entrapped phage cocktail. A significant enhancement of 2 log was observed in LCP mice, clearly indicating that drop in initial titer and phage viability could be prevented by phage entrapment within liposomes. Also, as noted, workers in the past have shown that use of DDS improves the pharmacokinetics and bio-distribution of the associated drug (Allen and Cullis, 2004; Zhang et al., 2013). In addition, efficient uptake of encapsulated bacteriophage by eukaryotic cells has also been reported (Nieth et al., 2015; Singla et al., 2016).

Faster Wound Healing

Wound contraction also demonstrated comparatively rapid healing (measured in terms of wound size) in all the treated groups as compared to infection control mice. Less number of days required for healing and obtaining sterile wounds was due to increased phage titer at wound site in LCP treated mice. Liposomes provided a depot effect and prevented phages from getting cleared off rapidly from the site. This rapid wound healing by day 9 also correlated well with the maximum deposition of mature collagen fiber in wound tissue by day 5 in animals treated with LCP. Mature collagen is an essential marker of wound healing and represents later stages of wound healing (Braiman-Wilksman et al., 2007; Suvik and Effendy, 2012). Histopathological examination of wound tissue of animals also supported these findings, and confirmed that those mice that received LCP showed minimal tissue damage and inflammation as compared to other groups. Epidermal healing and good amount of granulation tissue indicated significant wound healing by day 5. Besides this, maximum decrease in tissue MPO levels was also seen in group receiving LCP. This could be due to the broad spectrum effect of phage cocktail against MRSA, which efficiently arrested growth of invading bacteria at the site of injury, leading to decrease in neutrophil accumulation that correlated well with tissue healing.

From these observations it is concluded that although FCPs is a better option than monophage therapy, rapid inactivation of phages subsequently affects their ability in clearing the infectious agent. Liposomes are suitable delivery systems that help to increase the therapeutic efficacy of phages by improving their stability and delayed clearance by allowing timely release of phages at the infection site, leading to faster healing. The findings of this study thus provide new insights in the treatment of diabetic wound infection not explored by past workers. The use of liposome entrapped phage preparation is an attractive option.

AUTHOR CONTRIBUTIONS

SC: conceived and designed the experiments/contributed reagents/materials/analysis tools. JK and SK: performed the experiments. SC and SK: analyzed the data. SC, JK, and SK: wrote the paper.

FUNDING

This work was supported by Department of Microbiology, Panjab University, Chandigarh, DST-PURSE and UGC-SAP, New Delhi.

REFERENCES

Abedon, S. T., Kuhl, S. J., Blasdel, B. G., and Kutter, E. M. (2014). Phage treatment of human infections. *Bacteriophage* 1, 66–85. doi: 10.4161/bact.1.2.15845

Allen, T. M., and Cullis, P. R. (2004). Drug delivery systems: entering the mainstream. *Science* 303, 1818–1822. doi: 10.1126/science.1095833

Axelrod, L. (1985). Infections in the diabetic patients. *Clin. Diabetes* 3:98.

Bader, M. S. (2008). Diabetic foot infection. *Am. Fam. Physician* 78, 71–79.

Barenholz, Y. (1998). "Design of liposome-based drug carriers: from basic research to application as approved drugs," in *Medical Applications of Liposomes*, eds D. D. Lasic and D. Papahadjopoulos (New York, NY: Elsevier Science BV), 545–565.

Barrow, P. A., and Soothill, J. S. (1997). Bacteriophage therapy and prophylaxis: rediscovery and renewed assessment of potential. *Trends Microbiol.* 5, 268–271. doi: 10.1016/S0966-842X(97)01054-8

Bhatia, A., Kumar, R., and Katare, O. P. (2004). Tamoxifen in topical liposomes: development, characterization and in-vitro evaluation. *J. Pharm. Pharm. Sci.* 7, 252–259.

Braiman-Wilksman, L., Solomonik, R. S., and Tennenbaum, T. (2007). Novel insights into wound healing sequence of events. *Toxicol. Pathol.* 35, 767–779. doi: 10.1080/01926230701584189

Brans, T. A., Dutrieux, R. P., Hoekstra, M. J., Kreis, R. W., and du Pont, J. S. (1994). Histopathological evaluation of scalds and contact burns in the pig model. *Burns* 20, 48–51. doi: 10.1016/0305-4179(94)90090-6

Bull, J. J., Levin, B. R., DeRouin, T., Walker, N., and Bloch, C. A. (2002). Dynamics of success and failure in phage and antibiotic therapy in experimental infections. *BMC Microbiol.* 2:35. doi: 10.1186/1471-2180-2-35

Capparelli, R., Parlato, M., Borriello, G., Salvatore, P., and Iannelli, D. (2007). Experimental phage therapy against *Staphylococcus aureus* in mice. *Antimicrob. Agents Chemother.* 51, 2765–2773. doi: 10.1128/AAC.01513-06

Carlton, R. M., Noordman, W. H., Biswas, B., de Meester, E. D., and Loessner, M. J. (2005). Bacteriophage P100 for control of *Listeria monocytogenes* in foods: genome sequence, bioinformatic analyses, oral toxicity study, and application. *Regul. Toxicol. Pharmacol.* 43, 301–312. doi: 10.1016/j.yrtph.2005.08.005

Chadha, P., Katare, O. P., and Chhibber, S. (2016). In vivo efficacy of single phage versus phage cocktail in resolving burn wound infection in BALB/c mice. *Microb. Pathog* 99, 68–77. doi: 10.1016/j.micpath.2016.08.001

Chadha, P., Katare, O. P., and Chhibber, S. (2017). Liposome loaded phage cocktail: enhanced therapeutic potential in resolving *Klebsiella pneumoniae* mediated burn wound infections. *Burns* 43, 1532–1543. doi: 10.1016/j.burns.2017.03.029

Chan, B. K., Abedon, S. T., and Loc-Carrillo, C. (2013). Phage cocktails and the future of phage therapy. *Future Microbiol.* 8, 769–783. doi: 10.2217/fmb.13.47

Chhibber, S., Kaur, T., and Kaur, S. (2013). Co-therapy using lytic bacteriophage and linezolid: effective treatment in eliminating methicillin resistant *Staphylococcus aureus* (MRSA) from diabetic foot infections. *PLoS One* 8:e56022. doi: 10.1371/journal.pone.0056022

Colom, J., Cano-Sarabia, M., Otero, J., Cortés, P., Maspoch, D., and Llagostera, M. (2015). Liposome-encapsulated bacteriophages for enhanced oral phage therapy against *Salmonella* spp. *Appl. Environ. Microbiol.* 81, 4841–4849. doi: 10.1128/AEM.00812-15

Fish, R., Kutter, E., Wheat, G., Blasdel, B., Kutateladze, M., and Kuhl, S. (2016). Bacteriophage treatment of intransigent diabetic toe ulcers: a case series. *J. Wound Care* 25, 27–33. doi: 10.12968/jowc.2016.25.Sup7.S27

Fukui, T., Kawaguchi, A. T., Takekoshi, S., Miyasaka, M., and Tanaka, R. (2012). Liposome-encapsulated hemoglobin accelerates skin wound healing in mice. *Artif. Organs* 36, 161–169. doi: 10.1111/j.1525-1594.2011.01371.x

Goodridge, L., Gallacci, A., and Griffiths, M. W. (2003). Morphological, host range and genetic characterization of two coliphages. *Appl. Environ. Microbiol.* 69, 5364–5371. doi: 10.1128/AEM.69.9.5364-5371.2003

Greenberger, M. J., Strieter, R. M., Kunkel, S. L., Danforth, J. M., Laichalk, L. L., McGillicuddy, D. C., et al. (1996). Neutralization of macrophage inflammatory protein-2 attenuates neutrophil recruitment and bacterial clearance in murine *Klebsiella pneumonia*. *J. Infect. Dis.* 173, 159–165. doi: 10.1093/infdis/173.1.159

Gregoriadis, G. (1995). Engineering liposomes for drug delivery: progress and problems. *Trends Biotechnol.* 13, 527–537. doi: 10.1016/S0167-7799(00)89017-4

Gulati, M., Grover, M., Singh, M., and Singh, S. (1998). Study of azathioprine encapsulation into liposomes. *J. Microencapsul.* 15, 485–494. doi: 10.3109/02652049809006875

Hanlon, G. W. (2007). Bacteriophages: an appraisal of their role in the treatment of bacterial infections. *Int. J. Antimicrob. Agents* 30, 118–128. doi: 10.1016/j.ijantimicag.2007.04.006

Hsieh, S. E., Lo, H. H., Chen, S. T., Lee, M. C., and Tseng, Y. H. (2011). Wide host range and strong lytic activity of *Staphylococcus aureus* lytic phage Stau2. *Appl. Environ. Microbiol.* 77, 756–761. doi: 10.1128/AEM.01848-10

Hua, S. (2015). Lipid-based nano-delivery systems for skin delivery of drugs and bioactives. *Front. Pharmacol.* 6:219. doi: 10.3389/fphar.2015.00219

Kaur, S., Harjai, K., and Chhibber, S. (2012). Methicillin-resistant *Staphylococcus aureus* phage plaque size enhancement using sublethal concentrations of antibiotics. *Appl. Environ. Microbiol.* 78, 8227–8233. doi: 10.1128/AEM.02371-12

Kaur, S., Harjai, K., and Chhibber, S. (2014). Bacteriophage mediated killing of *Staphylococcus aureus in vitro* on orthopaedic K wires in presence of linezolid prevents implant colonization. *PLoS One* 9:e90411. doi: 10.1371/journal.pone.0090411

Keen, E. C. (2012). Phage therapy: concept to cure. *Front. Microbiol.* 3:238. doi: 10.3389/fmicb.2012.00238

King, L. (2001). Impaired wound healing in patients with diabetes. *Nurs. Stand.* 15, 39–45. doi: 10.7748/ns2001.06.15.38.39.c3039

Kumari, S., Harjai, K., and Chhibber, S. (2009). Efficacy of bacteriophage treatment in murine burn wound infection induced by *Klebsiella pneumoniae*. *J. Microbiol. Biotechnol.* 19, 622–628.

Kumari, S., Harjai, K., and Chhibber, S. (2011). Bacteriophage versus antimicrobial agents for the treatment of murine burn wound infection caused by *Klebsiella pneumoniae* B5055. *J. Med. Microbiol.* 60, 205–210. doi: 10.1099/jmm.0.018580-0

Kurilko, N. L., Kiiamov, A. K. Ivanova, M. A., Pashkov, E. P., Aleksandrov, M. T., Sorokoumova, G. M., et al. (2009). Impact of liposomes and ceftriaxone-entrapped liposomes on skin wound healing in rats. *Antibiot. Khimioter.* 54, 25–30.

Labrie, S. J., Samson, J. E., and Moineau, S. (2010). Bacteriophage resistance mechanisms. *Nat. Rev. Microbiol.* 8, 317–327. doi: 10.1038/nrmicro2315

Langley, R., Kenna, D. T., Vandamme, P., Ure, R., and Govan, J. R. W. (2003). Lysogeny and bacteriophage host range within the *Burkholderia cepacia* complex. *J. Med. Microbiol.* 52, 483–490. doi: 10.1099/jmm.0.05099-0

Loghmani, E. (2005). Diabetes mellitus: type 1 and type 2. *Diabetelogia* 27, 998–1010.

Mathera, C. D., and Loncar, D. (2006). Projections of global mortality and burden of disease from 2002 to 2030. *PLoS Med.* 3:e442. doi: 10.1371/journal.pmed.0030442

Mendes, J. J., Leandro, C. I., Bonaparte, D. P., and Pinto, A. L. (2012). A rat model of diabetic wound infection for the evaluation of topical antimicrobial therapies. *Comp. Med.* 62, 37–48.

Merril, C. R., Biswas, B., Carlton, R., Jensen, N. C., Creed, G. J., Zullo, S., et al. (1996). Long-circulating bacteriophage as antibacterial agents. *Proc. Natl. Acad. Sci. U.S.A.* 93, 3188–3192. doi: 10.1073/pnas.93.8.3188

Nallamothu, R., Wood, G. C., Kiani, M. F., Moore, B. M., Horton, F. P., and Thoma, L. A. (2006). A targeted liposome delivery system for combretastatin A4: formulation optimization through drug loading and *in vitro* release studies. *PDA. J. Pharm. Sci. Technol.* 60, 144–155.

Nieth, A., Verseux, C., Barnert, S., Süss, R., and Römer, W. (2015). A first step toward liposome-mediated intracellular bacteriophage therapy. *Expert Opin. Drug Deliv.* 12, 1411–1424. doi: 10.1517/17425247.2015.1043125

Oladeinde, F. O., Kinyua, A. M., Laditan, A. A., Michellin, R., Bryant, J. L., Denaro, F., et al. (2007). Effect of *Cnidoscolus aconitifolius* leaf extract on the blood glucose and insulin levels of inbred type 2 diabetic mice. *Cell. Mol. Biol.* 53, 34–41.

Pan, D., and Liu, H. (2008). Preventive effect of ordinary and hyperimmune bovine colostrums on mice diabetes induced by alloxan. *Afr. J. Biotechnol.* 7, 4369–4375.

Park, S., Rich, J., Hanses, F., and Lee, J. C. (2009). Defects in innate immunity predispose C57BL/6J-Leprdb/Leprdb mice to infection by *Staphylococcus aureus*. *Infect. Immun.* 77, 1008–1014. doi: 10.1128/IAI.00976-08

Parmar, J. J., Singh, D. J., Hegde, D. D., Lohade, A. A., Soni, P. S., Samad, A., et al. (2010). Development and evaluation of inhalational liposomal system of budesonide for better management of asthma. *Indian J. Pharm. Sci.* 72, 442–448. doi: 10.4103/0250-474X.73916

Pendsey, S. P. (2010). Understanding diabetic foot. *Int. J. Diabetes Dev. Ctries.* 30, 75–79. doi: 10.4103/0973-3930.62596

Powlson, A. S., and Coll, A. P. (2010). The treatment of diabetic foot infections. *J. Antimicrob. Chemother.* 65, 3–9. doi: 10.1093/jac/dkq299

Roesken, F., Uhl, E., Curri, S. B., Menger, M. D., and Messmer, K. (2000). Acceleration of wound healing by topical drug delivery via liposomes. *Langenbecks Arch. Surg.* 385, 42–49. doi: 10.1007/s004230050010

Rogers, L. C., and Bevilacqua, N. J. (2009). *MRSA in Diabetic Foot. Podiatry Managment*. Available at: http://www.podiatrym.com/cme/Nov09CME1.pdf

Scott, A. E., Timms, A. R., Connerton, P. L., El-Shibiny, A., and Connerton, I. F. (2007). Bacteriophage influence *Campylobacter jejuni* types populating broiler chickens. *Environ. Microbiol.* 9, 2341–2353. doi: 10.1111/j.1462-2920.2007.01351.x

Singla, S., Harjai, K., Katare, O. P., and Chhibber, S. (2015). Bacteriophage-loaded nanostructured lipid carrier: improved pharmacokinetics mediates effective resolution of *Klebsiella pneumoniae*-induced lobar pneumonia. *J. Infect. Dis.* 212, 325–334. doi: 10.1093/infdis/jiv029

Singla, S., Harjai, K., Katare, O. P., and Chhibber, S. (2016). Encapsulation of bacteriophage in liposome accentuates its entry in to macrophage and shields it from neutralizing antibodies. *PLoS One* 11:e0153777. doi: 10.1371/journal.pone.0153777

Sunagar, R., Patil, S. A., and Chandrakanth, R. K. (2010). Bacteriophage therapy for *Staphylococcus aureus* bacteremia in streptozotocin-induced diabetic mice. *Res. Microbiol.* 161, 854–860. doi: 10.1016/j.resmic.2010.09.011

Suvik, A., and Effendy, A. W. (2012). The use of modified masson's trichrome staining in collagen evaluation in wound healing study. *Malays. J. Vet. Res.* 3, 39–47.

Verma, D. D., Verma, S., Blume, G., and Fahr, A. (2003). Particle size of liposomes influences dermal delivery of substances into skin. *Int. J. Pharm.* 258, 141–151. doi: 10.1016/S0378-5173(03)00183-2

VinodKumar, C. S., Srinivasa, H., Basavarajappa, K. G., Patil, U., Bandekar, N., and Patil, R. (2011). Abrogation of *Staphylococcus aureus* wound infection by bacteriophage in diabetic rats. *Int. J. Pharm. Sci. Drug Res.* 3, 202–207.

Wild, S., Roglic, G., Green, A., Sicree, R., and King, H. (2004). Global prevalence of diabetes: estimates for the year 2000 and projections for 2030. *Diabetes Care* 27, 1047–1053. doi: 10.2337/diacare.27.5.1047

Wills, Q., Kerrigan, C., and Soothill, J. (2005). Experimental bacteriophage protection against *Staphylococcus aureus* abscesses in a rabbit model. *Antimicrob. Agents Chemother.* 49, 1220–1221. doi: 10.1128/AAC.49.3.1220-1221.2005

Xavier, W., Sukumaran, M. T., Varma, A. K., Kumar, H., and Chellan, G. (2014). Emergence of multi drug resistant bacteria in diabetic patients with lower limb wounds. *Indian J. Med. Res.* 140, 435–437.

Zhang, Y., Chan, H. F., and Leong, K. W. (2013). Advanced materials and processing for drug delivery: the past and the future. *Adv. Drug Deliv. Rev.* 65, 104–120. doi: 10.1016/j.addr.2012.10.003

Zylberberg, C., and Matosevic, S. (2016). Pharmaceutical liposomal drug delivery: a review of new delivery systems and a look at the regulatory landscape. *Drug Deliv.* 23, 3319–3329. doi: 10.1080/10717544.2016.1177136

18

Emerging Strategies to Combat ESKAPE Pathogens in the Era of Antimicrobial Resistance

*Mansura S. Mulani, Ekta E. Kamble, Shital N. Kumkar, Madhumita S. Tawre and Karishma R. Pardesi**

Department of Microbiology, Savitribai Phule Pune University, Pune, India

Correspondence:
Karishma R. Pardesi
karishma@unipune.ac.in

The acronym ESKAPE includes six nosocomial pathogens that exhibit multidrug resistance and virulence: *Enterococcus faecium, Staphylococcus aureus, Klebsiella pneumoniae, Acinetobacter baumannii, Pseudomonas aeruginosa*, and *Enterobacter* spp. Persistent use of antibiotics has provoked the emergence of multidrug resistant (MDR) and extensively drug resistant (XDR) bacteria, which render even the most effective drugs ineffective. Extended spectrum β-lactamase (ESBL) and carbapenemase producing Gram negative bacteria have emerged as an important therapeutic challenge. Development of novel therapeutics to treat drug resistant infections, especially those caused by ESKAPE pathogens is the need of the hour. Alternative therapies such as use of antibiotics in combination or with adjuvants, bacteriophages, antimicrobial peptides, nanoparticles, and photodynamic light therapy are widely reported. Many reviews published till date describe these therapies with respect to the various agents used, their dosage details and mechanism of action against MDR pathogens but very few have focused specifically on ESKAPE. The objective of this review is to describe the alternative therapies reported to treat ESKAPE infections, their advantages and limitations, potential application *in vivo,* and status in clinical trials. The review further highlights the importance of a combinatorial approach, wherein two or more therapies are used in combination in order to overcome their individual limitations, additional studies on which are warranted, before translating them into clinical practice. These advances could possibly give an alternate solution or extend the lifetime of current antimicrobials.

Keywords: ESKAPE, multidrug resistance, alternative therapy, combination therapy, phage therapy, antimicrobial peptides, silver nanoparticles, photodynamic light therapy

INTRODUCTION

Wonder drug penicillin started the era of antibiotics in 1928 and since then it has tremendously developed modern medicine. Persistent use of antibiotics, self-medication, and exposure to infections in hospitals has provoked the emergence of multidrug resistant (MDR) bacteria responsible for 15.5% Hospital Acquired Infection (HAIs) in the world (Rice, 2008; Allegranzi et al., 2011; Ibrahim et al., 2012; Pendleton et al., 2013). The term "ESKAPE" encompasses six such pathogens with growing multidrug resistance and virulence: *Enterococcus faecium, Staphylococcus aureus, Klebsiella pneumoniae, Acinetobacter baumannii, Pseudomonas aeruginosa,* and *Enterobacter* spp. (Rice, 2008). ESKAPE pathogens are responsible for majority of nosocomial infections and are capable of "escaping" the biocidal action of antimicrobial agents (Rice, 2008; Navidinia, 2016).

A systematic review of clinical and economic impact of antibiotic resistance reveals that, ESKAPE pathogens are associated with the highest risk of mortality thereby resulting in increased health care costs (Founou et al., 2017). World Health Organization (WHO) has also recently listed ESKAPE pathogens in the list of 12 bacteria against which new antibiotics are urgently needed (Tacconelli et al., 2018). They describe three categories of pathogens namely critical, high and medium priority, according to the urgency of need for new antibiotics. Carbapenem resistant *A. baumannii* and *P. aeruginosa* along with extended spectrum β-lactamase (ESBL) or carbapenem resistant *K. pneumoniae* and *Enterobacter* spp. are listed in the critical priority list of pathogens; whereas, vancomycin resistant *E. faecium (VRE)* and methicillin and vancomycin resistant *S. aureus* (MRSA and VRSA) are in the list of high priority group. The mechanisms of multidrug resistance exhibited by ESKAPE are broadly grouped into three categories namely, drug inactivation commonly by an irreversible cleavage catalyzed by an enzyme, modification of the target site where the antibiotic may bind, reduced accumulation of drug either due to reduced permeability or by increased efflux of the drug (Santajit and Indrawattana, 2016). They are also able to form biofilms that physically prevent the immune response cells of host as well as antibiotics to inhibit the pathogen. Moreover, biofilms protect specialized dormant cells called persister cells that are tolerant to antibiotics which cause difficult-to-treat recalcitrant infections (Lewis, 2007).

The general antimicrobial therapy to effectively treat infections involves the use of antibiotics either singly or in combination. With every passing year, the overall number of antibiotics effective against ESKAPE is declining, which is predisposing us toward a future with antibiotics that are ineffective. Analysis of the antibiotic lists recommended in the Clinical & Laboratory Standards Institute (CLSI) guidelines revealed that many antibiotics suggested against ESKAPE since 2010 have been deleted with addition of relatively few antibiotics/antibiotic combinations. Furthermore, there are incidences of resistance reported against some of these newly added antibiotics (**Table 1**). It is, therefore, imperative to find alternative ways to treat infections especially those caused by ESKAPE pathogens.

Alternative therapies that are currently in practice or under trial include the use of antibiotics in combination or with adjuvants, bacteriophage therapy, use of antimicrobial peptides, photodynamic therapy, antibacterial antibodies, phytochemicals and nanoparticles as antibacterial agents (Mandal et al., 2014; Kaur, 2016). There are several reviews published which describe alternative/novel therapies against MDR pathogens, however, not many have specifically focused on the ESKAPE group as a whole. These reviews describe the various therapeutic agents used with respect to their dosage, mode of action, pharmacokinetics and pharmacodynamics, stability, and toxicity. Although many alternative therapies reported have shown promising results *in vitro*, their efficacy when applied *in vivo* may not be the same due to one or several limitations. It therefore, becomes necessary to understand the action of these therapeutic agents *in vivo*. This review highlights therapies used to treat ESKAPE infections namely, antibiotics in combination or with adjuvants, bacteriophage therapy, antimicrobial peptides, photodynamic light therapy, and nanoparticles which have received significant attention in the last 5 years. Hereby, we have also tried to include studies especially focusing on *in vivo* efficacy of above mentioned therapy/therapeutic agents, their advantages and limitations. **Figure 1** summarizes the major limitations of each alternative therapy which has been elaborately discussed in the following sections. To improve the efficiency and/or minimize the limitations of any therapy/therapeutic agents, combinatorial approaches are suggested. It involves use of two or more monotherapies together (co-administered, functionalized, or conjugated) which is also further described. Altogether, combinatorial approach could be a prospect for exploring novel alternate solutions against ESKAPE.

ANTIBIOTICS IN COMBINATION

Antibiotics in combination have been tested as a treatment method by a number of researchers because the possibility of a pathogen to develop resistance against a combination of two drugs is much less than that against a single drug. Similarly, the synergistic effect of combined antibiotics is more than that of the individual antibiotic. A combination of drugs also increases the spectrum of coverage (Vazquez-grande and Kumar, 2015) and has been found to be beneficial in severe infections caused by multiple pathogens (Ahmed et al., 2014). Some of these combinations tested against the ESKAPE are listed in **Table 2**. The problem of antibiotic resistance is so severe that it has become necessary to try combinations of the most recently synthesized antibiotics and/or last resort antibiotics to study their potential in antimicrobial therapy. The Gram positive members of the ESKAPE, *E. faecium* and *S. aureus*, have been tested against a combination of fosfomycin and daptomycin which has shown to successfully clear infection (Hall Snyder et al., 2016; Coronado-Álvarez et al., 2018). The former is a broad spectrum antibiotic that has shown promising results against Gram negative bacteria while the latter is a last resort antibiotic used to treat infections caused by *E. faecium* and *S. aureus*. Despite being a resistant pathogen there is a lack of substantial research in antibiotic combination therapy against *E. faecium* over the last 5 years. Most combinations tested against *S. aureus in vitro* include daptomycin or vancomycin with other antibiotics including ceftaroline, a newly added antibiotic to the CLSI guidelines. The effect of these and other such combinations have also been tested in various mouse models which cleared away the *S. aureus* infection with minimal to no toxicity. Colistin (polymyxin E) is the last resort antibiotic prescribed against Gram negative bacilli. In recent years, research has been conducted to treat infections caused by *K. pneumoniae* and *A. baumannii* using a combination of colistin or tigecycline with other antibiotics and has shown promising results *in vitro* and in cohort studies.

Some molecules when combined with antibiotics make an ineffective drug effective. These molecules, named "adjuvants" or "resistance breakers," have little to no antimicrobial activity of their own (González-Bello, 2017) but inhibit the mechanism

TABLE 1 | Antibiotics added/revised and eliminated against ESKAPE from CLSI document M100 since 2010.

Antibiotics added/with revised breakpoint	Tested against pathogen					
	Ef	S	K	A	P	E
Amikacin, Amoxicillin-clavulanate, Ampicillin-sulbactam, Cefaclor, Cefamandole, Cefdinir, Cefmetazole, Cefonicid, Cefotetan, Cefpodoxime, Cefprozil, Cefuroxime, Kanamycin, Loracarbef, Netilmicin, Oxacillin, Tobramycin		0				
Aztreonam			1			1
Cefazolin, Cefepime, Ceftazidime		0	1			1
Cefoperazone, Moxalactam		0			0	
Cefotaxime, Ceftizoxime, Ceftriaxone		0	1		0	1
Ceftaroline		1	1			1
Ceftazidime-avibactam, Ceftolozane-tazobactam			1			1
Cephalothin		0	0			0
Colistin, Piperacillin					1	
Dalbavancin, Telavancin, Oritavancin, Tedizolid	1	1				
Doripenem, Imipenem, Meropenem		0	1	1	1	1
Ertapenem		0	1	1		1
Mezlocillin				0		
Nalidixic acid			0			0
Piperacillin-tazobactam, Ticarcillin-clavulanate		0			1	
Ticarcillin			0	0	0	0

Please note that the table includes ONLY those antibiotics which are deleted or newly added since 2010.

0 = Antibiotics deleted from CLSI guidelines between 2010 and 2018; 1, New antibiotics added in the CLSI guidelines since 2010; 1 = No resistance reported till date; 1 = Resistance reported; Ef, E. faecium; S, S. aureus; K, K. pneumoniae; A, A. baumannii; P, P. aeruginosa; E= Enterobacter spp.

S = (Long et al., 2014; Chan et al., 2015; Nigo et al., 2017); K = (Zowawi et al., 2015; Vuotto et al., 2017; Stanley et al., 2018); A = (Göttig et al., 2014; Goic-Barisic et al., 2017; Nowak et al., 2017; Caio et al., 2018; Chuang and Ratnayake, 2018); P = (Prakash et al., 2014; Gill et al., 2016; Alipour et al., 2017; Mohapatra et al., 2018; Palavutitotai et al., 2018); E = (Lee et al., 2015; Babouee Flury et al., 2016; Zeng et al., 2016; Kulengowski et al., 2018).

of resistance by increasing the uptake of the antibiotic through the bacterial membrane, blocking of efflux pumps, and changing the physiology of resistant cells (i.e., dispersal of biofilms to planktonic cells) (Kalan and Wright, 2011; Bernal et al., 2013). Essential oils and phenothiazines enhance the antimicrobial activity of drugs and also inhibit the transmission of resistance to other populations (Bueno, 2016).

The most popularly known adjuvants are β-lactamase inhibitors while the most recent adjuvant tested to restore meropenem activity is vaborbactam which inhibits *K. pneumoniae* carbapenemase activity (Jorgensen and Rybak, 2018). It has also undergone a clinical trial; registered on ClinicalTrials.gov under identifier NCT02020434; which proved the combination to be safe after testing 41 subjects (Rubino et al., 2018). However, it has a limited inhibition activity as it has been unable to do so with class B and class D β-lactamases. Other β-lactamase inhibitors include avibactam, nacubactam, and tazobactam (Monogue et al., 2018a,b). Metal chelators like EDTA, deferasirox, and deferoxamine also inhibit β-lactamases as these enzymes require metal ions for their activity (Aoki et al., 2010; Santos et al., 2012; Yoshizumi et al., 2013). These chelators have been tested in combination with antibiotics like imipenem, tobramycin, and vancomycin against *S. aureus*, *P. aeruginosa*, and *E. coli* in murine models with successful decrease in bacterial load. Quorum quenchers, molecules that inhibit quorum sensing thereby inhibiting biofilm formation, have also shown potential to cure infection in combination with certain antibiotics (Balamurugan et al., 2015; Chatterjee et al., 2016). 1-[(2,4-Dichlorophenethyl)amino]-3-Phenoxypropan-2-ol is so far the most promising antimicrobial agent as it has been reported to kill not only persister cells of *P. aeruginosa* but also non-persister cells of all the other ESKAPE members. It has also been shown to enhance killing of antibiotic resistant strains in both planktonic and biofilm forms. Its combination with a variety of antibiotics is shown to kill all of the ESKAPE making it an ideal candidate as an adjuvant (Defraine et al., 2017).

Even though there is increased activity of antibiotics when used in combination against pathogens *in vitro*, there are limited studies demonstrating the same *in vivo* and some among those have proven disadvantageous. If monotherapy selects for a narrow spectrum of resistance, a combination of two or more antibiotics selects for a broad spectrum of resistance defeating the purpose of combination therapy entirely (Vestergaard et al., 2016). Certain combinations that are meant to treat infections tend to have the opposite effect resulting in far worse damage. One antibiotic can lead to the induction of a resistance mechanism against a second antibiotic administered in combination leading to antagonistic effect (Fallah, 2018). A clinical trial conducted in Italy in which infections caused by XDR *A. baumannii* were treated with a combination of colistin and rifampin showed no improvement in survival rates. In fact, this combination led

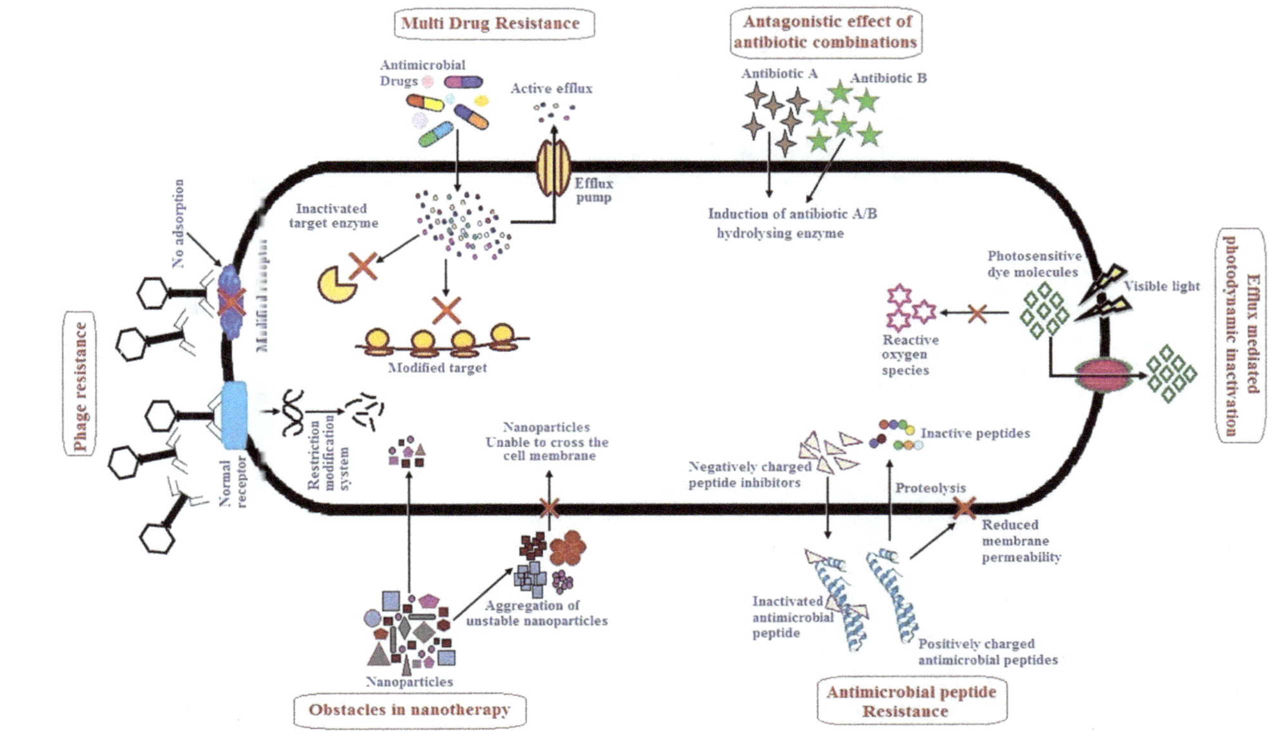

FIGURE 1 | Major challenges of antibacterial monotherapies.

to increased hepatic toxicity (Durante-Mangoni et al., 2013). A similar study using a combination of colistin, tigecycline and carbapenems against *A. baumannii* showed futile results (López-Cortés et al., 2014). Metal chelators have shown to sequester ions not only from bacterial cells but also from host tissue cells (Yoshizumi et al., 2013).

The most recent alternative to antibiotics or their combination that shows a promising future is antibiotic hybrids which have been defined by Domalaon et al. (2018) as synthetic constructs of two or more pharmacophores belonging to an established agent known to elicit a desired antimicrobial effect. This method provides the advantage of combination therapy through the mono therapy approach, where chances of resistance are curbed, while overcoming the problem of non-complementary pharmacodynamic profiles of the individual antibiotics.

The ESKAPE tend to become resistant to either or both antibiotics used in combination with every passing year due not only to natural selection of resistant strains but also horizontal gene transfer from them to sensitive strains. This warrants testing of still new combinations. The result is a never-ending cycle from which there is no escape. It can therefore be concluded that antibiotics in combination may not always be effective and that there is a need for extensive research of alternative strategies.

BACTERIOPHAGE THERAPY

Phages are century old therapeutic agents that were used for the treatment of bacterial infections. The discovery of antibiotics was an influential factor in side-lining this ambition (Mann, 2005). The focus on phage therapy has sharpened ever since antimicrobial resistance has been on a dramatic rise. Lytic phages against ESKAPE pathogens have been isolated from hospital wastewater, making them easily available therapeutic agents (Latz et al., 2016). Bacteriophages used for therapy present many advantages such as high host specificity (prevent damage to normal flora, do not infect the eukaryotic cells), low dosages for treatment, rapid proliferation inside the host bacteria, etc. that make them ideal candidates to treat bacterial infections (Domingo-Calap and Delgado-Martínez, 2018). Unlike antibiotics, the advantage of using phages is that, they develop new infectivity and regain an upper hand over bacteria as they mutate alongside their host (Pirnay et al., 2018).

Several studies carried out *in vitro* have proven phages to be effective as antibacterial agents against biofilm and planktonic cells of ESKAPE (Pallavali et al., 2017; Dvořáčková et al., 2018; Jamal et al., 2019). **Table 2** gives information of phage therapy studied in various animal models as well as recent case studies and case reports of patients infected with ESKAPE pathogens. Phage therapy carried out in animal wound infection models have shown reduced mortality and enhanced wound healing. Additional studies carried out *in vivo* have also demonstrated efficacy and safety (non-toxic with reduced inflammatory responses) of phages used in treatment of bacterial infections.

Phage therapy, though promising, comes with some limitations. It can, however, be overcome by appropriate modifications (Wittebole et al., 2014; El-Shibiny and El-Sahhar,

TABLE 2 | Alternative strategies against ESKAPE pathogens.

Target ESKAPE	Model used	Agent used and dosage details	Route of administration	*In vivo* efficacy: log reduction of pathogen; % survival of host	Other advantages	References
ANTIBIOTICS IN COMBINATION						
Ef	*Galleria mellonella* larvae infection model	Rifampin (0.5–2) μg/ml+Tigecycline (0.03 μg/ml)/Vancomycin (64, 128 μg/ml)/Linezolid (2 μg/ml)	Injection into hemocoel	20–73% survival	–	Skinner et al., 2017
S	Retrospective study 2011–2017	Fosfomycin+Daptomycin/ Oxacillin/Vancomycin	–	Successful treatment in 81% patients	–	Coronado-Álvarez et al., 2018
S	Wistar mouse	Rifampin (20 mg/kg) + Flucloxacillin (200 mg/kg)/ Moxifloxacin (10 mg/mg)	Intraperitoneal (IP)	4 log decrease with both combinations	Antibiofilm	Greimel et al., 2017
S	Wistar rats	Gentamicin (8, 50 mg/kg) + 4-(Benzylamino) cyclohexyl 2-hydroxycinnamate (16, 64 mg/kg)	–	4 log reduction; 100% survival	Antibiofilm	Balamurugan et al., 2015
K	Murine complicated urinary tract infection model	Meropenem (400 mg/kg) + Nacubactam (150 mg/kg)	–	>3 log reduction in isolates resistant to meropenem-nacubactam	–	Monogue et al., 2018a
A	Murine Thigh and Lung Infection Models	Colistin + Tazobactam/Avibactam	IP	No effect	–	Monogue et al., 2018b
P	Murine thigh infection model	Imipenem (4 or 5 g/day with a 1-g loading dose)+ Tobramycin (7 mg/kg)	–	≥2.5 or ≥1.50 log reduction	–	Yadav et al., 2017
P	Murine infection model	Colistin (2.5–5 mg/kg) + Rifampicin (10 mg/kg)	Subcutaneous	~5 log reduction	–	Cai et al., 2018
E	*G.mellonella* infection model	Colistin (2.5 mg/kg) + Imipenem (15 mg/kg)	Injection into hemocoel	80–90% survival	–	Yang et al., 2018a
PHAGE THERAPY						
Ef	Murine bacteraemia model	Phage ENB6 and C3 (A2 morphotype group), of 3×10^8 PFU	IP	Single dose: 50% survival; Multiple doses: 100% survival	Immunocompatible	Biswas et al., 2002
S	65-year-old woman with Corneal abscess	SATA-8505 (ATCC PTA-9476)	Topical (eye drops and nasal spray) and intravenous (IV)	Eradication of pathogen and stabilization of ocular signs	-	Fadlallah et al., 2015
S	Case series (six human subjects suffering from diabetic foot ulcer)	Commercial staphylococcal phage Sb-1; (0.05–0.4 ml of 10^7-10^8 PFU/ml)	Topical	–	Wound healing within 7 weeks	Fish et al., 2016
S	Rabbit osteomyelitis model	Cocktail of phages (SA-BHU1, 2, 8, 15, 21, 37 and 47); 15 μl of 5×10^{12} PFU/ml of each	Intramuscular (IM)	100% survival	Viruses with stable genomic structure	Kishor et al., 2016
S	Murine bacteraemia model	Phage SLPW Podoviridae; 0.2 mL of 1×10^9 PFU	IP	~100% decrease in bacterial count; up to 80% survival	Stable up to 45°C, pH 6-10; Immunocompatible	Wang et al., 2016
S	Murine wound infection model	MR 5 and MR 10, Myoviridae; free phage 10^9 PFU/50 μl and its liposomal formulation	Topical	Up to 3 log reduction on day 10	Wound healing within 7 days	Chhibber et al., 2018

(Continued)

TABLE 2 | Continued

Target ESKAPE	Model used	Agent used and dosage details	Route of administration	*In vivo* efficacy: log reduction of pathogen; % survival of host	Other advantages	References
K	Murine burn wound infection model	Five phages KØ1 to 5 (10^7 PFU/ml) in equal proportion as a cocktail or loaded in liposomes	IP	>4 log reduction; 100% survival	Enhanced wound healing	Chadha et al., 2017
A	Case study 77-year-old man with post-operative infection	Five phages active against 104 *A. baumannii* from the NMRC's phage-Biolog system 2.14×10^7 PFU/mL	Intravenous (IV)	No effect	–	LaVergne et al., 2018
A	Murine wound infection model	Cocktail of AB-Army 1 and AB-Navy 1 to 4 (~4×10^9 PFU)	Topical, IP or loaded on TegadermTM bandage	3 log tested *in vitro*; ND	Antibiofilm; Reduction in wound bio-burden and size (loss of capsule production in phage infected *Acinetobacter*)	Regeimbal et al., 2016
A	Murine wound infection model	Acinetobacter phage- Siphoviridae; (400 µl of 3×10^9 PFU/ml)	Topical	100% clearance of infection in 8 days	Reduction in wound bio-burden but no difference in time required for wound healing	Shivaswamy et al., 2015
A	*G.mellonella* infection model	Phage WCHABP1 and WCHABP12 Myoviridae; 10^4 PFU/larva	Injection into hemocoel	75% survival	No integrase and repressor genes were identified in both bacteriophages	Zhou et al., 2018
A	Case study (68 year old patient with infected diabetic patient)	Cocktails of AB Phage ΦPC (AB-Navy1, 4, 71, 97, and AbTP3Φ1); ~10^9 PFU/dose	Percutaneous catheter, IV	Clearance of infection	–	Schooley et al., 2017
P	Murine infected model	Phage PEV20, Podoviridae; Inhalable powder 2×10^7 PFU/mg	Intranasal and intratracheal	5 log reduction	Non-toxic	Chang et al., 2018
P	Case study (2-year-old boy with a history of DiGeorge syndrome)	Cocktail from US Navy library of bacteriophages 3.5×10^5 every 6 h. six doses total and resumed after 11 days	IV	Blood cultures negative After phage treatment	-	Duplessis et al., 2018
P	Case study (61 year old male patient with acute septicaemia and large necrotic pressure sores)	Phage BFC1 50 µl IV infusion every 6 h for 10 days; Wounds irrigation-50 ml BFC1 every 8 h for 10 days	IV infusion and Topical	Clearance of septicaemia immediately after therapy; pressure sores remained infected with several bacterial species, including *P. aeruginosa*	No adverse effects	Jennes et al., 2017
P	*G.mellonella* infection model	Phage KTN4; MOI100	Injection into hemocoel	4–7 log reduction; 100% survival	Antibiofilm; Stable up to 40–70°C	Danis-Wlodarczyk et al., 2016
E & P	Case series (9 UTI patients)	Pyophage	Pyophage instillation by suprapubic catheter	bacterial titers decreased after bacteriophage treatment in six out of nine patients (67%).	No bacteriophage-associated adverse events detected	Ujmajuridze et al., 2018
S, A, & P	Murine sepsis model	Phage against *A. baumanni*, *P. aeruginosa,* and *S. aureus*	IP	100% reduction in A and P; 100% survival	–	Soothill, 1992; Lin et al., 2017

(Continued)

TABLE 2 | Continued

Target ESKAPE	Model used	Agent used and dosage details	Route of administration	*In vivo* efficacy: log reduction of pathogen; % survival of host	Other advantages	References
K & E	*G. mellonella* infection model	Cocktail of Escherichia phage ECP311, Klebsiella phage KPP235, and Enterobacter phage ELP140	–	100% reduction after 5 doses; 90% survival	–	Manohar et al., 2018
SILVER NANOPARTICLES						
S	Infected *Daniorerio*-Zebrafish model	Sunlight mediated AgNP synthesized using plantextract (HWP AgNP) (10–40 nm)	–	>1 log reduction	Antibiofilm; Non-toxic	Lotha et al., 2018
S	Murine wound infection model	Chitosan-coated AgNPs (10–30 nm) (50 μg/g·bw)	Topical	–	Wound healing within 14 days; Non-toxic	Peng et al., 2017
S	Rabbit flexor tendon rupture model	Core-shell nanofibrous membranes with embedded AgNPs in PEG/poly (caprolactone) shell and hyaluronic acid/ibuprofen in the core	AgNP Coated implant	–	Antibacterial activity; Prevention of peritendinous adhesion after tendon surgery; Non-toxic	Shalumon et al., 2018
S	Murine model	Wound dressing containing nanosilver nanohydrogels (nSnH) along with *Aloe vera*	Topical	–	Antibacterial; Wound healing within 16 days; Non-toxic	Anjum et al., 2016
S	Murine wound infection model	Sodium carboxymethylcellulose hydrogel loaded with PEG-coated-AgNPs (19.2 ± 3.6 nm) (500 μg AgNPs/g of hydrogel)	Topical	97.30% reduction; 100% survival	Wound healing within 10 days	Mekkawy et al., 2017
S	Murine model	Mesoporous silica nanoparticles coated with AgNPs (Ag-MSNs)	Topical	–	Antibacterial; Wound healing within 5 weeks; Anti-inflammatory	Dong et al., 2016
S	Rabbit flexor tendon model	AgNPs embedded in electrospun hyaluronic acid (HA)/polycaprolactone (PCL) nanofibrous membranes (NFMs)	AgNP Coated implant	–	Antibacterial; Prevention of peritendinous adhesion after tendon surgery	Chen et al., 2015
S & P	Murine wound infection model	AgNPs (20 nm)/chitosan composite dressing (0.5 mM)	Topical	–	Wound healing within 8 days; Non-toxic	Liang et al., 2016
S & P	*G. mellonella* model	Electrochemically synthesized AgNPs (8–10 nm) (6.8 and 3.4 mg/mL)	Injected into hemocoel	–	Antibiofilm; Non-toxic	Pompilio et al., 2018
S & P	Murine model	Bilayer composite of Chitosan-AgNPs (5–50 nm) (CS-AgG) on CSGB (*Bletilla striata* polysaccharide) both linked with genipin	Topical	–	Antibacterial; Wound healing; Non toxic	Ding et al., 2017
S & P	Murine model	NanoAg (<50 nm) wound dressings; 100 μL of 1 mg/mL	Topical	–	Antibacterial; Antibiofilm; Biocompatible	Radulescu et al., 2016
S & P	Murine model	Collagen nanofiber mats containing AgNPs (25–55 nm)	Topical	–	Antibacterial; Wound healing within 14 weeks; No hypersensitive; Anti-inflammatory	Rath et al., 2016

(Continued)

TABLE 2 | Continued

Target ESKAPE	Model used	Agent used and dosage details	Route of administration	*In vivo* efficacy: log reduction of pathogen; % survival of host	Other advantages	References
S & P	Gottingen minipigs femur model	Nanocomposite coating formed by polysaccharide 1-deoxylactit-1-yl chitosan (Chitlac) and AgNPs on methacrylate thermosets	AgNP Coated implant	–	Antibiofilm; Anti-inflammatory; Non-toxic	Marsich et al., 2013
ANTIMICROBIAL PEPTIDE (AMP)						
A	Murine infection model	Chex1-Arg20 amide; 2 and 5 mg/kg	IM	>2 log reduction; >50% survival	Anti-inflammatory	Ostorhazi et al., 2018
A	Murine wound infection model	K11, a hybrid peptide of melittin, cecropin A1, and magainin 2	Topical	~100% pathogen clearance; 100% survival	Wound healing (21 days)	Rishi et al., 2018
P	Murine infection model	Feleucin-K3 analogs; 5 mg/kg	IP	~ 1 log reduction	Stable; Low toxicity; Antibiofilm	Xie et al., 2018
S	*G. mellonella* infection model	PT-13, Plant derived crude extract; 64 μM	Injection into hemocoel	60% survival	–	Al Akeel et al., 2018
P	*G. mellonella* infection model	SP-E, a proline-rich pig saliva derived peptide; 6.1 μmol/kg	Injection into hemocoel	~50% survival	Non-toxic	Ciociola et al., 2018
S & A	*S. aureus* murine sepsis model, *A. baumannii* infected murine lung model	D-150–177C, peptide modified by attaching C-terminal Cysteine; 5 and 10 mg/kg	IP	70% survival	Non-toxic	Chen et al., 2018
S & A	Murine skin infection model	SAAP-148, a LL-37 human cathelicidin inspired peptide used to prepare ointment; 0.125 to 0.5% (w/w)	Topical	87% and complete clearance of *S. aureus* and *A. baumannii*, respectively After a single treatment with 2% (w/w) SAAP-148 ointment	Antibiofilm; Kills persister cells; Reducing bioburden and wound healing; Non-toxic	de Breij et al., 2018
P	Murine lung infection model	Esc (1–21)-1c, frog skin derived AMP; 0.1 mg/kg	Intra-tracheal injection	2 log reduction	Anti-inflammatory	Chen et al., 2017
ANTIMICROBIAL LIGHT THERAPY						
S	Murine burn infection model	Laser light-50 J/cm^2; PS-PS-sinoporphyrin sodium (DVDMS)- 2, 5, and 10 μM, 75 min	Topical	4 log reduction at 5 μM of DVDMS with 50 J/cm^2 light	DVDMS promoted wound healing after burn infections	Mai et al., 2017
S	Murine ulcer infection model	Laser light-LED 410 nm, 50 J/cm^2; PS-5-ALA; 200 mg/kg	Topical	2 log reduction	–	Morimoto et al., 2014
S	Murine infection model	Light: 660 nm- 45 J/cm^2- 10 min exposure; household light- 7.5 J/cm^2- 10 min exposure; PS pentalysine-β-carbonylphthalocyanine Zinc (ZnPc(Lys)5)- 5 μl at 1 mM	Topical	44.3% clearance of infection at 7.5 J/cm^2	Improved wound healing	Ullah et al., 2018
A	Murine burn infection model	Light- LED 415 nm 72–360 J/cm^2	Topical	3 log reduction	Antibiofilm	Wang et al., 2017
P	Murine skin abrasion model	Light- 415 nm, 48 J/cm^2	Topical	5 log reduction	–	Amin et al., 2016

Ef, Enterococcus faecium; S, Staphylococcus aureus; K, Klebsiella pneumonia; A, Acinetobacter baumannii; P, Pseudomonas aeruginosa; and E, Enterobacter spp.

2017; Domingo-Calap and Delgado-Martínez, 2018). High specificity of the phages can be considered as both advantageous and a limiting factor. Monophage therapy involves the need to check the efficacy of the phage by testing it *in vitro* against the disease-causing bacteria before applying it to a patient which can be a difficult process. The use of phage cocktails, comprising of a combination of phages acting against different bacterial species or strains, can avoid these problems (Chan et al., 2013). International experts believe that an ideal phage cocktail should be prepared using phages belonging to different families or groups such as having broad host range, high adsorption ability to the highly conserved cell wall structures in bacteria. Using such phage cocktails may reduce the emergence of phage resistant bacterial population. However, others advocate strategies wherein individual active phages are applied sequentially to the patient. In clinical practice, however, it appears to be difficult (Rohde et al., 2018).

Genomic characterization of phages is very important so as to predict their "safety" in therapeutic applications as demonstrated by several experts in this field. Phages can be vectors for horizontal gene transfer in bacteria, sometimes being involved in exchange of virulence or antibiotic resistance genes making a microbe more pathogenic or resistant to an antibiotic (Chen and Novick, 2009). Phages reported for therapeutic applications should not harbor virulence or antibiotic resistance genes as well as integrases, site-specific recombinases, and repressors of the lytic cycle that may accelerate the transfer/integration of these genes in the host bacterial genome. Algorithms that can be used for predicting lifestyle of a phage, and its virulent traits are available but their database needs to be updated with more genome sequences of phages (Mcnair et al., 2012). Two recent reviews excellently describe the work flow to select ideal phage candidates for therapeutic purposes (Casey et al., 2018; Philipson et al., 2018). Recent studies demonstrating *in vivo* efficacy of phages against ESKAPE infections have used fully characterized phages that show no virulence or antibiotic resistance genes, are considered safe as they do not exhibit any allergic or immune response, and are also reported to remain stable at varied pH and temperature which make them ideal candidates for therapy (Fish et al., 2016; Kishor et al., 2016; Wang et al., 2016; Zhou et al., 2018).

Similarly, it has also been reported that the bacterial strains used for phage production should ideally be free of functional prophages. These prophages may get induced and contaminate the phage preparation. However, a recent report discusses the risk benefit evaluation that needs to be done in highly experimental treatments of patients infected with MDR pathogens such as ESKAPE (Rohde et al., 2018).

Another limitation reported is the stability of phages and their proper administration in order to reach the site of action. Phage formulations are ingested orally, administered nasally or applied topically (Malik et al., 2017; Cooper et al., 2018). Studies have shown improved efficacy of phage when entrapped with liposomes (Singla et al., 2016; Chadha et al., 2017; Malik et al., 2017; Chhibber et al., 2018). Phages can be targeted at the infection site in the form of powdered formulations (Chang et al., 2018). Phage derived product like phage encoded lytic enzymes showing function similar to lysozyme can also be used as an antibacterial agent or can be combined with other antimicrobials like antibiotics to improve efficacy of treatment (Lin et al., 2017). A phage derived protein, "endolysin" is reported for its antibacterial and antibiofilm activity against ESKAPE (Viertel et al., 2014; Gong et al., 2016; Rios et al., 2016; Lin et al., 2017; Zhang et al., 2018). V12CBD a recombinant protein derived from bacteriophage lysine, PlyV12, was able to attenuate virulence of *S. aureus,* and enhance its phagocytosis in mice (Yang et al., 2018b).

Several commercial phage preparations which can be used against ESKAPE are available some of which include, "Stafal," "Sextaphage," "PhagoBioDerm," and "Pyophage". Stafal (Bohemia Pharmaceuticals, Slovakia) is an antistaphylococcal phage preparation, Sextaphage (Microgen, ImBio Nizhny Novgorod, Russia) is a cocktail against *P. aeruginosa and E. coli* while, Pyophage (Georgian Eliava Institute of Bacteriophage, Microbiology, and Virology) contains bacteriophages specifically eliminating causative agents of pyoinflammatory and enteric diseases. PhagoBioDerm, a polymeric bandage impregnated with cocktail of phages, ciprofloxacin, and other active ingredients ensured for sustained release of phages to treat ulcers or wound infections caused by *S. aureus* and *P. aeruginosa* (Markoishvili et al., 2002). Clinical potential of these preparations has been investigated further to determine their broad spectrum activity against other strains *in vitro*, *in vivo* efficacy in animal models as well as through several case studies or clinical trials described below.

Recent human case studies involving treatment of ESKAPE associated infections with different phages are described in **Tables 2, 3**. Readers may refer to previous reviews published on phage therapy which have described in numerous studies (Abedon et al., 2011; Chan et al., 2013; Górski et al., 2017; Lin et al., 2017; Sybesma et al., 2018). Most of the case studies report phage therapy given to patients on a compassionate care basis where antibiotic treatment fails.

Several case studies have demonstrated the efficacy of phage therapy in treating patients suffering from eye infections (Fadlallah et al., 2015), pancreatitis (Schooley et al., 2017), diabetic foot ulcer (Fish et al., 2016), and urinary tract infection (Ujmajuridze et al., 2018). Fadlallah et al. (2015), reported a case study of a 65 year old woman suffering from a secondary eye infection by VRSA, treated with a well-characterized commercially available lytic phage, SATA-8505 (ATCC PTA-9476) against MRSA. After 6 months of treatment, the patient was diagnosed as negative for cultures of VRSA. This case study suggests that bacteriophage eye-drops can be used as an alternative treatment of infectious keratitis by MDR pathogens. Fish et al. (2016), reported a case involving nine patients suffering from diabetic foot ulcer, who were treated with a preparation of anti-staphylococcal phages (Sb-1) on a compassionate care basis. The average healing time reported was ~7 weeks. However, one ulcer, with poor vascularity required 18 weeks of treatment. Similarly, Ujmajuridze et al. (2018), reported a preclinical pilot study for a double blind RCT registered at ClinicalTrials: NCT03140085 (Leitner et al., 2017). Pyophage were used in this study to treat nine patients suffering from UTI infections. The first phase

TABLE 3 | Alternative strategies used in combination against ESKAPE pathogens.

Target ESKAPE member	Study model	Agent used and dosage details	Efficacy: log reduction of pathogen using combination; % survival of host, additional advantage	References
PHAGE + ANTIBIOTIC				
P	Case study (76 year old male with postoperative infection after arch replacement surgery)	Phage OMKO1 titer of 10^7 PFU/ml + Ceftazidime (0.2 gm/ml)—10 ml of this combination was injected into the mediastinal fistula which was in continuity with the perigraft collection	Eradication of *the P. aeruginosa* infection	Chan et al., 2018
K	*in vitro*–antibiofilm assay, *in vivo*—murine model (for raising antibodies)	KPO1K2, Podoviridae; free and liposome encapsulated (1.2×10^{13} in 200 µl, MOI = 1) + amikacin (40 µg/ml)	*in vitro*: 94.6% reduction in intracellular pathogen load; Antibiofilm activity (liposome entrapped phage -7 ± 0.1 logs reduction in bacterial count upto day 4 of biofilm formation)	Singla et al., 2016
P	*in vitro*–antibiofilm assay	NP1 and NP3 phages + ceftazidime, ciprofloxacin, colistin, gentamicin or tobramycin	Synergy between phage and ciprofloxacin/ tobramycin reduced bioburden within the biofilm	Chaudhry et al., 2017
P	*in vitro*	Phage PEV20 (10^{10} PFU/mL; MOI 0.1 and 100) + ciprofloxacin, amikacin, aztreonam, colistin or tobramycin	No obvious growth of pathogen throughout 24 h of incubation for ciprofloxacin or amikacin in combination with phage PEV20	Lin Q. et al., 2018
SILVER NANOPARTICLES + ANTIBIOTICS				
A	*in vivo* (murine peritonitis model)	Citrate capped AgNPs (5–12 nm, 2 mg/kg) + Polymyxin B (10 µg/kg)	60% survival; Non-toxic; Anti-inflammatory	Wan et al., 2016
S	*in vitro*	AgNPs (synthesized using two actinobacteria, 5–50 and 5–20 nm) + ampicillin, kanamycin /tetracycline	Antibiofilm; Non toxic	Wypij et al., 2018
A	*in vitro*	AgNPs (synthesized using *A. calcoaceticus*, 8–12 nm) + tetracycline, erythromycin or doxycycline	MBEC of combination with AgNPs was 0.5 mg/ml for doxycycline and 4 mg/mL for erythromycin	Singh et al., 2018
S & P	*in vitro*	AgNPs (synthesized using *Garcinia indica* fruit extract, 5 and 30 nm) + tetracycline	Increase in zone of inhibition in S and P with combination	Sangaonkar and Pawar, 2018
P	*in vitro*	Citrate-capped silver nanoparticles (10 nm and 20 nm) + tobramycin	Antibiofilm activity observed using combination	Habash et al., 2017
S, K, & P	*in vitro*	AgNPs (synthesized using Actinomycetes, 59 and 28 nm) + kanamycin,ampicillin or tetracycline	Increase in zone of inhibition using combination	Golińska et al., 2016
ANTIMICROBIAL PEPTIDES (AMP) + NPS;				
Ef	*in vitro*	Synthetic peptide-immobilized gold nanoparticles; 250 µg/ml	Reduced bacterial load (by 0.4 OD units)	Kuo et al., 2016
S	*in vitro*	AMP TP359 covalently linked to silver coated single walled carbon nanotubes	100% reduction	Chaudhari et al., 2016

(Continued)

TABLE 3 | Continued

Target ESKAPE member	Study model	Agent used and dosage details	Efficacy: log reduction of pathogen using combination; % survival of host, additional advantage	References
S & P	*in vitro*	Paenipeptin analog (synthetic linear lipopeptide analogs) + rifampicin, clarithromycin, or erythromycin	Reduction in cell count of biofilms- *S. aureus*–5 logs and *P. aeruginosa*–3 logs	Moon et al., 2017
K	*in vitro*	SPR741, a cationic peptide derived from Polymyxin B + antibiotics	128-fold reduction in MIC with rifampin and clarithromycin –	Corbett et al., 2017
ANTIMICROBIAL PHOTODYNAMIC LIGHT THERAPY (aPDT) + ANTIBIOTIC				
Ef	*in vivo* (G. mellonella infection model)	Light- 660 ± 15 nm, 0.9 J/cm^2 PS: Methylene blue (MB); Time 30 s + vancomycin-50 mg/kg	100% reduction; ~60% survival	Chibebe Junior et al., 2013
S	*in vitro*	UVC light–254 nm, 6.4 mW + vancomycin (16 μg/mL) or quinupristin/ dalfopristin (32 μg/mL) or linezolid (64 μg/mL)	40% reduction in bacterial load with vancomycin or quinupristin/ dalfopristin and 20% in with linezolid; Synergy reduced viability of cells within the biofilm considerably	El-Azizi and Khardori, 2016
S	*in vitro*	LED light 650 nm, 2.8–22.4 J/cm^2. PS-MB 6.25–400 μg/mL, ciprofloxacin (0.5 μg/mL)	5 log reduction in bacterial load; 4 log reduction in bacterial cell count in biofilm	Ronqui et al., 2016
aPDT + EFFLUX PUMP INHIBITOR				
S	*in vitro*	Light- 22 J/cm^2; PS- MB-200 μg/mL + EPI- verapamil 312 μg/mL	3.38 log reduction in biofilm	de Aguiar Coletti et al., 2017
S	*in vitro and in vivo* (Murine wound infection model)	aPDT using NorA EPI-MB hybrid, INF55-(Ac)en-MB	*in vitro*: 6 log reduction; *in vivo*: 100% reduction within 4 days; enhanced wound healing	Rineh et al., 2017
A	*in vitro* and *in vivo* (Murine wound infection model)	*in vitro*: aPDT using NorA EPI-MB hybrid, INF55-(Ac)en-MB	*in vitro*: 5 log reduction; *in vivo*: 100% reduction within 6 days; enhanced wound healing	Rineh et al., 2018
ANTIBACTERIAL BLUE LIGHT (aBL) + AgNP				
S & P	*in vitro*, *in vivo* (murine burn wound infection model) and Case study (chronic wound infection of horse)	AgNP- chemically synthesized (15–20 nm) + Light-aBL- 460 nm, 2 h exposure after AgNP application	*in vitro*: 10 log reduction in bacterial count in biofilms; *in vivo*: 100% reduction in 2 h in mice; Reduction in wound bioburden; Case study: Wound healed completely within 4 weeks in the horse	Nour El Din et al., 2016
P	*in vitro*	Light- 650 nm, PS: Sodium salt of tetrasulfonated hydroxyaluminum phthalocyanine [Al(OH)Pc(SO3Na)4] + A. pullulans synthesized Au-AgNPs- 14 nm (20 ppm)	3 log reduction	Maliszewska et al., 2018

(Continued)

TABLE 3 | Continued

Target ESKAPE member	Study model	Agent used and dosage details	Efficacy: log reduction of pathogen using combination; % survival of host, additional advantage	References
BL + AgNP + ANTIBIOTICS				
S	*in vitro*	Light-aBL-460 nm, 250 mW, 1 h, various antibiotics + AgNP- chemically synthesized (15–20 nm). Double combination- AgNP at sub MIC + antibiotics/ aBL; Triple combination- AgNP+ antibiotic+ aBL	100% reduction in 8 h, synergistic activities of AgNP when used in double or triple combinations.	Akram et al., 2016
aPDT + AMP				
S, A, Ef	*in vitro*	MB, MB-PDT at 45 J/cm² or Chlorin 6, Ce6-PDT at 30 J/cm² + AMP- aurein 1.2, AU at 16 μM	*S. aureus*- 6 log reduction, *A. baumannii*- 5 log reduction, *E. faecium*-2.5 log reduction	de Freitas et al., 2018
P	*in vitro*	Rose Bengal (RB)-antimicrobial peptide conjugate to enhance the sonodynamic therapy	7 log reduction, increase in diffusion of RB 2.6 fold through the biofilm	Costley et al., 2017
P	*in vitro*	AMP (CAMEL or pexiganan) aPDT RB at 15–60 J/cm^2. aPDT with RB and PEX at 5μM each OR RB and CAM at 10μM each	5 log reduction	Nakonieczna et al., 2018
aPDT + ADJUVANT				
P	*in vitro* and *in vivo* (murine wound infection model)	*in vitro*: green light 0, 10, and 20 J/cm^2; PS- RB- 100 nM; KI- 0–100 mM; *in vivo*: green light-20 J/cm^2; PS - 500 μM RB alone or mixed with 1M KI	*in vitro*: 7 log reduction; *in vivo*-100% reduction; Inhibition of wound bioburden	Wen et al., 2017
P	*in vitro* and *in vivo* (murine cutaneous ulcer infection model)	*in vitro*: LED 410 nm, 6 and 9 J/cm^2; PS- 5-Aminolevulinic acid (ALA)-0.05–0.5%, EDTA-2Na 0.001–0.005%; *in vivo*: LED 410 nm, 6 and 9 J/cm^2; KY jelly with 5-ALA-0.1 and 0.5%, EDTA-2Na 0.001 and 0.005%.	*in vitro*: Combination was less efficient than EDTA-2Na in biofilm inhibition; *in vivo:* 6 log reduction in wound bioburden with 60% healing within 13 days	Katayama et al., 2018
S & A	*in vitro* and *in vivo* (murine skin abrasion model)	*in vitro*: UVA Light 360 ± 20 nm- 0–20 J/cm^2-exposure; white light- 400–700 nm, 0–120 J/cm^2; PS- C60-fullerene (LC16)- 20 μM with or without KI (1 M–30 μl); *in vivo*: UVA Light 360 ± 20 nm- 20 J/cm^2-exposure; white light- 400–700 nm 120 J/cm^2; PS- C60-fullerene (LC16)- 200 μM with or without KI (10 mM)	*in vitro*: 1–2 log reduction; *in vivo*: 1–2 log reduction in *A. baumannii* only	Zhang et al., 2015

Ef, Enterococcus faecium; S, Staphylococcus aureus; K, Klebsiella pneumonia; A, Acinetobacter baumannii; P, Pseudomonas aeruginosa; and E, Enterobacter spp.

of this study involved adaptation cycles of the commercial Pyophage preparation to increase its sensitivity toward the uropathogens. In the second phase, six of the nine patients responded to the adapted bacteriophage showing up to five log reduction in CFU of the infecting bacteria. Another study by Schooley et al. (2017) described the case of a 68 year old male diabetic patient having necrotizing pancreatitis which was complicated by an MDR *A. baumannii.* The patient responded to a phage therapy which consisted of a cocktail of nine phages against *A. baumannii.*

Few cases showing partial success of phage therapy in treating the infection are also reported (Jennes et al., 2017; Duplessis et al., 2018). Jennes et al. (2017) reported a case study of 61-year-old man diagnosed with septicaemia caused by a colistin-only-sensitive *P. aeruginosa.* Blood cultures turned negative immediately after BFC1 phage therapy but sores remained infected. No adverse side effects were observed during this therapy. In another study, a 2-year-old boy with a history of DiGeorge syndrome and complex congenital heart disease developed post-operative recalcitrant *P. aeruginosa* bacteraemia. A cocktail of two phages were used to target the infecting pathogen turning the blood cultures negative. However, the bacteraemia re-occurred after the discontinuation of phage therapy (Duplessis et al., 2018). It is however felt that commonly approved guidelines for application of phages is warranted in order to compare the efficacies of various phage treatments.

Several clinical trials have demonstrated the safety of phages and phage lytic enzymes which are in agreement with the studies carried out in animal models or as reported in numerous case studies. Although, many phase I and/or phase II clinical trials to demonstrate the efficacy of phages against ESKAPE infections have been registered in the past few years, the number of well-documented and completed trials are too low to draw meaningful conclusions (Sybesma et al., 2018). Moreover, the number of patients enrolled for the trials have severely limited the conclusions. A notable example of this is "PhagoBurn," a multicentric randomized single blind and controlled clinical study on phage therapy to treat burn wound infections caused by *P. aeruginosa* and *E. coli* (ClinicalTrials.gov registry, NCT02116010). Twenty seven patients were enrolled for the trial which resulted in being too low from the pre-calculated 220 patients expected to give statistically significant results. Restrictive patient inclusion criteria, shorter duration of patient enrolment, and low incidence of burn wound infection during the period of study were described as possible reasons for the very few eligible patients (Servick, 2016). The 27 patients were randomly assigned to the phage treatment group and safety control group for further investigation. A cocktail of 12 phages (PP1131) with lytic activity against *P. aeruginosa* were added to an alginate template that was applied directly to the wound of the treated group. A diluted phage cocktail was used due to its high endotoxin content. The control group received a topical application of the standard care treatment (1% sulfadiazine silver). Few adverse events were reported both in phage treated and safety control group. The trial, however, was terminated prematurely due to insufficient efficacy of PP1131. A supporting study showed that the bacteria isolated from patients with the failed treatment were resistant to low phage doses used for this study. This, however, was the first Randomised Clinical Trial (RCT) performed following both good manufacturing practices as well as good clinical practices and was approved by three national health regulators (Belgium, France, and Switzerland). Further studies with increased phage concentration and higher number of participants are needed (Jault et al., 2019). In case of phage lytic enzymes, the first-in-human phase I clinical trial study for phage endolysin-based candidate drug SAL200, after a single intravenous administration among healthy volunteers showed no clinically significant detrimental effect (Youn Jun et al., 2017).

The other recent ongoing trial includes a randomized placebo controlled double blind clinical trial (ClinicalTrials.gov registry, NCT03140085) to study the efficacy and safety of commercially available Pyophages for treating UTI infections in patients planned for transurethral resection of prostate. Eighty-one patients were expected to enroll for this interventional study design planned between Nov 2015–Dec 2018 that may provide necessary insights into this potentially transforming alternative treatment option (Leitner et al., 2017). Similarly, another multicentric, randomized, two-parallel group, double blind controlled trial expected to enroll 60 patients was registered (ClinicalTrials.gov registry, NCT02664740) to compare efficacy of anti-staphylococcal phages verses standard treatment and placebo for diabetic foot ulcers infected by *S. aureus.* This study has not yet begun recruiting patients.

To further overcome limitations of phage therapy, phages can be combined with antibiotics which may show synergistic action by making either a phage or antibiotic or both to act more effectively (**Table 3**). Reduction in the formation of bacterial biofilms has also been reported when antibiotic treatment is used in combination with phages (Jo et al., 2016; Chaudhry et al., 2017). Endolysin produced by bacteriophages, proves to be more beneficial than lysing cell wall and facilitating entry of the antibiotic inside the bacteria (Rios et al., 2016). Phage PEV20 and ciprofloxacin exhibited a synergistic effect *in vitro* against *P. aeruginosa* (Lin Y. et al., 2018). Another interesting study reported that *P. aeruginosa,* while developing phage resistance when under attack by OMKO1 phage, changed the efflux pump mechanism which ultimately increased the sensitivity of *P. aeruginosa* to antibiotics. Such an approach creates a win-win situation causing the killing of the bacteria either through phage or by antibiotic action (Chan et al., 2016). Similarly, it has been reviewed that such changes in the surface receptors of any bacterium may also reduce its virulence (Rios et al., 2016). A case study reported OMKO1 phage in combination with ceftazidime could successfully treat a complicated postoperative *P. aeruginosa* infection in a patient who underwent an aortic arch replacement surgery (Chan et al., 2018). The success or failure of phage antibiotic combination therapy is still in a state of immaturity as the mechanisms involved in synergy have not been fully understood and the data of *in vivo* models and case reports is scarce. Further investigations are warranted in order to make any conclusive remarks.

ANTIMICROBIAL PEPTIDES (AMPs) IN THERAPY

Antimicrobial peptides (AMPs) are short, positively charged, diverse host defense oligopeptides produced by all living forms including protozoa, bacteria, archaea, fungi, plants, and animals (Wang et al., 2010). They show a broad spectrum of activity against a wide range of pathogens. The capacity of AMPs to interact with bacterial cell membrane and thereby cause cell lysis makes them a potential alternative to combat MDR pathogens (Berglund et al., 2015). Furthermore, in contrast to conventional antibiotics, AMPs physically damage the bacterial cell through electrostatic interactions thereby making it difficult for bacteria to develop resistance against AMPs (Pfalzgraff et al., 2018).

Considering the critical status of ESKAPE pathogens, several attempts have been made to find out AMP based effective therapeutics. To date, there are numerous natural as well as bioengineered AMPs reported to show *in vitro* (Björn et al., 2016; Cappiello et al., 2016; Liu et al., 2017; Gandt et al., 2018; Irani et al., 2018; Téllez et al., 2018) as well as *in vivo* (Björn et al., 2016; Liu et al., 2017) antimicrobial, antibiofilm, anti-inflammatory, and wound healing abilities with minimum cytotoxicity. Histatin 5, a natural histidine rich cationic human salivary peptide, is an example. This peptide shows a strong *in vitro* anti-biofilm as well as potent bactericidal activity (≥70%) against ESKAPE (Du et al., 2017). Similarly, a *de novo*-engineered cationic peptide, WLBU-2, and a natural AMP LL-37 at 1/3X MIC has demonstrated 90% biofilm inhibition as compared to that shown by antibiotics such as tobramycin, ciprofloxacin, ceftazidime, and vancomycin at 1X MIC (Lin Q. et al., 2018). In 2017, Gaglione et al. examined human ApoB derived recombinant peptides namely r(P)ApoB$_L$ and r(P)ApoB$_S$. Both peptides showed effective *in vitro* wound healing, anti-inflammatory, antimicrobial, and antibiofilm properties against MDR strains of *S. aureus* and *P. aeruginosa*.

Similar to their remarkable *in vitro* properties, AMPs also exhibit promising *in vivo* activity against ESKAPE. For example, peptide HLR1r, a structural derivative of human milk protein, lactoferrin, at very low concentration (5 mg/kg) was found to show anti-infectivity against MRSA infected wound excision model in rat along with *in vitro* anti-inflammatory and non-cytotoxic effects suggesting use of HLR1r in topical formulation to treat skin infections (Björn et al., 2016). PT-13 a peptide derived from seeds and leaves of *Populus trichocarpa* crude extract also demonstrated effective *in vivo* antibacterial activity in *S. aureus* infected *G. mellonella* model (Al Akeel et al., 2018). In another instance, a synthetic analog of Feleucin-K3 has shown to clear *P. aeruginosa* induced bacteremia in mice model with good stability and very low cytotoxicity (Xie et al., 2018). Also, a hydrogelformulation containing K-11, a hybrid peptide of melittin, cecropin A1 and magainin-2 has shown to possess wound healing ability against *A. baumannii* infected murine excision model proposing its possible use as a topical anti-infective therapeutic agent (Rishi et al., 2018).

Over the past decades, intense efforts taken by the scientific community and pharmaceutical industries together has made it possible to introduce certain peptides such as vancomycin, telavancin, telaprevir, teicoplanin, enfuvirtide, daptomycin, dalbavancin, bacitracin etc. for clinical use (Gomes et al., 2018). A clinical trial conducted on rabbits and humans using the peptide melamine proved it to be a stable and safe antibacterial coating for eye lenses (Dutta et al., 2014). Similarly, Pexiganan (analog of magainin), LL-37 (analog of human cathelicidin peptide), hLF1-11, and PXL-01 (derivatives of human milk protein), Novexatin (derivative of human defense peptide), Iseganan (derivative of porcine leukocytes), PAC-113 (derivative of human saliva histatin-3 peptide) etc. are few examples of AMPs which also are under clinical trials (Mahlapuu et al., 2016).

Unfortunately, such a low number of AMPs seeking clinical approval is quite discouraging. Despite their successful *in vitro* and/or *in vivo* broad-spectrum activities, numerous AMPs have not yet crossed the hurdle of clinical trial. Amongst the few challenges that hamper the *in vivo* efficacy of AMPs are their cytotoxicity to mammalian cells, liability to degradation by tissue proteases, loss of activity at low salt concentrations or in presence of plasma proteins and higher production cost (Mahlapuu et al., 2016; Rios et al., 2016). The issue of peptide degradation can be solved by structural modification of AMPs such as addition of non-natural amino acids or their D-isomers, peptide cyclisation, acetylation, and amidation of N-terminus. Introduction of peptide mimetics or the use of suitable delivery system like liposome encapsulation can be done to improve their stability and reduce toxicity (Seo et al., 2012; Reinhardt and Neundorf, 2016). Additionally, efficiency of AMPs can be enhanced by combining AMPs with antibiotics (Gaglione et al., 2017; Zheng et al., 2017; Pletzer et al., 2018) or nanoparticles (Chaudhari et al., 2016; Kuo et al., 2016). Otvos et al. (2018), reported a synergestic effect of A3-APO, a proline-rich AMP, and colistin when studied in a *K. pneumoniae* infected bacteremia mice model. The basis for *in vitro* decrease in MIC of A3-APO when combined with colistin can be explained by considering the fact that colistin kills bacteria by interfering with bacterial membrane assembly and, therefore, slight reductions in bacterial membrane integrity potentiate A3-APO antibacterial action. Surprisingly, the same combination also showed a 100% survival in mice. This observation can be a direct consequence of A3-APO ability to induce immune augmentation or the deactivation of bacterial toxins. Enhanced *in vitro* bactericidal activity against *S. aureus* was also found in the case where LL-37, a human cathelicidin peptide, combined with gold nanoparticles as compared to vancomycin alone (Wang et al., 2018). In this case, gold nanoparticles increased the local density of positive charges and peptide mass and thereby enhanced the bactericidal properties of LL-37.

To summarize, owing to their *in vitro* and *in vivo* broad-spectrum antibacterial activities AMPs offer a hopeful alternative to conventional therapeutics. However, to overcome challenges in developing a safe, stable and efficient commercial product, a thorough understanding of their structure and interaction with bacterial as well as host cells is still needed. It will also be helpful to find better AMP formulation strategies to obtain maximum therapeutic actions. Overall, considering the extensive research being carried out on different AMPs against various infectious agents, the future of peptide based commercial drug formulations looks hopeful.

PHOTODYNAMIC LIGHT THERAPY

Antimicrobial light therapy, either alone or combined with a photosensitizer (PS), results in a photooxidative stress response that leads to microbial death. Excitation of PS with light of an appropriate wavelength leads to formation of an excited triplet state. An excited PS can transfer electrons or energy to biomolecules or molecular oxygen, resulting in the formation of reactive oxygen species (ROS) or singlet oxygen radicals, which are toxic to cellular targets such as nucleic acids, proteins and lipids (Mai et al., 2017; Yang M.-Y. et al., 2018). Some of the most frequently used PSs include phenothiazinium derivatives (methylene blue, toluidine blue), xanthine derivatives (rose bengal), porphyrin, chlorin, or fullerene derivatives amongst many others (Abrahamse and Hamblin, 2016; Cieplik et al., 2018). Antimicrobial photodynamic therapy is widely used for treating dental, skin, and soft tissue infections. For a more detailed description of the current state and future prospects of light therapy with respect to the various photosensitisers, light sources, and methods used, mechanism of antimicrobial action or antibiofilm potential, the reader may be referred to the excellent reviews published recently (Cieplik et al., 2018; Hu et al., 2018; Tomb et al., 2018; Wozniak and Grinholc, 2018). However, none of these reviews have especially focused on *in vivo* studies of aPDT against ESKAPE pathogens.

There has been extensive research on designing the PSs so as to improve their pharmaceutical potential. An ideal PS used for antimicrobial therapy should have greater permeability to cross the microbial cell wall/cell membrane, selective toxicity toward the microbial cell with minimal or no damage to the host tissue and an absorption coefficient appropriate for effective penetration at the site of action. The PS chosen should not have a long half-life which causes prolonged photosensitization in the host cells even after the infection is cured. It should also not be effluxed out by the microbial efflux systems (Cieplik et al., 2018; Hu et al., 2018; Tomb et al., 2018; Wozniak and Grinholc, 2018). Efficacy of aPDT also depends on the light fluence, PS concentration and treatment time (Tomb et al., 2017; Sueoka et al., 2018; Ullah et al., 2018).

PSs chosen preferably have a large absorption coefficient in the visible spectrum, especially in the long wavelength (red near infrared) region, to allow effective penetration of light in the infected tissue (**Table 2**). Many researchers have attempted to improve the availability of PS by potentiating or functionalizing it with other molecules including galactose, amino acids, efflux pump inhibitors, potassium iodide, EDTA etc. A variety of PSs functionalized with addends are used to target ESKAPE pathogens. A boron-dipyrrolemethene (BODIPY)-based polygalactose, named pGEMA-I (7.3 kDa) with increased water solubility was used to demonstrate antibacterial and antibiofilm activity against *P. aeruginosa*, without much affecting the viability of normal cells. It was demonstrated that the selective recognition of the pathogen was due its carbohydrate binding lectin protein (LecA) which interacted with the galactose moiety of the PS (Zhao et al., 2018). C60-fullerene (LC16) bearing deca-quaternary chain and deca-tertiary-amino groups facilitates electron-transfer reactions via the photoexcited fullerene for antimicrobial effect studied in *A. baumannii* and *S. aureus* (Huang et al., 2014; Zhang et al., 2015). Another drawback of aPDT is that the ROS generation may cease after the light irradiation is turned off thus allowing un-killed bacteria to re-grow. Potentiating aPDT with potassium iodide allows the formation of iodine/tri-iodide that may remain active in the wound for a longer duration sufficient enough to prevent bacterial re-growth (Zhang et al., 2015; Wen et al., 2017).

In vitro studies have shown that blue light (aBL) has a broad spectrum antibacterial and antibiofilm activity against all six ESKAPE members (Halstead et al., 2016). *In vivo* data also corroborated this finding and further confirmed that using a low penetrating blue light of 415 ± 10 nm should be a preferred choice of treatment in case of topical wound infections as it causes minimal damage to the uninfected tissue cells below (Amin et al., 2016; Wang et al., 2017; Katayama et al., 2018). Some studies additionally report that an exogenous PS may not be required (Amin et al., 2016; Wang et al., 2017). Their finding was supported by experimental data showing that the endogenous porphyrins present in the bacterial cell membrane play a role in triggering the photoxidative response (Amin et al., 2016). aBL using 5-aminolevulinic acid with disodium EDTA (ALA-EDTA/2Na) had antibacterial and antibiofilm potential thus showing significant wound healing of *P. aeruginosa* infected cutaneous ulcers in mice model (Katayama et al., 2018). However, the role of EDTA in increasing the antibacterial action of aBL needs further investigation. The physiological mechanism behind wound healing was studied in a *S. aureus* infected burn model in mice revealing that the enhanced levels of factors promoting angiogenesis and epithelial regeneration (bFGF, TGFβ1, and VEGF) led to the inhibition of inflammatory factors (TNFα and IL6) in the aPDT treated group as compared to the control (Mai et al., 2017).

Sueoka et al. (2018) studied the time dependant effect of aPDT-TON 504 on *P. aeruginosa* and showed that a repeated exposure to light emitting diode (LED) enhanced the inhibitory effect on bacterial growth. This enhanced effect was possibly because the bacteria that survived the initial aPDT were injured by singlet oxygen generated due to excitation of remaining photosensitizer. On the contrary there are also a few reports investigating the development of resistance/tolerance to aBL. It was observed that initial exposure to low doses of aBL increased the tolerance of methicillin susceptible *S. aureus* (MSSA) to subsequent doses of high intensity aBL-405 nm. It is likely that increased tolerance to high intensity light may be due to up-regulation of bacterial stress responses which needs detailed investigations. However, a second set of experiment showed that repeated sub-lethal exposures of 405 nm light indicate no evidence of tolerance in *S. aureus* (Tomb et al., 2017).

A considerable amount of literature has been published on combined efficacy of aPDT and antibiotics demonstrated *in vitro* (El-Azizi and Khardori, 2016; Ronqui et al., 2016). Synergistic effects of aPDT-antibiotic combination resulted in inactivation of several virulence factors in *P. aeruginosa* isolates (Fila et al., 2017). aPDT when used in combination with vancomycin prolonged the survival of *Galleria mellonella* infected with a vancomycin resistant strain of *E. faecium* as compared to either of the two therapies used alone (Chibebe Junior et al., 2013). Wozniak and Grinholc (2018) in their comprehensive review analysis have, however, pointed out that most of the aPDT carried out in combination with antibiotics lack a standard methodology followed to evaluate the synergistic effect.

One of the strategies for improved PS delivery involves the use of nanoparticles which are co-administered to allow the PS entry across the membrane or for a synergistic ROS response resulting in an antimicrobial action. A combination of tetrasulfonated hydroxyl aluminum phthalocyanine ($AlPcS_4$) and bimetallic gold/silver nanoparticles (Au/Ag-NPs) synthesized using a cell-free filtrate of *Aureobasidium pullulans* showed significantly higher killing as compared to the agents used individually (Maliszewska et al., 2018). Au/Ag-NPs possibly disrupted the cell membrane allowing enhanced uptake of the PS, $AlPcS_4$. *In vitro* and *in vivo* studies demonstrated that AgNPs used in combination with blue light showed synergistic antimicrobial and antibiofilm activities against *P. aeruginosa* infection. Interestingly, this combination was also effective for the treatment of a chronic wound caused by mixed infection in a horse (Nour El Din et al., 2016). More recently, an *in vitro* study carried out using *A. baumannii* isolates, demonstrated that the antibacterial action of ZnO-NPs with blue light irradiation was due to their ability to damage the cytomembrane but not DNA (Yang M.-Y. et al., 2018).

Over expressing multidrug efflux pumps, commonly found in resistant pathogens, are reported to affect the intracellular concentration of PS used in aPDT, thus limiting its action (Tegos and Hamblin, 2006). Tegos et al. (2008) carried out *in vitro* experiments by co-incubating various combinations of PS with efflux pump inhibitors to select the best combination showing antibacterial activity. Photodynamic killing mediated by toluidine blue (TBO), when used in combination with PaβN, or INF271 (as EPIs) was most effective against *P. aeruginosa* and *S. aureus* isolates, respectively. Similarly, an *in vitro* study demonstrated that verapamil, an efflux pump inhibitor, when combined with aPDT, required a lower light dose for effective antibacterial, and antibiofilm action against *S. aureus* (de Aguiar Coletti et al., 2017). In further development of such an approach, it was recently demonstrated that INF55-(Ac)en–MB, synthetic antimicrobial hybrids designed by covalently linking a PS (methylene blue) to efflux pump inhibitors (INF55 and INF271) were more effective in treating wound infections caused by *S. aureus* or *A. baumannii* studied in mice models (Rineh et al., 2017, 2018).

It is also worth noting that synergistic effect of aPDT when used in combination with antimicrobial peptide was also demonstrated recently (de Freitas et al., 2018; Nakonieczna et al., 2018). Aurein 1.2 augmented the aPDT activity mediated by methylene blue or chlorin-e6 against strains of *S. aureus, A. baumannii* and more importantly against vancomycin resistant *E. faecium*, whereas the AMP aPDT combination with curcumin (as PS) had no effect thus revealing a PS-dependent mechanism (de Freitas et al., 2018). Later, Nakonieczna et al. (2018) carried out a similar study showing synergistic effect of rose bengal-aPDT with two synthetic AMPs, CAMEL, and pexiganan against 35 isolates of *P. aeruginosa.* Notably, it was also shown that this combination was non-toxic to human keratinocytes. Conjugates such as $ZnPc(Lys)_5$ (a zinc phthalocyanine derivative coupled with pentalysine) also showed a synergistic antibacterial action which was sufficient to heal *S. aureus* wound infection in mice models (Ullah et al., 2018).

Overall, photodynamic therapy appears to be a promising option for treatment of infections caused due to ESKAPE pathogens, particularly effective in topical applications. aPDT co administered or conjugated with antibiotics, antimicrobial peptides, nanoparticles, or efflux pump inhibitors show a synergistic effect. However, it is difficult to compare efficacy between different combinatorial approaches due to lack of uniform methodologies. More studies on investigation of toxicity and biocompatibility of various combinations should be investigated using *in vivo* models for translating them into clinical practice.

SILVER NANOPARTICLES IN THERAPY

Nanomedicine is one of the emerging branches for treating drug resistant pathogens. Metal nanoparticles have wide biomedical applications as antimicrobial agents due to their unique physical and chemical properties (Beyth et al., 2015; Hemeg, 2017). Amongst metal nanoparticles, silver nanoparticles (AgNPs) synthesized using physical, chemical or biological methods have shown promising antibacterial activity due to their multi-targeted approach which reduces the probability of resistance (Möhler et al., 2018; Siddiqi et al., 2018). AgNPs act by releasing Ag^+ ions which results in disruption of electron transport or signal transduction pathway or leads to generation of ROS, ultimately damaging important biomolecules such as cell wall, cell membrane, cellular DNA, and/or proteins (Dakal et al., 2016; Qayyum et al., 2017).

AgNPs act by inhibiting or disrupting planktonic cells as well as biofilms of MDR pathogens. Even though earlier reports have suggested the cytotoxic effects of AgNPs (Mohanty et al., 2012), recently *in vitro* and *in vivo* studies have demonstrated the safe usage of AgNPs (Möhler et al., 2018). AgNPs synthesized using aqueous leaf extract of *Corchorus capsularis* exhibited antibacterial activity against *S. aureus* and *P. aeruginosa* and were found to be non-toxic to mouse fibroblast cells (Kasithevar et al., 2017). Electrochemically synthesized AgNPs showing antimicrobial activity against planktonic and biofilm forming *P. aeruginosa* strain were non-toxic to *G. mellonella* larvae model (Pompilio et al., 2018). Recently, sunlight mediated AgNPs synthesized using *Capsicum annuum* was tested in *S. aureus* infected zebra fish model which proved to be effective in inhibiting biofilm formation. Histological studies revealed that they are non-toxic and hence can be tested for efficacy in higher mammalian *in vivo* models (Lotha et al., 2018). A single-blind clinical trial (Clinical Trial Registration: NCT01243320 and NCT01405794) carried out in 60 healthy human volunteers, showed that commercial AgNPs when administered orally at dose of 10 and 32 ppm and monitored over 14 days were found to be non-toxic. The study revealed no significant changes in metabolic, hematologic and pro-inflammatory responses as well as no morphological changes in vital organs (Munger et al., 2014).

One of the widely explored applications of AgNPs is their use in the form of composite dressings or hydrogels for treatment of topical wound infections. AgNPs incorporated in chitosan composite dressings offer sustained release of Ag^+ ions at low dosage which are non-toxic to fibroblast cells. Studies in mice models suggested that AgNPs/chitosan composite dressings and low molecular weight chitosan-coated silver nanoparticles were effective in reducing bacterial load, were non-toxic and biocompatible, had low absorption in body and promoted better wound healing against *S. aureus* and *P. aeruginosa* (Liang et al., 2016; Peng et al., 2017). Similarly, studies using three other polymer dressings made of chitosan, nylon, and collagen incorporated with AgNPs exhibited *in vitro* antibacterial activities against ESKAPE pathogens (Radulescu et al., 2016; Rath et al., 2016; Ding et al., 2017). These dressings did not exhibit inflammatory responses, showed re-epithelization of cells and better wound contraction leading to accelerated wound healing in mice models. Sodium carboxymethyl cellulose hydrogel loaded with polyethylene glycol coated AgNPs showed antibacterial activity, re-epithelization, and wound healing in MRSA infected mice model (Mekkawy et al., 2017). Similarly, topical application of nanosilvernanohydrogels in combination with *Aloe vera* accelerated wound contraction and enhanced wound healing due to the moist environment provided by *Aloe vera* (Anjum et al., 2016). In yet another formulation, AgNPs coated on to MCM-41 type mesoporous silica nanoparticles prevented their aggregation and allowed sustained release of Ag^+ ions displaying a long-term antibacterial activity against *S. aureus*. These antibacterial nanofibrous membranes could reduce inflammatory response and accelerate wound healing in wistar rats (Dong et al., 2016). A randomized clinical trial was carried out to test the antibacterial effect of two silver dressings and their healing time in burn patients. It was demonstrated that the hydrofiber silver dressing (Aquacel^R) was preferred over the nanocrystalline silver dressing (Acticoat^{TM}) due to reduction of bioburden, quick wound healing, ease of using, comfort to the patients, and low cost (Verbelen et al., 2014). On the other hand Acticoat^{TM} showed complete wound healing within 12 weeks in 64% of the patients with leg ulcers as compared to those who were treated with Iodosorb dressings (cadexomer iodine) (Miller et al., 2010).

Polymer-based nanomaterials and metal NPs are used in antimicrobial coatings on surface of medical devices, such as catheters and implants for prevention of infections. AgNPs when embedded in electrospun hyaluronic acid/polycaprolactonenanofibrous membranes coated on flexor tendon animal models prevented bacterial infection during the early postsurgical period (Chen et al., 2015; Shalumon et al., 2018). Likewise, implants coated with nanocomposite layer of polysaccharide 1-deoxylactit-1-yl chitosan and AgNPs in a mini-pig animal model showed good biocompatibility with the bone tissue (Marsich et al., 2013). All these studies demonstrated that the entrapped AgNPs allowed controlled release of Ag^+ ions displaying prolonged antibacterial and antibiofilm action as well as reduced inflammatory responses. A randomized clinical trial demonstrated the efficacy of triple-lumen central venous catheters impregnated with AgNPs (AgTive) which showed reduced bacterial colonization as compared to conventional catheters in intensive care unit patients (Antonelli et al., 2012).

Repeated exposure of AgNPs at sub inhibitory concentrations may lead to resistance in bacterial pathogens. To overcome this limitation, a combination of AgNPs with antibiotics has been suggested in order to increase the therapeutic efficacy of either, resulting in reduction of dose and hence toxicity. *In vitro* studies demonstrating AgNPs co-incubated with different antibiotics showed synergistic antibacterial activities against ESKAPE (Ghosh et al., 2012; Panáček et al., 2015; Golińska et al., 2016; Habash et al., 2017; Singh et al., 2018; Wypij et al., 2018). Synergistic antibacterial activity of AgNPs in combination with polymyxin B was demonstrated in *A. baumannii* infected mouse model with 60% survival rate as compared to the controls treated with antibiotic or AgNPs alone (Wan et al., 2016).

Despite the use of AgNPs as a potential therapeutic agent, literature survey indicates a paucity of data obtained from *in vivo* studies carried out to test the toxicity, efficacy, pharmacokinetic, and immuno-modulatory response of the AgNPs. Further investigations through well-defined studies and clinical trials will lead to applications of AgNPs in wound dressings or medical devices.

CONCLUDING REMARKS

There is an urgent need to restock our armamentarium of antimicrobials in order to stay ahead of the ever rising drug resistant ESKAPE pathogens. There is an insufficiency of effective antibiotic combinations in addition to the dry pipeline of new drugs. Huge efforts have been taken to use antibiotics in combination with adjuvants targeting important metabolic mechanisms/pathways contributing to drug resistance (permeablisers, lactamase inhibitors, efflux pump inhibitors, quorum sensing inhibitors, toxin inhibitors etc.) The modest success received to date with such antibiotic-adjuvant combinations has paved way to explore other alternative strategies to combat drug resistance. There is a significant rise in the interest shown by the scientific community to use novel therapeutic agents such as phages, antimicrobial peptides, metal nanoparticles, and photodynamic light which, although, have some limitations as discussed above. Some of the commonly described limitations of these therapies include stability and toxicity of the therapeutic agent, its targeted delivery at the site of infection, or immune response developed by the host against the therapeutic agent. Ongoing research has therefore led to further develop or modify these novel therapeutic agents or therapies so as to surmount the limitations as well as to overcome the barriers of bacterial resistance.

This review summarizes studies that demonstrate potential alternative therapies using *in vivo* models some of which have extended further to the level of clinical trials. The interest in phage therapy to treat bacterial infections is fast growing leading to development of commercial preparations such as "Stafal," "Sextaphage," "PhagoBioDerm," and "Pyophage" against MDR pathogens. Similarly, use of silver nanoparticles as antibiofilm coatings in surgical implants, antimicrobial agents in topical applications or as formulations in wound dressings has shown promising activities in animal models. Clinical trials using commercially available nanosilver coated dressings (Acticoat^{TM}, Acquacel^{R}) or catheters (AgTive) is another noteworthy advancement. AMPs have received great attention due to their broad spectrum activity; however, they have shown limited pharmaceutical potential due to their toxicity, stability, and production costs. Photodynamic light therapy which is widely used for cancer therapy has also been demonstrated to be an effective strategy for clearing wound infections. However, additional studies demonstrating the efficacy and safety of these therapeutic agents against ESKAPE infections are desired. Similarly, randomized clinical trials would enable these therapeutic agents to cross the regulatory hurdles and find application in clinical practice.

It was observed that, majority of these studies have used animal models infected by *S. aureus, A. baumannii,* and *P. aeruginosa* to test the efficacy of the therapeutic agent. The probable reason for this could be that these pathogens mostly cause topical infections (wound, burn and abscess) and because majority of the limitations (targeted delivery, stability, immune response, toxicity etc.) described for each therapy can be minimized though not avoided in such models. It would be important to study the effect of these therapeutic agents against systemic infections caused by ESKAPE members. It was also observed that, the methods used for estimating efficacy of any therapeutic agent were not uniform. **Table 2** reveals that, the *in vivo* efficacy of various therapies is given either in terms of log or percent reduction of microbial load or as percent survival of the infected host (animal model). The methods followed to estimate the reduced pathogen loads as well as dosages used for treatment also vary. It is therefore not appropriate to compare these studies to identify the best therapeutic agent/therapy against any ESKAPE member.

In addition to the growing concern in searching and evaluating the clinical potential of the above discussed alternative therapies, research on combinatorial approach, based on the synergistic action of two or more therapies is also gaining attention. Most commonly studied combinations involve use of a therapeutic agent/ therapy (phage, aPDT, AMP, or AgNP) in combination with antibiotic/s or in some cases with an efflux pump inhibitor or quorum sensing inhibitor. Another interesting option used was the combination of the therapeutic agents in a conjugate or hybrid (antibiotic-antibiotic, antibiotic-EPI, PS-AMP, PS-EPI etc.) for an increased efficacy against the pathogen. Most of these studies demonstrated that the combinatorial approach helped overcome the limitation caused by individual therapeutic agent. For example, an antibiotic combined with an efflux pump inhibitor or a photosensitizer conjugated with an AMP improved their entry and retention into the target pathogen for enhanced antimicrobial action. Similarly, combinations of antibiotics with nanoparticles or AMPS reduced the toxicity caused by these agents which were required at high dosages when used alone. The synergistic action allows for an increased bioavailability of the drug or therapeutic agent, broad antimicrobial spectrum, reduced toxicity, and decreased chances of development of resistance. However, **Table 3** shows that most of the studies demonstrating potential of combinatorial approach are currently based on *in vitro* evaluation only. Data supporting the potential of a combinatorial therapy with respect to the mechanism of synergy, its *in vivo* efficacy, toxicity, and immune response is scarce and needs further investigation.

Finally, cost effectiveness of the above described therapeutic agents/therapy over the conventional antimicrobial agents also play a crucial role in their clinical application. Production cost for any therapeutic agent will strongly depend on the various regulatory hurdles they pass to come into clinical practice. An agent or therapy which is too expensive may not be a preferred choice for treatment in under developed countries or weaker economies thus leading to over-use of conventional antimicrobials thus contributing to the growing drug resistance.

To conclude, a uniform research methodology used to test the efficacy of these therapeutic agents in accordance with well-defined standards will make it possible to reliably compare the data presented by various research groups. Well-performed clinical trials of these therapeutic agents used as monotherapy or as a combinatorial approach will allow us to derive the real potential of these therapeutic combinations for being translated into clinical practice.

AUTHOR CONTRIBUTIONS

KP conceived the concept and edited. MM, EK, SK, and MT wrote and edited the manuscript and agreed for submission.

FUNDING

MT is a Project Assistant under UPE-Phase II (UGC-262-A-2); EK is a recipient of CSIR-SRF; SK is a Project Assistant DST-PURSE (GOI-A-670).

REFERENCES

Abedon, S. T., Kuhl, S. J., Blasdel, B. G., and Kutter, E. M. (2011). Phage treatment of human infections. *Bacteriophage* 1, 66–85. doi: 10.4161/bact.1.2.15845

Abrahamse, H., and Hamblin, M. R. (2016). New photosensitizers for photodynamic therapy. *Biochem. J.* 473, 347–364. doi: 10.1042/BJ20150942

Ahmed, A., Azim, A., Gurjar, M., and Baronia, A. K. (2014). Current concepts in combination antibiotic therapy for critically ill patients. *Indian J. Crit. Care Med.* 18, 310–314. doi: 10.4103/0972-5229.132495

Akram, F. E., El-Tayeb, T., Abou-Aisha, K., and El-Azizi, M. (2016). A combination of silver nanoparticles and visible blue light enhances the antibacterial efficacy of ineffective antibiotics against methicillin-resistant *Staphylococcus aureus* (MRSA). *Ann. Clin. Microbiol. Antimicrob.* 15, 48. doi: 10.1186/s12941-016-0164-y

Al Akeel, R., Mateen, A., Syed, R., Alqahtani, M. S., and Alqahtani, A. S. (2018). Alanine rich peptide from *Populus trichocarpa* inhibit growth of *Staphylococcus aureus* via targetting its extracellular domain of Sensor Histidine Kinase YycGex protein. *Microb. Pathog.* 121, 115–122. doi: 10.1016/j.micpath.2018.05.010

Alipour, N., Karagoz, A., Taner, A., Gaeini, N., Alipour, N., Zeytin, H., et al. (2017). Outbreak of hospital infection from biofilm-embedded pan drug-resistant *Pseudomonas aeroginosa*, due to a contaminated bronchoscope. *J. Prev. Med.* 2:1. doi: 10.21767/2572-5483.100014

Allegranzi, B., Nejad, S. B., Combescure, C., Graafmans, W., Attar, H., Donaldson, L., et al. (2011). Burden of endemic health-care-associated infection in developing countries: systematic review and meta-analysis. *Lancet* 377, 228–241. doi: 10.1016/S0140-6736(10)61458-4

Amin, R. M., Bhayana, B., Hamblin, M. R., and Dai, T. (2016). Antimicrobial blue light inactivation of *Pseudomonas aeruginosa* by photo-excitation of endogenous porphyrins: *in vitro* and *in vivo* studies. *Lasers Surg. Med.* 48, 562–568. doi: 10.1002/lsm.22474

Anjum, S., Gupta, A., Sharma, D., Gautam, D., Bhan, S., Sharma, A., et al. (2016). Development of novel wound care systems based on nanosilver nanohydrogels of polymethacrylic acid with *Aloe vera* and curcumin. *Mater. Sci. Eng. C. Mater. Biol. Appl.* 64, 157–166. doi: 10.1016/j.msec.2016.03.069

Antonelli, M., De Pascale, G., Ranieri, V. M., Pelaia, P., Tufano, R., Piazza, O., et al. (2012). Comparison of triple-lumen central venous catheters impregnated with silver nanoparticles (AgTive®) vs. conventional catheters in intensive care unit patients. *J. Hosp. Infect.* 82, 101–107. doi: 10.1016/j.jhin.2012.07.010

Aoki, N., Ishii, Y., Tateda, K., Saga, T., Kimura, S., Kikuchi, Y., et al. (2010). Efficacy of calcium-EDTA as an inhibitor for metallo-β-lactamase in a mouse model of *Pseudomonas aeruginosa* pneumonia. *Antimicrob. Agents Chemother.* 54, 4582–4588. doi: 10.1128/AAC.00511-10

Babouee Flury, B., Ellington, M. J., Hopkins, K. L., Turton, J. F., Doumith, M., Loy, R., et al. (2016). Association of novel nonsynonymous single nucleotide polymorphisms in ampD with cephalosporin resistance and phylogenetic variations in ampC, ampR, ompF, and ompC in *Enterobacter cloacae* isolates that are highly resistant to carbapenems. *Antimicrob. Agents Chemother.* 60, 2383–2390. doi: 10.1128/AAC.02835-15

Balamurugan, P., Hema, M., Kaur, G., Sridharan, V., Prabu, P. C., Sumana, M. N., et al. (2015). Development of a biofilm inhibitor molecule against multidrug resistant *Staphylococcus aureus* associated with gestational urinary tract infections. *Front. Microbiol.* 6:832. doi: 10.3389/fmicb.2015.00832

Berglund, N. A., Piggot, T. J., Jefferies, D., Sessions, R. B., Bond, P. J., and Khalid, S. (2015). Interaction of the antimicrobial peptide polymyxin B1 with both membranes of *E. coli*: a molecular dynamics study. *PLoS Comput. Biol.* 11:e1004180. doi: 10.1371/journal.pcbi.1004180

Bernal, P., Molina-Santiago, C., Daddaoua, A., and Llamas, M. A. (2013). Highlight Antibiotic adjuvants: identification and clinical use. *Microb. Biotechnol.* 6, 445–449. doi: 10.1111/1751-7915.12044

Beyth, N., Houri-Haddad, Y., Domb, A., Khan, W., and Hazan, R. (2015). Alternative antimicrobial approach: nano-antimicrobial materials. *Evid. Based Complement. Altern. Med.* 2015:246012. doi: 10.1155/2015/246012

Biswas, B., Adhya, S., Washart, P., Paul, B., Trostel, A. N., Powell, B., et al. (2002). Bacteriophage therapy rescues mice bacteremic from a clinical isolate of vancomycin-resistant *Enterococcus faecium*. *Infect. Immun.* 70, 204–210. doi: 10.1128/IAI.70.1.204-210.2002

Björn, C., Mahlapuu, M., Mattsby-Baltzer, I., and Håkansson, J. (2016). Anti-infective efficacy of the lactoferrin-derived antimicrobial peptide HLR1r. *Peptides* 81, 21–28. doi: 10.1016/j.peptides.2016.04.005

Bueno, J. (2016). Antimicrobial adjuvants drug discovery, the challenge of avoid the resistance and recover the susceptibility of multidrug-resistant strains. *J. Microb. Biochem. Technol.* 8, 169–176. doi: 10.4172/1948-5948.1000281

Cai, Y., Yang, D., Wang, J., and Wang, R. (2018). Activity of colistin alone or in combination with rifampicin or meropenem in a carbapenem-resistant bioluminescent *Pseudomonas aeruginosa* intraperitoneal murine infection model. *J. Antimicrob. Chemother.* 73, 456–461. doi: 10.1093/jac/dkx399

Caio, C., Maugeri, G., Zingali, T., Gona, F., Stefani, S., and Mezzatesta, M. L. (2018). Extensively drug-resistant ArmA-producing *Acinetobacter baumannii* in an Italian intensive care unit. *N. Microbiol.* 41, 159–161.

Cappiello, F., Di Grazia, A., Segev-Zarko, L.-A., Scali, S., Ferrera, L., Galietta, L., et al. (2016). Esculentin-1a-derived peptides promote clearance of *Pseudomonas aeruginosa* internalized in bronchial cells of cystic fibrosis patients and lung cell migration: biochemical properties and a plausible mode of action. *Antimicrob. Agents Chemother.* 60, 7252–7262. doi: 10.1128/AAC.00904-16

Casey, E., van Sinderen, D., and Mahony, J. (2018). *In vitro* characteristics of phages to guide 'real life' phage therapy suitability. *Viruses* 10:E163. doi: 10.3390/v10040163

Chadha, P., Katare, O. P., and Chhibber, S. (2017). Liposome loaded phage cocktail: enhanced therapeutic potential in resolving *Klebsiella pneumoniae* mediated burn wound infections. *Burns* 43, 1532–1543. doi: 10.1016/j.burns.2017.03.029

Chan, B. K., Abedon, S. T., and Loc-Carrillo, C. (2013). Phage cocktails and the future of phage therapy. *Future Microbiol.* 8, 769–783. doi: 10.2217/fmb.13.47

Chan, B. K., Sistrom, M., Wertz, J. E., Kortright, K. E., Narayan, D., and Turner, P. E. (2016). Phage selection restores antibiotic sensitivity in MDR *Pseudomonas aeruginosa*. *Sci. Rep.* 6:26717. doi: 10.1038/srep26717

Chan, B. K., Turner, P. E., Kim, S., Mojibian, H. R., Elefteriades, J. A., and Narayan, D. (2018). Phage treatment of an aortic graft infected with *Pseudomonas aeruginosa*. *Evol. Med. Public Heal.* 2018, 60–66. doi: 10.1093/emph/eoy005

Chan, L. C., Basuino, L., Diep, B., Hamilton, S., Chatterjee, S. S., and Chambers, H. F. (2015). Ceftobiprole- and ceftaroline-resistant methicillin-resistant *Staphylococcus aureus*. *Antimicrob. Agents Chemother.* 59, 2960–2963. doi: 10.1128/AAC.05004-14

Chang, R. Y. K., Chen, K., Wang, J., Wallin, M., Britton, W., Morales, S., et al. (2018). Proof-of-principle study in a murine lung infection model of antipseudomonal activity of phage PEV20 in a dry-powder formulation. *Antimicrob. Agents Chemother.* 62:e01714-17. doi: 10.1128/AAC.01714-17

Chatterjee, M., Anju, C. P., Biswas, L., Anil Kumar, V., Gopi Mohan, C., and Biswas, R. (2016). Antibiotic resistance in *Pseudomonas aeruginosa* and alternative therapeutic options. *Int. J. Med. Microbiol.* 306, 48–58. doi: 10.1016/j.ijmm.2015.11.004

Chaudhari, A. A., Ashmore, D., Nath, S., deb, Kate, K., Dennis, V., Singh, S. R., et al. (2016). A novel covalent approach to bio-conjugate silver coated single walled carbon nanotubes with antimicrobial peptide. *J. Nanobiotechnol.* 14:58. doi: 10.1186/s12951-016-0211-z

Chaudhry, W. N., Concepcion-Acevedo, J., Park, T., Andleeb, S., Bull, J. J., and Levin, B. R. (2017). Synergy and order effects of antibiotics and phages in killing *Pseudomonas aeruginosa* biofilms. *PLoS ONE* 12:e0168615. doi: 10.1371/journal.pone.0168615

Chen, C., Mangoni, M. L., and Di, Y. P. (2017). *In vivo* therapeutic efficacy of frog skin-derived peptides against *Pseudomonas aeruginosa*-induced pulmonary infection. *Sci. Rep.* 7:8548. doi: 10.1038/s41598-017-08361-8

Chen, C. H., Chen, S. H., Shalumon, K. T., and Chen, J. P. (2015). Dual functional core-sheath electrospun hyaluronic acid/polycaprolactone nanofibrous membranes embedded with silver nanoparticles for prevention of peritendinous adhesion. *Acta Biomater.* 26, 225–235. doi: 10.1016/j.actbio.2015.07.041

Chen, H. L., Su, P. Y., Kuo, S. C., Lauderdale, T. L. Y., and Shih, C. (2018). Adding a C-terminal cysteine (CTC) can enhance the bactericidal activity of three different antimicrobial peptides. *Front. Microbiol.* 9:1440. doi: 10.3389/fmicb.2018.01440

Chen, J., and Novick, R. P. (2009). Phage-mediated intergeneric transfer of toxin genes. *Science* 323, 139–141. doi: 10.1126/science.1164783

Chhibber, S., Kaur, J., and Kaur, S. (2018). Liposome entrapment of bacteriophages improves wound healing in a diabetic mouse MRSA infection. *Front. Microbiol.* 9:561. doi: 10.3389/fmicb.2018.00561

Chibebe Junior, J., Fuchs, B. B., Sabino, C. P., Junqueira, J. C., Jorge, A. O. C., Ribeiro, M. S., et al. (2013). Photodynamic and antibiotic therapy impair the pathogenesis of *Enterococcus faecium* in a whole animal insect model. *PLoS ONE* 8:e55926. doi: 10.1371/journal.pone.0055926

Chuang, L., and Ratnayake, L. (2018). Overcoming challenges of treating extensively drug-resistant *Acinetobacter baumannii* bacteraemic urinary tract infection. *Int. J. Antimicrob. Agents.* 52, 521–522. doi: 10.1016/j.ijantimicag.2018.07.016

Cieplik, F., Deng, D., Crielaard, W., Buchalla, W., Hellwig, E., Al-Ahmad, A., et al. (2018). Antimicrobial photodynamic therapy – what we know and what we don't. *Crit. Rev. Microbiol.* 44, 571–589. doi: 10.1080/1040841X.2018.1467876

Ciociola, T., Giovati, L., Giovannelli, A., Conti, S., Castagnola, M., and Vitali, A. (2018). The activity of a mammalian proline-rich peptide against Gram-negative bacteria, including drug-resistant strains, relies on a nonmembranolytic mode of action. *Infect. Drug Resist.* 11, 969–979. doi: 10.2147/IDR.S165179

Cooper, C. J., Koonjan, S., and Nilsson, A. S. (2018). Enhancing whole phage therapy and their derived antimicrobial enzymes through complex formulation. *Pharmaceuticals* 11:E34. doi: 10.3390/ph11020034

Corbett, D., Wise, A., Langley, T., Skinner, K., Trimby, E., Birchall, S., et al. (2017). Potentiation of antibiotic activity by a novel cationic peptide: potency and spectrum of activity of SPR741. *Antimicrob. Agents Chemother.* 61, e00200–e00217. doi: 10.1128/AAC.00200-17

Coronado-Álvarez, N. M., Parra, D., and Parra-Ruiz, J. (2018). Clinical efficacy of fosfomycin combinations against a variety of gram-positive cocci. *Enferm. Infecc. Microbiol. Clin.* 37, 4–10. doi: 10.1016/j.eimc.2018.05.009

Costley, D., Nesbitt, H., Ternan, N., Dooley, J., Huang, Y. Y., Hamblin, M. R., et al. (2017). Sonodynamic inactivation of gram-positive and gram-negative bacteria using a rose bengal-antimicrobial peptide conjugate. *Int. J. Antimicrob. Agents* 49, 31–36. doi: 10.1016/j.ijantimicag.2016.09.034

Dakal, T. C., Kumar, A., Majumdar, R. S., and Yadav, V. (2016). Mechanistic basis of antimicrobial actions of silver nanoparticles. *Front. Microbiol.* 7:1831. doi: 10.3389/fmicb.2016.01831

Danis-Wlodarczyk, K., Vandenheuvel, D., Jang, H. B., Briers, Y., Olszak, T., Arabski, M., et al. (2016). A proposed integrated approach for the preclinical evaluation of phage therapy in Pseudomonas infections. *Sci. Rep.* 6:28115. doi: 10.1038/srep28115

de Aguiar Coletti, T. M. S. F., de Freitas, L. M., Almeida, A. M. F., and Fontana, C. R. (2017). Optimization of antimicrobial photodynamic therapy in biofilms by inhibiting efflux pump. *Photomed. Laser Surg.* 35, 378–385. doi: 10.1089/pho.2016.4246

de Breij, A., Riool, M., Cordfunke, R. A., Malanovic, N., de Boer, L., Koning, R. I., et al. (2018). The antimicrobial peptide SAAP-148 combats drug-resistant bacteria and biofilms. *Sci. Transl. Med.* 10:eaan4044. doi: 10.1126/scitranslmed.aan4044

de Freitas, L. M., Lorenzón, E. N., Santos-Filho, N. A., Zago, L. H. P., Uliana, M. P., de Oliveira, K. T., et al. (2018). Antimicrobial photodynamic therapy enhanced by the peptide aurein 1.2. *Sci. Rep.* 8:4212. doi: 10.1038/s41598-018-22687-x

Defraine, V., Verstraete, L., Van Bambeke, F., Anantharajah, A., Townsend, E. M., Ramage, G., et al. (2017). Antibacterial activity of 1-[(2,4-Dichlorophenethyl)amino]-3-Phenoxypropan-2-ol against antibiotic-resistant strains of diverse bacterial pathogens, biofilms and in pre-clinical infection models. *Front. Microbiol.* 8:2585. doi: 10.3389/fmicb.2017.02585

Ding, L., Shan, X., Zhao, X., Zha, H., Chen, X., Wang, J., et al. (2017). Spongy bilayer dressing composed of chitosan-Ag nanoparticles and chitosan-*Bletilla striata* polysaccharide for wound healing applications. *Carbohydr. Polym.* 157, 1538–1547. doi: 10.1016/j.carbpol.2016.11.040

Domalaon, R., Idowu, T., Zhanel, G. G., and Schweizer, F. (2018). Antibiotic hybrids: the next generation of agents and adjuvants against gram-negative pathogens? *Clin. Microbiol. Rev.* 31, e00077–e00017. doi: 10.1128/CMR.00077-17

Domingo-Calap, P., and Delgado-Martínez, J. (2018). Bacteriophages: protagonists of a post-antibiotic era. *Antibiotics* 7:66. doi: 10.3390/antibiotics7030066

Dong, R. H., Jia, Y. X., Qin, C. C., Zhan, L., Yan, X., Cui, L., et al. (2016). *In situ* deposition of a personalized nanofibrous dressing via a handy electrospinning device for skin wound care. *Nanoscale* 8, 3482–3488. doi: 10.1039/C5NR08367B

Du, H., Puri, S., McCall, A., Norris, H. L., Russo, T., and Edgerton, M. (2017). Human salivary protein histatin 5 has potent bactericidal activity against ESKAPE pathogens. *Front. Cell. Infect. Microbiol.* 7:41. doi: 10.3389/fcimb.2017.00041

Duplessis, C., Biswas, B., Hanisch, B., Perkins, M., Henry, M., Quinones, J., et al. (2018). Refractory *Pseudomonas* bacteremia in a 2-year-old sterilized by bacteriophage therapy. *J. Pediatric Infect. Dis. Soc.* 7, 253–256. doi: 10.1093/jpids/pix056

Durante-Mangoni, E., Signoriello G., Andini, R., Mattei, A., De Cristoforo, M., Murino, P., et al. (2013). Colistin and rifampicin compared with colistin alone for the treatment of serious infections due to extensively drug-resistant *Acinetobacter baumannii*: a multicenter, randomized clinical trial. *Clin. Infect. Dis.* 57, 349–358. doi: 10.1093/cid/cit253

Dutta, D., Ozkan, J., and Willcox, M. D. P. (2014). Biocompatibility of antimicrobial melimine lenses. *Optom. Vis. Sci.* 91, 570–581. doi: 10.1097/OPX.0000000000000232

Dvořáčková, M., Růžička, F., Benešík, M., Pantůček, R., and Dvořáková-Heroldová, M. (2018). Antimicrobial effect of commercial phage preparation Stafal® on biofilm and planktonic forms of methicillin-resistant *Staphylococcus aureus*. *Folia Microbiol.* 64, 121–126. doi: 10.1007/s12223-018-0622-3

El-Azizi, M., and Khardori, N. (2016). Efficacy of ultraviolet C light at sublethal dose in combination with antistaphylococcal antibiotics to disinfect catheter biofilms of methicillin-susceptible and methicillin-resistant *Staphylococcus aureus* and *Staphylococcus epidermidis in vitro*. *Infect. Drug Resist. Volume* 9, 181–189. doi: 10.2147/IDR.S109343

El-Shibiny, A., and El-Sahhar, S. (2017). Bacteriophages: the possible solution to treat infections caused by pathogenic bacteria. *Can. J. Microbiol.* 63, 865–879. doi: 10.1139/cjm-2017-0030

Fadlallah, A., Chelala, E., and Legeais, J. M. (2015). Corneal infection therapy with topical bacteriophage administration. *Open Ophthalmol. J.* 9, 167–168. doi: 10.2174/1874364101509010167

Fallah, K. N. (2018). *The Effects of Combination Antibiotic Therapy on Methicillin-Resistant Staphylococcus aureus.* Doctoral dissertation.

Fila, G., Kawiak, A., and Grinholc, M. S. (2017). Blue light treatment of *Pseudomonas aeruginosa*: strong bactericidal activity, synergism with antibiotics and inactivation of virulence factors. *Virulence* 8, 938–958. doi: 10.1080/21505594.2016.1250995

Fish, R., Kutter, E., Wheat, G., Blasdel, B., Kutateladze, M., and Kuhl, S. (2016). Bacteriophage treatment of intransigent diabetic toe ulcers: a case series. *J. Wound Care* 25, S27–S33. doi: 10.12968/jowc.2016.25.Sup7.S27

Founou, R. C., Founou, L. L., and Essack, S. Y. (2017). Clinical and economic impact of antibiotic resistance in developing countries: a systematic review and meta-analysis. *PLoS ONE* 12:e0189621. doi: 10.1371/journal.pone.0189621

Gaglione, R., Dell'Olmo, E., Bosso, A., Chino, M., Pane, K., Ascione, F., et al. (2017). Novel human bioactive peptides identified in Apolipoprotein B: evaluation of their therapeutic potential. *Biochem. Pharmacol.* 130, 34–50. doi: 10.1016/j.bcp.2017.01.009

Gandt, A., Griffith, E. C., Lister, I. M., Billings, L. L., Han, A., Tangallapally, R., et al. (2018). *In vivo* and *in vitro* effects of a ClpP-activating antibiotic against vancomycin-resistant *Enterococci*. *Antimicrob. Agents Chemother.* 62, e00424–e00418. doi: 10.1128/AAC.00424-18

Ghosh, S., Patil, S., Ahire, M., Kitture, R., Kale, S., Pardesi, K., et al. (2012). Synthesis of silver nanoparticles using *Dioscorea bulbifera* tuber extract and evaluation of its synergistic potential in combination with antimicrobial agents. *Int. J. Nanomed.* 7, 483–96. doi: 10.2147/IJN.S24793

Gill, J. S., Arora, S., Khanna, S. P., and Kumar, K. H. (2016). Prevalence of multidrug-resistant, extensively drug-resistant, and pandrug-resistant *Pseudomonas aeruginosa* from a tertiary level intensive care unit. *J. Glob. Infect. Dis.* 8, 155–159. doi: 10.4103/0974-777X.192962

Goic-Barisic, I., Seruga Music, M., Kovacic, A., Tonkic, M., and Hrenovic, J. (2017). Pan drug-resistant environmental isolate of *Acinetobacter baumannii* from croatia. *Microb. Drug Resist.* 23, 494–496. doi: 10.1089/mdr.2016.0229

Golińska, P., Wypij, M., Rathod, D., Tikar, S., Dahm, H., and Rai, M. (2016). Synthesis of silver nanoparticles from two acidophilic strains of *Pilimelia columellifera* subsp. pallida and their antibacterial activities. *J. Basic Microbiol.* 56, 541–556. doi: 10.1002/jobm.201500516

Gomes, B., Augusto, M. T., Felício, M. R., Hollmann, A., Franco, O. L., Gonçalves, S., et al. (2018). Designing improved active peptides for therapeutic approaches against infectious diseases. *Biotechnol. Adv.* 36, 415–429. doi: 10.1016/j.biotechadv.2018.01.004

Gong, P., Cheng, M., Li, X., Jiang, H., Yu, C., Kahaer, N., et al. (2016). Characterization of *Enterococcus faecium* bacteriophage IME-EFm5 and its endolysin LysEFm5. *Virology* 492, 11–20. doi: 10.1016/j.virol.2016.02.006

González-Bello, C. (2017). Antibiotic adjuvants – a strategy to unlock bacterial resistance to antibiotics. *Bioorg. Med. Chem. Lett.* 27, 4221–4228. doi: 10.1016/j.bmcl.2017.08.027

Górski, A., Jończyk-Matysiak, E., Łusiak-Szelachowska, M., Międzybrodzki, R., Weber-Dąbrowska, B., and Borysowski, J. (2017). The potential of phage therapy in sepsis. *Front. Immunol.* 8:1783. doi: 10.3389/fimmu.2017.01783

Göttig, S., Gruber, T. M., Higgins, P. G., Wachsmuth, M., Seifert, H., and Kempf, V. A. J. (2014). Detection of pan drug-resistant *Acinetobacter baumannii* in Germany. *J. Antimicrob. Chemother.* 69, 2578–2579. doi: 10.1093/jac/dku170

Greimel, F., Scheuerer, C., Gessner, A., Simon, M., Kalteis, T., Grifka, J., et al. (2017). Efficacy of antibiotic treatment of implant-associated *Staphylococcus aureus* infections with moxifloxacin, flucloxacillin, rifampin, and combination therapy: an animal study. *Drug Des. Devel. Ther.* 11, 1729–1736. doi: 10.2147/DDDT.S138888

Habash, M. B., Goodyear, M. C., Park, A. J., Surette, M. D., Vis, E. C., Harris, R. J., et al. (2017). Potentiation of tobramycin by silver nanoparticles against *Pseudomonas aeruginosa* Biofilms. *Antimicrob. Agents Chemother.* 61: e00415-17. doi: 10.1128/AAC.00415-17

Hall Snyder, A. D., Werth, B. J., Nonejuie, P., McRoberts, J. P., Pogliano, J., Sakoulas, G., et al. (2016). Fosfomycin enhances the activity of daptomycin against vancomycin-resistant *Enterococci* in an *in vitro* pharmacokinetic-pharmacodynamic model. *Antimicrob. Agents Chemother.* 60, 5716–5723. doi: 10.1128/AAC.00687-16

Halstead, F. D., Thwaite, J. E., Burt, R., Laws, T. R., Raguse, M., Moeller, R., et al. (2016). Antibacterial activity of blue light against nosocomial wound pathogens growing planktonically and as mature biofilms. *Appl. Environ. Microbiol.* 82, 4006–4016. doi: 10.1128/AEM.00756-16

Hemeg, H. (2017). Nanomaterials for alternative antibacterial therapy. *Int. J. Nanomed. Vol.* 12, 8211–8225. doi: 10.2147/IJN.S132163

Hu, X., Huang, Y. Y., Wang, Y., Wang, X., and Hamblin, M. R. (2018). Antimicrobial photodynamic therapy to control clinically relevant biofilm infections. *Front. Microbiol.* 9, 1–24. doi: 10.3389/fmicb.2018.01299

Huang, L., Wang, M., Dai, T., Sperandio, F. F., Huang, Y. Y., Xuan, Y., et al. (2014). Antimicrobial photodynamic therapy with decacationic monoadducts and bisadducts of [70]fullerene: *in vitro* and *in vivo* studies. *Nanomedicine* 9, 253–266. doi: 10.2217/nnm.13.22

Ibrahim, M. E., Bilal, N. E., and Hamid, M. E. (2012). Increased multi-drug resistant *Escherichia coli* from hospitals in Khartoum state, Sudan. *Afr. Health Sci.* 12, 368–375. doi: 10.4314/ahs.v12i3.19

Irani, N., Basardeh, E., Samiee, F., Fateh, A., Shooraj, F., Rahimi, A., et al. (2018). The inhibitory effect of the combination of two new peptides on biofilm formation by *Acinetobacter baumannii*. *Microb. Pathog.* 121, 310–317. doi: 10.1016/j.micpath.2018.05.051

Jamal, M., Andleeb, S., Jalil, F., Imran, M., Nawaz, M. A., Hussain, T., et al. (2019). Isolation, characterization and efficacy of phage MJ2 against biofilm forming multi-drug resistant *Enterobacter cloacae*. *Folia Microbiol.* 64, 101–111. doi: 10.1007/s12223-018-0636-x

Jault, P., Leclerc, T., Jennes, S., Pirnay, J. P., Que, Y. A., Resch, G., et al. (2019). Efficacy and tolerability of a cocktail of bacteriophages to treat burn wounds infected by *Pseudomonas aeruginosa* (PhagoBurn): a randomised, controlled, double-blind phase 1/2 trial. *Lancet Infect. Dis.* 19, 35–45. doi: 10.1016/S1473-3099(18)30482-1

Jennes, S., Merabishvili, M., Soentjens, P., Pang, K. W., Rose, T., Keersebilck, E., et al. (2017). Use of bacteriophages in the treatment of colistin-only-sensitive *Pseudomonas aeruginosa* septicaemia in a patient with acute kidney injury-a case report. *Crit. Care* 21:129. doi: 10.1186/s13054-017-1709-y

Jo, A., Ding, T., and Ahn, J. (2016). Synergistic antimicrobial activity of bacteriophages and antibiotics against *Staphylococcus aureus*. *Food Sci. Biotechnol.* 25, 935–940. doi: 10.1007/s10068-016-0153-0

Jorgensen, S. C. J., and Rybak, M. J. (2018). Meropenem and vaborbactam: stepping up the battle against carbapenem-resistant Enterobacteriaceae. *Pharmacotherapy* 38, 444–461. doi: 10.1002/phar.2092

Kalan, L., and Wright, G. D. (2011). Antibiotic adjuvants: multicomponent anti-infective strategies. *Expert Rev. Mol. Med.* 13:e5. doi: 10.1017/S1462399410001766

Kasithevar, M., Periakaruppan, P., Muthupandian, S., and Mohan, M. (2017). Antibacterial efficacy of silver nanoparticles against multi-drug resistant clinical isolates from post-surgical wound infections. *Microb. Pathog.* 107, 327–334. doi: 10.1016/j.micpath.2017.04.013

Katayama, B., Ozawa, T., Morimoto, K., Awazu, K., Ito, N., Honda, N., et al. (2018). Enhanced sterilization and healing of cutaneous pseudomonas infection using 5-aminolevulinic acid as a photosensitizer with 410-nm LED light. *J. Dermatol. Sci.* 90, 323–331. doi: 10.1016/j.jdermsci.2018.03.001

Kaur, I. (2016). Novel strategies to combat antimicrobial resistance. *J. Infect. Dis. Ther.* 4:292. doi: 10.4172/2332-0877.100029

Kishor, C., Mishra, R. R., Saraf, S. K., Kumar, M., Srivastav, A. K., and Nath, G. (2016). Phage therapy of staphylococcal chronic osteomyelitis in experimental animal model. *Indian J. Med. Res.* 143, 87–94. doi: 10.4103/0971-5916.178615

Kulengowski, B., Rutter, W. C., Campion, J. J., Lee, G. C., Feola, D. J., and Burgess, D. S. (2018). Effect of increasing meropenem MIC on the killing activity of meropenem in combination with amikacin or polymyxin B against MBL- and KPC-producing *Enterobacter cloacae*. *Diagn. Microbiol. Infect. Dis.* 92, 262–266. doi: 10.1016/j.diagmicrobio.2018.06.013

Kuo, Y. L., Wang, S. G., Wu, C. Y., Lee, K. C., Jao, C. J., Chou, S. H., et al. (2016). Functional gold nanoparticle-based antibacterial agents for nosocomial and antibiotic-resistant bacteria. *Nanomedicine* 11, 2497–2510. doi: 10.2217/nnm-2016-0232

Latz, S., Wahida, A., Arif, A., Häfner, H., Hoß, M., Ritter, K., et al. (2016). Preliminary survey of local bacteriophages with lytic activity against multi-drug resistant bacteria. *J. Basic Microbiol.* 56, 1117–1123. doi: 10.1002/jobm.201600108

LaVergne, S., Hamilton, T., Biswas, B., Kumaraswamy, M., Schooley, R. T., and Wooten, D. (2018). Phage therapy for a multidrug-resistant *Acinetobacter baumannii* craniectomy site infection. *Open Forum Infect. Dis.* 5:ofy064. doi: 10.1093/ofid/ofy064

Lee, N. Y., Lee, C. C., Li, C. W., Li, M. C., Chen, P. L., Chang, C. M., et al. (2015). Cefepime therapy for monomicrobial *Enterobacter cloacae* bacteremia: unfavorable outcomes in patients infected by cefepime-susceptible dose-dependent isolates. *Antimicrob. Agents Chemother.* 59, 7558–7563. doi: 10.1128/AAC.01477-15

Leitner, L., Sybesma, W., Chanishvili, N., Goderdzishvili, M., Chkhotua, A., Ujmajuridze, A., et al. (2017). Bacteriophages for treating urinary tract infections in patients undergoing transurethral resection of the prostate: a randomized, placebo-controlled, double-blind clinical trial. *BMC Urol.* 17:90. doi: 10.1186/s12894-017-0283-6

Lewis, K. (2007). Persister cells, dormancy and infectious disease. 5, 48–56. doi: 10.1038/nrmicro1557

Liang, D., Lu, Z., Yang, H., Gao, J., and Chen, R. (2016). Novel asymmetric wettable AgNPs/Chitosan wound dressing: *in vitro* and *in vivo* evaluation. *ACS Appl. Mater. Interfaces* 8, 3958–3968. doi: 10.1021/acsami.5b11160

Lin, D., Koskella, B., and Lin, H. C. (2017). Phage therapy: An alternative to antibiotics in the age of multi-drug resistance. *World J. Gastrointest. Pharmacol. Ther.* 8, 162–173. doi: 10.4292/wjgpt.v8.i3.162

Lin, Q., Deslouches, B., Montelaro, R. C., and Di, Y. P. (2018). Prevention of ESKAPE pathogen biofilm formation by antimicrobial peptides WLBU2 and LL37. *Int. J. Antimicrob. Agents.* 52, 667–672. doi: 10.1016/j.ijantimicag.2018.04.019

Lin, Y., Chang, R. Y. K., Britton, W. J., Morales, S., Kutter, E., and Chan, H.-K. (2018). Synergy of nebulized phage PEV20 and ciprofloxacin combination against *Pseudomonas aeruginosa*. *Int. J. Pharm.* 551, 158–165. doi: 10.1016/j.ijpharm.2018.09.024

Liu, S., Long, Q., Xu, Y., Wang, J., Xu, Z., Wang, L., et al. (2017). Assessment of antimicrobial and wound healing effects of Brevinin-2Ta against the bacterium *Klebsiella pneumoniae* in dermally-wounded rats. *Oncotarget* 8, 111369–111385. doi: 10.18632/oncotarget.22797

Long, S. W., Olsen, R. J., Mehta, S. C., Palzkill, T., Cernoch, P. L., Perez, K. K., et al. (2014). PBP2a mutations causing high-level Ceftaroline resistance in clinical methicillin-resistant *Staphylococcus aureus* isolates. *Antimicrob. Agents Chemother.* 58, 6668–6674. doi: 10.1128/AAC.03622-14

López-Cortés, L. E., Cisneros, J. M., Fernández-Cuenca, F., Bou, G., Tomás, M., Garnacho-Montero, J., et al. (2014). Monotherapy versus combination therapy for sepsis due to multidrug-resistant *Acinetobacter baumannii*: analysis of a multicentre prospective cohort. *J. Antimicrob. Chemother.* 69, 3119–3126. doi: 10.1093/jac/dku233

Lotha, R., Shamprasad, B. R., Sundaramoorthy, N. S., Ganapathy, R., Nagarajan, S., and Sivasubramanian, A. (2018). Zero valent silver nanoparticles capped with capsaicinoids containing *Capsicum annuum* extract, exert potent anti-biofilm effect on food borne pathogen *Staphylococcus aureus* and curtail planktonic growth on a zebrafish infection model. *Microb. Pathog.* 124, 291–300. doi: 10.1016/j.micpath.2018.08.053

Mahlapuu, M., Håkansson, J., Ringstad, L., and Björn, C. (2016). Antimicrobial peptides: an emerging category of therapeutic agents. *Front. Cell. Infect. Microbiol.* 6:194. doi: 10.3389/fcimb.2016.00194

Mai, B., Gao, Y., Li, M., Wang, X., Zhang, K., Liu, Q., et al. (2017). Photodynamic antimicrobial chemotherapy for *Staphylococcus aureus* and multidrug-resistant bacterial burn infection *in vitro* and *in vivo*. *Int. J. Nanomed.* 12, 5915–5931. doi: 10.2147/IJN.S138185

Malik, D. J., Sokolov, I. J., Vinner, G. K., Mancuso, F., Cinquerrui, S., Vladisavljevic, G. T., et al. (2017). Formulation, stabilisation and encapsulation of bacteriophage for phage therapy. *Adv. Colloid Interface Sci.* 249, 100–133. doi: 10.1016/j.cis.2017.05.014

Maliszewska, I., Kałas, W., Wysokińska, E., Tylus, W., Pietrzyk, N., Popko, K., et al. (2018). Enhancement of photo-bactericidal effect of tetrasulfonated hydroxyaluminum phthalocyanine on *Pseudomonas aeruginosa*. *Lasers Med. Sci.* 33, 79–88. doi: 10.1007/s10103-017-2337-0

Mandal, S. M., Roy, A., Ghosh, A. K., Hazra, T. K., Basak, A., and Franco, O. L. (2014). Challenges and future prospects of antibiotic therapy: from peptides to phages utilization. *Front. Pharmacol.* 5:105. doi: 10.3389/fphar.2014.00105

Mann, N. H. (2005). The third age of phage. *PLoS Biol.* 3:182. doi: 10.1371/journal.pbio.0030182

Manohar, P., Nachimuthu, R., and Lopes, B. S. (2018). The therapeutic potential of bacteriophages targeting gram-negative bacteria using *Galleria mellonella* infection model. *BMC Microbiol.* 18:97. doi: 10.1186/s12866-018-1234-4

Markoishvili, K., Tsitlanadze, G., Katsarava, R., Morris, J. G., and Sulakvelidze, A. (2002). A novel sustained-release matrix based on biodegradable poly(ester amide)s and impregnated with bacteriophages and an antibiotic shows promise in management of infected venous stasis ulcers and other poorly healing wounds. *Int. J. Dermatol.* 41, 453–458. doi: 10.1046/j.1365-4362.2002.01451.x

Marsich, E., Travan, A., Donati, I., Turco, G., Kulkova, J., Moritz, N., et al. (2013). Biological responses of silver-coated thermosets: an *in vitro* and *in vivo* study. *Acta Biomater.* 9, 5088–5099. doi: 10.1016/j.actbio.2012.10.002

Mcnair, K., Bailey, B. A., and Edwards, R. A. (2012). PHACTS, a computational approach to classifying the lifestyle of phages. *Bioinformatics* 28, 614–618. doi: 10.1093/bioinformatics/bts014

Mekkawy, A. I., El-Mokhtar, M. A., Nafady, N. A., Yousef, N., Hamad, M. A., El-Shanawany, S. M., et al. (2017). *In vitro* and *in vivo* evaluation of biologically synthesized silver nanoparticles for topical applications: effect of surface coating and loading into hydrogels. *Int. J. Nanomedicine* 12, 759–777. doi: 10.2147/IJN.S124294

Miller, C. N., Newall, N., Kapp, S. E., Lewin, G., Karimi, L., Carville, K., et al. (2010). A randomized-controlled trial comparing cadexomer iodine and nanocrystalline silver on the healing of leg ulcers. *Wound Repair Regen.* 18, 359–367. doi: 10.1111/j.1524-475X.2010.00603.x

Mohanty, S., Mishra, S., Jena, P., Jacob, B., Sarkar, B., and Sonawane, A. (2012). An investigation on the antibacterial, cytotoxic, and antibiofilm efficacy of starch-stabilized silver nanoparticles. *Nanomedicine* 8, 916–924. doi: 10.1016/j.nano.2011.11.007

Mohapatra, D. P., Debata, N. K., and Singh, S. K. (2018). Extensively drug-resistant and pan-drug resistant Gram-negative bacteria in a tertiary-care hospital in Eastern India: A 4 year retrospective study. *J. Glob. Antimicrob. Resist.* 15, 246–249. doi: 10.1016/j.jgar.2018.08.010

Möhler, J. S., Sim, W., Blaskovich, M. A. T., Cooper, M. A., and Ziora, Z. M. (2018). Silver bullets: a new lustre on an old antimicrobial agent. *Biotechnol. Adv.* 36, 1391–1411. doi: 10.1016/j.biotechadv.2018.05.004

Monogue, M. L., Giovagnoli, S., Bissantz, C., Zampaloni, C., and Nicolau, D. P. (2018a). *In vivo* efficacy of meropenem, with a novel non-β-lactam β-lactamase inhibitor, nacubactam, against gram-negative organisms exhibiting various resistance mechanisms in a murine complicated urinary tract infection model. *Antimicrob. Agents Chemother.* 62:e02596-17. doi: 10.1128/AAC.02596-17

Monogue, M. L., Sakoulas, G., Nizet, V., and Nicolau, D. P. (2018b). Humanized exposures of a β-lactam-β-lactamase inhibitor, tazobactam, versus non-β-lactam-β-lactamase inhibitor, avibactam, with or without colistin, against *Acinetobacter baumannii* in murine thigh and lung infection models. *Pharmacology* 101, 255–261. doi: 10.1159/000486445

Moon, S. H., Zhang, X., Zheng, G., Meeker, D. G., Smeltzer, M. S., and Huang, E. (2017). Novel linear lipopeptide paenipeptins with potential for eradicating biofilms and sensitizing gram-negative bacteria to rifampicin and clarithromycin. *J. Med. Chem.* 60, 9630–9640. doi: 10.1021/acs.jmedchem.7b01064

Morimoto, K., Ozawa, T., Awazu, K., Ito, N., Honda, N., Matsumoto, S., et al. (2014). Photodynamic therapy using systemic administration of 5-aminolevulinic acid and a 410-nm wavelength light-emitting diode for methicillin-resistant *Staphylococcus aureus*-infected ulcers in mice. *PLoS ONE* 9:e105173. doi: 10.1371/journal.pone.0105173

Munger, M. A., Radwanski, P., Hadlock, G. C., Stoddard, G., Shaaban, A., Falconer, J., et al. (2014). *In vivo* human time-exposure study of orally dosed commercial silver nanoparticles. *Nanomed. Nanotechnol. Biol. Med.* 10, 1–9. doi: 10.1016/j.nano.2013.06.010

Nakonieczna, J., Wolnikowska, K., Ogonowska, P., Neubauer, D., Bernat, A., and Kamysz, W. (2018). Rose bengal-mediated photoinactivation of multidrug resistant *Pseudomonas aeruginosa* is enhanced in the presence of antimicrobial peptides. *Front. Microbiol.* 9:1949. doi: 10.3389/fmicb.2018.01949

Navidinia, M. (2016). The clinical importance of emerging ESKAPE pathogens in nosocomial infections. *J. Paramed. Sci.* 7, 2008–4978. doi: 10.22037/jps.v7i3.12584

Nigo, M., Diaz, L., Carvajal, L. P., Tran, T. T., Rios, R., Panesso, D., et al. (2017). Ceftaroline-resistant, daptomycin-tolerant, and heterogeneous vancomycin-intermediate methicillin-resistant *Staphylococcus aureus* causing infective endocarditis. *Antimicrob. Agents Chemother.* 61:e01235-16. doi: 10.1128/AAC.01235-16

Nour El Din, S., El-Tayeb, T. A., Abou-Aisha, K., and El-Azizi, M. (2016). *In vitro* and *in vivo* antimicrobial activity of combined therapy of silver nanoparticles and visible blue light against *Pseudomonas aeruginosa*. *Int. J. Nanomed.* 11, 1749–1758. doi: 10.2147/IJN.S102398

Nowak, J., Zander, E., Stefanik, D., Higgins, P. G., Roca, I., Vila, J., et al. (2017). High incidence of pandrug-resistant *Acinetobacter baumannii* isolates collected from patients with ventilator-associated pneumonia in Greece, Italy and Spain as part of the magicbullet clinical trial. *J. Antimicrob. Chemother.* 72, 3277–3282. doi: 10.1093/jac/dkx322

Ostorhazi, E., Hoffmann, R., Herth, N., Wade, J. D., Kraus, C. N., and Otvos, L. (2018). Advantage of a narrow spectrum host defense (Antimicrobial) peptide over a broad spectrum analog in preclinical drug development. *Front. Chem.* 6:359. doi: 10.3389/fchem.2018.00359

Otvos, L., Ostorhazi, E., Szabo, D., Zumbrun, S. D., Miller, L. L., Halasohoris, S. A., et al. (2018). Synergy between proline-rich antimicrobial peptides and small molecule antibiotics against selected gram-negative pathogens *in vitro* and *in vivo*. *Front. Chem.* 6:309. doi: 10.3389/fchem.2018.00309

Palavutitotai, N., Jitmuang, A., Tongsai, S., Kiratisin, P., and Angkasekwinai, N. (2018). Epidemiology and risk factors of extensively drug-resistant *Pseudomonas aeruginosa* infections. *PLoS ONE* 13:e0193431. doi: 10.1371/journal.pone.0193431

Pallavali, R. R., Degati, V. L., Lomada, D., Reddy, M. C., and Durbaka, V. R. P. (2017). Isolation and *in vitro* evaluation of bacteriophages against MDR-bacterial isolates from septic wound infections. *PLoS ONE* 12:e0179245. doi: 10.1371/journal.pone.0179245

Panáček, A., Smékalová, M., Kilianová, M., Prucek, R., Bogdanová, K., Večeřová, R., et al. (2015). Strong and nonspecific synergistic antibacterial efficiency of antibiotics combined with silver nanoparticles at very low concentrations showing no cytotoxic effect. *Molecules* 21:26. doi: 10.3390/molecules21010026

Pendleton, J. N., Gorman, S. P., and Gilmore, B. F. (2013). Clinical relevance of the ESKAPE pathogens. *Expert Rev. Anti. Infect. Ther.* 11, 297–308. doi: 10.1586/eri.13.12

Peng, Y., Song, C., Yang, C., Guo, Q., and Yao, M. (2017). Low molecular weight chitosan-coated silver nanoparticles are effective for the treatment of MRSA-infected wounds. *Int. J. Nanomed.* 12, 295–304. doi: 10.2147/IJN.S122357

Pfalzgraff, A., Brandenburg, K., and Weindl, G. (2018). Antimicrobial peptides and their therapeutic potential for bacterial skin infections and wounds. *Front. Pharmacol.* 9:281. doi: 10.3389/fphar.2018.00281

Philipson, C., Voegtly, L., Lueder, M., Long, K., Rice, G., Frey, K., et al. (2018). Characterizing phage genomes for therapeutic applications. *Viruses* 10:188. doi: 10.3390/v10040188

Pirnay, J. P., Verbeken, G., Ceyssens, P. J., Huys, I., De Vos, D., Ameloot, C., et al. (2018). The magistral phage. *Viruses* 10:64. doi: 10.3390/v10020064

Pletzer, D., Mansour, S. C., and Hancock, R. E. W. (2018). Synergy between conventional antibiotics and anti-biofilm peptides in a murine, sub-cutaneous abscess model caused by recalcitrant ESKAPE pathogens. *PLoS Pathog.* 14:e1007084. doi: 10.1371/journal.ppat.1007084

Pompilio, A., Geminiani, C., Bosco, D., Rana, R., Aceto, A., Bucciarelli, T., et al. (2018). Electrochemically synthesized silver nanoparticles are active against planktonic and biofilm cells of *Pseudomonas aeruginosa* and other cystic fibrosis-associated bacterial pathogens. *Front. Microbiol.* 9:1349. doi: 10.3389/fmicb.2018.01349

Prakash, V., Mishra, P., Premi, H., Walia, A., Dhawan, S., and Kumar, A. (2014). Increasing incidence of multidrug resistant *Pseudomonas aeruginosa* in inpatients of a tertiary care hospital. *Int. J. Res. Med. Sci.* 2:1302. doi: 10.5455/2320-6012.ijrms20141111

Qayyum, S., Oves, M., and Khan, A. U. (2017). Obliteration of bacterial growth and biofilm through ROS generation by facilely synthesized green silver nanoparticles. *PLoS ONE* 12:0181363. doi: 10.1371/journal.pone.0181363

Radulescu, M., Andronescu, E., Dolete, G., Popescu, R. C., Fufă, O., Chifiriuc, M. C., et al. (2016). Silver nanocoatings for reducing the exogenous microbial colonization of wound dressings. *Materials* 9:345. doi: 10.3390/ma9050345

Rath, G., Hussain, T., Chauhan, G., Garg, T., and Goyal, A. K. (2016). Collagen nanofiber containing silver nanoparticles for improved wound-healing applications. *J. Drug Target.* 24, 520–529. doi: 10.3109/1061186X.2015.1095922

Regeimbal, J. M., Jacobs, A. C., Corey, B. W., Henry, M. S., Thompson, M. G., Pavlicek, R. L., et al. (2016). Personalized therapeutic cocktail of wild environmental phages rescues mice from *Acinetobacter baumannii* wound infections. *Antimicrob. Agents Chemother.* 60, 5806–5816. doi: 10.1128/AAC.02877-15

Reinhardt, A., and Neundorf, I. (2016). Design and application of antimicrobial peptide conjugates. *Int. J. Mol. Sci.* 17:E701. doi: 10.3390/ijms17050701

Rice, L. B. (2008). Federal funding for the study of antimicrobial resistance in nosocomial pathogens: no ESKAPE. *J. Infect. Dis.* 197, 1079–1081. doi: 10.1086/533452

Rineh, A., Bremner, J. B., Hamblin, M. R., Ball, A. R., Tegos, G. P., and Kelso, M. J. (2018). Attaching NorA efflux pump inhibitors to methylene blue enhances antimicrobial photodynamic inactivation of *Escherichia coli* and *Acinetobacter baumannii in vitro* and *in vivo*. *Bioorg. Med. Chem. Lett.* 28, 2736–2740. doi: 10.1016/j.bmcl.2018.02.041

Rineh, A., Dolla, N. K., Ball, A. R., Magana, M., Bremner, J. B., Hamblin, M. R., et al. (2017). Attaching the NorA efflux pump inhibitor INF55 to methylene blue enhances antimicrobial photodynamic inactivation of methicillin-resistant *Staphylococcus aureus in vitro* and *in vivo*. *ACS Infect. Dis.* 3, 756–766. doi: 10.1021/acsinfecdis.7b00095

Rios, A. C., Moutinho, C. G., Pinto, F. C., Del Fiol, F. S., Jozala, A., Chaud, M. V., et al. (2016). Alternatives to overcoming bacterial resistances: state-of-the-art. *Microbiol. Res.* 191, 51–80. doi: 10.1016/j.micres.2016.04.008

Rishi, N. P., Vashist, T., Sharma, A., Kaur, A., Kaur, A., Kaur, N., et al. (2018). Efficacy of designer K11 antimicrobial peptide (a hybrid of melittin, cecropin A1 and magainin 2) against *Acinetobacter baumannii* infected wounds. *Pathog. Dis.* 76:fty072. doi: 10.1093/femspd/fty072

Rohde, C., Resch, G., Pirnay, J. P., Blasdel, B., Debarbieux, L., Gelman, D., et al. (2018). Expert opinion on three phage therapy related topics: bacterial phage resistance, phage training and prophages in bacterial production strains. *Viruses* 10:178. doi: 10.3390/v10040178

Ronqui, M. R., de Aguiar Coletti, T. M. S. F., de Freitas, L. M., Miranda, E. T., and Fontana, C. R. (2016). Synergistic antimicrobial effect of photodynamic therapy and ciprofloxacin. *J. Photochem. Photobiol. B Biol.* 158, 122–129. doi: 10.1016/j.jphotobiol.2016.02.036

Rubino, C. M., Bhavnani, S. M., Loutit, J. S., Lohse, B., Dudley, M. N., and Griffith, D. C. (2018). Single-dose pharmacokinetics and safety of meropenem-vaborbactam in subjects with chronic renal impairment. *Antimicrob. Agents Chemother.* 62:e02103-17. doi: 10.1128/AAC.02103-17

Sangaonkar, G. M., and Pawar, K. D. (2018). Garcinia indica mediated biogenic synthesis of silver nanoparticles with antibacterial and antioxidant activities. *Colloids Surf. B. Biointerfaces* 164, 210–217. doi: 10.1016/j.colsurfb.2018.01.044

Santajit, S., and Indrawattana, N. (2016). Mechanisms of antimicrobial resistance in ESKAPE pathogens. *Biomed Res. Int.* 2016:2475067. doi: 10.1155/2016/2475067

Santos, A., L., Sodre, C. L., Valle, R. S., Silva, B. A., Souza-Goncalves, A. L., Sangenito, L. S., et al. (2012). Antimicrobial action of chelating agents: repercussions on the microorganism development, virulence and pathogenesis. *Curr. Med. Chem.* 19, 2715–2737. doi: 10.2174/092986712800609788

Schooley, R. T., Biswas, B., Gill, J. J., Hernandez-Morales, A., Lancaster, J., Lessor, L., et al. (2017). Development and use of personalized bacteriophage-based therapeutic cocktails to treat a patient with a disseminated resistant *Acinetobacter baumannii* Infection. *Antimicrob. Agents Chemother.* 61:e00954-17. doi: 10.1128/AAC.00954-17

Seo, M. D., Won, H. S., Kim, J. H., Mishig-Ochir, T., Lee, B. J., Seo, M. D., et al. (2012). Antimicrobial peptides for therapeutic applications: a review. *Molecules* 17, 12276–12286. doi: 10.3390/molecules171012276

Servick, K. (2016). Beleaguered phage therapy trial presses on. *Science* 352, 1506–1506. doi: 10.1126/science.352.6293.1506

Shalumon, K. T., Sheu, C., Chen, C. H., Chen, S. H., Jose, G., Kuo, C. Y., et al. (2018). Multi-functional electrospun antibacterial core-shell nanofibrous membranes for prolonged prevention of post-surgical tendon adhesion and inflammation. *Acta Biomater.* 72, 121–136. doi: 10.1016/j.actbio.2018.03.044

Shivaswamy, V. C., Kalasuramath, S. B., Sadanand, C. K., Basavaraju, A. K., Ginnavaram, V., Bille, S., et al. (2015). Ability of bacteriophage in resolving wound infection caused by multidrug-resistant *Acinetobacter baumannii* in uncontrolled diabetic rats. *Microb. Drug Resist.* 21, 171–177. doi: 10.1089/mdr.2014.0120

Siddiqi, K. S., Husen, A., and Rao, R. A. K. (2018). A review on biosynthesis of silver nanoparticles and their biocidal properties. *J. Nanobiotechnol.* 16:14. doi: 10.1186/s12951-018-0334-5

Singh, R., Vora, J., Nadhe, S. B., Wadhwani, S. A., Shedbalkar, U. U., and Chopade, B. A. (2018). Antibacterial activities of bacteriagenic silver nanoparticles against nosocomial *Acinetobacter baumannii*. *J. Nanosci. Nanotechnol.* 18, 3806–3815. doi: 10.1166/jnn.2018.15013

Singla, S., Harjai, K., Katare, O. P., and Chhibber, S. (2016). Encapsulation of bacteriophage in liposome accentuates its entry in to macrophage and shields it from neutralizing antibodies. *PLoS ONE* 11:e0153777. doi: 10.1371/journal.pone.0153777

Skinner, K., Sandoe, J. A. T., Rajendran, R., Ramage, G., and Lang, S. (2017). Efficacy of rifampicin combination therapy for the treatment of enterococcal infections assessed *in vivo* using a *Galleria mellonella* infection model. *Int. J. Antimicrob. Agents* 49, 507–511. doi: 10.1016/j.ijantimicag.2016.12.006

Soothill, J. S. (1992). Treatment of experimental infections of mice with bacteriophages. *J. Med. Microbiol.* 37, 258–261. doi: 10.1099/00222615-37-4-258

Stanley, I. J., Kajumbula, H., Bazira, J., Kansiime, C., Rwego, I. B., and Asiimwe, B. B. (2018). Multidrug resistance among *Escherichia coli* and *Klebsiella pneumoniae* carried in the gut of out-patients from pastoralist communities of Kasese district, Uganda. *PLoS ONE* 13:e0200093. doi: 10.1371/journal.pone.0200093

Sueoka, K., Chikama, T., Latief, M. A., Ko, J. A., Kiuchi, Y., Sakaguchi, T., et al. (2018). Time-dependent antimicrobial effect of photodynamic therapy with TONS 504 on *Pseudomonas aeruginosa*. *Lasers Med. Sci.* 33, 1455–1460. doi: 10.1007/s10103-018-2490-0

Sybesma, W., Rohde, C., Bardy, P., Pirnay, J. P., Cooper, I., Caplin, J., et al. (2018). Silk route to the acceptance and re-implementation of bacteriophage therapy—part II. *Antibiotics* 7:35. doi: 10.3390/antibiotics7020035

Tacconelli, E., Carrara, E., Savoldi, A., Harbarth, S., Mendelson, M., Monnet, D. L., et al. (2018). Discovery, research, and development of new antibiotics: the WHO priority list of antibiotic-resistant bacteria and tuberculosis. *Lancet Infect. Dis.* 18, 318–327. doi: 10.1016/S1473-3099(17)30753-3

Tegos, G. P., and Hamblin, M. R. (2006). Phenothiazinium antimicrobial photosensitizers are substrates of bacterial multidrug resistance pumps. *Antimicrob. Agents Chemother.* 50, 196–203. doi: 10.1128/AAC.50.1.196-203.2006

Tegos, G. P., Masago, K., Aziz, F., Higginbotham, A., Stermitz, F. R., and Hamblin, M. R. (2008). Inhibitors of bacterial multidrug efflux pumps potentiate antimicrobial photoinactivation. *Antimicrob. Agents Chemother.* 52, 3202–3209. doi: 10.1128/AAC.00006-08

Téllez, G. A., Zapata, J. A., Toro, L. J., Henao, D. C., Bedoya, J. P., Rivera, J. D., et al. (2018). Identification, characterization, immunolocalization, and biological activity of lucilin peptide. *Acta Trop.* 185, 318–326. doi: 10.1016/j.actatropica.2018.06.003

Tomb, R. M., Maclean, M., Coia, J. E., MacGregor, S. J., and Anderson, J. G. (2017). Assessment of the potential for resistance to antimicrobial violet-blue light in *Staphylococcus aureus*. *Antimicrob. Resist. Infect. Control* 6:100. doi: 10.1186/s13756-017-0261-5

Tomb, R. M., White, T. A., Coia, J. E., Anderson, J. G., MacGregor, S. J., and Maclean, M. (2018). Review of the comparative susceptibility of microbial species to photoinactivation using 380–480 nm violet-blue light. *Photochem. Photobiol.* 94, 445–458. doi: 10.1111/php.12883

Ujmajuridze, A., Chanishvili, N., Goderdzishvili, M., Leitner, L., Mehnert, U., Chkhotua, A., et al. (2018). Adapted bacteriophages for treating urinary tract infections. *Front. Microbiol.* 9:1832. doi: 10.3389/fmicb.2018.01832

Ullah, A., Zhang, Y., Iqbal, Z., Zhang, Y., Wang, D., Chen, J., et al. (2018). Household light source for potent photo-dynamic antimicrobial effect and wound healing in an infective animal model. *Biomed. Opt. Express* 9, 1006–1019. doi: 10.1364/BOE.9.001006

Vazquez-grande, G., and Kumar, A. (2015). Optimizing antimicrobial therapy of sepsis and septic shock : focus on antibiotic combination therapy. *Semin Respir Crit Care Med.* 1, 154–166. doi: 10.1055/s-0034-1398742

Verbelen, J., Hoeksema, H., Heyneman, A., Pirayesh, A., and Monstrey, S. (2014). Aquacel® Ag dressing versus Acticoat™ dressing in partial thickness burns: a prospective, randomized, controlled study in 100 patients. Part 1: burn wound healing. *Burns* 40, 416–427. doi: 10.1016/j.burns.2013.07.008

Vestergaard, M., Paulander, W., Marvig, R. L., Clasen, J., Jochumsen, N., Molin, S., et al. (2016). Antibiotic combination therapy can select for broad-spectrum multidrug resistance in *Pseudomonas aeruginosa*. *Int. J. Antimicrob. Agents* 47, 48–55. doi: 10.1016/j.ijantimicag.2015.09.014

Viertel, T. M., Ritter, K., and Horz, H. P. (2014). Viruses versus bacteria-novel approaches to phage therapy as a tool against multidrug-resistant pathogens. *J. Antimicrob. Chemother.* 69, 2326–2336. doi: 10.1093/jac/dku173

Vuotto, C., Longo, F., Pascolini, C., Donelli, G., Balice, M. P., Libori, M. F., et al. (2017). Biofilm formation and antibiotic resistance in *Klebsiella* pneumoniae urinary strains. *J. Appl. Microbiol.* 123, 1003–1018. doi: 10.1111/jam.13533

Wan, G., Ruan, L., Yin, Y., Yang, T., Ge, M., and Cheng, X. (2016). Effects of silver nanoparticles in combination with antibiotics on the resistant bacteria *Acinetobacter baumannii*. *Int. J. Nanomed. Vol.* 11, 3789–3800. doi: 10.2147/IJN.S104166

Wang, G., Li, X., and Zasloff, M. (2010). "A database view of naturally occurring antimicrobial peptides: nomenclature, classification and amino acid sequence analysis," in *Antimicrobial Peptides: Discovery, Design and Novel Therapeutic Strategies* (Oxfordshire: CABI), 1–21. doi: 10.1079/9781845936570.0001

Wang, S., Yan, C., Zhang, X., Shi, D., Chi, L., Luo, G., et al. (2018). Antimicrobial peptide modification enhances the gene delivery and bactericidal efficiency of gold nanoparticles for accelerating diabetic wound healing. *Biomater. Sci.* 6, 2757–2772. doi: 10.1039/C8BM00807H

Wang, Y., Harrington, O. D., Wang, Y., Murray, C. K., Hamblin, M. R., and Dai, T. (2017). *In vivo* investigation of antimicrobial blue light therapy for multidrug-resistant *Acinetobacter baumannii* burn infections using bioluminescence imaging. *J. Vis. Exp.* 122:e54997. doi: 10.3791/54997

Wang, Z., Zheng, P., Ji, W., Fu, Q., Wang, H., Yan, Y., et al. (2016). SLPW: a virulent bacteriophage targeting methicillin-resistant *Staphylococcus aureus* in vitro and *in vivo*. *Front. Microbiol.* 7:934. doi: 10.3389/fmicb.2016.00934

Wen, X., Zhang, X., Szewczyk, G., El-Hussein, A., Huang, Y.-Y., Sarna, T., et al. (2017). Potassium iodide potentiates antimicrobial photodynamic inactivation mediated by rose bengal in *in vitro* and *in vivo* studies. *Antimicrob. Agents Chemother.* 61:e00467-17. doi: 10.1128/AAC.00467-17

Wittebole, X., De Roock, S., and Opal, S. M. (2014). A historical overview of bacteriophage therapy as an alternative to antibiotics for the treatment of bacterial pathogens. *Virulence* 5, 226–235. doi: 10.4161/viru.25991

Wozniak, A., and Grinholc, M. (2018). Combined antimicrobial activity of photodynamic inactivation and antimicrobials-state of the art. *Front. Microbiol.* 9:930. doi: 10.3389/fmicb.2018.00930

Wypij, M., Świecimska, M., Czarnecka, J., Dahm, H., Rai, M., and Golinska, P. (2018). Antimicrobial and cytotoxic activity of silver nanoparticles synthesized from two haloalkaliphilic actinobacterial strains alone and in combination with antibiotics. *J. Appl. Microbiol.* 124, 1411–1424. doi: 10.1111/jam.13723

Xie, J., Li, Y., Li, J., Yan, Z., Wang, D., Guo, X., et al. (2018). Potent effects of amino acid scanned antimicrobial peptide Feleucin-K3 analogs against both multidrug-resistant strains and biofilms of *Pseudomonas aeruginosa*. *Amino Acids* 50, 1471–1483. doi: 10.1007/s00726-018-2625-4

Yadav, R., Bulitta, J. B., Wang, J., Nation, R. L., and Landersdorfer, C. B. (2017). Evaluation of pharmacokinetic/ pharmacodynamic model-based optimized combination regimens against multidrug-resistant *Pseudomonas aeruginosa* in a murine thigh infection model by using humanized dosing schemes. *Antimicrob. Agents Chemother.* 61:e01268-17. doi: 10.1128/AAC.01268-17

Yang, H., Chen, G., Hu, L., Liu, Y., Cheng, J., Ye, Y., et al. (2018a). Enhanced efficacy of imipenem-colistin combination therapy against multiple-drug-resistant *Enterobacter cloacae*: *in vitro* activity and a *Galleria mellonella* model. *J. Microbiol. Immunol. Infect.* 51, 70–75. doi: 10.1016/j.jmii.2016.01.003

Yang, H., Xu, J., Li, W., Wang, S., Li, J., Yu, J., et al. (2018b). *Staphylococcus aureus* virulence attenuation and immune clearance mediated by a phage lysin-derived protein. *EMBO J.* 37:e98045. doi: 10.15252/embj.201798045

Yang, M. Y., Chang, K. C., Chen, L. Y., Wang, P. C., Chou, C. C., Wu, Z. B., et al. (2018). Blue light irradiation triggers the antimicrobial potential of ZnO nanoparticles on drug-resistant *Acinetobacter baumannii*. *J. Photochem. Photobiol. B.* 180, 235–242. doi: 10.1016/j.jphotobiol.2018.02.003

Yoshizumi, A., Ishii, Y., Livermore, D. M., Woodford, N., Kimura, S., Saga, T., et al. (2013). Efficacies of calcium-EDTA in combination with imipenem in a murine model of sepsis caused by *Escherichia coli* with NDM-1 β-lactamase. *J. Infect. Chemother.* 19, 992–995. doi: 10.1007/s10156-012-0528-y

Youn Jun, S., Jin Jang, I., Yoon, S., Jang, K., Yu, K. S., Youn Cho, J., et al. (2017). Pharmacokinetics and tolerance of the phage endolysin-based candidate drug SAL200 after a single intravenous administration among healthy volunteers. *Antimicrob. Agents Chemother.* 61:e02629-16. doi: 10.1128/AAC.02629-16

Zeng, K. J., Doi, Y., Patil, S., Huang, X., and Tian, G. B. (2016). Emergence of the plasmid-mediated mcr-1 gene in colistin-resistant *Enterobacter aerogenes* and *Enterobacter cloacae*. *Antimicrob. Agents Chemother.* 60, 3862–3863. doi: 10.1128/AAC.00345-16

Zhang, J., Xu, L. L., Gan, D., and Zhang, X. (2018). *In vitro* study of bacteriophage AB3 endolysin LysAB3 activity against *Acinetobacter baumannii* biofilm and biofilm-bound *A. baumannii*. *Clin. Lab.* 64, 1021–1030. doi: 10.7754/Clin.Lab.2018.180342

Zhang, Y., Dai, T., Wang, M., Vecchio, D., Chiang, L. Y., and Hamblin, M. R. (2015). Potentiation of antimicrobial photodynamic inactivation mediated by a cationic fullerene by added iodide: *in vitro* and *in vivo* studies. *Nanomedicine* 10, 603–614. doi: 10.2217/nnm.14.131

Zhao, Y., Lu, Z., Dai, X., Wei, X., Yu, Y., Chen, X., et al. (2018). Glycomimetic-conjugated photosensitizer for specific *Pseudomonas aeruginosa* recognition and targeted photodynamic therapy. *Bioconjug. Chem.* 29, 3222–3230. doi: 10.1021/acs.bioconjchem.8b00600

Zheng, Z., Tharmalingam, N., Liu, Q., Jayamani, E., Kim, W., Fuchs, B. B., et al. (2017). Synergistic efficacy of *Aedes aegypti* antimicrobial peptide cecropin A2 and tetracycline against *Pseudomonas aeruginosa*. *Antimicrob. Agents Chemother.* 61:e00686-17. doi: 10.1128/AAC.00686-17

Zhou, W., Feng, Y., and Zong, Z. (2018). Two new lytic bacteriophages of the myoviridae family against carbapenem-resistant *Acinetobacter baumannii*. *Front. Microbiol.* 9:850. doi: 10.3389/fmicb.2018.00850

Zowawi, H. M., Forde, B. M., Alfaresi, M., Alzarouni, A., Farahat, Y., Chong, T. M., et al. (2015). Stepwise evolution of pandrug-resistance in *Klebsiella pneumoniae*. *Sci. Rep.* 5:15082. doi: 10.1038/srep15082

19

In silico Evolution and Comparative Genomic Analysis of IncX3 Plasmids Isolated From China Over Ten Years

Baomo Liu[1,2†], Yingyi Guo[1†], Ningjing Liu[1], Jiong Wang[1], Feifeng Li[1], Likang Yao[1] and Chao Zhuo[1*]

[1] State Key Laboratory of Respiratory Disease, The First Affiliated Hospital of Guangzhou Medical University, Guangzhou, China,

[2] Department of Respiratory Medicine, The First Affiliated Hospital of Sun Yat-sen University, Guangzhou, China

***Correspondence:**
Chao Zhuo
chao_sheep@263.net

† These authors have contributed equally to this work

IncX3 plasmids are correlated with the dissemination and acquisition of carbapenem resistance in *Enterobacteriaceae* and have been prevalent in China over the last 10 years. Since the distribution characteristics of IncX3 plasmids across China as well as their evolutionary traits for 10 years remain unclear, here we conducted a retrospective literature review and *in silico* comparative analysis of IncX3 plasmids in publicly available IncX3 plasmid genomes. IncX3 plasmids distributed in 17 provinces or cities were extracted for analysis, which tend to be specifically associated with hospital-isolated *Escherichia coli* ST410 from phylogroup A. Although the backbones of IncX3 plasmids have remained highly conservative over the last 10 years, the bla_{NDM} resistance genetic contexts on these plasmids could fall into five subtypes, among which AR_N1_I has been identified in *Enterobacter cloacae174* chromosome and AR_N5_I was simultaneously located on IncF and IncA/C plasmids. This suggests that the bla_{NDM} resistance gene environment can spread between different plasmids, between different bacterial genera, or between strains and plasmids, highlighting that it is imperative to adopt more stringent infection control measures targeting IncX3 plasmid spread.

Keywords: IncX3 plasmid, bla_{NDM}, carbapenem, *Escherichia coli*, genome

INTRODUCTION

IncX3 plasmids were discovered 10 years ago, since Ho et al. (2012) first isolated the bla_{NDM}/IncX3 plasmid pNDM-HN380 in China in 2011. IncX3 seems to be the most common plasmid-incompatible type for carrying bla_{NDM} in China and even the world (Ma et al., 2020). However, no previous research has investigated the distribution characteristics of IncX3 plasmids across China as well as their evolutionary traits over the last 10 years. A substantial number of plasmid whole genome sequences from China have been reported over the last few decades, which make it possible to conduct long-term and large-scale plasmid comparison and evolutionary analysis.

Therefore, the current study using published literature about IncX3 plasmids isolated from China and the IncX3 plasmid complete gene sequence deposited in NCBI was presented (i) to describe the prevalence of IncX3 plasmids across China over approximately 10 years, (ii) to identify the genetic context of IncX3 plasmids to further clarify the mechanisms related to antibiotic resistance gene transfer, and (iii) to explore the diversity of IncX3 plasmids and refine the IncX3 subgroup. This project provided an excellent opportunity to facilitate the understanding of the mechanisms of IncX3 plasmids' high prevalence in China and the mechanism of the wide dissemination of carbapenem-resistant strains.

MATERIALS AND METHODS

Search Strategy

We searched the PubMed database for published research of IncX3 separated in China before August 15, 2020. There was no language restriction. Keywords included ("China" and "IncX3").

Article inclusion criteria: (1) the strain containing the IncX3 plasmid was isolated from China; and (2) the basic information of the strain can be queried in the article, including strain species, isolation dates, cities, and specimen sources.

Exclusion criteria: (1) the strains and plasmids were not isolated from China; (2) there was no bacterial species information of the plasmid host; and (3) all other basic information except the plasmid name is missing.

Referring to selected literature and GenBank online information, we collected the basic information of all IncX3 plasmids including specimen sources, isolation dates, cities, and MLST types (see section "Results" in detail).

Plasmid Replicon Verification and Database Construction

We took the Rep sequence of the IncX3 plasmid deposited in the PlasmidFinder database as a reference and used BLASTN to verify the incompatibility group of the extracted plasmid sequence (homology >90% coverage >90%). The hit rate of BLASTN was manually reviewed, and only published sequences were included in our IncX3 plasmid database.

Antibiotic Resistance Gene Annotation

We used Mega-BLAST (*e* value ≤0.0001, identity ≥70%) against the ResFinder database to compare and annotate antibiotic resistance genes located in plasmids and then performed a manual inspection.

Comparative Genomics Analysis of IncX3 Plasmids

The *bla*$_{NDM}$/IncX3 plasmid pNDM-HN380 (GenBank accession number: JX104760.1) in *Klebsiella pneumoniae* strain HN380 was adopted as a reference plasmid for comparison. BLAST was used to compare all completely sequenced IncX3 plasmids with pNDM-HN380. We counted the number of hits in different regions of pNDM-HN380 to determine the conserved regions. Annotation of the complete gene sequence was performed using Prokka for all collected plasmids.

Plasmid Backbone Recognition, Multiple Sequence Alignment, and Visualization

Mauve was used to perform multiple sequence alignment of plasmid DNA sequences to identify backbone genes. Plasmid backbone genes were defined as regions of plasmid DNA whose sequences were highly conserved in all aligned genomes.

The local blast + method was used for pairwise comparison to determine the plasmid group. Snippy software was applied to identify single-nucleotide polymorphism (SNP), insertion, or deletion changes between the reference plasmid pNDM-HN380 and other plasmids. Visualization of the comparison results was generated by Easyfig software, and the produced pictures were marked with gene names using Adobe Illustrator CC 2019 software.

RESULTS

The Distribution and Host Characteristics of IncX3 Plasmids Reported in China

By searching "China and IncX3" in the PubMed database, the genome sequences and basic information of 84 IncX3 plasmids involving 60 documents were collected (see **Supplementary Table 1** for all collected plasmid information).

From 2011 to 2021, a total of 84 non-duplicate collected IncX3 plasmids were reported in 13 provinces or cities across China, namely, Shandong, Jiangsu, Zhejiang, Guangdong, Shaanxi, Chongqing, Sichuan, Henan, Hong Kong, Beijing, Shanghai, Hunan, and Jiangxi. In this collection, the reported IncX3 plasmid-containing strains were isolated from clinical specimens (60.7%, 51/84, blood, urine, or sputum), livestock animals (17.9%, 15/84), life environment (such as sewage samples and surface of subway instruments), anal swab screening of admitted patients, and retail food meat.

The collected isolates carrying IncX3 plasmids were inspected further. The hosts of IncX3 plasmids involved 15 species. *Escherichia coli* (51.2%, 43/84), *K. pneumoniae* (23.8%, 20/84), and *Enterobacter cloacae* (7.1%, 6/84) were the most common hosts. The IncX3 plasmid was also sporadically distributed in 12 other species of *Enterobacteriaceae*, namely, *Citrobacter freundii, Salmonella Typhimurium, Cronobacter sakazakii, K. aerogenes, K. quasipneumoniae, Klebsiella oxytocin, Klebsiella oxytoca, Kluyvera cryocrescens, M. morganii, Proteus mirabilis, Raoultella planticola, Raoultella ornithinolytica*, and *Salmonella Lomita*.

A remarkable diversity of sequence types (STs) was identified among IncX3 plasmid-containing *E. coli* isolates. Among the 43 *E. coli* isolates, 17 different STs were noted. The preferred STs seemed to be ST48 (6/33), ST410 (4/33), ST156 (4/33), ST167 (3/33), ST1114 (2/33), ST10 (2/33), ST617 (2/33), and ST641 (2/33). The other *E. coli* isolates belonged to single diverse STs (including ST46, ST3835, ST224, ST-744, ST44, ST1236, ST448, ST3076, and ST8809). It is worth noting that all ST48 *E. coli* were isolated from animals and ST410s were from clinical patients and hospital environments.

We also obtained phylotype data of 16 *E. coli* strains in our collection. Phylotype data suggested that more than half (68.8%, 11/16) belonged to non-pathogenic phylogroup A. Phylogroup B included three strains, and the remaining two strains belong to group C. Phylogroup A strains have been isolated from various sources, including clinical specimens, animals, human colonization, and environment. Four types of *bla*$_{NDM}$

variants (bla_{NDM-1}, bla_{NDM-5}, bla_{NDM-7}, and bla_{NDM-21}) were identified in IncX3 plasmid-carrying phylogroup A strains.

Carbapenem Resistance Genes Carried on IncX3 Plasmids

All the collected IncX3 plasmids were positive for carbapenemase genes, among which 81 (96.4%) of them were NDM-positive and 3 (3.6%) were OXA181-positive. The IncX3 plasmid carried eight types of NDM variants, namely, NDM-1 (22.2%, 18/81), NDM-5 (67.9%, 55/81), NDM-7 (3/81), NDM-21 (1.2%, 1/81), NDM-13 (1.2%, 1/81), NDM-17 (1.2%, 1/81), NDM-19 (1.2%, 1/81), and NDM-20 (1.2%, 1/81). No bla_{KPC}-carrying IncX3 plasmid was recorded in China.

Notably, bla_{NDM-5} was the most prevalent carbapenemase gene in the IncX3 plasmids, followed by the bla_{NDM-1} subtype. The bla_{NDM-5}-carrying IncX3 plasmids included plasmids from clinical specimens, livestock animals, life environment, anal swab screening of admitted patients, and retail food, indicating the wide dissemination of NDM-5-producing carbapenem-resistant isolates mediated by quick transfer of IncX3 plasmids. Interestingly, IncX3 plasmids containing the bla_{NDM-1} gene could be recovered from patient clinical specimens, rectal swabs, and hospital environments, which showed a preferred in-hospital spread for this gene subtype.

Whole Genome Sequence Grouping of IncX3 Plasmids

Among the 84 plasmids collected, a total of 76 IncX3 plasmid complete genome sequences were finally obtained. The analysis using Mauve and BlastN software identified that all 76 plasmids could be divided into nine subgroups by comparing sequences, that is, pNDM-HN380 (group1), pNDM_MGR194 (group2), pOXA181_EC14828 (group3), MH10T (group4), pNDM-BJ03 (group5), pGZ2-NDM (group6), pWLK-NDM (group7), pNDM5-LDR (group8), and pNDM5-GZ04_A (group9).

Comparison of plasmid sequences revealed nine distinct types, mainly because of the variety of the genetic load region (**Table 1**). Researchers have referred to "the gene load region" as the fragments containing inserted sequences and different resistance genetic context (Ho et al., 2012). For example, for the first featured IncX3 plasmid pNDM-HN380, the gene load region was between the *resolvase* gene and *hns* gene, and involved bla_{SHV}, bla_{NDM}, and their surrounding mobile genetic elements (*IS26*, *Tn3*, and *tnpA*).

The gene load region of the nine subgroups differed in resistance gene composition and mobile genetic elements. Most of the gene load regions (6/9) included resistance genes, more than just the carbapenemase gene as shown in **Table 1**.

IncX3 Plasmid Backbone Region Was Highly Conserved

The gene organization of the IncX3 plasmid backbones was nearly identical to that of plasmid pNDM-HN380, and the counterparts shared >95% amino acid identities (**Figure 1** and **Supplementary Table 2**). Among 75 plasmids compared with pNDM-HN380, only 21 plasmid backbones had a single-nucleotide change, or insertion/deletion of a single nucleotide, indicating that the IncX3 backbone has been highly conserved for 10 years.

TABLE 1 | IncX3 plasmid gene load regions.

Name	Carbapenemase	Size (bp)	Other resistance genes
pNDM-HN380	NDM-1	23,031	bla_{SHV-12}
pNDM-BJ03	NDM-1	31,079	bla_{SHV-12}
pWLK-NDM	NDM-1	45,279	*ampC*[f], *tetA*, *tetR*
pMGR194	NDM-5	15,157	–
MH10T	NDM-5	12,803	–
pGZ2-NDM	NDM-5	39,545	*tmrB*[a], *tap*[b], *ant1*[c], *emrE*[d],
pNDM5-LDR	NDM-5	19,975	–
pNDM5-GZ04_A	NDM-5	26,207	*mphA*[e], *tap*
pOXA181_EC14828	OXA-181	15,371	*qnrS1*

[a] *Tunicamycin resistance protein, which is a nucleotide antibiotic produced by the actinomycete Streptomyces lysosuperficus. It can inhibit the reproduction of viruses with envelopes (glycoproteins). It can inhibit the formation of glycoprotein by inhibiting the transfer of N-acetylglucosamine-1-phosphate to monophosphate long alcohol.*
[b] *Scaini et al. (2019).*
[c] *Prabhu et al. (2017).*
[d] *Saleh et al. (2018).*
[e] *Fong et al. (2017).*
[f] *Cephalosporinase.*

Subtype of bla_{NDM} Genetic Contexts Located in IncX3 Plasmids and Exploring the Mechanisms of Resistance Gene Transfer

The bla_{NDM} genetic contexts identified fell into five groups according to the comparison analysis, including AR_N1_I–AR_N1_III and AR_N5_I–AR_N5_II (**Figure 2**). Among them, AR_N1 corresponds to bla_{NDM-1} genetic context and AR_N5 means bla_{NDM-5} genetic context. Deletion or insertion of mobile gene elements (i.e., IS5 or IS125) and ORFs of unknown functions (i.e., *groL* and *groS*) accounted for the majority of the variations of these gene environments.

To detect the location of all bla_{NDM} genetic contexts other than IncX3 plasmids to discover the potential of transposon transfer, we searched all identified genetic context subtypes in the NCBI database. Surprisingly, we found that the genetic structure of AR_N1_I was nearly identical to a chromosome-encoded fragment containing bla_{NDM-1} in *Enterobacter cloacae174* (accession number: CP020528, 1628321...1645166, **Figure 3**), whose gene composition of the chromosome-encoded fragment was flanked by *IS26*, in addition to holding AR_N1_I genetic context.

DISCUSSION

Previous studies have sporadically reported that the presence of IncX3 plasmids mediated the dissemination of carbapenem-resistant *Enterobacteriaceae* strains in China (Yang et al., 2020; Zhai et al., 2020; Zhou et al., 2020). However, no previous

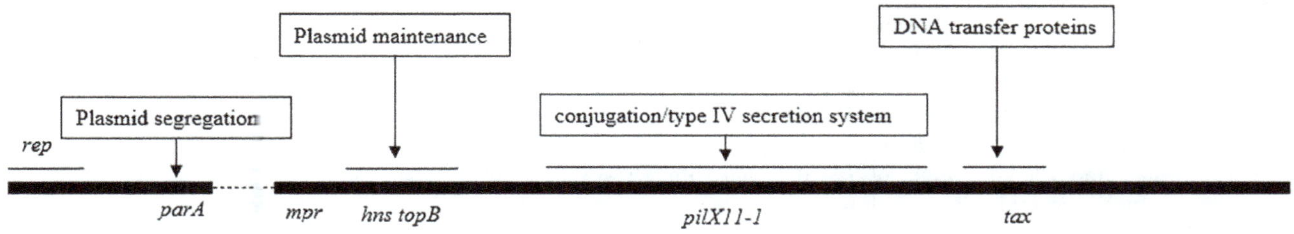

FIGURE 1 | Plasmid backbone region map (dotted line indicates gene load region).

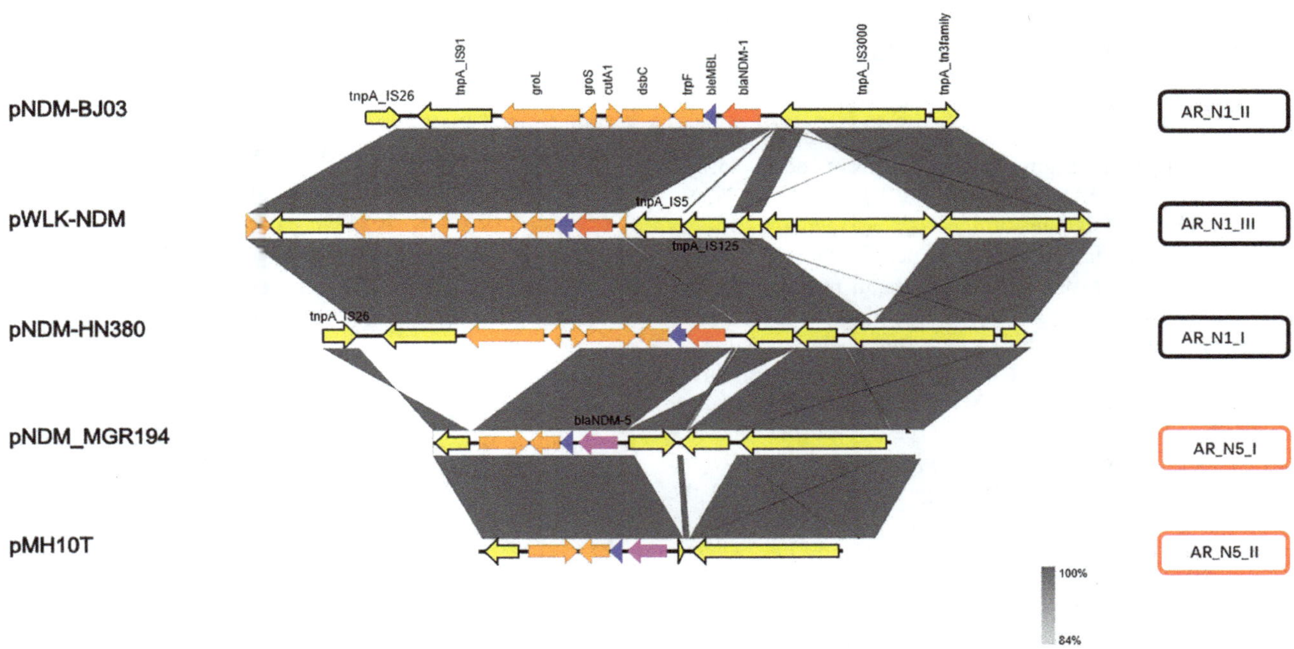

FIGURE 2 | Summary of sub-classifications of resistance gene environment.

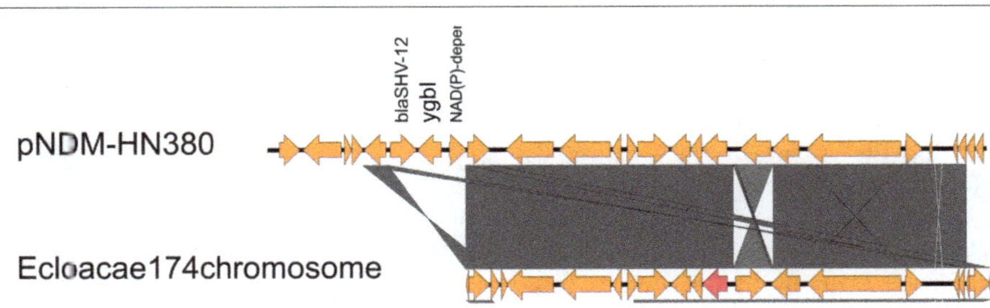

FIGURE 3 | Comparison of AR_N1_I structure of pNDM-HN380 with the *Enterobacter cloacae 174* chromosome gene fragment in NCBI.

research has investigated the distribution characteristics of IncX3 plasmids across China as well as their evolutionary traits over the last 10 years. This study provided a comprehensive and updated prevalence and sequence characteristic profile of carbapenem-resistant IncX3 plasmids isolated from various sources in China. We have performed large-scale and long-term *in silico* analyses of reported IncX3 plasmids to elucidate IncX3 plasmid structural features over 10 years.

IncX3 plasmids are the most prevalent in *E. coli* and *K. pneumoniae* but sparse in other *Enterobacteriaceae*, where phylogroup A and ST410 *E. coli* isolated from patients seems to be the preferred host for IncX3 plasmids, highlighting that more infection control measures should be the target at these emerging specific associations between plasmids and bacterial clones. Consistently, Ma et al. (2020) demonstrated that IncX3 plasmids could often transfer to phylogroup A *E. coli* successfully and maintain high stability. The study of Huang et al. (2021) published in 2021 has found that bla_{NDM}/IncX3 plasmids tend to be concentrated in ST410 *E. coli*, which also belongs to phylotype A. Our team also found a large number of ST410 *E. coli* with bla_{NDM}-carrying IncX3 plasmids (data not shown).

The IncX3 plasmid carries at least eight kinds of bla_{NDM} gene variants, among which bla_{NDM-5} is dominant. The bla_{NDM-5}-carrying IncX3 plasmids were recovered from diverse sources, indicating the wide dissemination of NDM-5-producing carbapenem-resistant isolates mediated by quick transfer of IncX3 plasmids. However, bla_{NDM-1}-carrying IncX3 plasmids were mainly distributed in the hospital, which show more limited dissemination compared with $bla_{\mathrm{NDM}-5}$.

We further divided carbapenem resistance genes and surrounding structural fragments obtained from IncX3 plasmid into five subtypes, AR_N1_I–AR_N1_III and AR_N5_I–AR_N5_II. The sub-classification of bla_{NDM} genetic contexts can help researchers understand the structural characteristics of resistance genes and explore its transmission mechanism. Our results found that AR_N1_I is highly homologous to bla_{NDM-1} surrounding fragments encoded by *Enterobacter cloacae174* chromosome, indicating that bla_{NDM-1} surrounding fragments could transfer between the IncX3 plasmid and *Enterobacter* chromosome. In 2020, Zou et al. (2020) reported that the genetic environment containing bla_{NDM-5} could be divided into five subtypes. Among them, Type A corresponds to the AR_N5_I genetic environment in our study. The Type A genetic environment has been the most common (50%) genetic environment containing bla_{NDM}, suggesting that the AR_N5_I genetic environment has an advantage in assisting the wide spread of bla_{NDM-5}. Besides, the AR_N5_I genetic environment is also distributed on the IncF and IncA/C plasmids, and the IncA/C plasmid is a well-known broad host plasmid (Douarre et al., 2020), suggesting that the dissemination of bla_{NDM} gene will cross genus, not only limited to *Enterobacteriaceae* bacteria.

Therefore, the bla_{NDM-5} genetic context carried by IncX3 plasmids can spread between different plasmids, between different bacterial genera, or between strains and plasmids. This suggests that controlling the spread of IncX3 plasmids has significant meaning for controlling the quick occurrence of carbapenem-resistant bacteria.

The genes on the backbone are responsible for maintaining the basic functions of the plasmid, including conjugation transfer and plasmid progeny distribution. The comparative analysis of the plasmid backbone region shows that the IncX3 backbone genes have been highly conservative for the last 10 years. This suggests that the IncX3 plasmid backbone gene itself has the advantage of mediating the wide spread of bla_{NDM}. The theory of plasmid biology shows that high conjugation efficiency, powerful distribution system, and low fitness cost are three factors to ensure the long-term existence and wide spread of plasmids (Zwanzig, 2021). The T4SS system in the backbone region guarantees the efficiency of plasmid self-conjugation (Costa et al., 2020); the *parAB* distribution system ensures that progeny plasmids can be assigned to the offspring host, promoting plasmid stability (Sheng et al., 2020). Further research into backbone gene function will facilitate the deep investigation of IncX3 plasmid fitness mechanisms in China.

CONCLUSION

In this study, our data indicate that carbapenem-resistant gene-carrying IncX3 plasmids tend to be specifically associated with hospital-isolated *E. coli* ST410 from phylogroup A. Although the backbones of IncX3 plasmids remained highly conservative over the last 10 years, the bla_{NDM} resistance genetic contexts on plasmid could fall into five subtypes, among which AR_N1_I has been identified in *Enterobacter cloacae174* chromosome and AR_N5_I was simultaneously located on IncF and IncA/C plasmids. This suggests that the bla_{NDM} resistance gene environment can spread between different plasmids, between different bacterial genera, or between strains and plasmids, highlighting that it is imperative to adopt more stringent infection control measures targeting IncX3 plasmid spread.

AUTHOR CONTRIBUTIONS

CZ, BL, and YG conceived and designed the experiments and wrote the manuscript. NL, JW, FL, and LY searched PubMed and collected IncX3 plasmid information. BL and YG performed the bioinformatic analysis. All authors provide critical input to the manuscript and endorsed the final version.

FUNDING

The research was supported by the National Natural Science Foundation of China (Project Nos. 81772238 and 81861138056) and the Guangzhou Municipal Science and Technology Bureau (Project No. 201607020044).

ACKNOWLEDGMENTS

We thank Jingjie Song from Shenzhen People's Hospital for helping us to analyze the WGS data.

REFERENCES

Costa, T. R. D., Harb, L., Khara, P., Zeng, L., Hu, B., and Christie, P. J. (2020). Type IV secretion systems: advances in structure, function, and activation. *Mol. Microbiol.* 115, 436–452. doi: 10.1111/mmi.14670

Douarre, P. E., Mallet, L., Radomski, N., Felten, A., and Mistou, M. Y. (2020). Analysis of COMPASS, a new comprehensive plasmid database revealed prevalence of multireplicon and extensive diversity of IncF plasmids. *Front. Microbiol.* 11:483. doi: 10.3389/fmicb.2020.00483

Fong, D. H., Burk, D. L., Blanchet, J., Yan, A. Y., and Berghuis, A. M. (2017). Structural basis for kinase-mediated macrolide antibiotic resistance. *Structure* 25, 750.e5–761.e5. doi: 10.1016/j.str.2017.03.007

Ho, P. L., Li, Z., Lo, W. U., Cheung, Y. Y., Lin, C. H., Sham, P. C., et al. (2012). Identification and characterization of a novel incompatibility group X3 plasmid carrying bla NDM-1 in *Enterobacteriaceae* isolates with epidemiological links to multiple geographical areas in China. *Emerg. Microbes. Infect.* 1:e39. doi: 10.1038/emi.2012.37

Huang, Y. S., Tsai, W. C., Li, J. J., Chen, P. Y., Wang, J. T., Chen, Y. T., et al. (2021). Increasing New Delhi metallo-beta-lactamase-positive *Escherichia coli* among carbapenem non-susceptible *Enterobacteriaceae* in Taiwan during 2016 to 2018. *Sci. Rep.* 11:2609. doi: 10.1038/s41598-021-82166-8

Ma, T., Fu, J., Xie, N., Ma, S. Lei, L., Zhai, W., et al. (2020). Fitness Cost of bla_{NDM-5}-Carrying p3R-IncX3 Plasmids in Wild-Type NDM-Free *Enterobacteriaceae. Microorganisms* 8:377. doi: 10.3390/microorganisms8030377

Prabhu, D., Vidhyavathi, R., and Jeyakanthan, J. (2017). Computational identification of potent inhibitors for Streptomycin 3′′-adenylyltransferase of *Serratia marcescens. Microb. Pathog.* 103, 94–106. doi: 10.1016/j.micpath.2016.12.015

Saleh, M., Bay, D. C., and Turner, R. J. (2018). Few conserved amino acids in the small multidrug resistance transporter EmrE influence drug polyselectivity. *Antimicrob. Agents Chemother.* 62:e00461-18. doi: 10.1128/AAC.00461-18

Scaini, J. L. R., Camargo, A. D., Seus, V. R., von Groll, A., Werhli, A. V., da Silva, P. E. A., et al. (2019). Molecular modelling and competitive inhibition of a *Mycobacterium tuberculosis* multidrug-resistance efflux pump. *J. Mol. Graph. Model.* 87, 98–108. doi: 10.1016/j.jmgm.2018.11.016

Sheng, D., Chen, X., Li, Y., Wang, J., Zhuo, L., and Li, Y. (2020). ParC, a new partitioning protein, is necessary for the active form of ParA From Myxococcus pMF1 plasmid. *Front. Microbiol.* 11:623699. doi: 10.3389/fmicb.2020.623699

Yang, L., Li, J., Zha, L., Wang, K., Qi, K., Qiu, S., et al. (2020). OXA-181-producing extraintestinal pathogenic *Escherichia coli* sequence Type 410 Isolated from a dog in portugal. *Infect. Drug. Resist.* 64:e02298-19. doi: 10.1128/AAC.02298-19

Zhai, R., Fu, B., Shi, X., Sun, C., Liu, Z., Wang, S., et al. (2020). Contaminated in-house environment contributes to the persistence and transmission of NDM-producing bacteria in a Chinese poultry farm. *Environ. Int.* 139:105715. doi: 10.1016/j.envint.2020.105715

Zhou, H., Zhang, K., Chen, W., Chen, J., Zheng, J., Liu, C., et al. (2020). Epidemiological characteristics of carbapenem-resistant *Enterobacteriaceae* collected from 17 hospitals in Nanjing district of China. *Antimicrob. Agents. Chemother.* 9:15. doi: 10.1186/s13756-019-0674-4

Zou, H., Jia, X., Liu, H., Li, S., Wu, X., and Huang, S. (2020). Emergence of NDM-5-Producing *Escherichia coli* in a teaching hospital in chongqing, China: IncF-Type plasmids may contribute to the prevalence of bla NDM- 5. *Front. Microbiol.* 11:334. doi: 10.3389/fmicb.2020.00334

Zwanzig, M. (2021). The ecology of plasmid-coded antibiotic resistance: a basic framework for experimental research and modeling. *Comput. Struct. Biotechnol. J.* 19, 586–599. doi: 10.1016/j.csbj.2020.12.027

20

Boeravinone B, A Novel Dual Inhibitor of NorA Bacterial Efflux Pump of *Staphylococcus aureus* and Human *P*-Glycoprotein, Reduces the Biofilm Formation and Intracellular Invasion of Bacteria

Samsher Singh[1,2], Nitin P. Kalia[1†], Prashant Joshi[2,3], Ajay Kumar[4], Parduman R. Sharma[2,4], Ashok Kumar[2,4], Sandip B. Bharate[2,3] and Inshad A. Khan[1,2]*

[1] Clinical Microbiology Division, Indian Institute of Integrative Medicine (CSIR), Jammu, India, [2] Academy of Scientific and Innovative Research (AcSIR), Indian Institute of Integrative Medicine (CSIR), Jammu, India, [3] Medicinal Chemistry Division, Indian Institute of Integrative Medicine (CSIR), Jammu, India, [4] Cancer Pharmacology Division, Indian Institute of Integrative Medicine (CSIR), Jammu, India

***Correspondence:**
Inshad A. Khan
inshad@rediffmail.com;
iakhan@iiim.ac.in

†Present address:
Nitin P. Kalia,
Lee Kong Chian School of Medicine,
Nanyang Technological University,
Singapore, Singapore

This study elucidated the role of boeravinone B, a NorA multidrug efflux pump inhibitor, in biofilm inhibition. The effects of boeravinone B plus ciprofloxacin, a NorA substrate, were evaluated in NorA-overexpressing, wild-type, and knocked-out *Staphylococcus aureus* (SA-1199B, SA-1199, and SA-K1758, respectively). The mechanism of action was confirmed using the ethidium bromide accumulation and efflux assay. The role of boeravinone B as a human *P*-glycoprotein (*P*-gp) inhibitor was examined in the LS-180 (colon cancer) cell line. Moreover, its role in the inhibition of biofilm formation and intracellular invasion of *S. aureus* in macrophages was studied. Boeravinone B reduced the minimum inhibitory concentration (MIC) of ciprofloxacin against *S. aureus* and its methicillin-resistant strains; the effect was stronger in SA-1199B. Furthermore, time–kill kinetics revealed that boeravinone B plus ciprofloxacin at subinhibitory concentration (0.25 × MIC), is as equipotent as that at the MIC level. This combination also had a reduced mutation prevention concentration. Boeravinone B reduced the efflux of ethidium bromide and increased the accumulation, thus strengthening the role as a NorA inhibitor. Biofilm formation was reduced by four–eightfold of the minimal biofilm inhibitory concentration of ciprofloxacin, effectively preventing bacterial entry into macrophages. Boeravinone B effectively inhibited *P*-gp with half maximal inhibitory concentration (IC_{50}) of 64.85 μM. The study concluded that boeravinone B not only inhibits the NorA-mediated efflux of fluoroquinolones but also considerably inhibits the biofilm formation of *S. aureus*. Its *P*-gp inhibition activity demonstrates its potential as a bioavailability and bioefficacy enhancer.

Keywords: NorA, *P*-glycoprotein, biofilm, *Staphylococcus aureus*, efflux inhibition

INTRODUCTION

The development of multidrug resistance (MDR) upon chronic exposure to chemotherapeutic agents is considered the major reason for the failure of chemotherapy in cancer and infectious diseases (Poole, 2005; Leitner et al., 2011; Joshi et al., 2014). Efflux pumps are transmembrane proteins, which are the major contributors to multidrug resistance (MDR) in patients with cancer and infectious diseases. *P*-glycoprotein (gp), a multidrug-resistance protein (also called MDR1), accounts for the development of resistance to various drugs as well as for the transport of endogenous and exogenous substrate ligands, such as various toxins, hormones, and drugs (Chen et al., 1986; Joshi et al., 2014). Moreover, *P*-gp alters the pharmacokinetics and pharmacodynamics of its substrates by modulating their absorption, distribution, metabolism, elimination, and toxicity properties (Lin, 2003). Bacterial multidrug efflux pumps are the major contributors to microbial resistance to several classes of antibiotics (Kaatz et al., 2003; Tegos et al., 2011; Kalia et al., 2012).

Presence or augmented expression of efflux pumps is responsible for reduced drug availability to inhibit the specific target. Due to continuous efflux, comparatively lower concentration of antimicrobial agent reaches the target, which may increase the rate of new mutations thus generating newer types resistant mutants exhibiting novel resistance mechanisms (Poole, 2005; Piddock, 2006; Sun et al., 2014). With the continuous emergence of pathogenic resistance to conventional drugs because of efflux through MDR pumps, increasing efforts are directed toward discovering efflux inhibitory molecules. NorA efflux pump is the most widely studied among efflux pumps of *Staphylococcus aureus*. According to a study NorA efflux pump was found to be overexpressed in 43% of resistant strains of *S. aureus* (Patel et al., 2010; Astolfi et al., 2017). NorA, an established multidrug efflux pump model in *S. aureus*, accounts for extruding quinolones, quaternary ammonium salts, acridines, rhodamines, verapamil, and ethidium bromide (Kaatz et al., 2003; Khan et al., 2006; Leitner et al., 2011; Tegos et al., 2011; Holler et al., 2012; Schindler et al., 2013; Fontaine et al., 2015; Tintino et al., 2016). Recently some non-antibiotics derivatives as potent NorA efflux pump inhibitors have been reported utilizing pharmacophore based modeling and drug repurposing utilizing *in silico* approach (Astolfi et al., 2017; Sabatini et al., 2017). In addition, some less toxic benzochromene derivatives and dithiazole thione derivatives have also been reported as NorA efflux inhibitors (Ganesan et al., 2016; Lowrence et al., 2016). A recently published comprehensive review summarized the applications of nanoparticles are also being explored for efflux inhibitory activity in addition to biofilm inhibition (Gupta et al., 2017).

Despite their varying structures, the efflux pumps of bacterial and mammalian systems have sufficient substrate homology. Studies have reported many dual types of natural plant products that act as inhibitors, such as verapamil, reserpine, piperine, and capsaicin (**Figure 1**), as well as osthol and curcumin (Bhardwaj et al., 2002; Khan et al., 2006; Kalia et al., 2012; Joshi et al., 2014). These inhibitors offer advantages, such as enhanced gastrointestinal absorption, improved permeation through the blood–brain barrier, increased drug concentrations in mammalian cells for improved killing of invasive pathogens, and the use of lower concentrations of drugs to eliminate side effects (Khan et al., 2006).

In addition to drug efflux, a critical problem is biofilm formation, which poses a major hindrance in the evolution of novel chemotherapeutic agents (Bjarnsholt et al., 2013). Nearly 80% of human bacterial infections are caused by biofilm formation, and 60% of nosocomial infections are caused by biofilm formation on medical devices and implants (Darouiche, 2004; Hou et al., 2012). Biofilm eradication requires a much higher concentration, namely 10–1000 times the minimum inhibitory concentration (MIC), of antibiotics. Active efflux has been reported to contribute to increased resistance in bacterial biofilms (Lewis, 2001; Kvist et al., 2008; Baugh et al., 2014; Van Acker and Coenye, 2016; Sabatini et al., 2017). Biofilms have slow metabolism and growth, the main reasons for increased resistance, because most antibiotics target metabolic or cell division pathways (Lewis, 2007, 2008). Researchers have reported that the synergistic action of molecules abolishes biofilm formation (Baugh et al., 2012).

Staphylococcus aureus is considered an extracellular pathogen, but there are accumulating evidences to reveal that *S. aureus* causes severe intracellular infections, such as endocarditis and septic shock (Hooper, 2005). This organism, on getting an opportunity to invade, survives and promotes diseases. Hirakata et al. (2009) and Kalia et al. (2012) concluded that efflux pump-overexpressing strains can easily invade cells.

Several natural plant products act as efflux pump inhibitors (Stavri et al., 2007). Boeravinone B, the compound of interest in the present study, was isolated from the roots of *Boerhavia diffusa*, a plant belonging to the Nyctaginaceae family (Patil and Bhalsing, 2016). This plant is also known as Punarnava in the Indian traditional system of medicine, Ayurveda, and is established for its medicinal properties. In ancient times, plants were used to cure various physiological conditions, such as inflammation, jaundice, dyspepsia, nephrotic syndrome, convulsions, spleen enlargement, abdominal pain and stress, nematodal and microbial infections, and asthma (Ahmed-Belkacem et al., 2007; Khan et al., 2013; Bairwa et al., 2014). Boeravinone C and G have been reported to possess *P*-gp

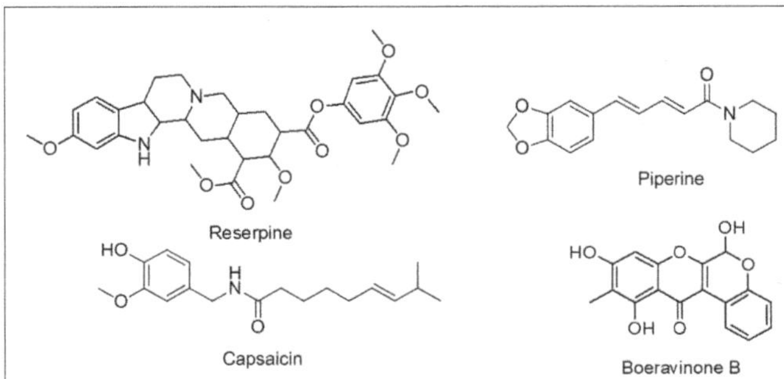

FIGURE 1 | Reserpine, piperine, capsaicin and boeravinone B (molecule used in this study).

TABLE 1 | Characteristics of *Staphylococcus aureus* strains used in this study.

Strain code	Characteristic	Origin
SA-1199	Wild type	Clinical isolate (endocarditis)
SA-1199B	NorA overexpressing	Ciprofloxacin resistant derivative of SA-1199
SA-K1758	NorA knockout	Derivative of NCTC-8325-4
MT23142	NorA overexpressing	Derivative of NCTC-8325
MRSA15187	MRSA	MRSA
ATCC 29213	MSSA	Standard strain; methicillin sensitive

inhibitory activity (Ahmed-Belkacem et al., 2007; Stacy et al., 2013).

In this study, we described the role of boeravinone B in ciprofloxacin potentiating activity against NorA-overexpressing strains of *S. aureus* and *P*-gp inhibition in the colon cancer cell line.

MATERIALS AND METHODS

Chemicals

All fluoroquinolones, ethidium bromide reserpine, piperine, fluorescein isothiocyanate (FITC) and 4′,6-diamidino- 2-phenylindole (DAPI) were purchased from Sigma Chemical Co. (St. Louis, MO, United States). Microbiological media were purchased BD Microbiology Products (Sparks, MD, United States). All other chemicals were of analytical grade.

Bacterial Strains

Staphylococcus aureus ATCC 29213, SA-1199B, SA-1199, SA-K1758, MT23142, and MRSA15187 were cultivated on trypticase soya agar (TSA). Important characteristics are described in **Table 1**.

Boeravinone B Isolation

Authentic samples of *B. diffusa* roots were collected from Jammu region (Voucher Specimen No. 21713), dried and powdered followed by solvent extraction in dichloromethane: methanol mixture (1:1 v/v) using cold maceration method. Crude extract was concentrated and purified by repeated silica gel column chromatography using hexane: ethyl acetate (95: 5 to 75: 25 v/v).

Drug Potentiation by Broth Checkerboard Microdilution

Drug potentiation or synergistic action of compound was assessed by broth checkerboard microdilution technique, which is most known method (Eliopoulos and Wennersten, 2002). Combination of ciprofloxacin and boeravinone B was tested in Mueller Hinton Broth (MHB; pH 7.0) against all bacterial strains using 96 well microtitre plates at a concentration range of 0.06–32 μg/ml and 0.8–50 μM, respectively. Additionally, combination of ethidium bromide and boeravinone B was assessed in similar way using *S. aureus* SA-1199B. Cell suspension of a density of 0.5 McFarland ($\approx 1.5 \times 10^8$ cfu per ml of *Escherichia coli*) was used as inoculum after diluting 1:100, a volume of 0.1 ml (5×10^5) was added to plates. The plates were incubated at 37°C for 18–20 h. Reserpine and piperine (known efflux pump blocker) were used as the control in this study. Minimum effective concentration (MEC) of boeravinone B was determined which is defined as concentration at which there is atleast fourfold reductions in MIC of ciprofloxacin. In a similar way various other fluoroquinolones and ethidium bromide were also assessed for synergistic potential of boeravinone B.

Time Kill Curve

Time-kill study of ciprofloxacin alone and in combination with boeravinone B was performed in 50 ml volume conical flasks containing 25 ml of MHB using the previously described method (Eliopoulos and Moellering, 1996). Ciprofloxacin at 2 μg/ml (0.25 × MIC) was tested alone and in combination with boeravinone B at the MEC concentration (12.5 μM) as determined above. Ciprofloxacin was also tested alone at an MIC of 8 μg/ml. NorA overexpressing *S. aureus* SA-1199B was used as the test bacterium. Ten folds serial dilutions of these aliquots were spotted on TSA plates.

Impact on Frequency of Resistance

Frequency of resistance (FOR) or Mutation prevention concentration (MPC) of ciprofloxacin against *S. aureus* ATCC 29213 was determined by method described elsewhere (Drugeon et al., 1999). MHA plates were supplemented with MIC, 2×, 4×, and 8× MIC of ciprofloxacin's concentrations with or without boeravinone B at MEC. A bacterial suspension of 0.1 mL (10^9 cfu) was plated on to each ciprofloxacin containing plates without and with boeravinone B. MPC was determined as the ratio of colonies appearing on ciprofloxacin or ciprofloxacin with boeravinone B combination to total colonies plated on a drug free plate.

Ethidium Bromide Efflux and Accumulation Studies

Fluorescence based method as described by Brenwald et al. (1998) was used to determine the ethidium bromide efflux inhibitory as well accumulation studies. For this purpose a freshly grown NorA overexpressing *S. aureus* SA-1199B was suspended to an optical density of 0.2 in uptake buffer (110 mM NaCl, 7 mM KCl, 50 mM NH_4Cl, 0.4 mM Na_2HPO_4, 52 mM Tris base and 0.2% glucose, adjusted to pH 7.5 with HCl). Cells were loaded with 10 μg/ml ethidium bromide for 30 min at 37°C. Extracellular ethidium bromide was removed by centrifugation and pellet was resuspended in same volume of uptake buffer with and without boeravinone B (12.5 μM). Reserpine at 25 μg/ml was used as a known efflux pump inhibitor. For accumulation studies bacterial cells loaded with ethidium bromide for 30 min after which EPIs (boeravinone B and reserpine) were added. Loss or gain of fluorescence in presence of compound and known EPI was deduced at 530 and 600 nm for excitation and emission wavelength, respectively, using multimode reader Infinite 200 Pro (Tecan Mannedorf, Switzerland).

Biofilm Inhibition

Effect of boeravinone B on the biofilm inhibitory potential of ciprofloxacin was studied with drug combination on biofilm formation, as previously described (Schillaci et al., 2010). For biofilm formation, cultures (S. *aureus* SA-1199 and SA-1199B) were grown overnight using TSB supplemented with 2% glucose (TSBG) and diluted to an optical density (570 nm) of 0.015 after diluting 1:200 (1×10^9 cells/mL). Microtitre plates for inhibitory studies were prepared as described for synergistic activity with ciprofloxacin by checkerboard microdilution method. After 24 h, wells were washed thrice with PBS followed by fixation with methanol for 15 min and finally air-dried in inverted position at 37°C. The wells of the dried plates were stained with 0.1% (w/v) crystal violet for 10 min and rinsed thoroughly with water until the negative control wells (without biofilms) appeared colorless. To quantify biofilm formation, 0.2 mL of 95% ethanol was added to wells of plate that were stained with crystal violet. Immediately absorbance read at 595 nm using microplate reader. In a separate plate the contents were decanted and washed with PBS to remove the planktonic cells and again filled with fresh TSB. After incubation for 30 min, 15 μl of 0.04% resazurin and 12.5 μl of 20% Tween80 were added in each well of the plate to access the viability of the cells within biofilm. The plates were incubated for 15 min and fluorescence was determined at an excitation at 560 nm and emission at 590 nm (Tecan Infinite M200 microplate reader) as described previously (Bauer et al., 2013). Minimal biofilm inhibitory concentration (MBIC) is defined as the concentration at which absorbance was reduced by ≥90% or was nearly equivalent to media control wells.

Confocal Microscopic Studies for Biofilm Inhibition

The potentiating effect of boeravinone B was further confirmed by staining the biofilms with FITC and DAPI which stains protein (amine reactive) and nucleic acid (DNA), respectively, by modified method as described by Yang (using DAPI in place of Hoechst) followed by visualization by confocal laser scanning microscopy (Yang et al., 2015). The biofilm of *S. aureus* ATCC 29213 was grown in six well poly styrene plate (Nunc) containing sterile 18 mm glass cover slips. Ciprofloxacin was used at 4 μg/ml which is MBIC and at 1 μg/ml which is subMBIC (0.25× MBIC) as determined above. Boeravinone B at 12.5 μM (MBIC) was added to sub-inhibitory concentration of ciprofloxacin (0.25× MBIC). The plates were incubated for 24 h at 37°C. PBS washes were given to eliminate planktonic cells followed by fixation of biofilm with 5% para-formaldehyde for 1 h at 50°C. Fixed biofilm was flooded with 0.001% (w/v) FITC and 1 μg/ml DAPI at kept at room temperature for 1 h. Images were seen and captured on 40× oil immersion lens using CLSM (Olympus flou View 1000).

In Vitro Screening of *P*-Glycoprotein Inhibitory Activity

P-glycoprotein inhibitory activity was assessed by the method described earlier using colorectal cell line LS180 (Jin et al., 2012; Joshi et al., 2014). Cell monolayer was prepared in 96 well plate using Dulbecco's Modified Eagle's medium (DMEM) media. The media was decanted and replaced with Hank's buffer containing 10 mM of Rh123 as a *P*-gp substrate. Twofold serial dilutions of boeravinone B (80–5 μM) were added and plate was incubated at 37°C in CO_2 incubator for 90 min. A known *P*-gp inhibitor elacridar (10 μM) was used as positive control. The contents of the wells were decanted and washed four times with cold PBS followed by cell lysis for 1 h using 200 μl of lysis buffer (0.1% Triton X 100 and 0.2 N NaOH). A total of 100 μl of lysate was used for reading fluorescence of Rh123 at an excitation at 485 nm and emission at 590 nm. All samples were normalized by dividing fluorescence of each sample with total protein present in the lysate. Half minimal inhibitory concentration (IC_{50}) value of boeravinone B was calculated using Graphpad Prism 5 software (GraphPad Software, Inc., La Jolla, CA, United States). Data is expressed as mean ± SD or representative of one of three similar experiments. Comparisons were made between control and treated groups or the entire intra group using one way ANOVA with post Bonferroni test through GraphPad Prism 5.00.288 statistical analysis software. **p*-values <0.05 were considered significant.

Molecular Docking Studies against *P*-Glycoprotein and NorA Efflux Pumps

Due to unavailability of crystal structures of human *P*-gp and *S. aureus* NorA, molecular docking studies were carried out using the homology models. The homology models for human *P*-gp (Jin et al., 2012) was prepared from *Caenorhabditis elegans* *P*-gp (PDB ID: 4AZF) and *S. aureus* NorA efflux pump (Aller et al., 2009) was prepared from glycerol 3-phosphate transporter pump from *E. coli* (PDB ID: IPW4) using Glide Induced Fit Docking in default setting. For Nor A docking studies, ciprofloxacin/reserpine binding site was used to construct grid file whereas for *P*-gp docking, verapamil binding site was used (Aller et al., 2009).

Macrophage Invasion Assay

To assess the impact of boeravinone B on invasion of *S. aureus* in macrophage, previously described method was used (Cheung and Bayles, 2007). Murine macrophage cell line J774 maintained on Roswell Park Memorial Institute medium (RPMI) supplemented with 10% (v/v) fetal calf serum was used as host. The macrophages were grown in monolayer to a density to 10^5 cells/well in 24 well plate in physiological conditions, i.e., 37°C and 5% CO_2 for 24 h. 10^6 cfu/well of overnight grown *S. aureus* strains SA-1199B, SA-1199, and SA-K1758 were used to infect macrophages (MOI of 10) in presence and absence of boeravinone B at its MEC (12.5 μM) for 2 h. Extracellular and adherent bacteria washed with PBS (pH 7.4) followed by treatment with 50 μg/ml gentamicin for 30 min. Intracellular bacteria were quantified by host cell lysis by brief treatment of 0.07% SDS which followed neutralization with 6% BSA. Viable bacteria were counted by plating on TSA. In a similar experiment RPMI devoid of FCS was used to assess the role of FCS.

TABLE 2 | Ciprofloxacin potentiation by boeravinone B against various strains of *S. aureus* with different levels of NorA expressions and MRSA.

Compounds	EPI# μg/ml (μM)	MIC (μg/ml) of ciprofloxacin					
		SA1199	SA-1199B	SA-K 1758	ATCC 29213	MT-23142	MRSA-15187
Ciprofloxacin	0	0.25	8	0.12	0.25	0.25–0.5	32
Boeravinone B	8 (25)	0.12	1	0.12	0.12	0.03	8
Piperine	50 (88)	0.12	4	0.12	0.06	ND	16
Reserpine	25 (41)	0.06	2	0.12	0.12	ND	ND

#*All EPIs tested have no self-antimicrobial activity up to 100 μM.*

TABLE 3 | Activity of boeravinone B on the MICs of ethidium bromide and other fluoroquinolones in susceptible and resistant *S. aureus* strains.

Antibacterial agents	Boeravinone B concentration in μg/ml (μM)	MIC (μg/ml) for given *S. aureus* strain			
		SA-1199B	SA-1199	SA-K1758	MT23142
EtBr	0	32	1	0.5	2
	8 (25)	2	0.25	0.12	0.12
Norfloxacin	0	32	0.25	0.12	32
	8 (25)	4	0.12	0.12	4
Ofloxacin	0	1	1	1	0.5
	8 (25)	0.5	1	0.5	0.5
Moxifloxacin	0	0.25	0.06	0.12	0.06
	8 (25)	0.12	0.06	0.12	0.06
Gatifloxacin	0	1	1	0.12	0.06
	8 (25)	0.25	0.5	0.12	0.06

RESULTS

Isolation and Purity of Boeravinone B

By using the cold maceration method, 6,9,11-trihydroxy-10-methylchromeno[3,4-b]chromen-12(6H)-one (boeravinone B; **Figure 1**) was isolated from the roots of *B. diffusa*. It is a yellow solid compound, with a melting point of 201°C–203°C. The structure was confirmed through high-resolution mass spectroscopy (m/z 313.0708 [M + H$^+$], as calculated for $C_{17}H_{12}O_6$ + H$^+$: 313.0707) and comparison of the ^{1}H and ^{13}C NMR data. Boeravinone B used in this study had 96% purity, as determined through high performance liquid chromatography. Data related to the purity and structure of the isolated boeravinone B was characterized by comparison of spectral data with described reported values (Kadota et al., 1989) (Supplementary Data S1).

Effect of NorA Efflux Pump Inhibition on MIC of Fluoroquinolones and Ethidium Bromide

The resistance reversal activity of boeravinone B was quantified by calculating the fold reduction in the MIC of ciprofloxacin. Boeravinone B lack anti-staphylococcal activity when assessed up to 100 μM against all tested strains. This MIC of ciprofloxacin alone and in combination with boeravinone B was determined (**Table 2**). Boeravinone B reduced the MIC of ciprofloxacin by twofold in *S. aureus* SA-1199 and ATCC 29213, whereas the effect was stronger in the NorA-overexpressing *S. aureus* strains SA-1199B and MT-23142, where the MIC was reduced by eightfold. Conversely, SA-K1758 (NorA knocked out) did not show any reduction in the MIC of ciprofloxacin. Boeravinone B was also active against a methicillin-resistant *S. aureus* (MRSA) strain, which showed a fourfold reduction in the ciprofloxacin MIC.

In addition to ciprofloxacin, spectrum of activity was also assessed using other fluoroquinolones like ofloxacin and norfloxacin which are well known substrates for NorA efflux pump and newer fluoroquinolones like gatifloxacin and moxifloxacin which are poor efflux substrates for NorA. Boeravinone B was used at 4× MEC for ethidium bromide (6.25 μM or 2 μg/ml). Potential of boeravinone B to inhibit the efflux of other fluoroquinolones was investigated using *S. aureus* strains SA-1199B, SA-1199, SA-K1758, and MT23142 (**Table 3**). MIC potentiation using ethidium bromide yielded similar effects of eightfold reduction in the MIC of ethidium bromide (2 μg/mL) compared with that of ethidium bromide alone, which exhibited an MIC of 16 μg/mL against SA-1199B. In NorA overexpressing strains (SA-1199B and MT23142), boeravinone B reduced the MIC of norfloxacin by eightfold while only twofold reduction in MIC of ofloxacin, moxifloxacin, and gatifloxacin was observed. It was observed that ciprofloxacin MIC reduction was relatively less (two-fourfold) in case of wild type *S. aureus* SA-1199 against these fluoroquinolones. There was no synergistic effect against *S. aureus* SA-K1758 due to absence of NorA efflux pump. Significant reduction in MICs against NorA overexpressing strains of *S. aureus* concludes that ciprofloxacin and norfloxacin

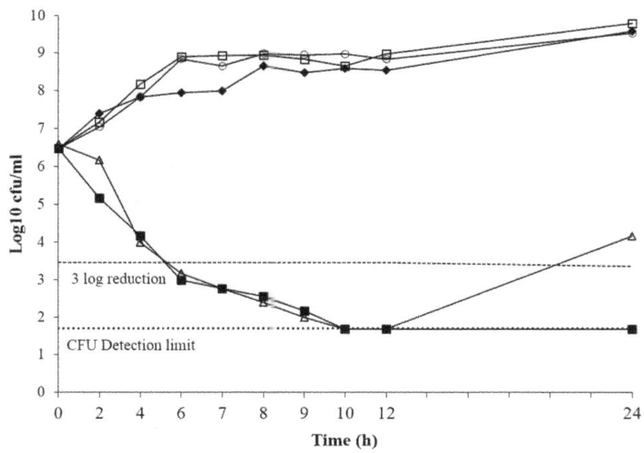

FIGURE 2 | Time kill curve of *Staphylococcus aureus* SA-1199B showing the bactericidal effect of ciprofloxacin alone (open triangle), subMIC alone (closed diamond) and ciprofloxacin at subMIC in combination with boeravinone B at MEC (closed square) including boeravinone B alone (Open circle). Growth control having plain media without ciprofloxacin or EPI served control (Open square). Each time point is mean Log_{10} of three independent readings.

TABLE 4 | Mutation prevention concentration (MPC) of ciprofloxacin with boeravinone B against *S. aureus* ATCC 29213.

Boeravinone	Mutation frequency with ciprofloxacin			
B conc. (μM)	**2 × MIC**	**4 × MIC**	**8 × MIC**	**16 × MIC**
0	5×10^{-8}	8×10^{-9}	4×10^{-9}	$<10^{-9}$
12.5	2.2×10^{-9}	$<10^{-9}$	$<10^{-9}$	$<10^{-9}$
25.0	$<10^{-9}$	$<10^{-9}$	$<10^{-9}$	$<10^{-9}$

have stronger affinity for NorA and efflux can be inhibited using boeravinone B.

Effect of Boeravinone B on Time–Kill Kinetics of Ciprofloxacin

The effect of boeravinone B on the time–kill kinetics of ciprofloxacin was assessed in *S. aureus* SA-1199B. Ciprofloxacin alone (MIC: 8 μg/mL) showed 3-log reduction in growth, whereas the same was accomplished at a subinhibitory concentration of the ciprofloxacin (0.25 × MIC) in combination with boeravinone B at a minimum effective concentration (MEC; 12.5 μM). The sub MIC of ciprofloxacin alone could not reduce the growth. Ciprofloxacin alone at an MIC effectively reduced the colony-forming units (CFU) in 6 h, but cell growth reoccurred after 24 h. The combination of ciprofloxacin (at subinhibitory concentration) and boeravinone B prevented the growth of resistant colonies (**Figure 2**).

Frequency of Ciprofloxacin Resistance in Presence of Boeravinone B

For effective clinical applications, drugs should be able to suppress mutations and resistance mechanisms. A resistant mutant selection study was performed on wild-type *S. aureus* ATCC 29213 because this strain does not have any known mutations in the regulatory region of NorA and drug targets (DNA gyrase and topoisomerase IV). The minimum concentration of a drug at which no resistant mutant is selected is defined as its MPC. Ciprofloxacin alone showed an MPC of 4 μg/ml whereas, in combination with 12.5 and 25 μg/ml of boeravinone B, the MPC of ciprofloxacin reduced to 2 and 1 μg/ml, respectively (**Table 4**). The MPC of this combination was lower than the C_{max} of ciprofloxacin (3–4 μg/ml) in human plasma, indicating the clinical relevance of these combinations in restricting the selection of resistant mutants.

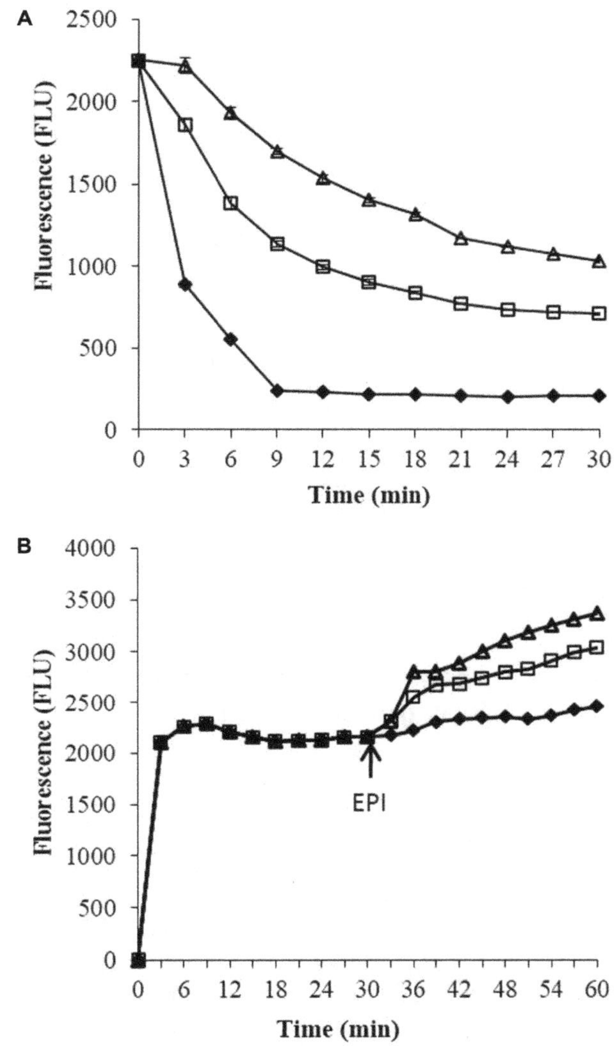

FIGURE 3 | Ethidium bromide studies efflux **(A)** and accumulation **(B)** studies against *S. aureus* SA-1199B. Symbols represents control which have no addition of any EPI (closed diamond), in presence of boeravinone B (open square) and in presence of known EPI, i.e., reserpine (open triangle).

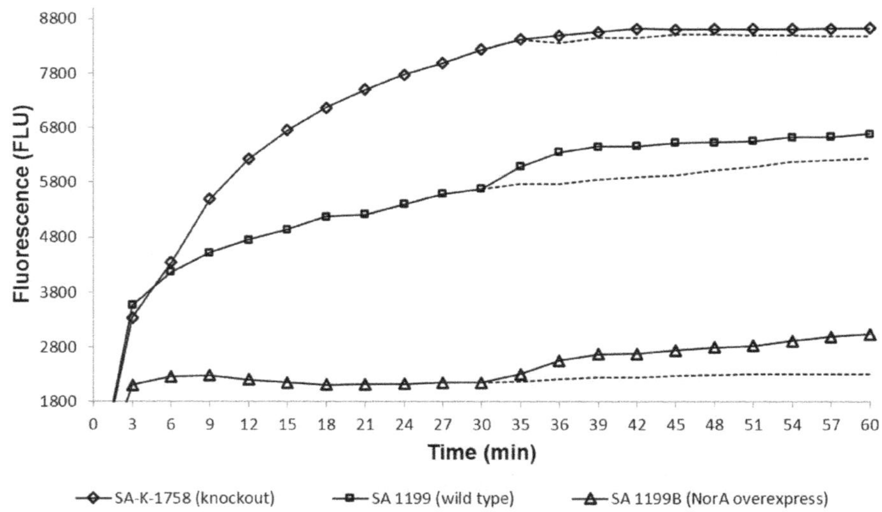

FIGURE 4 | Comparative accumulation of EtBr in presence of Boeravinone B against *S. aureus* SA-1199B (triangle), SA-1199 (square) and SA-K1758 (diamond) having different levels of NorA expressions, i.e., overexpression, wild type and knockout, respectively. Dotted lines after 30 min indicates the respective controls in absence of boeravinone B.

Effect of Boeravinone B on Ethidium Bromide Efflux Inhibition and Accumulation

Ethidium bromide is a well-known substrate for the NorA MDR efflux pump. SA-1199B cells were allowed to be loaded with ethidium bromide with and without boeravinone B and placed in a fluorometer cuvette containing fresh medium. Ethidium bromide fluoresces only when bound to nucleic acids in cells; therefore, a rapid decrease occurred in the fluorescence because of the NorA-mediated efflux of ethidium bromide. As shown in **Figure 3**, only the control cells without boeravinone B maximally extruded ethidium bromide, resulting in significantly decreased fluorescence in the assay period. Conversely, in cells treated with boeravinone B, the efflux of ethidium bromide was prevented, resulting in the prolonged retention of fluorescence. In the accumulation studies, ethidium bromide uptake was allowed in bacterial cells for 30 min. A counterbalance effect occurred because of the simultaneous efflux of ethidium bromide, which effectively increased the fluorescence. The addition of boeravinone B at this stage resulted in a surge in the fluorescence because of the inhibition of efflux pumps, resulting in a higher retention of fluorescence (**Figure 3**). Reserpine, a known efflux pump inhibitor, was used as the positive control in both studies. When compared, ethidium bromide accumulation in SA-1199B, SA-1199, and SA-K1758, accumulation was maximum in knockout followed by wild type and overexpressing which is in correlation with the phenotypes of the tested strains. In presence of boeravinone B, accumulation was significantly increased in NorA overexpressing, while minor effect was seen for wild type. *S. aureus* SA-1199. There was no effect on the accumulation efficiency of SA-K1758 which is devoid of functional *norA* gene (**Figure 4**).

TABLE 5 | Effect on biofilm inhibitory potential of ciprofloxacin when combined with boeravinone B at different concentrations against various strains of *S. aureus*.

Boeravinone B (μM)	MBIC (μg/ml) of ciprofloxacin		
	SA-1199	SA1199B	*S. aureus* ATCC 29213
0	4	16	4
6.25	2	8	2
12.5	1	4	1
25	1	2	1

Biofilm Inhibition

The minimum concentration of a drug for inhibiting a biofilm is defined and expressed as its MBIC. The MBIC of a drug is typically higher than its MIC because of the lesser permeability of the drug within the matrix of a biofilm. In this study, ciprofloxacin showed an MBIC of 4 and 16 μg/mL for *S. aureus* SA-1199 and SA-1199B, respectively. A concentration-dependent decrease occurred in the MBIC of ciprofloxacin against both strains in the presence of boeravinone B (6.25–25 μM; **Table 5**). To ascertain that the biofilm inhibition was caused by the killing of the bacteria embedded in the matrix of biofilm, the resazurin staining of a parallel set of plates was performed. The change in the color of this redox dye from blue to red indicated the viability of the cells in the well. The biofilm inhibition correlated well with the cell viability (Supplementary Figure S1).

Microscopic Studies

Effect of boeravinone B plus ciprofloxacin was evaluated by microscopic studies of the *S. aureus* ATCC 29213-generated biofilm. Fluorescein isothiocyanate stains proteins

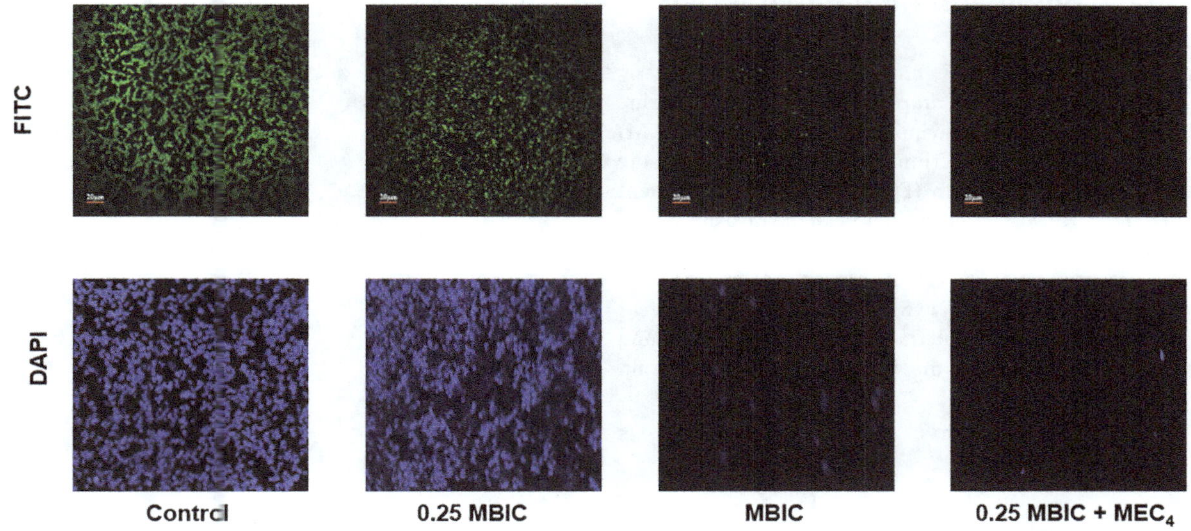

FIGURE 5 | CLSM of biofilm; untreated, treated with ciprofloxacin at subMBIC (0.25 × MBIC) and MBIC alone. Last column shows the presence of boeravinone B combined with subMBIC of ciprofloxacin. Upper line is stained with FITC and lower with DAPI.

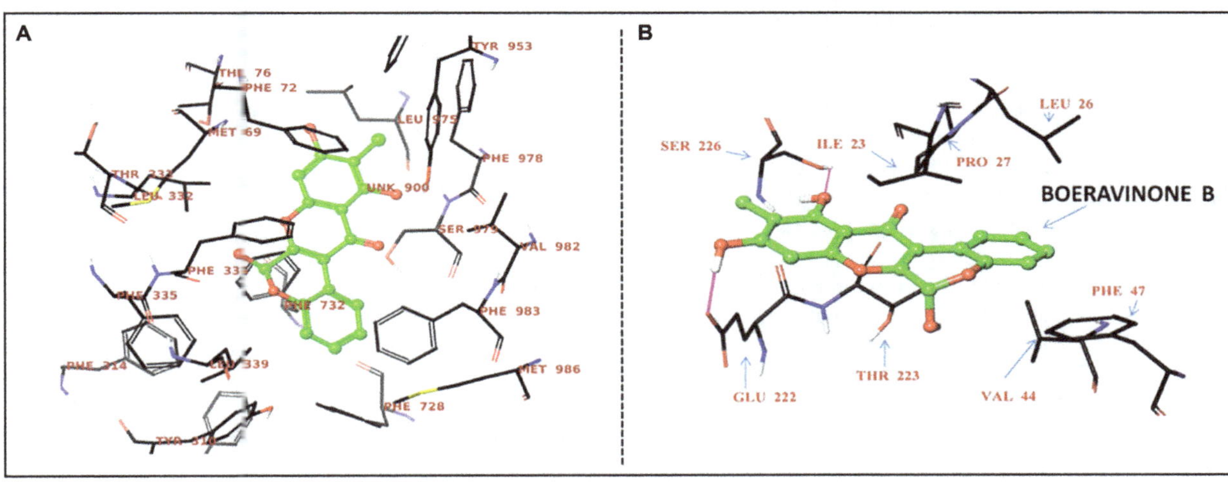

FIGURE 6 | Proposed binding site of boeravinone B with human *P*-gp **(A)** and *S. aureus* NorA efflux pumps **(B)**.

and imparts green fluorescence, whereas 4′,6-diamidino-2-phenylindole binds to nucleic acids and yields blue fluorescence when observed in the whole image field. As shown in **Figure 5**, the untreated biofilms were associated with a large amount of proteins and DNA. The sub MBIC of ciprofloxacin did not inhibit the biofilms; however, in combination with the MEC of boeravinone B, ciprofloxacin inhibited the biofilm, as did the MBIC of ciprofloxacin, as evident by the reduced intensity of green and blue fluorescence.

Molecular Docking on *P*-gp

Boeravinone B was observed to interact with *P*-gp at the verapamil binding site, particularly with the residues Met69, Phe72, Tyr307, Tyr310, Phe314, Leu332, Phe335, Phe336, Leu339, Phe728, Phe759, Phe957, Phe978, and Val982 through hydrophobic π–π interactions (**Figure 6A**). Consequently, it led to an increase in the intracellular accumulation of the substrate Rh123. Similarly, the NorA efflux pump is a transmembrane pump, in which ciprofloxacin or reserpine optimally bind to site 1 through strong hydrogen bonding of carboxyl functionality with the Arg98 cationic guanido group. The hydrophobic and hydrogen interactions of ciprofloxacin were mimicked by boeravinone B. Molecular modeling studies with the bacterial NorA efflux pump homology model revealed that boeravinone B binds to the Ile23 and Glu222 residues of the pump through strong hydrogen bonding formed by phenolic hydroxyl groups and thus block the interaction of substrate quinolones with the efflux binding cavity (**Figure 6B**).

Invasion Inhibition and Role of Fetal Calf Serum

The intracellular invasion of *S. aureus* SA-1199B was nearly 1.5 $\log_{10}$ higher than that of *S. aureus* SA-1199 in the murine macrophage cell line J774. Boeravinone B at its MEC (12.5 μM) was not active when the experiment was performed in the presence of 10% fetal calf serum (FCS). When the experiment was repeated using RPMI media without FCS, the invasiveness of *S. aureus* had reduced, suggesting the binding of boeravinone B to FCS. The invasiveness of SA-1199B showed greater reduction (1.6 $\log_{10}$) than did that of *S. aureus* SA-1199 (0.5 $\log_{10}$). *S. aureus* SA-K1758 exhibited the least penetration into macrophages, and boeravinone B did not affect the invasiveness of this strain (**Figure 7**).

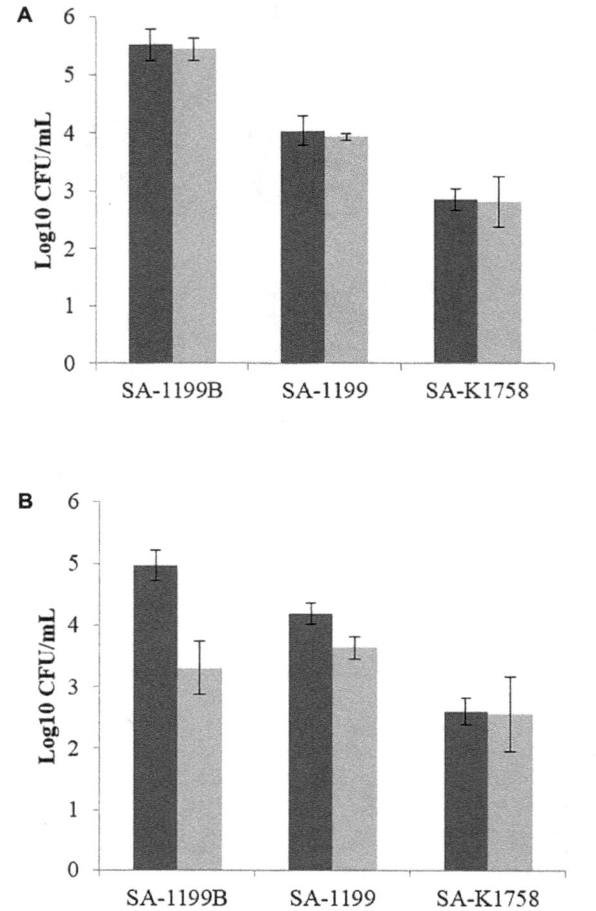

FIGURE 7 | Macrophage invasiveness by various strains of *S. aureus* in presence (gray bars) and absence (black bars) of boeravinone B. Assay was performed using standard RPMI media with **(A)** and without FCS **(B)**.

DISCUSSION

Efflux pumps are membrane-bound proteinaceous transporters known for extruding chemotherapeutic agents or xenobiotics, which are otherwise harmful for bacterial survival. During evolution, microbes were selected and evolved through antibiotic pressure with the overexpression of efflux pumps, which renders the antibiotics inefficient and hence results in the poor efficacy of chemotherapeutic agents. Efflux pumps can export a large pool of structurally unrelated substrates out of cells, which hampers their clinical efficacy. NorA is an MDR efflux pump of the major facilitator superfamily pumps and has 12 transmembrane segments. It is established for expelling various fluoroquinolones. NorA has been well established as a model system for studying efflux pump inhibition in Gram-positive pathogens (Kaatz, 2005; Kumar et al., 2008).

In the present study, boeravinone B obtained from *B. diffusa* was assessed for its NorA inhibitory activity in SA-1199B, which is a model organism for NorA inhibition studies because it mimics the resistance induced by fluoroquinolone pressure. Ethidium bromide MIC potentiation by 16-fold in NorA overexpressing strains in presence of boeravinone B shows inhibition of efflux mediated resistance. Presence of boeravinone B also exhibited two–eightfold reduction in MIC of ciprofloxacin and norfloxacin in these strains. The potentiating effect was less prominent (twofold) in wild type strain *S. aureus* SA-1199. Additionally there was no reduction in MIC of *S. aureus* SA-K1758 which is lacking functional *norA* gene. This concludes that ciprofloxacin and norfloxacin fluoroquinolone are favorable substrate for NorA. Similar observation about the enhanced affinity of NorA for these fluoroquinolones have been reported previously (Gibbons et al., 2003; Mullin et al., 2004). Boeravinone B increased the intrinsic susceptibility of *S. aureus* to ciprofloxacin and significantly reduced the emergence of ciprofloxacin-resistant *S. aureus*. A subinhibitory concentration of ciprofloxacin (2 μg/ml) with the MEC of boeravinone B (12.5 μM) exhibited a bactericidal effect and a 3-$\log_{10}$ reduction in CFU in 6 h, with no emergence of mutants even after 24 h. Conversely, ciprofloxacin alone exhibited the same effect at 8 μg/mL, but resistant mutants were observed after 24 h (**Figure 2**). Ethidium bromide efflux inhibition and accumulation are well-known mechanism-based descriptors for the specificity of NorA inhibition. The fluorescence-based efflux accumulation studies of ethidium bromide-preloaded NorA-overproducing *S. aureus* cells revealed reduced efflux in the presence of boeravinone B, indicating the inhibition of the ethidium bromide efflux mechanism. Furthermore, its effect on the retention of Rh123 in *P*-gp-overexpressing human adenocarcinoma LS-180 cells confirmed its role as a dual inhibitor of *P*-gp and the *S. aureus* efflux pump inhibitor. Studies have reported several similar dual inhibitors, such as osthol, curcumin, piperine, and capsaicin (Khan et al., 2006; Kalia et al., 2012). Docking results with the NorA homologous structure and *P*-gp obtained using Glide clearly elaborated that boeravinone B interacts with both pumps through core hydrophobic $\pi-\pi$ interactions and hydrogen bonding.

Both methicillin susceptible *S. aureus* and MRSA are common pathogenic concerns in the hospital environment (Livermore et al., 2015). MRSA remains a major concern in the clinical treatment of *S. aureus*-related infections since half a century. Vancomycin was the only drug of choice for treating the increased incidence of MRSA, but resistance abolished the drug's mechanism of action. With time, novel candidates were observed to be active against these strains, such as daptomycin, linezolid, and some glycopeptides, but resistance to these drugs was reported (Nannini et al., 2010). Because of frequent reports on resistance to antimicrobials, researchers are now using adjuvant therapy as a treatment strategy (Drugeon et al., 1999).

Active efflux has been reported to be associated with increased resistance in bacterial biofilms (Lewis, 2007; Van Acker and Coenye, 2016). The treatment of biofilm-related infections is a major unmet clinical concern because currently used antibiotics are insufficient to treat these highly persistent infections; some candidate molecules are under early development. Evidently, biofilms have slow metabolism and cell growth, which contribute to increased resistance because most currently used antibiotics have been discovered by targeting metabolic or cell division pathways. The synergistic action of molecules was reported to abolish the formation of biofilms (Baugh et al., 2014). These ideas prompted the assessment of the role of boeravinone B in the prevention and eradication of biofilms, a major clinical problem in the current era of anti-infective drug discovery (Bharate et al., 2015). Current studies have revealed that in combination with boeravinone B, the sub MBIC of ciprofloxacin inhibited the formation of biofilms through enhanced drug accumulation. Therefore, boeravinone B could penetrate the complex matrix of *S. aureus*-generated biofilms to inhibit viable bacteria, as observed in the resazurin assay (Supplementary Figure S1). The involvement of efflux pump inhibitors, such as certain diamines, was reported in reducing the invasiveness of *Pseudomonas aeruginosa* in eukaryotic cells (Hirakata et al., 2009). We obtained the similar results for capsaicin in a previous study (Kalia et al., 2012). This observation shows similar effects of boeravinone B, as expected, after the removal of FCS from the assay media (RPMI).

CONCLUSION

Boeravinone B is a novel dual inhibitor of bacterial NorA efflux pump and human *P*-gp. Such inhibitors play potential role in drug combinations by retaining higher concentrations of drugs in bacterial and host cells.

AUTHOR CONTRIBUTIONS

SS and NK performed microbiological studies. PJ performed isolation of compound and *in silico* studies. AsK and PS performed microscopic studies. SS and IK participated in design and execution of microbiological studies. SB participated in isolation and identification of compound used in this study. PJ and AjK participated in *P*-glycoprotein efflux inhibition studies. IK and SS prepared the manuscript and all authors participated in revising manuscript. All authors approved the study. All authors are accountable for all aspects of work in ensuring that questions related to the accuracy or integrity of the part of work are appropriately investigated and resolved.

FUNDING

SS received a Senior Research Fellowship from the Indian Council of Medical Research, New Delhi, India (80/993/2015-ECD-1). This work was supported by Council of Scientific and Industrial Research (CSIR), New Delhi, India (Grant no. BSC0205).

ACKNOWLEDGMENTS

We are grateful to Professor G. W. Kaatz (Wayne State University School of Medicine, Detroit, MI, United States) for providing *S. aureus* SA-1199, SA-1199B and SA-K1758. MT23142, a NorA over expressing strain was a kind gift from Professor David Hooper (Harvard Medical School, Boston, MA, United States).

REFERENCES

Ahmed-Belkacem, A., Macalou, S., Borrelli, F., Capasso, R., Fattorusso, E., Taglialatela-Scafati, O., et al. (2007). Nonprenylated rotenoids, a new class of potent breast cancer resistance protein inhibitors. *J. Med. Chem.* 50, 1933–1938. doi: 10.1021/jm061450q

Aller, S. G., Yu, J., Ward, A., Weng, Y., Chittaboina, S., Zhuo, R., et al. (2009). Structure of P-glycoprotein reveals a molecular basis for poly-specific drug binding. *Science* 323, 1718–1722. doi: 10.1126/science.1168750

Astolfi, A., Felicetti, T., Iraci, N., Manfroni, G., Massari, S., Pietrella, D., et al. (2017). Pharmacophore-based repositioning of approved drugs as novel *Staphylococcus aureus* NorA efflux pump inhibitors. *J. Med. Chem.* 60, 1598–1604. doi: 10.1021/acs.jmedchem.6b01439

Bairwa, K., Srivastava, A., and Jachak, S. M. (2014). Quantitative analysis of boeravinones in the roots of *Boerhavia diffusa* by UPLC/PDA. *Phytochem. Anal.* 25, 415–420. doi: 10.1002/pca.2509

Bauer, J., Siala, W., Tulkens, P. M., and Van Bambeke, F. (2013). A combined pharmacodynamic quantitative and qualitative model reveals the potent activity of daptomycin and delafloxacin against *Staphylococcus aureus* biofilms. *Antimicrob. Agents Chemother.* 57, 2726–2737. doi: 10.1128/AAC.00181-13

Baugh, S., Ekanayaka, A. S., Piddock, L. J., and Webber, M. A. (2012). Loss of or inhibition of all multidrug resistance efflux pumps of *Salmonella enterica* serovar Typhimurium results in impaired ability to form a biofilm. *J. Antimicrob. Chemother.* 67, 2409–2417. doi: 10.1093/jac/dks228

Baugh, S., Phillips, C. R., Ekanayaka, A. S., Piddock, L. J., and Webber, M. A. (2014). Inhibition of multidrug efflux as a strategy to prevent biofilm formation. *J. Antimicrob. Chemother.* 69, 673–681. doi: 10.1093/jac/dkt420

Bharate, J. B., Singh, S., Wani, A., Sharma, S., Joshi, P., Khan, I. A., et al. (2015). Discovery of 4-acetyl-3-(4-fluorophenyl)-1-(p-tolyl)-5-methylpyrrole as a dual inhibitor of human P-glycoprotein and *Staphylococcus aureus* NorA efflux pump. *Org. Biomol. Chem.* 13, 5424–5431. doi: 10.1039/c5ob00246j

Bhardwaj, R. K., Glaeser, H., Becquemont, L., Klotz, U., Gupta, S. K., and Fromm, M. F. (2002). Piperine, a major constituent of black pepper, inhibits human P-glycoprotein and CYP3A4. *J. Pharmacol. Exp. Ther.* 302, 645–650. doi: 10.1124/jpet.102.034728

Bjarnsholt, T., Ciofu, O., Molin, S., Givskov, M., and Hoiby, N. (2013). Applying insights from biofilm biology to drug development - can a new approach be developed? *Nat. Rev. Drug Discov.* 12, 791–808. doi: 10.1038/nrd4000

Brenwald, N. P., Gill, M. J., and Wise, R. (1998). Prevalence of a putative efflux mechanism among fluoroquinolone-resistant clinical isolates of *Streptococcus pneumoniae*. *Antimicrob. Agents Chemother.* 42, 2032–2035.

Chen, C. J., Chin, J. E., Ueda, K., Clark, D. P., Pastan, I., Gottesman, M. M., et al. (1986). Internal duplication and homology with bacterial transport proteins in the mdr1 (P-glycoprotein) gene from multidrug-resistant human cells. *Cell* 47, 381–389. doi: 10.1016/0092-8674(86)90595-7

Cheung, A. L., and Bayles, K. W. (2007). Tissue culture assays used to analyze invasion by *Staphylococcus aureus*. *Curr. Protoc. Microbiol.* 4, 9C.4.1–9C.4.7. doi: 10.1002/9780471729259.mc09c04s4

Darouiche, R. O. (2004). Treatment of infections associated with surgical implants. *N. Engl. J. Med.* 350, 1422–1429. doi: 10.1056/NEJMra035415

Drugeon, H. B., Juvin, M. E., and Bryskier, A. (1999). Relative potential for selection of fluoroquinolone-resistant *Streptococcus pneumoniae* strains by levofloxacin: comparison with ciprofloxacin, sparfloxacin and ofloxacin. *J. Antimicrob. Chemother.* 43(Suppl. C), 55–59. doi: 10.1093/jac/43.suppl_3.55

Eliopoulos, G. M., and Moellering, R. C. J. (1996). "Antimicrobial combinations," in *Antibiotics in Laboratory Medicine*, 4th Edn, ed. V. Lorian (Baltimore, MD: Williams & Wilkins), 330–336.

Eliopoulos, G. M., and Wennersten, C. B. (2002). Antimicrobial activity of quinupristin-dalfopristin combined with other antibiotics against vancomycin-resistant enterococci. *Antimicrob. Agents Chemother.* 46, 1319–1324. doi: 10.1128/AAC.46.5.1319-1324.2002

Fontaine, F., Hequet, A., Voisin-Chiret, A. S., Bouillon, A., Lesnard, A., Cresteil, T., et al. (2015). Boronic species as promising inhibitors of the *Staphylococcus aureus* NorA efflux pump: study of 6-substituted pyridine-3-boronic acid derivatives. *Eur. J. Med. Chem.* 95, 185–198. doi: 10.1016/j.ejmech.2015.02.056

Ganesan, A., Christena, L. R., Venkata Subbarao, H. M., Venkatasubramanian, U., Thiagarajan, R., Sivaramakrishnan, V., et al. (2016). Identification of benzochromene derivatives as a highly specific NorA efflux pump inhibitor to mitigate the drug resistant strains of *S. aureus*. *RSC Adv.* 6, 30258–30267. doi: 10.1039/C6RA01981A

Gibbons, S., Oluwatuyi, M., and Kaatz, G. W. (2003). A novel inhibitor of multidrug efflux pumps in *Staphylococcus aureus*. *J. Antimicrob. Chemother.* 51, 13–17. doi: 10.1093/jac/dkg044

Gupta, D., Singh, A., and Khan, A. U. (2017). Nanoparticles as efflux pump and biofilm inhibitor to rejuvenate bactericidal effect of conventional antibiotics. *Nanoscale Res. Lett.* 12, 454. doi: 10.1186/s11671-017-2222-6

Hirakata, Y., Kondo, A., Hoshino, K., Yano, H., Arai, K., Hirotani, A., et al. (2009). Efflux pump inhibitors reduce the invasiveness of *Pseudomonas aeruginosa*. *Int. J. Antimicrob. Agents* 34, 343–346. doi: 10.1016/j.ijantimicag.2009.06.007

Holler, J. G., Christensen, S. B., Slotved, H. C., Rasmussen, H. B., Guzman, A., Olsen, C. E., et al. (2012). Novel inhibitory activity of the *Staphylococcus aureus* NorA efflux pump by a kaempferol rhamnoside isolated from *Persea lingue* Nees. *J. Antimicrob. Chemother.* 67, 1138–1144. doi: 10.1093/jac/dks005

Hooper, D. C. (2005). Efflux pumps and nosocomial antibiotic resistance: a primer for hospital epidemiologists. *Clin. Infect. Dis.* 40, 1811–1817. doi: 10.1086/430381

Hou, W., Sun, X., Wang, Z., and Zhang, Y. (2012). Biofilm-forming capacity of *Staphylococcus epidermidis*, *Staphylococcus aureus*, and *Pseudomonas aeruginosa* from ocular infections. *Invest. Ophthalmol. Vis. Sci.* 53, 5624–5631. doi: 10.1167/iovs.11-9114

Jin, M. S., Oldham, M. L., Zhang, Q., and Chen, J. (2012). Crystal structure of the multidrug transporter P-glycoprotein from *Caenorhabditis elegans*. *Nature* 490, 566–569. doi: 10.1038/nature11448

Joshi, P., Singh, S., Wani, A., Sharma, S., Jain, S. K., Singh, B., et al. (2014). Osthol and curcumin as inhibitors of human Pgp and multidrug efflux pumps of *Staphylococcus aureus*: reversing the resistance against frontline antibacterial drugs. *MedChemComm* 5, 1540–1547. doi: 10.1039/C4MD00196F

Kaatz, G. W. (2005). Bacterial efflux pump inhibition. *Curr. Opin. Investig. Drugs* 6, 191–198.

Kaatz, G. W., Moudgal, V. V., Seo, S. M., and Kristiansen, J. E. (2003). Phenothiazines and thioxanthenes inhibit multidrug efflux pump activity in *Staphylococcus aureus*. *Antimicrob. Agents Chemother.* 47, 719–726. doi: 10.1128/AAC.47.2.719-726.2003

Kadota, S., Tezuka, N. Y., and Kikuchi, T. (1989). Constituents of the roots of *Boerhavia diffusa* L.I. examination of sterols and structures of new rotenoids, boeravinones A and B. *Chem. Pharm. Bull.* 37, 3214–3220. doi: 10.1248/cpb.37.3214

Kalia, N. P., Mahajan, P., Mehra, R., Nargotra, A., Sharma, J. P., Koul, S., et al. (2012). Capsaicin, a novel inhibitor of the NorA efflux pump, reduces the intracellular invasion of *Staphylococcus aureus*. *J. Antimicrob. Chemother.* 67, 2401–2408. doi: 10.1093/jac/dks232

Khan, I. A., Mirza, Z. M., Kumar, A., Verma, V., and Qazi, G. N. (2006). Piperine, a phytochemical potentiator of ciprofloxacin against *Staphylococcus aureus*. *Antimicrob. Agents Chemother.* 50, 810–812. doi: 10.1128/AAC.50.2.810-812.2006

Khan, M. S., Ansari, I. A., Ahmad, S., Ahmad, S., Akhter, F., Hashim, A., et al. (2013). Chemotherapeutic potential of *Boerhavia diffusa* Linn: a review. *J. Appl. Pharm. Sci.* 3, 133–139.

Kumar, A., Khan, I. A., Koul, S., Koul, J. L., Taneja, S. C., Ali, I., et al. (2008). Novel structural analogues of piperine as inhibitors of the NorA efflux pump of *Staphylococcus aureus*. *J. Antimicrob. Chemother.* 61, 1270–1276. doi: 10.1093/jac/dkn088

Kvist, M., Hancock, V., and Klemm, P. (2008). Inactivation of efflux pumps abolishes bacterial biofilm formation. *Appl. Environ. Microbiol.* 74, 7376–7382. doi: 10.1128/AEM.01310-08

Leitner, I., Nemeth, J., Feurstein, T., Abrahim, A., Matzneller, P., Lagler, H., et al. (2011). The third-generation P-glycoprotein inhibitor tariquidar may overcome bacterial multidrug resistance by increasing intracellular drug concentration. *J. Antimicrob. Chemother.* 66, 834–839. doi: 10.1093/jac/dkq526

Lewis, K. (2001). Riddle of biofilm resistance. *Antimicrob. Agents Chemother.* 45, 999–1007. doi: 10.1128/AAC.45.4.999-1007.2001

Lewis, K. (2007). Persister cells, dormancy and infectious disease. *Nat. Rev. Microbiol.* 5, 48–56. doi: 10.1038/nrmicro1557

Lewis, K. (2008). Multidrug tolerance of biofilms and persister cells. *Curr. Top. Microbiol. Immunol.* 322, 107–131. doi: 10.1007/978-3-540-75418-3_6

Lin, J. H. (2003). Drug-drug interaction mediated by inhibition and induction of P-glycoprotein. *Adv. Drug Deliv. Rev.* 55, 53–81. doi: 10.1016/S0169-409X(02)00171-0

Livermore, D. M., Mushtaq, S., Warner, M., James, D., Kearns, A., and Woodford, N. (2015). Pathogens of skin and skin-structure infections in the UK and their susceptibility to antibiotics, including ceftaroline. *J. Antimicrob. Chemother.* 70, 2844–2853. doi: 10.1093/jac/dkv179

Lowrence, R. C., Raman, T., Makala, H. V., Ulaganathan, V., Subramaniapillai, S. G., Kuppuswamy, A. A., et al. (2016). Dithiazole thione derivative as competitive NorA efflux pump inhibitor to curtail multi drug resistant clinical isolate of MRSA in a zebrafish infection model. *Appl. Microbiol. Biotechnol.* 100, 9265–9281. doi: 10.1007/s00253-016-7759-2

Mullin, S., Mani, N., and Grossman, T. H. (2004). Inhibition of antibiotic efflux in bacteria by the novel multidrug resistance inhibitors biricodar (VX-710) and timcodar (VX-853). *Antimicrob. Agents Chemother.* 48, 4171–4176. doi: 10.1128/AAC.48.11.4171-4176.2004

Nannini, E., Murray, B. E., and Arias, C. A. (2010). Resistance or decreased susceptibility to glycopeptides, daptomycin, and linezolid in methicillin-resistant *Staphylococcus aureus*. *Curr. Opin. Pharmacol.* 10, 516–521. doi: 10.1016/j.coph.2010.06.006

Patel, D., Kosmidis, C., Seo, S. M., and Kaatz, G. W. (2010). Ethidium bromide MIC screening for enhanced efflux pump gene expression or efflux activity in *Staphylococcus aureus*. *Antimicrob. Agents Chemother.* 54, 5070–5073. doi: 10.1128/AAC.01058-10

Patil, K. S., and Bhalsing, S. R. (2016). Ethnomedicinal uses, phytochemistry and pharmacological properties of the genus *Boerhavia*. *J. Ethnopharmacol.* 182, 200–220. doi: 10.1016/j.jep.2016.01.042

Piddock, L. J. (2006). Clinically relevant chromosomally encoded multidrug resistance efflux pumps in bacteria. *Clin. Microbiol. Rev.* 19, 382–402. doi: 10.1128/CMR.19.2.382-402.2006

Poole, K. (2005). Efflux-mediated antimicrobial resistance. *J. Antimicrob. Chemother.* 56, 20–51. doi: 10.1093/jac/dki171

Sabatini, S., Piccioni, M., Felicetti, T., De Marco, S., Manfroni, G., Pagiotti, R., et al. (2017). Investigation on the effect of known potent *S. aureus* NorA efflux pump inhibitors on the staphylococcal biofilm formation. *RSC Adv.* 7, 37007–37014. doi: 10.1039/C7RA03859C

Schillaci, D., Arizza, V., Parrinello, N., Di Stefano, V., Fanara, S., Muccilli, V., et al. (2010). Antimicrobial and antistaphylococcal biofilm activity from the sea urchin *Paracentrotus lividus*. *J. Appl. Microbiol.* 108, 17–24. doi: 10.1111/j.1365-2672.2009.04394.x

Schindler, B. D., Jacinto, P., and Kaatz, G. W. (2013). Inhibition of drug efflux pumps in *Staphylococcus aureus*: current status of potentiating existing antibiotics. *Future Microbiol.* 8, 491–507. doi: 10.2217/fmb.13.16

Stacy, A. E., Jansson, P. J., and Richardson, D. R. (2013). Molecular pharmacology of ABCG2 and its role in chemoresistance. *Mol. Pharmacol.* 84, 655–669. doi: 10.1124/mol.113.088609

Stavri, M., Piddock, L. J., and Gibbons, S. (2007). Bacterial efflux pump inhibitors from natural sources. *J. Antimicrob. Chemother.* 59, 1247–1260. doi: 10.1093/jac/dkl460

Sun, J., Deng, Z., and Yan, A. (2014). Bacterial multidrug efflux pumps: mechanisms, physiology and pharmacological exploitations. *Biochem. Biophys. Res. Commun.* 453, 254–267. doi: 10.1016/j.bbrc.2014.05.090

Tegos, G. P., Haynes, M., Strouse, J. J., Khan, M. M., Bologa, C. G., Oprea, T. I., et al. (2011). Microbial efflux pump inhibition: tactics and strategies. *Curr. Pharm. Des.* 17, 1291–1302. doi: 10.2174/138161211795703726

Tintino, S. R., Oliveira-Tintino, C. D., Campina, F. F., Silva, R. L., Costa Mdo, S., Menezes, I. R., et al. (2016). Evaluation of the tannic acid inhibitory effect against the NorA efflux pump of *Staphylococcus aureus*. *Microb. Pathog.* 97, 9–13. doi: 10.1016/j.micpath.2016.04.003

Van Acker, H., and Coenye, T. (2016). The role of efflux and physiological adaptation in biofilm tolerance and resistance. *J. Biol. Chem.* 291, 12565–12572. doi: 10.1074/jbc.R115.707257

Yang, H., Wang, M., Yu, J., and Wei, H. (2015). Aspartate inhibits *Staphylococcus aureus* biofilm formation. *FEMS Microbiol. Lett.* 362:fnv025. doi: 10.1093/femsle/fnv025

21

Mobile Plasmid Mediated Transition From Colistin-Sensitive to Resistant Phenotype in *Klebsiella pneumoniae*

Baoyue Zhang[1,2], Bing Yu[3], Wei Zhou[1,2], Yue Wang[4], Ziyong Sun[4], Xiaojun Wu[5], Shiyun Chen[1], Ming Ni[6] and Yangbo Hu[1]**

[1] CAS Key Laboratory of Special Pathogens and Biosafety, Center for Biosafety Mega-Science, Wuhan Institute of Virology, Chinese Academy of Sciences, Wuhan, China, [2] University of Chinese Academy of Sciences, Beijing, China, [3] Department of Pathogen Biology, School of Basic Medicine, Tongji Medical College, Huazhong University of Science and Technology, Wuhan, China, [4] Department of Laboratory Medicine, Tongji Hospital, Tongji Medical College, Huazhong University of Science and Technology, Wuhan, China, [5] Department of Respiratory and Critical Medicine, Renmin Hospital of Wuhan University, Wuhan, China, [6] Department of Infectious Diseases, Tongji Hospital, Tongji Medical College, Huazhong University of Science and Technology, Wuhan, China

***Correspondence:**
Ming Ni
niming@tjh.tjmu.edu.cn
Yangbo Hu
ybhu@wh.iov.cn

Multidrug-resistant bacteria, including carbapenem-resistant *Klebsiella pneumoniae* (CRKP), are becoming an increasing health crisis worldwide. For CRKP, colistin is regarded as "the last treatment option." In this study, we isolated a clinical CRKP strain named as *K. pneumoniae* R10-341. Phenotyping analysis showed that this strain could transit from a colistin-sensitive to a resistant phenotype by inserting an IS*4* family IS*Kpn72* element into the colistin-resistance associated *mgrB* gene. To investigate the mechanism of this transition, we performed genome sequencing analysis of the colistin-sensitive parental strain and found that 12 copies of IS*Kpn72* containing direct repeats (DR) are located on the chromosome and 1 copy without DR is located on a multidrug-resistant plasmid pR10-341_2. Both types of IS*Kpn72* could be inserted into the *mgrB* gene to cause colistin-resistance, though the plasmid-derived IS*Kpn72* without DR was in higher efficiency. Importantly, we demonstrated that colistin-sensitive *K. pneumoniae* strain transferred with the IS*Kpn72* element also obtained the ability to switch from colistin-sensitive to colistin-resistant phenotype. Furthermore, we confirmed that the IS*Kpn72*-containing pR10-341_2 plasmid was able to conjugate, suggesting that the ability of causing colistin-resistant transition is transferable through common conjugation. Our results point to new challenges for both colistin-resistance detection and CRKP treatment.

Keywords: multidrug resistance, CRKP, mgrB, colistin, phenotype transition

INTRODUCTION

Multidrug-resistant pathogenic bacteria, such as carbapenem-resistant *Klebsiella pneumoniae* (CRKP), are increasingly becoming a health crisis worldwide (Nordmann et al., 2011; Pitout et al., 2015). Polymyxins, including polymyxin B and polymyxin E (colistin), have been regarded as "the last treatment option" for CRKP (Biswas et al., 2012). Polymyxins are lipopeptide antibiotics targeting the lipopolysaccharide (LPS) of the bacterial outer membrane, the main component of the Gram-negative bacterial cell wall (Hancock, 1997; Li et al., 2006).

The increase in infections by polymyxin-resistant bacteria has become a great challenge to clinical treatment (Antoniadou et al., 2007; Bogdanovich et al., 2011; Macesic et al., 2020). In *K. pneumoniae*, the most common polymyxin-resistance mechanism is achieved by LPS modification, which decreases the negative charge of LPS and reduces its affinity to polymyxins (Velkov et al., 2014; Liu et al., 2017). The mobile colistin resistance gene (*mcr-1*) is the first reported plasmid-mediated colistin resistance gene (Liu et al., 2016), which encodes a phosphoethanolamine-lipid A transferase catalyzing the addition of phosphoethanolamine (PEtN) to lipid A (Liu et al., 2016, 2017). To date, 10 variants (*mcr*1-10) have been identified on a wide variety of transferable plasmids (Wang et al., 2018, 2020; Yang et al., 2018; Zhong et al., 2018; Lei et al., 2020), leading to the widespread diffusion of *mcr*-mediated colistin-resistance (Zhong et al., 2018; Nang et al., 2019). Chromosome-mediated colistin-resistance has also been characterized by the involvement of a small transmembrane protein MgrB and the two-component systems (TCSs) PhoPQ, PmrAB, and CrrAB (Gunn and Miller, 1996; Olaitan et al., 2014). To the best of our knowledge, in contrast to *mcr* genes, chromosome-mediated colistin-resistance mechanisms are considered to be stable and have not been reported to be transferred or mobile to other bacteria. However, inactivation of the *mgrB* gene has been widely identified from clinical colistin-resistant clinical *K. pneumoniae* strains (Cannatelli et al., 2013; Gaibani et al., 2014; Olaitan et al., 2014).

In this study, we isolated a multidrug resistant *K. pneumoniae* strain named R10-341 with high frequency ($\sim10^{-6}$) of colistin heteroresistance (El-Halfawy and Valvano, 2015; Halaby et al., 2016). Genetic and molecular analyses identified that insertion of an IS*Kpn72* element into the *mgrB* gene was responsible for the acquisition of colistin resistance. We further analyzed IS*Kpn72* copies in this strain and demonstrated that the IS*Kpn72* element is derived from a mobile plasmid and suggested that this mobile plasmid has the ability to render transition from colistin-sensitive to resistant phenotype in *K. pneumoniae*.

MATERIALS AND METHODS

Bacterial Strains, Plasmids, and Primers

The *K. pneumoniae* strains named R10-341 and 7097 used in this study were isolated from the sputum samples collected from the Tongji Hospital, Hubei Province, China. The *K. pneumoniae* strains were grown in LB medium with 100 μg/mL ampicillin at 37°C.

For plasmid constructions, the p15A *ori* from plasmid pACYC184 (Rose, 1988) and the streptomycin-resistance gene from pTargetF (Jiang et al., 2015) were PCR amplified, respectively. These two fragments were assembled as the linearized vector p15A-Sm by overlap PCR, which was then cloned with IS*pla* (IS fragment from pR10-341_2) or IS*chr* (IS fragment from chromosome) fragment using the ClonExpress II One Step Cloning Kit (Vazyme) to generate two plasmids named p15A-Sm-IS*pla* and p15A-Sm-IS*chr* respectively. All primers used in this study are listed in **Supplementary Table 1**.

Sequence Typing and Colistin Resistant Gene Detection

Multilocus sequence typing (MLST) for the *K. pneumoniae* R10-341 strain was performed as described (Diancourt et al., 2005).[1] Colistin resistance associated genes were detected by PCR. Each of the *mcr* genes was amplified using two pairs of primers. Genes encoding the two-component systems were amplified by PCR and confirmed by DNA sequencing in comparison with the *K. pneumoniae* HS11286 strain (Accession: NC_016845). All primers are listed in **Supplementary Table 1**.

Drug Susceptibility Test

MICs of antibiotics (except colistin) for *K. pneumoniae* R10-341 were determined using the broth microdilution method according to the Clinical and Laboratory Standards Institute (CLSI) guidelines (CLSI document M100-S28)[2]. The susceptibility to colistin was tested according to the guidelines of European Committee on Antimicrobial Susceptibility Testing (EUCAST)[3]. Briefly, 100 μL Cation-adjusted Mueller-Hinton Broth containing 2-fold diluted antibiotics was added to a 96-well plate, followed by the addition of 100 μL bacterial cells ($10^5\sim10^6$ CFU/mL) to each well. The 96-well plate was incubated at 37°C for 16–24 h. The lowest concentration of antibiotic with complete inhibition (clear broth) was regarded as the MIC.

Genome DNA Extraction, Whole Genome Sequencing, and Bioinformatics Analysis

The *K. pneumoniae* R10-341 strain was first spread onto a LB plate. A single colony was selected and cultured in LB medium at 37°C. Genomic DNA was extracted using a bacterial genomic DNA extraction Kit (Tiangen). Genome DNA sequencing was performed by both Hiseq X Ten (Illumina) and MinION (Oxford Nanopore Technologies) platforms according to a standard protocol provided by Illumina and Oxford Nanopore Technologies. The off-machine data of Nanopore sequencing is converted to fastq format through the Albacore software in the MinKNOW software package[4] (Payne et al., 2019). After filtering to obtain clean reads, these reads are randomly selected and aligned with the Nucleotide Sequence Database. *De novo* genome assembly was performed with Unicycler v0.4.7 (Wick et al., 2017). NCBI Prokaryotic Genomes Annotation Pipeline (PGAP) was used to annotate assembled genome sequence and to identify genes related to conjugation (Tatusova et al., 2016). Antibiotic resistance genes and plasmid replicons were respectively identified by ResFinder v3.0 (Zankari et al., 2012) and PlasmidFinder v2.0 (Carattoli et al., 2014) from the Center for Genomic Epidemiology website[5]. Sequence reads for the whole-genome sequencing are available from the NCBI Sequence Read Archive (PRJNA655367).

[1] https://bigsdb.pasteur.fr/klebsiella/

[2] https://clsi.org/standards/products/microbiology/documents/m100-preorder/

[3] https://www.eucast.org/fileadmin/src/media/PDFs/EUCAST_files/General_documents/Recommendations_for_MIC_determination_of_colistin_March_2016.pdf

[4] https://github.com/Albacore/albacore

[5] http://www.genomicepidemiology.org/

IS Element Analysis

For analyzing the IS elements in *K. pneumoniae* R10-341, the IS element inserted into the *mgrB* gene in colistin resistant colonies was first identified by PCR and DNA sequencing. This IS element sequence was analyzed in ISfinder database[6] and was named as IS*Kpn72* based on suggestion from ISfinder. The sequence of the ISKpn72 element was then aligned with the *K. pneumoniae* R10-341 genome sequence using BLASTn.

Amino acid sequences of transposases used in the phylogenetic tree analyses of the IS elements were downloaded from ISfinder database. Phylogenetic tree was constructed based on average distance using Jalview 2.11 (Waterhouse et al., 2009).

Conjugation Analysis

Since *K. pneumoniae* R10-341 is resistant to several antibiotics but is relatively sensitive to tetracycline, we constructed a tetracycline-resistant (TcR) *E. coli* K-12 strain as the recipient in conjugation experiment using a CRISPR/Cas9 system (Jiang et al., 2015). Briefly, the *E. coli* K-12 strain was first transformed with a Cas9 expressing plasmid pCas, and the sgRNA expressing plasmid pTargetF-EclacZ (targeting the *lacZ* gene) was then co-transformed with a DNA repairing fragment containing tetracycline-resistance gene from pACYC184 plasmid (Rose, 1988). The colonies resistant to tetracycline were screened. A single colony from 50 μg/ml tetracycline-containing LB agar plate was confirmed by DNA sequencing and was named as K12-TcR for subsequent conjugation tests.

Conjugation was performed by mixing an overnight donor (*K. pneumoniae* R10-341) and logarithmic phase recipient (K12-TcR) at a ratio of 4:1 in a total volume of 1 mL as described (Wu et al., 2019). The mixture was then concentrated and spotted onto LB agar without antibiotics at 37°C for 2–4 h to allow conjugation to occur. Since the pR10-341_2 plasmid contains streptomycin resistance gene (**Table 1**), the conjugated bacterial mixture was plated on LB agar containing 50 μg/ml tetracycline and 50 μg/ml streptomycin to screen for transconjugants carrying plasmid pR10-341_2. Transconjugants were confirmed by PCR using primers paired to *K. pneumoniae* R10-341 (Kpn-F-FR), K12-TcR (Ec-F-FR), and pR10-341_2 plasmid (P-F-FR), respectively.

[6]http://www-is.biotoul.fr

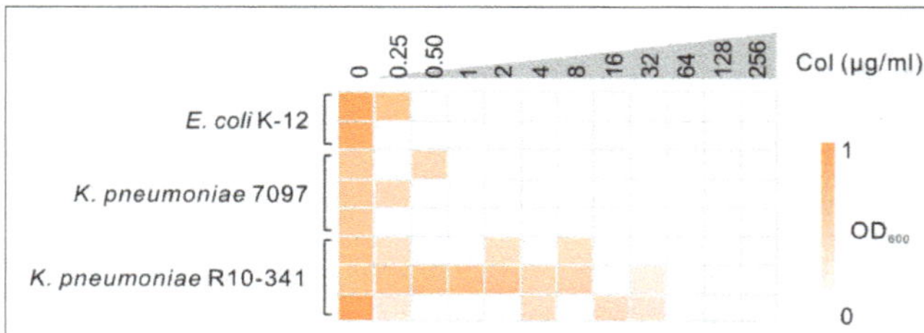

FIGURE 1 | Sensitivity test of the *K. pneumoniae* R10-341 strain to colistin. *E. coli* K-12 and *K. pneumoniae* 7097 were used as control strains. The depth of the color increases with the OD_{600} values.

RESULTS

Characterization of a Multi-Drug Resistant *Klebsiella pneumoniae* R10-341 Strain

The *K. pneumoniae* R10-341 strain was a clinical isolate from a sputum sample collected before antibiotic treatment from Tongji Hospital in Wuhan, China. This *K. pneumoniae* R10-341 strain was classified as ST11 and was resistant to different classes of antibiotics, including beta lactams, aminoglycosides, chloramphenicol, rifamycin, quinolones, sulfonamides and macrolides (summarized in **Table 1**). When testing the minimal inhibitory concentration (MIC) of colistin for this strain, we observed that some of the wells in the 96-well plate tested were resistant, while other wells showed colistin-sensitive phenotype (**Figure 1**). To exclude the possibility that the tested strain was a mixture of colistin sensitive and resistant, DNA sequences of known colistin resistance associated genes were tested in *K. pneumoniae* R10-341 parental strain. As summarized in **Table 2**, *phoPQ*, *pmrAB*, *crrAB*, and *mgrB* genes were the same as those in drug-sensitive strain, and the *mcr1-8* genes could not be successfully amplified in *K. pneumoniae* R10-341 strain. To further exclude the possibility of bacterial contamination, we streaked the R10-341 strain onto LB plate and selected different single colonies. Similar results were obtained for all these single colonies (data not shown), which suggested that the appearance of colistin resistant colonies for *K. pneumoniae* R10-341 strain was due to a colistin heteroresistance (CHR).

TABLE 1 | MIC values of different antibiotics to *K. pneumoniae* R10-341.

Antibiotic name	Antibiotic class	MIC (μg/ml)	Resistance gene	Gene location
Ampicillin	Beta lactams	>256	*bla*SHV-11 *bla*KPC-2 *bla*CTX-M-27	Chromosome pR10-341_2
Kanamycin	Aminoglycoside	128	–	–
Streptomycin	Aminoglycoside	256	*aadA*	pR10-341_2
Gentamicin	Aminoglycoside	>128	–	–
Rifampin	Rifamycin	>256	*arr-2*	pR10-341_2
Chloramphenicol	Chloramphenicol	128	*cat3*	Chromosome
Ciprofloxacin	Quinolones	>256	*qnrB*	pR10-341_2
Trimethoprim	Sulfonamides	>256	*dfrA12*	pR10-341_2
Tetracycline	Tetracyclines	16	–	–
Erythromycin	Macrolides	>256	–	–

TABLE 2 | Genes related to colistin resistance in *K. pneumoniae* R10-341.

Resistance mechanism	Gene	Gene functions	Detection results
Lipid A assembly PEtN	*mcr-1*	Phosphatidylethanolamine-lipid A transferase	No product
	mcr-2		No product
	mcr-3		No product
	mcr-4		No product
	mcr-5		No product
	mcr-6		No product
	mcr-7		No product
	mcr-8		No product
L-Ara4N and PEtN synthesis and modified LPS pathway	*mgrB*	PhoPQ negative-regulate protein	WT*
	phoPQ	TCS (Two-Component System)	WT*
	pmrAB	TCS	WT*
	crrAB	TCS	WT*

**WT indicates gene had the 100% DNA sequence identity in coding region and a ~150 bp promoter region as these in the reference strain K. pneumoniae HS11286.*

Insertion of an IS*4* Family Transposon Element Into *mgrB* Gene Generated Colistin-Resistant Colonies

To further characterize the *K. pneumoniae* R10-341 strain, we tested the growth of this strain on LB plates containing 100 μg/mL colistin. Consistent with MIC testing, some colonies (~10^{-6}) grew on the plate containing colistin, but no colonies were obtained from *E. coli* K-12 nor from another clinical isolate named *K. pneumoniae* 7097 on the colistin-containing plate (**Figure 2A**). To test the mechanism of this colistin resistance, we selected two colonies of the *K. pneumoniae* R10-341 strain from LB plate without colistin and then streaked onto LB plates containing 100 μg/mL colistin. Again, some colonies from both strains can grow on LB plates containing colistin. We then isolated four colonies from each of these two colistin-containing plates and sequenced the *phoPQ*, *pmrAB*, and *mgrB* genes (**Figure 2B**). Surprisingly, the amplified *mgrB* fragments from colistin-resistant colonies were all ~1.4 kb longer than that from parental colistin-sensitive strains (**Figures 2B,C**).

Next, we sequenced this ~1.4 kb inserted fragment. Sequence alignment in the NCBI database showed this fragment encodes an IS4 family transposase. Further analysis of this ~1.4 kb inserted fragment in ISfinder suggested that this insertion sequence could be named as IS*Kpn72* and classified into the IS*10* group in the IS4 family, as its sequence is >95% identical to IS*10R* (**Figure 2D**). In accordance with this analysis, we identified 22 bp inverted repeats (IR) at both the left and right ends of this insertion fragment and 9 bp direct repeats (DR) around the insertion site (**Figure 2C**).

K. pneumoniae R10-341 Carries the IS*Kpn72* Element Both in the Chromosome and Plasmid DNA

The R10-341 strain can become colistin-resistant by inserting the IS*Kpn72* element into the *mgrB* gene, but we do not know the source of the IS*Kpn72* element. We therefore sequenced the genome of the original colistin-sensitive *K. pneumoniae* R10-341 strain. We obtained a 5.3 Mb chromosome DNA and two plasmid sequences (named pR10-341_1 and pR10-341_2, respectively), which are 5.3Mb, 10.06 kb, and 236.3 kb with G + C contents of 57.46, 55.07, and 52.72%, respectively. According to the PlasmidFinder database, pR10-341_1 and pR10-341_2 harbored ColRNAI and IncR replicon sequence, respectively. Several antibiotic resistance genes were identified both on the chromosome and plasmids, which were in consistent with our drug resistance tests (**Table 1**). Genome sequencing analysis confirmed that colistin-resistance related genes, including *mgrB*, *phoPQ*, and *pmrAB*, were all the same as the *K. pneumoniae* reference strain HS11286 (Genome accession: NC_016845), which further supports our hypothesis that the colistin-sensitive strain acquired resistance in the presence of colistin.

In searching for the IS*Kpn72* element sequence in the whole genome we obtained, we found 12 copies of this IS*Kpn72* element on the chromosome, and 1 copy on the plasmid pR10-341_2. Similar to that observed in the colistin-resistant R10-341 strain, all copies of the IS*Kpn72* element contain a pair of 22 bp-length imperfect terminal inverted repeats (IR) (**Figure 3A**). Surrounding the 12 copies of the IS*Kpn72* element located on the chromosome are 9-bp direct repeated (DR) sequences. In contrast, the plasmid encoding the IS*Kpn72* element only contains IR sequences but not the 9 bp-DR sequences (**Figure 3A**). Therefore, we assumed that the copy without DR on pR10-341_2 might be the root of all the IS*Kpn72* copies on the chromosome. These analyses suggested that the IS*Kpn72* element had already been inserted into the chromosome in the parental colistin-sensitive strain.

Both the DR-Containing and DR-Missing IS*Kpn72* Elements Can Be Inserted Into the *mgrB* Gene

Whether these existing IS*Kpn72* elements could be inserted into the *mgrB* gene to cause colistin-resistance is the next question. We transformed plasmids cloned with either the IS*Kpn72* element from pR10-341_2 or an IS*Kpn72* element from the *K. pneumoniae* R10-341 chromosome (named as IS*pla* and IS*chr*, respectively) into the colistin-sensitive strain *K. pneumoniae* 7097 (**Figure 3B**). In contrast to the parental *K. pneumoniae* 7097 strain, the transformation of the plasmid containing either

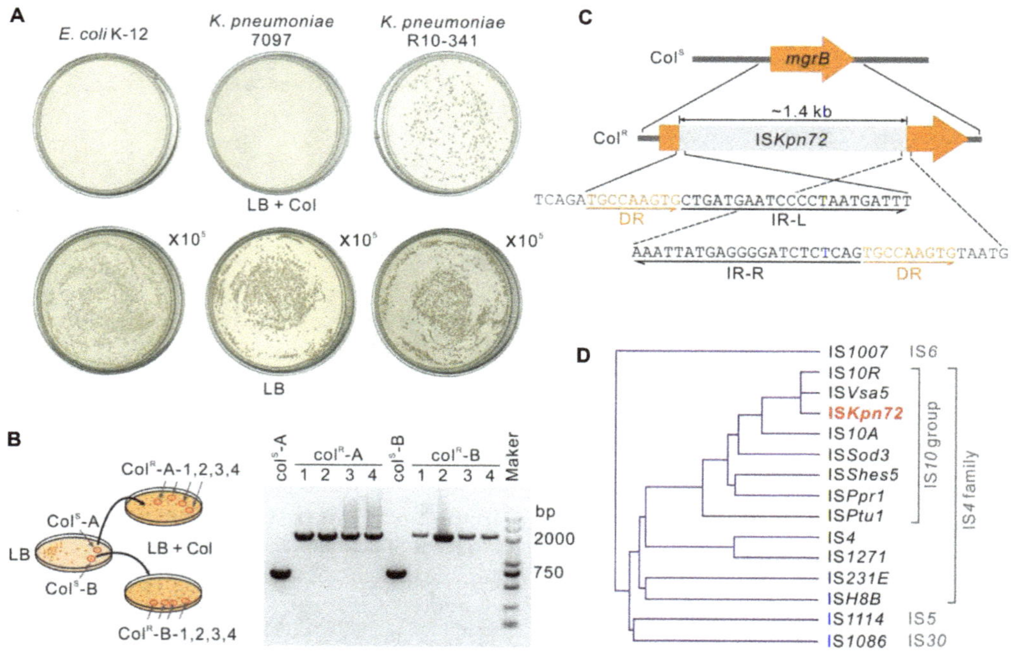

FIGURE 2 | Insertion of an IS*Kpn72* transposon element into the *mgrB* gene in colistin-resistant strain. **(A)** Colonies of *E. coli* K-12, *K. pneumoniae* 7097 and *K. pneumoniae* R10-341 streaked on LB plates containing 100 μg/mL colistin. Each plate was streaked with 100 μL of logarithmic phase bacteria. As a control, 100 μL of 10^5 diluted bacteria was also spread onto LB plates without colistin. **(B)** Confirmation of acquisition of colistin resistance for the *K. pneumoniae* R10-341 strain. Two separated colistin-sensitive colonies were spread onto two LB plates containing 100 μg/mL colistin. Fragment insertions of the *mgrB* gene in four colonies from each plate were tested by PCR. **(C)** Insertion of the IS*Kpn72* element into the *mgrB* gene in *K. pneumoniae* R10-341 colistin-resistant colonies. **(D)** Phylogenetic tree of the IS elements based on amino acid sequences of transposases.

IS*pla* or IS*chr* into this colistin-sensitive strain resulted in the growth of some colistin-resistant colonies. Colony forming units (CFU) on LB agar containing 100 μg/mL colistin revealed that the plasmid-derived IS*Kpn72* was more efficient than the chromosome-derived one in inserting into the *mgrB* gene to acquire colistin-resistance (**Figure 3C**). These data suggest that both IS*pla* and IS*chr* can be inserted into *mgrB* gene to acquire the colistin-resistance phenotype and IS*pla* without DRs had a higher efficiency.

The Resistance-Acquiring Mechanism May Be Potently Disseminated Among Bacteria

The next question is whether the IS*Kpn72* element on the pR10-341_2 plasmid could be horizontally transferred to acquire the colistin-resistant phenotype. Sequence alignment of the pR10-341_2 plasmid from the NCBI database showed high similarity to the conjugative multidrug resistant plasmid pR46-270 in a *K. pneumoniae* R46 isolate (GenBank: CP035776.1). Accordingly, a conjugative system consisting of *tra*, *trb*, and *finO* genes were encoded by the plasmid (**Figure 4A**). To confirm the transferability of the pR10-341_2, we used *K. pneumoniae* R10-341 as the donor and a tetracycline-resistant *E. coli* K12-TcR strain as the recipient to verify plasmid conjugation (**Figure 4B**). As expected, the *E. coli* K12-TcR strain containing the pR10-341_2 plasmid was successfully obtained (**Figure 4C**), suggesting the pR10-341_2 plasmid was transferable. Together, these results demonstrated that the *K. pneumoniae* R10-341 was able to disseminate the ability to switch from colistin-sensitive to resistant phenotype by transferring an IS containing plasmid.

DISCUSSION

Colistin-resistant bacteria are becoming an increasing threat to healthcare especially in hospitals (Antoniadou et al., 2007; Bogdanovich et al., 2011; Zhong et al., 2018; Nang et al., 2019). Previous studies have focused on mechanisms of drug-resistance and how to detect these resistant strains (Olaitan et al., 2014; Poirel et al., 2017). In this study, we identified a colistin-sensitive *K. pneumoniae* R10-341 strain with high frequency ($\sim 10^{-6}$) of colistin heteroresistance. The *K. pneumoniae* R10-341 strain was classified as ST11, which is the most widely prevalent CRKP genotype in China and contains the *bla*KPC-2 gene, which encodes the KPC family carbapenem-hydrolyzing class A beta-lactamase (Qi et al., 2011; Liu et al., 2018). We showed that this *K. pneumoniae* R10-341 strain could transit from a colistin-sensitive to a resistant phenotype by the insertion of an IS*Kpn72* element into the *mgrB* gene. Importantly, we characterized this IS*Kpn72* element in a mobile plasmid, which showed high similarity to the conjugative plasmid pR46-270 (Wu et al., 2019).

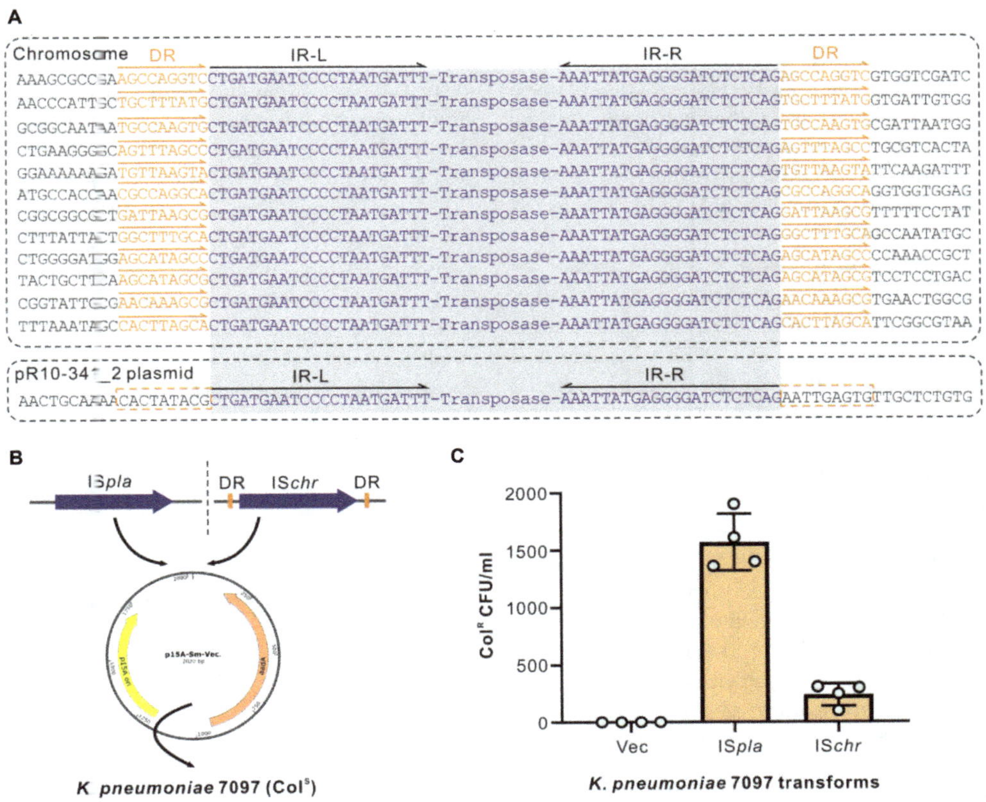

FIGURE 3 | Different types of ISs have different insertion efficiencies. **(A)** Schematic diagram of IS*Kpn72* elements located on chromosome and P2 plasmid. IR sequences are shown in blue and the DR sequences are indicated in orange. **(B)** Schematic diagram for cloning two forms of the IS*Kpn72* element into colistin-sensitive *K. pneumoniae* 7097 strain. **(C)** Acquired colistin-resistance for *K. pneumoniae* 7097 strain transformed with different IS*Kpn72* elements. Overnight grown bacteria were spread onto plates containing 100 μg/mL colistin, and bacterial colony forming unit (CFU) numbers were calculated. Representative data from two-independent experiments with four technique replicates are shown.

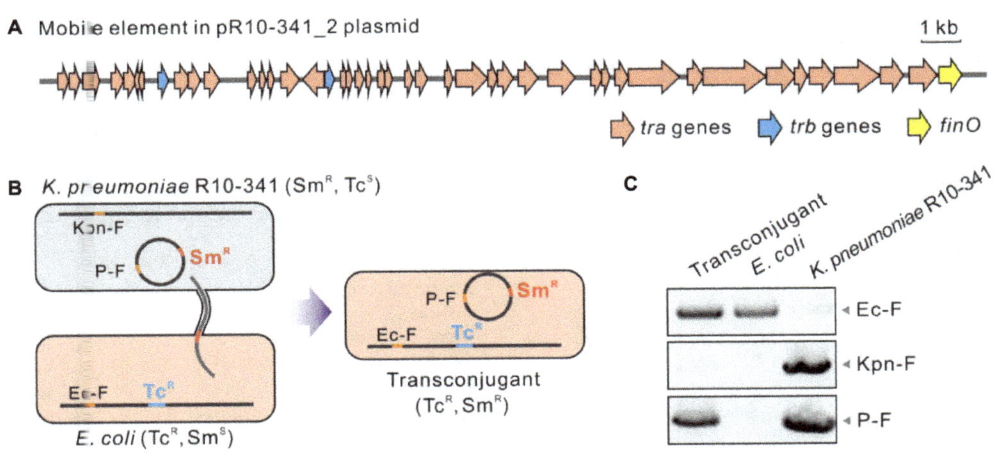

FIGURE 4 | Transconjugation of the pR10-341_2 plasmid from *K. pneumoniae* R10-341. **(A)** Genes involved in mobility of the pR10-341_2 plasmid. **(B)** Strategy used in conjugation transfer analysis. **(C)** PCR confirmation of transconjugant. Data of amplified products for Ec-F, Kpn-F, and P2-F are shown.

These analyses suggest that the ability of transiting from colistin-sensitive to resistant may be disseminated through plasmid transfer.

Heteroresistance has been reported to lead to failures in antibiotic treatment (Band et al., 2016; Band et al., 2019). In CRKP, colistin heteroresistance could be achieved by inserted inactivation and deletion or point mutations in *mgrB*, *phoP*, *phoQ*, *lpxM*, and *yciM* genes (Jayol et al., 2015; Halaby et al., 2016). Similar as previous studies, we found that the colistin heteroresistance in *K. pneumoniae* R10-341 was also caused by inactivation of chromosomal encoded *mgrB* gene, but we characterized that this inactivation was mediated by a mobile plasmid derived IS element. Therefore, our result is the first to report that the colistin heteroresistance is able to be transferred or spread via plasmid mobilization.

Colistin-resistance in *K. pneumoniae* can be achieved by chromosome- or plasmid-encoded genes (Ah et al., 2014; Olaitan et al., 2014; Rebelo et al., 2018). Chromosome-encoded mutations are considered to be stable (Gunn et al., 1998), while plasmid encoded *mcr* genes can be potentially transferred across bacterial species to cause direct colistin-resistance (Liu et al., 2016; Zhong et al., 2018). Being different from spreading of drug-resistance genes, we characterized the spread of the ability to become colistin-resistance via mobile plasmid. The IS*Kpn72*-containing mobile plasmid enables the strain to transit from colistin-sensitive to resistant phenotype by inactivating the *mgrB* gene, which may also explain the widespread of *mgrB* gene inactivation in clinical samples (Cannatelli et al., 2014; Gaibani et al., 2014). Interestingly, all copies of the IS*Kpn72* element contain a pair of 22 bp-length imperfect terminal inverted repeats (IR), which is a characteristic feature of the IS element in bacteria (Rezsöhazy et al., 1993; Mahillon and Chandler, 1998); but only the 12 copies of the IS*Kpn72* element located on the chromosome contain 9-bp direct repeated (DR) sequences, which are considered as a marker of IS insertion (Mahillon and Chandler, 1998). These observations indicate that the copies of IS*Kpn72* on the chromosome are probably inserted from the DR-missing IS*Kpn72* element on the pR10-341_2 plasmid. In addition, we observed a colistin-resistance acquirement of IS*chr* transformers (**Figure 3C**), which indicated that the bacteria also can store the ability to become colistin-resistance by inserting IS in chromosome. The ability to transit to colistin-resistant can be both stored at chromosome and disseminated through mobile plasmids.

The mechanism of a mobile plasmid-mediated transfer of the ability to transit from a colistin-sensitive to resistant phenotype brings not only challenges to colistin-resistance detection, but also raises concerns to the use of colistin in clinical treatment. which means the parental strain may be mis-classified as colistin-sensitive in drug-resistant genotyping or phenotyping assays. Secondly, the IS*Kpn72* and other IS elements widely exist in prokaryotes (Mahillon and Chandler, 1998; Frost et al., 2005), suggesting transition to colistin-resistance may be widely Firstly, this type of colistin-resistant phenotype was generated by the insertion of an IS*Kpn72* element into the *mgrB* gene, occurred (Cannatelli et al., 2013, 2014). Different methods have been deployed for antibiotic resistance analysis and prediction, including traditional antimicrobial susceptibility testing (AST) (Jorgensen and Ferraro, 1998) and bioinformatics tools (Zankari et al., 2012; Boolchandani et al., 2019). It is still a challenge to identify whether a strain is able to acquiring inheritable or transmissible antibiotic-resistance, or under specific conditions due to the wide existence of IS elements. Additionally, the frequency of the IS*Kpn72* insertion into the *mgrB* gene characterized in our study can reach $\sim 10^{-6}$, indicating that the IS insertion, especially the IS*4* family, should receive more attention in the clinical use of colistin.

AUTHOR CONTRIBUTIONS

MN and YH conceptualized and designed the study. BZ and BY performed the experiments. BZ, WZ, XW, and SC analyzed the data. YW and ZS provided the materials. BZ, MN, and YH drafted the manuscript. BY and SC critically revised the manuscript. All authors read and approved the final manuscript.

FUNDING

This work was supported by the Open Research Fund Program of National Biosafety Laboratory, Wuhan (2018SPCAS001 to MN and YH) and the Youth Innovation Promotion Association CAS (Y201750 to YH).

ACKNOWLEDGMENTS

We thank the Core Facility and Technical Support of Wuhan Institute of Virology for help in this study.

REFERENCES

Ah, Y. M., Kim, A. J., and Lee, J. Y. (2014). Colistin resistance in *Klebsiella pneumoniae*. *Int. J. Antimicrob. Agent.* 44, 8–15.

Antoniadou, A., Kontopidou, F., Poulakou, G., Koratzanis, E., Galani, I., Papadomichelakis, E., et al. (2007). Colistin-resistant isolates of *Klebsiella pneumoniae* emerging in intensive care unit patients: first report of a multiclonal cluster. *J. Antimicrob. Chemother.* 59, 786–790. doi: 10.1093/jac/dkl562

Band, V. I., Crispell, E. K., Napier, B. A., Herrera, C. M., Tharp, G. K., Vavikolanu, K., et al. (2016). Antibiotic failure mediated by a resistant subpopulation in *Enterobacter cloacae*. *Nat. Microbiol.* 1:16053.

Band, V. I., Hufnagel, D. A., Jaggavarapu, S., Sherman, E. X., Wozniak, J. E., Satola, S. W., et al. (2019). Antibiotic combinations that exploit heteroresistance to multiple drugs effectively control infection. *Nat. Microbiol.* 4, 1627–1635. doi: 10.1038/s41564-019-0480-z

Biswas, S., Brunel, J.-M., Dubus, J.-C., Reynaud-Gaubert, M., and Rolain, J.-M. (2012). Colistin: an update on the antibiotic of the 21st century. *Expert. Rev. Anti.Infect. Ther.* 10, 917–934. doi: 10.1586/eri.12.78

Bogdanovich, T., Adams-Haduch, J. M., Tian, G. B., Nguyen, M. H., Kwak, E. J., Muto, C. A., et al. (2011). Colistin-resistant, *Klebsiella pneumoniae* carbapenemase (KPC)-producing *Klebsiella pneumoniae* belonging to the international epidemic clone ST258. *Clin. Infec. Dis.* 53, 373–376. doi: 10.1093/cid/cir401

Boolchandani, M., D'souza, A. W., and Dantas, G. (2019). Sequencing-based methods and resources to study antimicrobial resistance. *Nat. Rev. Genet.* 20, 356–370.

Cannatelli, A., D'andrea, M. M., Giani, T., Di Pilato, V., Arena, F., Ambretti, S., et al. (2013). *In vivo* emergence of colistin resistance in *Klebsiella pneumoniae* producing KPC-type carbapenemases mediated by insertional inactivation of the PhoQ/PhoP mgrB regulator. *Antimicrob. Agent. Chemother.* 57, 5521–5526. doi: 10.1128/aac.01480-13

Cannatelli, A., Giani, T., D'andrea, M. M., Di Pilato, V., Arena, F., Conte, V., et al. (2014). MgrB inactivation is a common mechanism of colistin resistance in KPC-producing *Klebsiella pneumoniae* of clinical origin. *Antimicrob. Agent. Chemother.* 58, 5696–5703. doi: 10.1128/aac.03110-14

Carattoli, A., Zankari, E., García-Fernández, A., Voldby Larsen, M., Lund, O., Villa, L., et al. (2014). *In silico* detection and typing of plasmids using plasmidfinder and plasmid multilocus sequence typing. *Antimicrobial. Agent. Chemother.* 58, 3895–3903. doi: 10.1128/aac.02412-14

Diancourt, L., Passet, V., Verhoef, J., Grimont, P. A., and Brisse, S. (2005). Multilocus sequence typing of *Klebsiella pneumoniae* nosocomial isolates. *J. Clin. Microbiol.* 43, 4178–4182. doi: 10.1128/jcm.43.8.4178-4182.2005

El-Halfawy, O. M., and Valvano, M. A. (2015). Antimicrobial heteroresistance: an emerging field in need of clarity. *Clin. Microbiol. Rev.* 28, 191–207. doi: 10.1128/cmr.00058-14

Frost, L. S., Leplae, R., Summers, A. O., and Toussaint, A. (2005). Mobile genetic elements: the agents of open source evolution. *Nat. Rev. Microbiol.* 3, 722–732. doi: 10.1038/nrmicro1235

Gaibani, P., Lombardo, D., Lewis, R. E., Mercuri, M., Bonora, S., Landini, M. P., et al. (2014). *In vitro* activity and post-antibiotic effects of colistin in combination with other antimicrobials against colistin-resistant KPC-producing *Klebsiella pneumoniae* bloodstream isolates. *J. Antimicrobial. Chemother.* 69, 1856–1865. doi: 10.1093/jac/dku065

Gunn, J. S., Lim, K. B., Krueger, J., Kim, K., Guo, L., Hackett, M., et al. (1998). PmrA-PmrB-regulated genes necessary for 4-aminoarabinose lipid a modification and polymyxin resistance. *Mol. Microbiol.* 27, 1171–1182. doi: 10.1046/j.1365-2958.1998.00757.x

Gunn, J. S., and Miller, S. I. (1996). PhoP-PhoQ activates transcription of *pmrAB*, encoding a two-component regulatory system involved in *Salmonella typhimurium* antimicrobial peptide resistance. *J. Bacteriol.* 178, 6857–6864. doi: 10.1128/jb.178.23.6857-6864.1996

Halaby, T., Kucukkose, E., Janssen, A. B., Rogers, M. R. C., Doorduijn, D. J., Van Der Zanden, A. G. M., et al. (2016). Genomic characterization of colistin heteroresistance in *Klebsiella pneumoniae* during a nosocomial outbreak. *Antimicrobial. Agent. Chemother.* 60, 6837–6843. doi: 10.1128/aac.01344-16

Hancock, R. E. (1997). Peptide antibiotics. *Lancet* 349, 418–422.

Jayol, A., Nordmann, P., Brink, A., and Poirel, L. (2015). Heteroresistance to colistin in *Klebsiella pneumoniae* associated with alterations in the PhoPQ regulatory system. *Antimicrobial. Agent. Chemother.* 59, 2780–2784. doi: 10.1128/aac.05055-14

Jiang, Y., Chen, B., Duan, C., Sun, B., Yang, J., Yang, S. et al. (2015). Multigene editing in the *Escherichia coli* genome via the CRISPR-Cas9 system. *Appl. Environ. Microbiol.* 81, 2506–2514. doi: 10.1128/aem.04023-14

Jorgensen, J. H., and Ferraro, M. J. (1998). Antimicrobial susceptibility testing: general principles and contemporary practices. *Clin. Infect. Dis.* 26, 973–980. doi: 10.1086/513938

Lei, C. W., Zhang, Y., Wang, Y. T., and Wang, H. N. (2020). Detection of mobile colistin resistance gene mcr-10.1 in a conjugative plasmid from *Enterobacter* roggenkampii of chicken origin in china. *Antimicrob. Agent. Chemother.* 64, e1120–e1191.

Li, J., Nation, R. L., Turnidge, J. D., Milne, R. W., Coulthard, K., Rayner, C. R., et al. (2006). Colistin: the re-emerging antibiotic for multidrug-resistant Gram-negative bacterial infections. *Lancet Infect. Dis.* 6, 589–601. doi: 10.1016/s1473-3099(06)70580-1

Liu, L., Feng, Y., Tang, G., Lin, J., Huang, W., Qiao, F., et al. (2018). Carbapenem-resistant isolates of the *Klebsiella pneumoniae* complex in western china: the common ST11 and the surprising hospital-specific types. *Clin. Infect. Dis.* 67, S263–S265.

Liu, Y. Y., Chandler, C. E., Leung, L. M., Mcelheny, C. L., Mettus, R. T., Shanks, R. M. Q., et al. (2017). Structural modification of lipopolysaccharide conferred by in gram-negative ESKAPE pathogens. *Antimicrob. Agent. Chemother.* 61, e517–e580.

Liu, Y. Y., Wang, Y., Walsh, T. R., Yi, L. X., Zhang, R., Spencer, J., et al. (2016). Emergence of plasmid-mediated colistin resistance mechanism MCR-1 in animals and human beings in china: a microbiological and molecular biological study. *Lancet Infect. Dis.* 16, 161–168. doi: 10.1016/s1473-3099(15)00424-7

Macesic, N., Nelson, B., Mcconville, T. H., Giddins, M. J., Green, D. A., Stump, S., et al. (2020). Emergence of polymyxin resistance in clinical *Klebsiella pneumoniae* through diverse genetic adaptations: a genomic, retrospective cohort study. *Clin. Infect. Dis.* 70, 2084–2091. doi: 10.1093/cid/ciz623

Mahillon, J., and Chandler, M. (1998). Insertion sequences. *Microbiol. Mol. Biol. Rev.* 62, 725–774.

Nang, S. C., Li, J., and Velkov, T. (2019). The rise and spread of plasmid-mediated polymyxin resistance. *Crit. Rev. Microbiol.* 45, 131–161. doi: 10.1080/1040841x.2018.1492902

Nordmann, P., Naas, T., and Poirel, L. (2011). Global spread of carbapenemase-producing *enterobacteriaceae*. *Emerg. Infec. Dis.* 17, 1791–1798.

Olaitan, A. O., Morand, S., and Rolain, J. M. (2014). Mechanisms of polymyxin resistance: acquired and intrinsic resistance in bacteria. *Front. Microbiol.* 5:643. doi: 10.3389/fmicb.2014.00643

Payne, A., Holmes, N., Rakyan, V., and Loose, M. (2019). BulkVis: a graphical viewer for Oxford nanopore bulk FAST5 files. *Bioinformatics* 35, 2193–2198. doi: 10.1093/bioinformatics/bty841

Pitout, J. D. D., Nordmann, P., and Poirel, L. (2015). Carbapenemase-producing *Klebsiella pneumoniae*, a key pathogen set for global nosocomial dominance. *Antimicrob. Agent. Chemother.* 59, 5873–5884. doi: 10.1128/aac.01019-15

Poirel, L., Jayol, A., and Nordmann, P. (2017). Polymyxins: antibacterial activity, susceptibility testing, and resistance mechanisms encoded by plasmids or chromosomes. *Clin. Microbiol. Rev.* 30, 557–596. doi: 10.1128/cmr.00064-16

Qi, Y., Wei, Z., Ji, S., Du, X., Shen, P., Yu, Y. et al. (2011). ST11, the dominant clone of KPC-producing *Klebsiella pneumoniae* in China. *J. Antimicrob. Chemother.* 66, 307–312. doi: 10.1093/jac/dkq431

Rebelo, A. R., Bortolaia, V., Kjeldgaard, J. S., Pedersen, S. K., Leekitcharoenphon, P., Hansen, I. M., et al. (2018). Multiplex PCR for detection of plasmid-mediated colistin resistance determinants, *mcr*-1, *mcr*-2, *mcr*-3, *mcr*-4 and *mcr*-5 for surveillance purposes. *Euro. Surveill.* 23, 17–00672.

Rezsöhazy, R., Hallet, B., Delcour, J., and Mahillon, J. (1993). The IS4 family of insertion sequences: evidence for a conserved transposase motif. *Mol. Microbiol.* 9, 1283–1295. doi: 10.1111/j.1365-2958.1993.tb01258.x

Rose, R. E. (1988). The nucleotide sequence of pACYC184. *Nucleic Acids Res.* 16:355. doi: 10.1093/nar/16.1.355

Tatusova, T., Dicuccio, M., Badretdin, A., Chetvernin, V., Nawrocki, E. P., Zaslavsky, L., et al. (2016). NCBI prokaryotic genome annotation pipeline. *Nucleic Acids Res.* 44, 6614–6624. doi: 10.1093/nar/gkw569

Velkov, T., Deris, Z. Z., Huang, J. X., Azad, M. A., Butler, M., Sivanesan, S., et al. (2014). Surface changes and polymyxin interactions with a resistant strain of *Klebsiella pneumoniae*. *Innate. Immun.* 20, 350–363. doi: 10.1177/1753425913493337

Wang, C., Feng, Y., Liu, L., Wei, L., Kang, M., and Zong, Z. (2020). Identification of novel mobile colistin resistance gene. *Emerg. Microb. Infec.* 9, 508–516. doi: 10.1080/22221751.2020.1732231

Wang, X., Wang, Y., Zhou, Y., Li, J., Yin, W., Wang, S., et al. (2018). Emergence of a novel mobile colistin resistance gene, mcr-8, in NDM-producing *Klebsiella pneumoniae*. *Emerg. Microb. Infec.* 7:122.

Waterhouse, A. M., Procter, J. B., Martin, D. M. A., Clamp, M., and Barton, G. J. (2009). Jalview Version 2–a multiple sequence alignment editor and analysis workbench. *Bioinformatics* 25, 1189–1191. doi: 10.1093/bioinformatics/btp033

Wick, R. R., Judd, L. M., Gorrie, C. L., and Holt, K. E. (2017). Unicycler: Resolving bacterial genome assemblies from short and long sequencing reads. *PLoS comput. Biol.* 13:e1005595. doi: 10.1371/journal.pcbi.1005595

Wu, F., Ying, Y., Yin, M., Jiang, Y., Wu, C., Qian, C., et al. (2019). Molecular characterization of a multidrug-resistant strain R46 isolated from a rabbit. *Int. J. Genom.* 2019:5459190.

Yang, Y.-Q., Li, Y.-X., Lei, C.-W., Zhang, A.-Y., and Wang, H.-N. (2018). Novel plasmid-mediated colistin resistance gene mcr-7.1 in *Klebsiella pneumoniae*. *J. Antimicrob. Chemother.* 73, 1791–1795. doi: 10.1093/jac/dky111

Zankari, E., Hasman, H., Cosentino, S., Vestergaard, M., Rasmussen, S., Lund, O., et al. (2012). Identification of acquired antimicrobial resistance genes. *J. Antimicrob. Chemother.* 67, 2640–2644. doi: 10.1093/jac/dks261

Zhong, L. L., Phan, H. T. T., Shen, C., Vihta, K. D., Sheppard, A. E., Huang, X., et al. (2018). High rates of human fecal carriage of *mcr*-1-positive multidrug-resistant *Enterobacteriaceae* emerge in china in association with successful plasmid families. *Clin. Infect. Dis.* 66, 676–685. doi: 10.1093/cid/cix885

22

Defeating Antibiotic- and Phage-Resistant *Enterococcus faecalis* Using a Phage Cocktail *in Vitro* and in a Clot Model

Leron Khalifa[1], Daniel Gelman[1], Mor Shlezinger[1,2], Axel Lionel Dessal[1], Shunit Coppenhagen-Glazer[1], Nurit Beyth[1,2†] and Ronen Hazan[1*†]

[1] *Faculty of Dental Sciences, Hadassah School of Dental Medicine, Hebrew University of Jerusalem, Jerusalem, Israel,*
[2] *Department of Prosthodontics, Hadassah School of Dental Medicine, Hebrew University of Jerusalem, Jerusalem, Israel*

***Correspondence:**
Ronen Hazan
ronenh@ekmd.huji.ac.il

† These authors have contributed equally to this work.

The deteriorating effectiveness of antibiotics is propelling researchers worldwide towards alternative techniques such as phage therapy: curing infectious diseases using viruses of bacteria called bacteriophages. In a previous paper, we isolated phage EFDG1, highly effective against both planktonic and biofilm cultures of one of the most challenging pathogenic species, the vancomycin-resistant *Enterococcus* (VRE). Thus, it is a promising phage to be used in phage therapy. Further experimentation revealed the emergence of a mutant resistant to EFDG1 phage: EFDG1^r. This kind of spontaneous resistance to antibiotics would be disastrous occurrence, however for phage-therapy it is only a minor hindrance. We quickly and successfully isolated a new phage, EFLK1, which proved effective against both the resistant mutant EFDG1^r and its parental VRE, *Enterococcus faecalis* V583. Furthermore, combining both phages in a cocktail produced an additive effect against *E. faecalis* V583 strains regardless of their antibiotic or phage-resistance profile. An analysis of the differences in genome sequence, genes, mutations, and *tRNA* content of both phages is presented. This work is a proof-of-concept of one of the most significant advantages of phage therapy, namely the ability to easily overcome emerging resistant bacteria.

Keywords: bacteriophages, *Enterococcus faecalis*, antibiotic-resistance, phage therapy, phage-resistance, phage cocktail

INTRODUCTION

In 1967, William H. Stewart, the Surgeon General, said in the White House: "It's time to close the books on infectious diseases, declare the war against pestilence won...," expressing the general opinion, at the time, that antibiotics succeeded in solving all bacteria-related problems. Ironically, this very success has proved dangerous, as the frequent reliance on antibiotics has resulted in dissemination of resistant variants (Charles and Grayson, 2004; Davies and Davies, 2010).

One of the antibiotic – resistant, most frequently isolated species from hospital-associated infections, is vancomycin-resistant enterococci (VRE) (O'Driscoll and Crank, 2015; Khalifa et al., 2016). While mostly a commensal, when inhabiting the gastro-intestinal tract, Gram-positive *Enterococcus faecalis* bacterium can cause fatal infections (Rice, 2008; Orsi and Ciorba, 2013). In many cases, neither antibiotics (Erlandson et al., 2008; Chong et al., 2010) nor other antibacterial means like endodontic treatments and rinsing with calcium hydroxide, sodium hypochlorite, and chlorohexidine (Khalifa et al., 2016) have successfully prevented the morbidity or mortality resulting from *Enterococcus* infections especially in cases of biofilm (Donlan, 2001; de la Fuente-Nunez et al., 2013). The hazardous potential of these bacteria is exacerbated by the emergence of antibiotic-resistant strains, primarily VRE (Linden, 2002). So much so, that in 2013 the Center for Disease Control and Prevention (CDC) has declared VRE *enterococci* to be one amongst the top 18 drug-resistant threats to treat today[1].

With the limitations of chemical antibiotics and the emergence of antibiotic-resistant strains, the use of bacteriophages has been regaining interest (Golkar et al., 2014). Their effective potential is magnified as they are highly strain-specific, targeting only their pathogen and tend to only minimally disrupt normal flora (Loc-Carrillo and Abedon, 2011). Moreover, bacteriophages have evolved naturally to be become the most proficient bacterial killers (Srinivasiah et al., 2008) in all forms, including hard-to-eradicate biofilms (Donlan, 2009; Khalifa et al., 2016). Use of bacteriophages has numerous other advantages over antibiotics (Loc-Carrillo and Abedon, 2011; Khalifa et al., 2016), including ease of isolation. Additionally, recent human and animal trials have shown that phages are safe for use (Burrowes et al., 2011).

We recently demonstrated the treatment potential of phages against vancomycin-resistant *E. faecalis* infections. EFDG1, an anti-*E. faecalis* phage, was isolated from sewage and its genome was characterized. This phage proved highly effective against *E. faecalis* V583 in planktonic and biofilm cultures *in vitro* and in an *ex vivo* human root canal model (Khalifa et al., 2015a).

Successful though phage therapy may be, bacterial cells resistant to phages will no doubt emerge, just as in the case of antibiotics (Duerkop et al., 2016), as indeed has occurred in our case too. However, in contrast to the grave challenges facing antibiotics, phage therapy offers several simple approaches to combat phage-resistant bacteria. One strategy would be to isolate new phages and to use them in cocktails. Based on the number of previously isolated phages and phage sequences in microbiomes, it is estimated that a bacterial strain may have as many as several 100 phages capable of combating it Khalifa et al. (2016). A second approach is to improve current phages by random or directed mutagenesis: using UV radiation (Drake, 1966) or gamma rays (Bertram, 1988), by means of chemical mutagens such as methyl methanesulfonate (MMS) (Drake, 1982) or through genetic engineering (Kiro et al., 2014; Pires et al., 2016). In any case, multiple-phage cocktails are preferable to single-phage therapy, as they are better equipped to deal with phage-resistant bacterial mutants and multispecies bacterial cultures (polyphage therapy) (Chan and Abedon, 2012; Gu et al., 2012; Ormala and Jalasvuori, 2013).

In the current article, we demonstrate the first approach: isolating a new phage against phage-resistant bacteria, constructing a phage cocktail and then utilizing it successfully against both naïve and phage-resistant mutant strains in *in vitro* models. The phage EFLK1 was effective against the EFDG1 phage-resistant *E. faecalis* strain (EFDG1^r). Moreover, a cocktail of EFDG1 and EFLK1 phages had an additive effect on planktonic and biofilm cultures.

[1]https://www.cdc.gov/drugresistance/biggest_threats.html

MATERIALS AND METHODS

Emergence and Isolation of Phage-Resistant Bacteria

Following all experiments of EFV583 with phage, survivors were routinely tested for resistance to the phage. The survivors were plated and the resulting single colonies were collected and grown. The bacteria were then tested for susceptibility to the phage, by either spotting phages on them or by cross streak agar assay. For the spotting method, about 100–200 μl of bacterial culture was spread uniformly on a BHI agar plate and once it dried; 10 μl spots of phages were spotted, which was done in duplicates or triplicates. While the cross streak agar assays were performed by horizontally streaking the phage lysate in the middle of the plate and then vertically streaking the bacterial colonies over the phage in unidirectional streaks (Moore, 2011; Tiruvadi Krishnan et al., 2015).

Bacterial colonies that grew in presence of phage were considered to exhibit resistance to the phage. These colonies were then collected and grown at 37°C and checked numerous times for their resistant characteristics against the phage. Once their resistant property was confirmed, these bacteria were frozen with 25% glycerol at −80°C and store for future use.

Bacterial Strains and Materials

Enterococcus faecalis V583 (ATCC 700802) VRE and EFDG1^r, EFDG1 phage-resistant bacterial strain were grown in brain heart infusion (BHI) broth (Difco, Detroit, MI, United States) aerobically in an incubator shaker with shaking at 220 RPM at 37°C. BHI agar (1.5%) was used for isolation streaks and isolations of phage. For top agar, 0.6% of agar (soft agar) was used, with BHI as nutrient supplement.

Isolation and Storage of Phage

In order to combat the phage-resistant mutant strain, a new lytic phage was isolated from the sewage effluents collected from the "Nahal Sorek" decontamination facility located in West Jerusalem, as described previously (Khalifa et al., 2015a). The effluents were centrifuged using a 5430R centrifuge, and a fixed angle rotorFA-45-24-11HS; Eppendorf at 10,000 × *g* for 10 min, to pellet out the debris. The supernatant was filtered twice, initially through 0.45-μm-pore-size filters (Merck Millipore, Ltd., Ireland) to filter out larger particles and then through 0.22-μm-pore-size filters (Merck Millipore) to achieve lysate free from any residues. Different concentrations of the filtrates (between 0.1 and 1 ml) were then added to bacterial broth culture diluted 1:1000 in BHI. Once lysis was obtained, the lysate was centrifuged and filtered using the aforementioned method.

The phage lysate was then applied on bacterial lawn by the method of double layer agar to obtain clear plaques that symbolize the presence of phages. About 100 μl of bacteria was mixed with 100 μl of phage lysate and incubated for 20 min at 37°C to achieve better adsorption of the phage to the bacteria. The entire mixture was then added to 5 ml of melted 0.6% BHI top agar, poured evenly onto a BHI agar plate and incubated overnight at 37°C. The resultant single plaques were collected and added to 1 ml BHI and incubated at 4°C for diffusion. The liquid was centrifuged at 5000 RPM for 10 min and filtered through 0.22-μm-pore-size filters to obtain a clear phage lysate that was further used to grow large quantities of the phage. The phage was grown in BHI broth with EFV583 bacteria until a titer of 10^9 or higher was achieved. The phage titer of the phage lysate was determined by counting the Plaque forming units per ml (PFU/ml). For this; the phage lysate was serially diluted in BHI broth and 5 μl of these dilutions were spotted onto an overlayer of molten 0.6% agarose with 100 μl of bacteria. This plate was incubated overnight at 37°C and the numbers of plaques were counted to finally calculate the PFU/ml. A large volume of EFLK1 phage lysate with a high titer (10^{10}) was prepared and stored at 4°C.

Characterization of Phage Activity against *E. faecalis* Naïve and Phage-Resistant Form in Planktonic and Biofilm Cultures

To assess the phage effectiveness against planktonic bacteria, the growth kinetics were analyzed using a 96 well plate reader. The phage was added initially to both logarithmic cultures (10^4 to 10^5 CFU/ml) at MOI of 100–1000 (10^8 PFU/ml) and stationary cultures (10^8 to 10^9 CFU/ml) of *E. faecalis* at MOI of 0.1–1 (10^8 PFU/ml). Cell viability was also checked by determining CFU/ml for each well.

The biofilm eradication efficiency of the phage was tested by adding it in a MOI of 0.1 (10^8 PFU/ml) to a 2-week old stationary biofilm of *E. faecalis*. To obtain a 2-week old biofilm, overnight grown bacteria were diluted with BHI to obtain 10^4 to 10^5 CFU/ml of bacteria, which were then plated in a 96-well plate that was incubated for 2 weeks without any change of media or addition of new bacteria. Killing efficacy was validated using viable cell counting by calculating the CFU/ml of the biofilm as described previously (Khalifa et al., 2015a). Briefly, aspirated spent media was removed from the wells followed by washing the wells twice with sterile PBS (100 ul) carefully to not disrupt the biofilm. Sterile PBS (100 ul) was added and the biofilm was scraped and collected. The cells were sonicated in a water-bath for 5–10 min followed by several dilutions (1:10) and plating on BHI plates for CFU count.

One Step Growth

We based our protocol on the one step growth method of Ellis and Delbrück (Ellis and Delbrück, 1939). Briefly, phages were added to stationary-phase bacteria (10^9 CFU/ml) in a final concentration of 1×10^7 PFU/ml followed by incubation in 37°C for 10 min. The samples were diluted at a ratio of $1{:}10^4$ in fresh BHI medium, followed again by incubation at 37°C for 10 more minutes. Starting at 20 min after the introduction of the bacteriophages to the bacterial cultures, the diluted mixtures were enumerated through a double-layered agar plaque assay. To this end, 3 ml of Soft BHI Agar (0.6% Agar) were mixed with 100 μL of the diluted mixture and with 100 μL of stationary-phase bacteria, according to the tested bacterial strain. The plaque assays were conducted in the following time points after the introduction of the bacteriophages: 20, 35, 50, 60, 70, 85, 100, 120 min, in biological duplicates. Latent time and burst size were calculated from this growth curve for each of the bacteriophages described, with each of the bacterial hosts.

Genome Sequencing

To verify that the phage is indeed new, its DNA was isolated using the Norgen Biotek Phage DNA Isolation Kit (Cat. # 46800) and the resulting genome was sequenced and analyzed (Khalifa et al., 2015a,b). Analysis and comparison to other *E. faecalis* phages was performed using the GENIOUS 10.0.6 software and its plugins[2]. Annotation of genes was carried out using PHAST[3].

TEM Visualization

To observe the structure of the isolated phage accurately transmission electron microscopy (TEM) by the classic method of Gill as described in OpenWetWare[4], was conducted following the procedure mention in our previous paper (Khalifa et al., 2015a). Briefly, 1 ml of phage lysate with 10^9 PFU/ml was centrifuged at 19,283 × *g* (centrifuge 5430R, rotor FA-45-24-11HS; Eppendorf) for 2 h at room temperature. The supernatant was discarded, and the pellet was resuspended in 200 μl of 5 mM $MgSO_4$ and incubated overnight at 4°C. 30 μl of 5 mM $MgSO_4$ and 10 μl of the phage sample were mixed gently on a parafilm strip and 30 μl of 2% uranyl acetate was pipetted on it. On these drops of phage samples grids were then placed carefully using forceps, with the carbon side facing down. After about a minute the grids were dried and stored in the desiccator until further use. A TEM (Joel, TEM 1400 plus) with a charge-coupled device camera (Gatan Orius 600) was used to capture images.

Naïve and Resistant Bacterial Mixture

The naïve and resistant *E. faecalis* were mixed in 1:1 ratio (v/v) and the efficacy of phages was checked individually and in cocktail against them. The experiment mirrored the one described above (see section "Characterization of Phage Activity against *E. faecalis* Naïve and Phage-Resistant Form in Planktonic and Biofilm Cultures") for assessing phage activity on planktonic bacteria and on biofilm.

In Vitro Fibrin Clot Model

The *in vitro* fibrin clot model was prepared according to the protocol described by McGrath et al. (1994) and Entenza et al. (2009). Overnight cultures (10^9 CFU/ml) of *E. faecalis* individually or in a mixed cultures of naïve and resistant bacteria were diluted 1:10 with citrated plasma. Clots were formed by triggering coagulation by adding 20 μl bovine thrombin

[2]https://www.geneious.com
[3]http://www.phantome.org
[4]http://openwetware.org/wiki/Gill:Preparing_phage_specimens_for_TEM

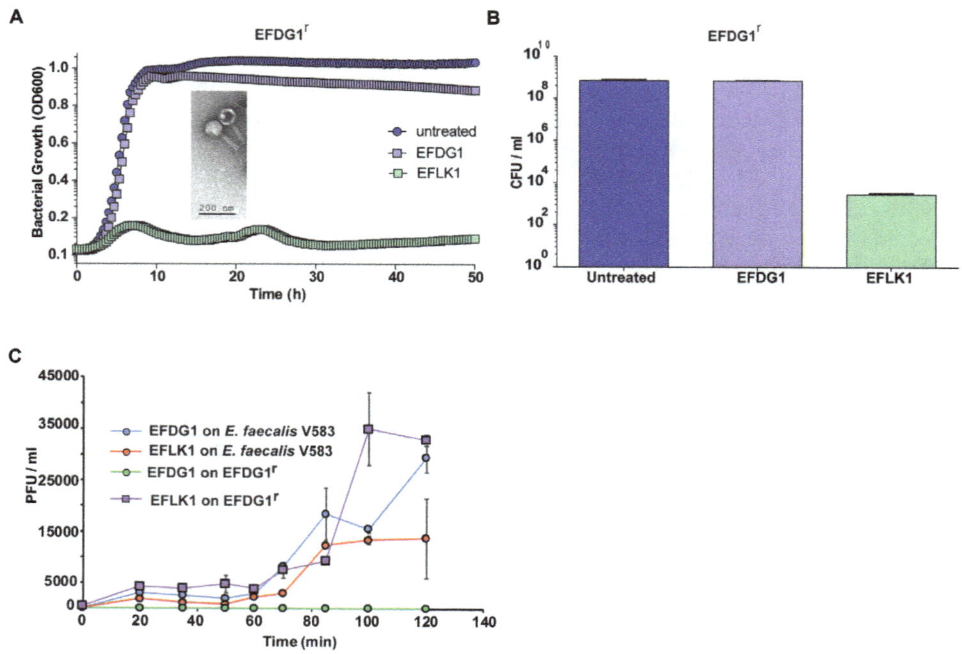

FIGURE 1 | Emergence of phage-resistant bacteria, EFDG1ʳ. The growth curve and CFU/ml values of EFDG1ʳ bacteria treated with EFDG1 phage resemble the untreated version of the same. Phage EFLK1 exhibited efficient lysis effect on the bacteria. **(A)** Logarithmic phase EFDG1ʳ bacteria without phage action (untreated) and with phages EFDG1 and EFLK1. The image inside the graph shows transmission electron microscopy (TEM) visualization image of the phage. **(B)** Colony counts revealing the CFU/ml of untreated and treated EFDG1ʳ bacteria after phage treatment. **(C)** One step growth curve of phages growing on and bacteria. Phages were added at 10^4 PFU/ml. One-step growth curve of EFDG1 and EFLK1 on *Enterococcus faecalis* V583 and EFDG1ʳ.

(5000 U/ml) and 20 μl $CaCl_2$ (50 mmol). The resultant clots were then re-suspended in 500 μl of bacteriophage lysate of 10^8 PFU/ml and for the control, 500 μl of BHI were added instead. The tubes were kept in an incubator-shaker for 6 h at 37°C. After incubation, the clots were washed with sterile PBS and lysed with 32 μl of 0.25% of Trypsin EDTA. After a 5-min centrifugation at 14,000 rpm, the cell pellet was re-suspended in 100 μl of PBS and used for calculating CFU/ml.

RESULTS

Emergence of the Phage-Resistant *E. faecalis* Mutant EFDG1ʳ and Isolation of EFLK1 Phage to Combat It

The lytic phage EFDG1 was isolated against vancomycin-resistant strains of *E. faecalis* V583 planktonic and biofilms cultures (Khalifa et al., 2015a). When strain EFDG1ʳ (resistant to EFDG1 phage) evolved during the experiments (**Figure 1A**), we screened various sewage effluent samples containing potential anti-*E. faecalis* phages. Within several weeks, a new lytic phage was isolated, EFLK1, from a sample collected from the sewage water of the "Nahal Sorek" decontamination facility. The new phage exhibited clear plaques on double-layered agar lawn of EFDG1ʳ. It also prevented the growth of EFDG1ʳ, as observed both in optical density growth curve (**Figure 1A**) and colony forming units (CFUs) count (**Figure 1B**). In agreement, a one-step growth experiment revealed that phage EFLK1 propagated on an EFDG1ʳ while EFDG1 phage did not (**Figure 1C**).

Phenotypic Differences Between EFDG1 and EFLK1 Phages

Despite the similarity between the two phages (32.187%), the efficiency and kinetics of EFLK1 phage infectivity against the parental strain V583 was distinct from that of EFDG1 phage. The lysis caused by EFDG1 phage during logarithmic growth was observed within 5 h (**Figure 1A**) and it reduced the viable cells number by four logs (**Figure 2A**) and (Khalifa et al., 2015a). In these conditions, EFLK1 phage was markedly slower; its lysis started after 12 h (**Figure 2A**) and it reduced cell viability by three logs (**Figure 2C**). In contrast, EFLK1 phage faired better against stationary cultures of V583 strain: EFLK1 phage lysis was observed after 10 h compared to much less significant lysis by EFDG1 phage (**Figure 2B**). These differences in lysis are reflected in the reduction of cell viability from 10^{11} to $\sim10^5$ by EFLK1 phage and only to $\sim10^8$ by EFDG1 phage (**Figure 2D**).

In Vitro Characterization of Combinatorial Cocktails of EFDG1 and EFLK1 Phages Aimed for Therapy

Since we aim to use EFDG1 and EFLK1 phages as therapeutic agents, we tested various combinations of phage cocktails,

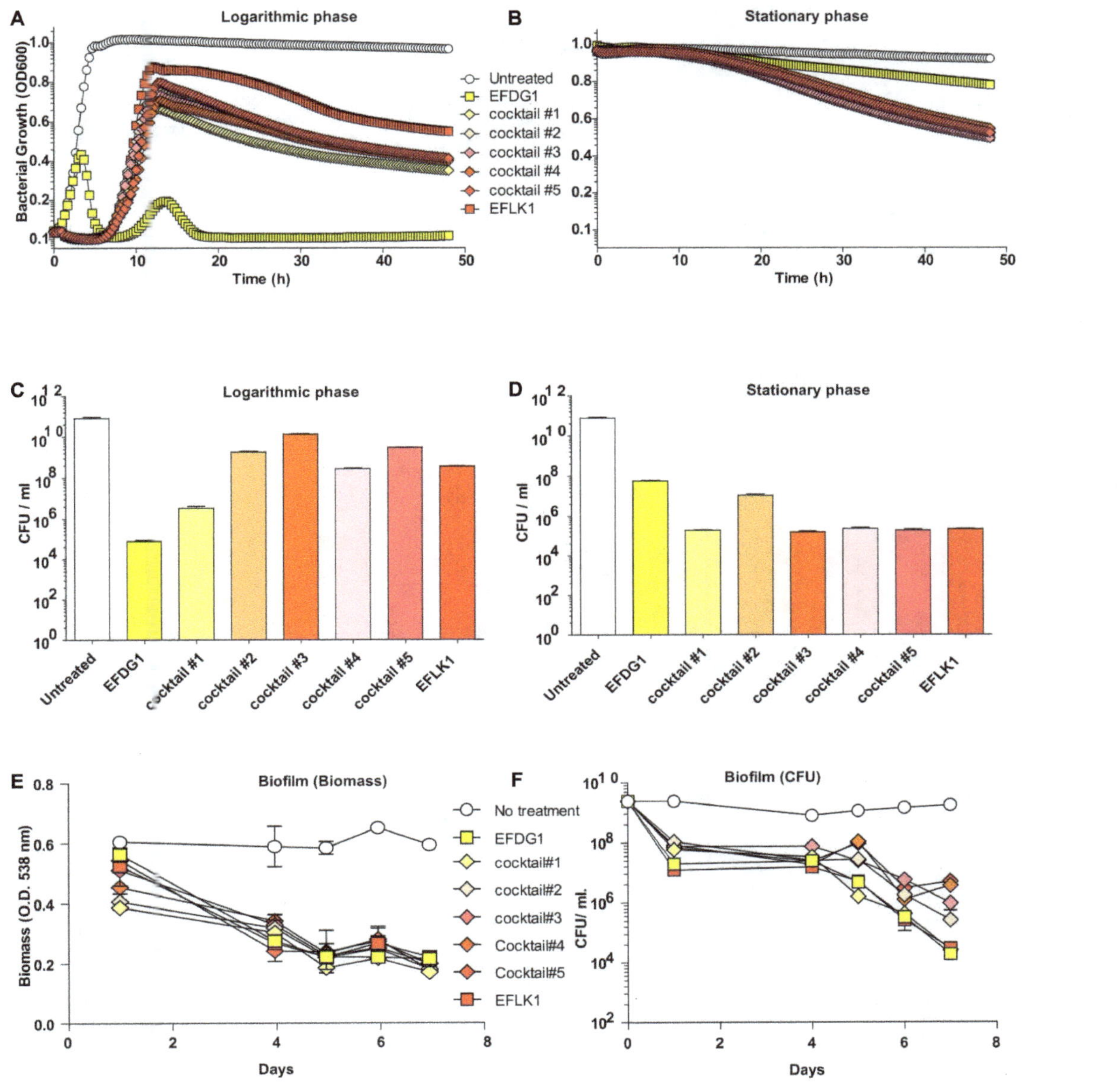

FIGURE 2 | Finding the most effective phage cocktail. **(A)** Logarithmic and **(B)** stationary phase *E. faecalis* V583 treated with EFDG1, EFLK1, and cocktails of these two phages in different ratios. Cocktail#1 (1:1), Cocktail#2 (1:2), Cocktail#3 (2:1), Cocktail#4 (1:3), and Cocktail#5 (3:1). Number of colony forming units per ml (CFU/ml) for logarithmic **(C)** and stationary phase **(D)** bacteria with and without treatment of the phages and their cocktails. **(E)** Biofilm biomass quantified by crystal violet staining of 2-weeks of *E. faecalis* V583 biofilm. **(F)** CFU/ml for phage treated and untreated 2-weeks old *E. faecalis* V583 biofilm.

initially on naïve *E. faecalis* V583. To this end, we combined EFDG1 and EFLK1 phages in various ratios: 1:1 (cocktail#1), 1:2 (cocktail#2), 2:1 (cocktail#3), 1:3 (cocktail#4), and 3:1 (cocktail#5) correspondingly (**Figure 2**). The best cocktail was found to be Cocktail#1 (1:1) as it killed the logarithmic culture of *E. faecalis* V583 as efficiently as EFDG1 phage (**Figures 2A–C**), and the stationary culture like EFLK1 phage (**Figures 2B–D**). Thus, cocktail#1 equaled the better phage in each case and outperformed the other cocktails against the challenging biofilm of *E. faecalis* V583 (**Figure 2E**).

When cocktail#1 was used against EFDG1^r mutants, it was found to be as effective as EFLK1 phage against logarithmic, stationary and biofilm cultures of the resistant mutants (**Figure 3**).

Finally, in order to simulate the evolution of resistant mutants within a culture, we mixed the WT *E. faecalis* V583 with its resistant mutant EFDG1^r and treated them with individual phages and cocktail #1, separately (**Figure 4**). We found that cocktail #1 and EFLK1 phage were effective against the bacterial mixture while EFDG1 phage was not.

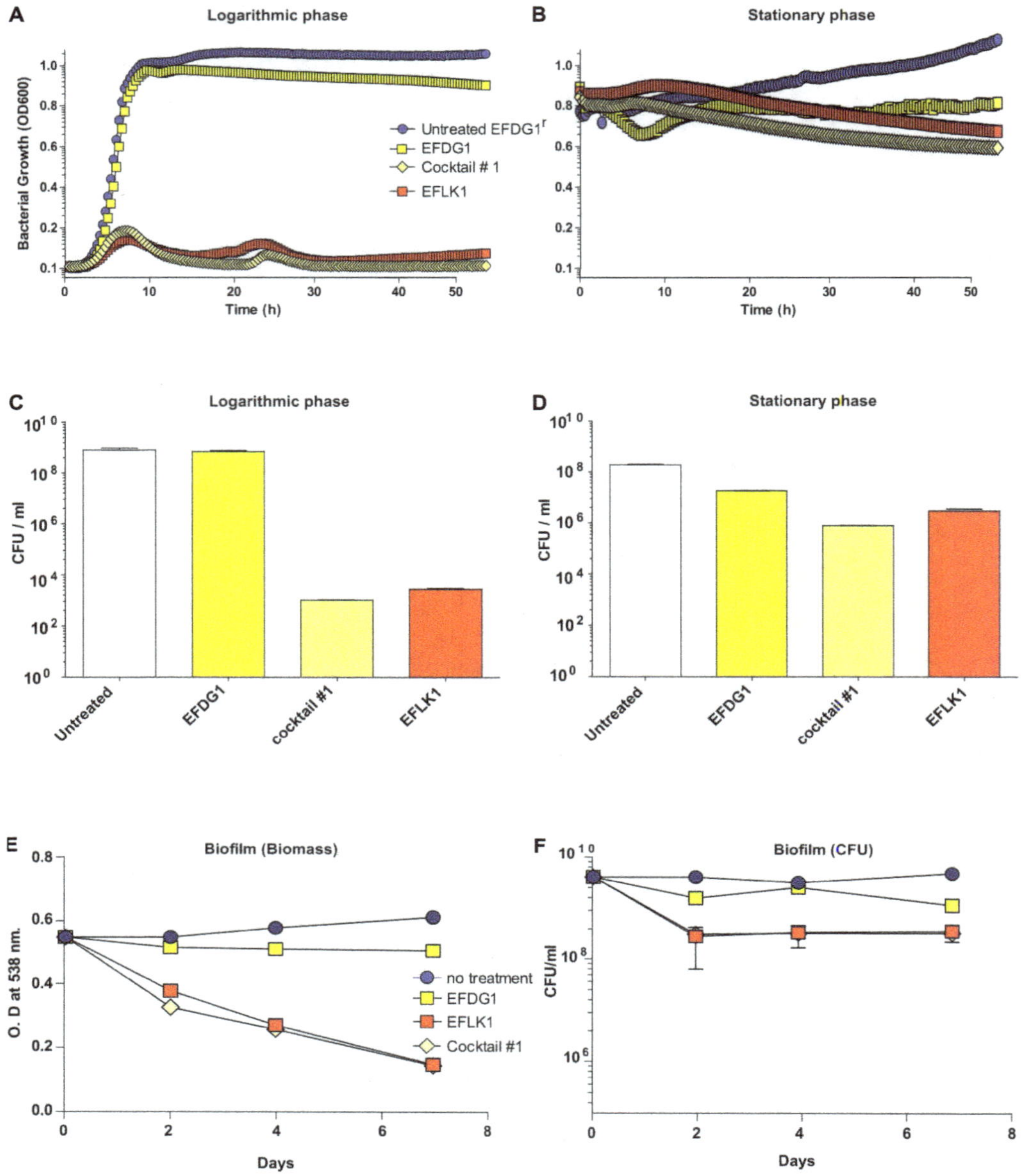

FIGURE 3 | Overcoming phage-resistance. **(A)** Logarithmic growth curve and their **(C)** CFU/ml along with **(B)** stationary growth curve and their **(D)** CFU/ml values depicting the lysis effect of EFLK1 phage and phage cocktail#1 (EFDG1:EFLK1 1:1) on EFDG1^r bacteria, whereas EFDG1 phage has no effect at all. Similarly, reduction is seen in the biofilm biomass **(E)** and the colony count **(F)** of a 2 week old biofilm of EFDG1^r bacteria only when treated with EFLK1 phage or phage cocktail#1.

Demonstrating Phage Efficacy in a Fibrin Clot Model

A recognized tool for the study of bacterial endocarditis (Hershberger et al., 2000), we used the *in vitro* fibrin-clot infection model (McGrath et al., 1994; Entenza et al., 2009) to assess the efficacy of the cocktail and the individual phages EFDG1 and EFLK1 against *E. faecalis* V583 and EFDG1^r (**Figure 5**). CFU/ml results following a 6-h incubation of *E. faecalis* V583 with EFLK1 phage and cocktail#1 showed a CFU reduction of three logs with EFDG1 phage and six logs with EFLK1 phage and cocktail#1. EFLK1 phage and the cocktail also reduced the CFU by five and six logs respectively, against EFDG1^r, while, EFDG1 phage failed as expected.

Genotypic Differences between EFDG1 and EFLK1 Phages

To explain the phenotypic differences between EFLK1 and EFDG1 phages, their genomes were compared (Khalifa et al., 2015a). In addition to EFLK1 phage, three additional *E. faecalis* phages of the Spounavirinae subfamily of the Myoviridae phage

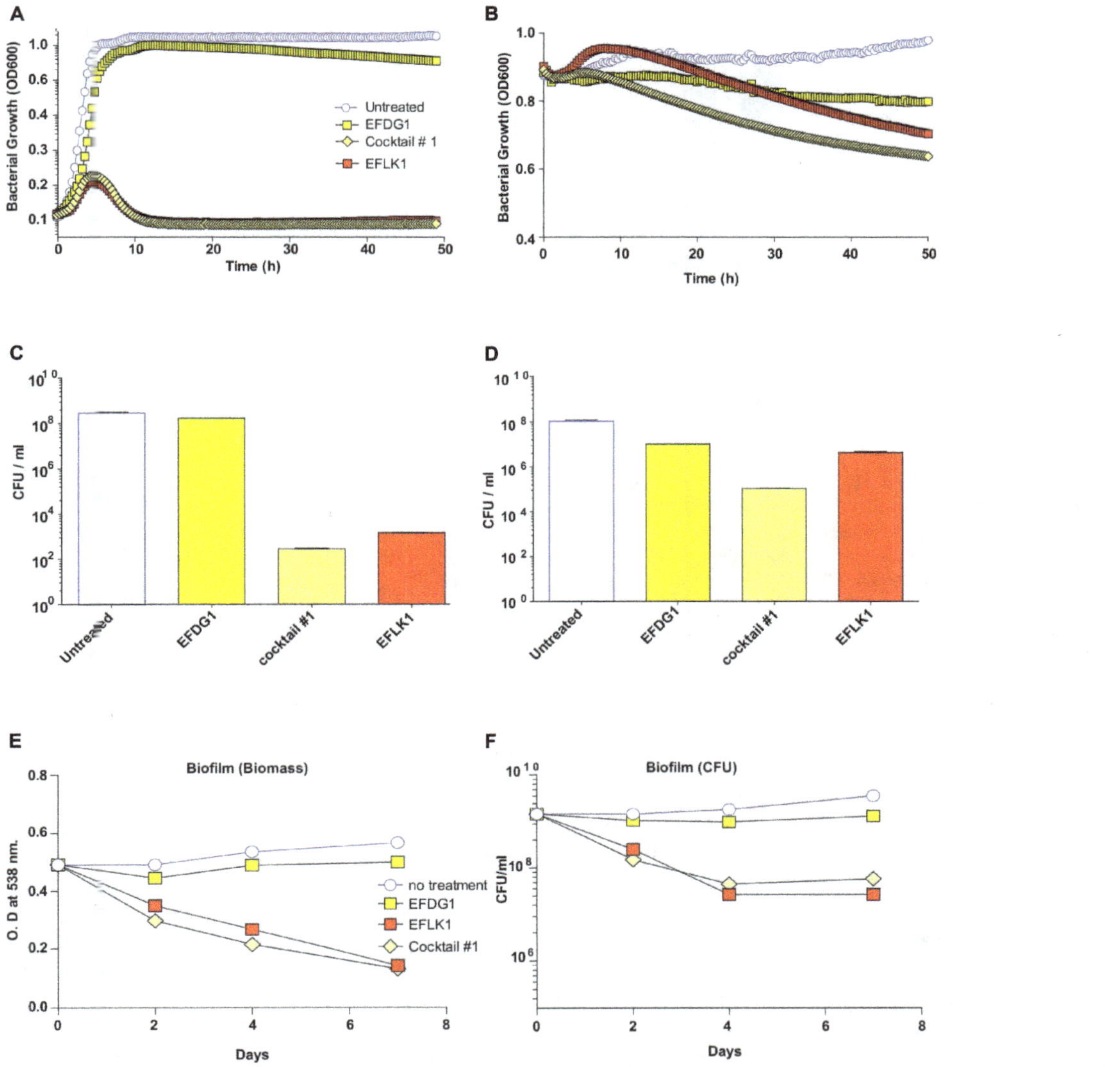

FIGURE 4 | Mixed bacterial population and Phage Cocktails. Similar to EFDG1^r bacteria; when the naïve *E. faecalis* V583 and mutant EFDG1^r are mixed in equal concentrations to get a mixed population; the growth curve **(A)** for logarithmic and **(B)** for stationary phase bacterial mixtures and their CFU/ml count counterparts **(C)** and **(D)** logarithmic and stationary respectively show desirable lysis by EFLK1 phage and its 1:1 phage cocktail. While EFDG1 phage has no significant effect in either case. **(E)** Crystal violet staining reveals a reduction in biofilm biomass and **(F)** CFU/ml also shows reduction in bacterial counts when treated with EFLK1 phage and phage cocktail.

family of lytic phages (Lavigne et al., 2009), were described. The highest resemblance (~45%) was found with EFDG1 phage, previously isolated by us (Khalifa et al., 2015a), and less with the other two phages phiEF24c and ECP3 (**Figures 6A–C**). All four phages share 60 core genes which are ~28% of their genes (**Figure 6A**).

The most significant difference between EFDG1 and EFLK1 phages genome sequences found was the number of *tRNA* genes (**Figure 6D**): EFDG1 phage contains 24 of them, EFLK1 phage carries none and the other two phages (phiEF24c and ECP3) contain five each which are all clustered in one region as in EFDG1 phage (**Figure 6D**). An analysis of the distribution of *tRNA* genes among all 2,053 fully sequenced tailed phages (NCBI, Caudovirales, taxid: 28883) revealed that nearly 60% (1,227) lacked *tRNA* genes as well (**Figure 6D**). Of the remainder, the majority carried only 1–5 genes, just like ECP3 and phiEF24c (**Figure 6D**). The highest number of *tRNA* genes (33) was found in the *Streptomyces* phage Jay2Jay (accession: KM652554.1). The cassette of five *tRNAs* in phiEF24c is identical to that in ECP3. EFDG1 phage contains the same five *tRNAs* and 19 more, all in a different order. Blast of these cassettes shows that they are unique and do not correspond to the ones on the *E. faecalis* genome.

One explanation for the presence of *tRNA* genes in phages is variance in codon usage between their own genome and that of the host. Consequently, one would expect EFDG1 phage codon usage to correlate less with that of its *E. faecalis* host than

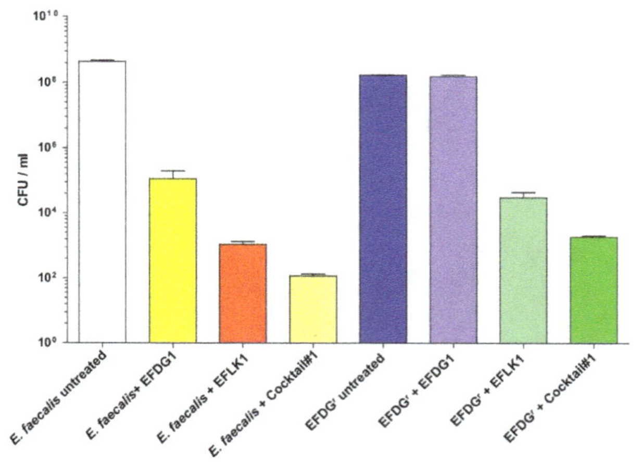

FIGURE 5 | *In vitro* fibrin clot model. The inset picture shows the clot model with phage (right) and without any phage treatment (left). The clot untreated by phage disintegrates due to the presence of *EFV583* bacteria while the treated clot is intact. The number of bacterial colonies in the clot before and after phage treatment were counted and CFU/ml was calculated for each sample after clot degradation.

the codon usage of the other phages and the large amount of *tRNAs* to compensate for that extra bias. However, COR function (R Bioconductor package) analysis disproved this theory, as no significant differences were found between the codon usage of the phages and *E. faecalis*. EFDG1 has 0.921 ECP3; 0.89522, EFLK1; 0.8954, and phiEF24c share 0.8948 correlation with the *E. faecalis* codon usage (**Supplementary Table S1**).

Next, we looked at the specific *tRNA* genes carried by these phages in accordance with their codon usage (**Supplementary Table S1**). The three anti-*E. faecalis* Spounavirinae phages with *tRNA's* (EFDG1, ECP3, and phiEF24c) carry *tRNA* genes corresponding to codons CTA, AGA, GAC, and TGG of leucine, arginine, aspartic acid, and tryptophan respectively. Besides these, EFDG1 phage encodes for two while ECP and phiEF24c phages for single *tRNA* corresponding to the initiation and sole methionine codon AUG. Indeed, in the three phages, the usage of all these codons is higher than their usage in *E. faecalis* (**Supplementary Table S1**), perhaps justifying the corresponding *tRNA* gene's existence. Surprisingly, the codon usage of these five codons is also higher in EFLK1 phage, which does not have any *tRNA* genes (**Supplementary Table S1**). Moreover, the codon usage should lead the four phages to carry the *tRNA* gene corresponding to codon TAC (tyrosine) while EFLK1, ECP3, and phiEF24c phages should carry *tRNA's* for AAG (lysine), AAC (asparagine), ACA (threonine) and GTA (valine) like EFDG1 phage, however this is not the case. On the other hand, EFDG1 phage carries several *tRNA* genes, such as TTA (leucine) which, according to the codon usage, seems to be not required. Thus, the question of the effect of codon usage on the presence of these *tRNA* and its relation to the phenotypic differences remains open.

We also analyzed the P2 mutation described by Uchiyama et al. (2011) in phage phiEF24c. The P2 mutation, located in Orf31, a conserved putative tail fiber, dramatically improves the ability of phiEF24c to adsorb and lyse the cells (Uchiyama et al., 2011). Nevertheless, EFDG1, EFLK1, and ECP3 phages harbor homologs for Orf31 but none of them has the P2 mutant allele (**Figure 6E**).

DISCUSSION

Phage therapy holds the promise of succeeding where antibiotics have failed against resistant bacteria. In some cases, phage resistance actually has led to loss of bacterial virulence (Scott et al., 2007; Zahid et al., 2008; Capparelli et al., 2010). In addition, while production of new antibiotics is slowing down (Silver, 2011; Laxminarayan et al., 2013), the rate of new phages isolation is increasing and new phages are being discovered daily as can be seen in phage databases such as the European Nucleotide Archive (ENA[5]). It is speculated that phages are the most prevalent replicating form on Earth and their number is estimated to be $\sim 10^{31}$, which is about 10 times more than prokaryotes (Diaz-Munoz and Koskella, 2014). Thus, in case of resistance, the likelihood of isolating an appropriate phage is indeed high. Furthermore, the variety of phages supports the construction of an almost unlimited number of combinations of cocktails to combat various strains or multispecies infections.

In this work, we demonstrated the isolation of a new phage when facing phage-resistant mutants and the advantages of a two-phage cocktail against VRE *E. faecalis* and its phage-resistant mutant.

Although similar, phages EFDG1 (Khalifa et al., 2015a) and EFLK1 have interesting phenotypic differences. While EFDG1 phage is more efficient against logarithmic *E. faecalis* V583 cultures, EFLK1 phage is a better killer of stationary (**Figure 2**). Joined in cocktail, they are even better at killing the bacteria than individually. Additionally, where EFDG1 phage failed to kill $EFDG1^r$, EFLK1 phage and the cocktail were effective against the WT and the phage-resistant mutant alone or in a mixed culture. This simulates the evolution of such mutants. We found the 1:1-ratio phage cocktail to be most effective, but we expect that ratios will vary and should therefore be determined on a case by case basis.

The reason for the phenotypic differences between EFDG1 and EFLK1 phages remains shrouded. One significant feature is the presence of 24 *tRNA* genes in EFDG1 phage, and their absence in EFLK1 phage. Theoretically, phages effective in the logarithmic stage (EFDG1), which benefits from elevated levels of host *tRNA*, should conceivably need to encode a small number of *tRNA* genes while phages effective in the stationary phage (EFLK1) should conceivably need a greater number. However, our findings indicated the opposite. The logarithmic efficient EFDG1 phage has more *tRNA* than the stationary efficient EFLK1 phage. Furthermore, the phages exhibited similar codon usage. In addition, the *tRNA* genes of EFDG1, ECP3, and phiEF24c phages are all encoded in a conserved region which is absent from EFLK1's genome. This suggests that the *tRNA*'s are required for the efficient translation of the proteins encoded in that region.

[5]http://www.ebi.ac.uk/genomes/phage.html

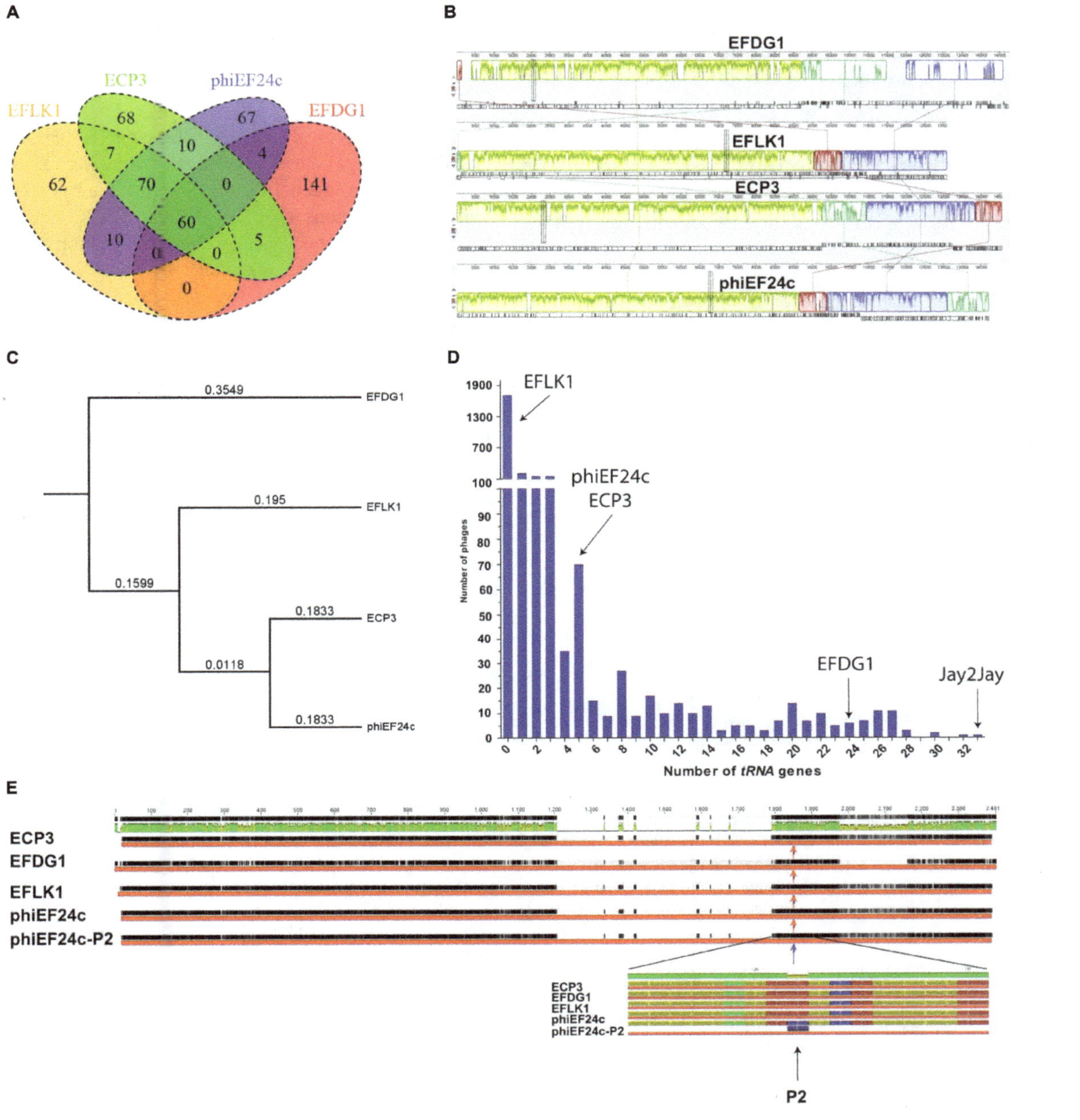

FIGURE 6 | Genomic analysis. **(A)** Venn diagram represents the number of similar *tRNA* between EFLK1, ECP3, phiEF24c, and EFDG1 phages (from left to right). **(B)** Comparative analysis of the genomes of EFDG1, EFLK1, ECP3, and phiEF24c phages (top to bottom). **(C)** Phylogenetic analysis depicting the similarity between the genomes of the four known phages of *E. faecalis*. **(D)** The number of *tRNA* genes present in the genomes of almost all known phages of *E. faecalis* V583 is shown here. With EFLK1 phage **(E)** P2 site mutation is known to be linked to enhanced adsorption as shown by Uchiyama et al., 2011. No differences were found in the P2 mutation site in all the cases.

Though one would expect to find a higher codon usage bias with respect to *E. faecalis* in this region, this is not the case. Despite a correlation between *tRNA* abundancy and virulence against bacteria (Bailly-Bechet et al. 2007) and evidence that deletion of *tRNA* genes reduced burst sizes and protein synthesis rates in the case of phage T4 of *E. coli* (Wilson, 1973), the role of *tRNA* in phages remains enigmatic.

P2 mutation in Orf31 (**Figure 6**), found to enhance adsorption in phiEF24c (Uchiyama et al., 2011), is absent in our phages. Nevertheless, Orf31 of EFDG1 phage appears to be less conserved in general compared to the other three phages of *E. faecalis*. This could mean that EFDG1 phage binds with a different affinity, or binds to another receptor all together. Further research is needed to determine whether the differences in Orf31 are responsible for the phenotypic differences between EFDG1 and EFLK1 phages. The effectiveness and complementary nature of EFDG1 and EFLK1 phages marks these phages as suitable for *in vivo* experiments toward the development of a high-efficacy anti-*E. faecalis* phage therapy.

AUTHOR CONTRIBUTIONS

RH initiated the research, designed the experiments, analyzed the data, and wrote the paper. LK designed and performed the experiments and wrote the paper. MS performed some of the experiments. AD performed the bioinformatic analysis. SC-G designed the experiments and wrote the paper. DG helped to perform some of the experiments. NB initiated the research, designed the experiments, analyzed the data, and wrote the paper.

FUNDING

We are grateful to the funding committee of the Rosetrees Trust for grant #0364821. Additionally, LK and MS are the recipients of the Ariane de Rothschild fellowship for women.

ACKNOWLEDGMENTS

We would like to thank the following: Hebrew University's interdepartmental core unit at the Ein Kerem Campus for help in deep sequencing, Dr. Violeta Temper of Hadassah Hospital's Infectious Diseases Unit at Ein Kerem for bacterial isolates; Nahal Sorek Sewage Decontamination Institute's Yuri Veinstein for samples for phage isolation, and finally to Dr. Dov Glazer and Elisheva Dorfman for critical editing of this manuscript.

SUPPLEMENTARY MATERIAL

TABLE S1 | *tRNA* codon usage in EFDG1, EFLK1 and the other two *E. faecalis* phages as compared to that in *E. faecalis*. This is depicted by the frequency occurrence of the amino acid codon and the number of *tRNA* encoded by them in each case.

REFERENCES

Bailly-Bechet, M., Vergassola, M., and Rocha, E. (2007). Causes for the intriguing presence of tRNAs in phages. *Genome Res.* 17, 1486–1495. doi: 10.1101/gr.6649807

Bertram, H. (1988). DNA damage and mutagenesis of lambda phage induced by gamma-rays. *Mutagenesis* 3, 29–33. doi: 10.1093/mutage/3.1.29

Burrowes, B., Harper, D. R., Anderson, J., Mcconville, M., and Enright, M. C. (2011). Bacteriophage therapy: potential uses in the control of antibiotic-resistant pathogens. *Expert Rev. Anti. Infect. Ther.* 9, 775–785. doi: 10.1586/eri.11.90

Capparelli, R., Nocerino, N., Iannaccone, M., Ercolini, D., Parlato, M., Chiara, M., et al. (2010). Bacteriophage therapy of *Salmonella enterica*: a fresh appraisal of bacteriophage therapy. *J. Infect. Dis.* 201, 52–61. doi: 10.1086/648478

Chan, B. K., and Abedon, S. T. (2012). Phage therapy pharmacology phage cocktails. *Adv. Appl. Microbiol.* 78, 1–23. doi: 10.1016/B978-0-12-394805-2.00001-4

Charles, P. G., and Grayson, M. L. (2004). The dearth of new antibiotic development: why we should be worried and what we can do about it. *Med. J. Aust.* 181, 549–553.

Chong, Y. P., Lee, S. O., Song, E. H., Lee, E. J., Jang, E. Y., Kim, S. H., et al. (2010). Quinupristin-dalfopristin versus linezolid for the treatment of vancomycin-resistant *Enterococcus faecium* bacteraemia: efficacy and development of resistance. *Scand. J. Infect. Dis.* 42, 491–499. doi: 10.3109/00365541003699623

Davies, J., and Davies, D. (2010). Origins and evolution of antibiotic resistance. *Microbiol. Mol. Biol. Rev.* 74, 417–433. doi: 10.1128/MMBR.00016-10

de la Fuente-Nunez, C., Reffuveille, F., Fernandez, L., and Hancock, R. E. (2013). Bacterial biofilm development as a multicellular adaptation: antibiotic resistance and new therapeutic strategies. *Curr. Opin. Microbiol.* 16, 580–589. doi: 10.1016/j.mib.2013.06.013

Diaz-Munoz, S. L., and Koskella, B. (2014). Bacteria-phage interactions in natural environments. *Adv. Appl. Microbiol.* 89, 135–183. doi: 10.1016/B978-0-12-800259-9.00004-4

Donlan, R. M. (2001). Biofilms and device-associated infections. *Emerg. Infect. Dis.* 7, 277–281. doi: 10.3201/eid0702.010226

Donlan, R. M. (2009). Preventing biofilms of clinically relevant organisms using bacteriophage. *Trends Microbiol.* 17, 66–72. doi: 10.1016/j.tim.2008.11.002

Drake, J. W. (1966). Ultraviolet mutagenesis in bacteriophage T-4. I. Irradiation of extracellular phage particles. *J. Bacteriol.* 91, 1775–1780.

Drake, J. W. (1982). Methyl methanesulfonate mutagenesis in bacteriophage T4. *Genetics* 102, 639–651.

Duerkop, B. A., Huo, W., Bhardwaj, P., Palmer, K. L., and Hooper, L. V. (2016). Molecular basis for lytic bacteriophage resistance in enterococci. *mBio* 7:e01304-16. doi: 10.1128/mBio.01304-16

Entenza, J. M., Haldimann, A., Giddey, M., Lociuro, S., Hawser, S., and Moreillon, P. (2009). Efficacy of iclaprim against wild-type and thymidine kinase-deficient methicillin-resistant *Staphylococcus aureus* isolates in an *in vitro* fibrin clot model. *Antimicrob. Agents Chemother.* 53, 3635–3641. doi: 10.1128/AAC.00325-09

Ellis, E. L., and Delbrück, M. (1939). The growth of bacteriophage. *J. Gen. Physiol.* 22, 365–384. doi: 10.1085/jgp.22.3.365

Erlandson, K. M., Sun, J., Iwen, P. C., and Rupp, M. E. (2008). Impact of the more-potent antibiotics quinupristin-dalfopristin and linezolid on outcome measure of patients with vancomycin-resistant *Enterococcus* bacteremia. *Clin. Infect. Dis.* 46, 30–36. doi: 10.1086/523588

Golkar, Z., Bagasra, O., and Pace, D. G. (2014). Bacteriophage therapy: a potential solution for the antibiotic resistance crisis. *J. Infect. Dev. Ctries.* 8, 129–136. doi: 10.3855/jidc.3573

Gu, J., Liu, X., Li, Y., Han, W., Lei, L., Yang, Y., et al. (2012). A method for generation phage cocktail with great therapeutic potential. *PLoS One* 7:e31698. doi: 10.1371/journal.pone.0031698

Hershberger, E., Coyle, E. A., Kaatz, G. W., Zervos, M. J., and Rybak, M. J. (2000). Comparison of a rabbit model of bacterial endocarditis and an in vitro infection model with simulated endocardial vegetations. *Antimicrob. Agents Chemother.* 44, 1921–1924. doi: 10.1128/AAC.44.7.1921-1924.2000

Khalifa, L., Brosh, Y., Gelman, D., Coppenhagen-Glazer, S., Beyth, S., Poradosu-Cohen, R., et al. (2015a). Targeting *Enterococcus faecalis* biofilms with phage therapy. *Appl. Environ. Microbiol.* 81, 2696–2705. doi: 10.1128/AEM.00096-15

Khalifa, L., Coppenhagen-Glazer, S., Shlezinger, M., Kott-Gutkowski, M., Adini, O., Beyth, N., et al. (2015b). Complete genome sequence of *Enterococcus* bacteriophage EFLK1. *Genome Announc.* 3, e1308-15. doi: 10.1128/genomeA.01308-15

Khalifa, L., Shlezinger, M., Beyth, S., Houri-Haddad, Y., Coppenhagen-Glazer, S., Beyth, N., et al. (2016). Phage therapy against *Enterococcus faecalis* in dental root canals. *J. Oral Microbiol.* 8, 32157. doi: 10.3402/jom.v8.32157

Kiro, R., Shitrit, D., and Qimron, U. (2014). Efficient engineering of a bacteriophage genome using the type I-E CRISPR-Cas system. *RNA Biol.* 11, 42–44. doi: 10.4161/rna.27766

Lavigne, R., Darius, P., Summer, E. J., Seto, D., Mahadevan, P., Nilsson, A. S., et al. (2009). Classification of *Myoviridae* bacteriophages using protein sequence similarity. *BMC Microbiol.* 9:224. doi: 10.1186/1471-2180-9-224

Laxminarayan, R., Duse, A., Wattal, C., Zaidi, A. K., Wertheim, H. F., Sumpradit, N., et al. (2013). Antibiotic resistance-the need for global solutions. *Lancet Infect. Dis.* 13, 1057–1098. doi: 10.1016/S1473-3099(13)70318-9

Linden, P. K. (2002). Treatment options for vancomycin-resistant enterococcal infections. *Drugs* 62, 425–441. doi: 10.2165/00003495-200262030-00002

Loc-Carrillo, C., and Abedon, S. T. (2011). Pros and cons of phage therapy. *Bacteriophage* 1, 111–114. doi: 10.4161/bact.1.2.14590

McGrath, B. J., Kang, S. L., Kaatz, G. W., and Rybak, M. J. (1994). Bactericidal activities of teicoplanin, vancomycin, and gentamicin alone and in combination against *Staphylococcus aureus* in an *in vitro* pharmacodynamic model of endocarditis. *Antimicrob. Agents Chemother.* 38, 2034–2040. doi: 10.1128/AAC.38.9.2034

Moore, S. D. (2011). Assembling new *Escherichia coli* strains by transduction using phage P1. *Methods Mol. Biol.* 765, 155–169. doi: 10.1007/978-1-61779-197-0_10

O'Driscoll, T., and Crank, C. W. (2015). Vancomycin-resistant enterococcal infections: epidemiology, clinical manifestations, and optimal management. *Infect. Drug Resist.* 8, 217–230. doi: 10.2147/IDR.S54125

Ormala, A. M., and Jalasvuori, M. (2013). Phage therapy: should bacterial resistance to phages be a concern, even in the long run? *Bacteriophage* 3:e24219.

Orsi, G. B., and Ciorba, V. (2013). Vancomycin resistant enterococci healthcare associated infections. *Ann. Ig.* 25, 485–492. doi: 10.7416/ai.2013.1948

Pires, D. P., Cleto, S., Sillankorva, S., Azeredo, J., and Lu, T. K. (2016). Genetically engineered phages: a review of advances over the last decade. *Microbiol. Mol. Biol. Rev.* 80, 523–543. doi: 10.1128/MMBR.00069-15

Rice, L. B. (2008). Federal funding for the study of antimicrobial resistance in nosocomial pathogens: no ESKAPE. *J. Infect. Dis.* 197, 1079–1081. doi: 10.1086/533452

Scott, A. E., Timms, A. R., Connerton, P. L., Loc Carrillo, C., Adzfa Radzum, K., and Connerton, I. F. (2007). Genome dynamics of *Campylobacter jejuni* in response to bacteriophage predation. *PLoS Pathog.* 3:e119. doi: 10.1371/journal.ppat.0030119

Silver, L. L. (2011). Challenges of antibacterial discovery. *Clin. Microbiol. Rev.* 24, 71–109. doi: 10.1128/CMR.00030-10

Srinivasiah, S., Bhavsar, J., Thapar, K., Liles, M., Schoenfeld, T., and Wommack, K. E. (2008). Phages across the biosphere: contrasts of viruses in soil and aquatic environments. *Res. Microbiol.* 159, 349–357. doi: 10.1016/j.resmic.2008.04.010

Tiruvadi Krishnan, S., Moolman, M. C., Van Laar, T., Meyer, A. S., and Dekker, N. H. (2015). Essential validation methods for *E. coli* strains created by chromosome engineering. *J. Biol. Eng.* 9:11. doi: 10.1186/s13036-015-0008-x

Uchiyama, J., Takemura, I., Satoh, M., Kato, S., Ujihara, T., Akechi, K., et al. (2011). Improved adsorption of an *Enterococcus faecalis* bacteriophage PhiEF24C with a spontaneous point mutation. *PLoS One* 6:e26648. doi: 10.1371/journal.pone.0026648

Wilson, J. H. (1973). Function of the bacteriophage T4 transfer RNA's. *J. Mol. Biol.* 74, 753–757. doi: 10.1016/0022-2836(73)90065-X

Zahid, M. S., Udden, S. M., Faruque, A. S., Calderwood, S. B., Mekalanos, J. J., and Faruque, S. M. (2008). Effect of phage on the infectivity of *Vibrio cholerae* and emergence of genetic variants. *Infect. Immun.* 76, 5266–5273. doi: 10.1128/IAI.00578-08

Permissions

All chapters in this book were first published by Frontiers; hereby published with permission under the Creative Commons Attribution License or equivalent. Every chapter published in this book has been scrutinized by our experts. Their significance has been extensively debated. The topics covered herein carry significant findings which will fuel the growth of the discipline. They may even be implemented as practical applications or may be referred to as a beginning point for another development.

The contributors of this book come from diverse backgrounds, making this book a truly international effort. This book will bring forth new frontiers with its revolutionizing research information and detailed analysis of the nascent developments around the world.

We would like to thank all the contributing authors for lending their expertise to make the book truly unique. They have played a crucial role in the development of this book. Without their invaluable contributions this book wouldn't have been possible. They have made vital efforts to compile up to date information on the varied aspects of this subject to make this book a valuable addition to the collection of many professionals and students.

This book was conceptualized with the vision of imparting up-to-date information and advanced data in this field. To ensure the same, a matchless editorial board was set up. Every individual on the board went through rigorous rounds of assessment to prove their worth. After which they invested a large part of their time researching and compiling the most relevant data for our readers.

The editorial board has been involved in producing this book since its inception. They have spent rigorous hours researching and exploring the diverse topics which have resulted in the successful publishing of this book. They have passed on their knowledge of decades through this book. To expedite this challenging task, the publisher supported the team at every step. A small team of assistant editors was also appointed to further simplify the editing procedure and attain best results for the readers.

Apart from the editorial board, the designing team has also invested a significant amount of their time in understanding the subject and creating the most relevant covers. They scrutinized every image to scout for the most suitable representation of the subject and create an appropriate cover for the book.

The publishing team has been an ardent support to the editorial, designing and production team. Their endless efforts to recruit the best for this project, has resulted in the accomplishment of this book. They are a veteran in the field of academics and their pool of knowledge is as vast as their experience in printing. Their expertise and guidance has proved useful at every step. Their uncompromising quality standards have made this book an exceptional effort. Their encouragement from time to time has been an inspiration for everyone.

The publisher and the editorial board hope that this book will prove to be a valuable piece of knowledge for researchers, students, practitioners and scholars across the globe.

List of Contributors

Divakar Sharma
Department of Biochemistry, National JALMA Institute for Leprosy and Other Mycobacterial Diseases, Agra, India
Interdisciplinary Biotechnology Unit, Aligarh Muslim University, Aligarh, India

Yogesh K. Dhuriya
Developmental Toxicology Laboratory, Systems Toxicology and Health Risk Assessment Group, CSIR-Indian Institute of Toxicology Research (CSIR-IITR), Lucknow, India

Nirmala Deo and Deepa Bisht
Department of Biochemistry, National JALMA Institute for Leprosy and Other Mycobacterial Diseases, Agra, India

Qixia Luo, Yuan Wang, Hao Fu, Xiao Yu, Beiwen Zheng, Yunbo Chen and Yonghong Xiao
State Key Laboratory for Diagnosis and Treatment of Infectious Diseases, National Clinical Research Center for Infectious Diseases, The First Affiliated Hospital, College of Medicine, Zhejiang University, Hangzhou, China

Björn Berglund
State Key Laboratory for Diagnosis and Treatment of Infectious Diseases, National Clinical Research Center for Infectious Diseases, The First Affiliated Hospital, College of Medicine, Zhejiang University, Hangzhou, China
Department of Clinical and Experimental Medicine, Linköping University, Linköping, Sweden

María E. Pachón-Ibáñez, Gema Labrador-Herrera, Tania Cebrero-Cangueiro and Younes Smani
Clinical Unit of Infectious Diseases, Microbiology, and Preventive Medicine, Institute of Biomedicine of Seville, University Hospital Virgen del Rocío/CSIC/University of Seville, Seville, Spain

Caridad Díaz and Jose P. del Palacio
Fundacion Centro de Excelencia en Investigación de Medicamentos Innovadores en Andalucía, MEDINA Foundation, Granada, Spain

Jesús Rodríguez-Baño
Clinical Unit of Infectious Diseases, Microbiology, and Preventive Medicine, Institute of Biomedicine of Seville, University Hospital Virgen de Macarena/CSIC/University of Seville, Seville, Spain
Department of Medicine, University of Seville, Seville, Spain

Alvaro Pascual
Clinical Unit of Infectious Diseases, Microbiology, and Preventive Medicine, Institute of Biomedicine of Seville, University Hospital Virgen de Macarena/CSIC/University of Seville, Seville, Spain
Department of Microbiology, University of Seville, Seville, Spain

Jerónimo Pachón
Clinical Unit of Infectious Diseases, Microbiology, and Preventive Medicine, Institute of Biomedicine of Seville, University Hospital Virgen del Rocío/CSIC/University of Seville, Seville, Spain
Department of Medicine, University of Seville, Seville, Spain

M. Carmen Conejo
Department of Microbiology, University of Seville, Seville, Spain

Higor Sette Pereira, Thaysa Leite Tagliaferri and Tiago Antônio de Oliveira Mendes
Laboratory of Synthetic Biology and Modelling of Biological Systems, Department of Biochemistry and Molecular Biology, Universidade Federal de Viçosa, Viçosa, Brazil

Bingyu Ding
Department of Laboratory Medicine, Shanghai General Hospital, Shanghai Jiao Tong University School of Medicine, Shanghai, China
Department of Laboratory Medicine, Ruijin Hospital, Shanghai Jiao Tong University School of Medicine, Shanghai, China

Qingtian Li
Department of Laboratory Medicine, Ruijin Hospital, Shanghai Jiao Tong University School of Medicine, Shanghai, China

Mingquan Guo, Ke Dong, Yan Zhang and Xiaokui Guo
Department of Immunology and Microbiology, Shanghai Jiao Tong University School of Medicine, Shanghai, China

Qingzhong Liu, Li Li and Zelin Cui
Department of Laboratory Medicine, Shanghai General Hospital, Shanghai Jiao Tong University School of Medicine, Shanghai, China

Sourabh Mehta
National Centre for Nanoscience and Nanotechnology, University of Mumbai, Mumbai, India

Kapil Punjabi, Vidushi Chitalia, Dhanashree Deogharkar and Sunita Deshpande
Department of Clinical Pathology, Haffkine Institute for Training, Research and Testing, Mumbai, India

Rujuta Chavan
Department of Microbiology, Guru Nanak Khalsa College, Mumbai, India

Heng Cai, Yiwei Zhu, Dandan Hu, Yue Li, Xiaoting Hua and Yunsong Yu
Department of Infectious Diseases, Sir Run Run Shaw Hospital, Zhejiang University School of Medicine, Hangzhou, China
Key Laboratory of Microbial Technology and Bioinformatics of Zhejiang Province, Hangzhou, China
Regional Medical Center for National Institute of Respiratory Diseases, Sir Run Run Shaw Hospital, Zhejiang University School of Medicine, Hangzhou, China

Sebastian Leptihn
Department of Infectious Diseases, Sir Run Run Shaw Hospital, Zhejiang University School of Medicine, Hangzhou, China
Zhejiang University-University of Edinburgh Institute, Zhejiang University, Haining, China

Belinda Loh
Zhejiang University-University of Edinburgh Institute, Zhejiang University, Haining, China

Min Lu, Tianhong Dai and Mei X. Wu
Wellman Center for Photomedicine, Massachusetts General Hospital, Harvard Medical School, Boston, MA, United States

Clinton K. Murray
First Area Medical Laboratory, JBSA-Fort Sam Houston, Houston, TX, United States

Yi-Jung Chang and Yi-Ching Chen
Department of Pediatrics, Chang Gung Memorial Hospital, College of Medicine, Chang Gung University, Taoyuan, Taiwan
Molecular Infectious Disease Research Center, Chang Gung Memorial Hospital, Taoyuan, Taiwan

Nai-Wen Chen, Ying-Jie Hsu and Hsiao-Han Chu
Department of Pediatrics, Chang Gung Memorial Hospital, College of Medicine, Chang Gung University, Taoyuan, Taiwan

Chyi-Liang Chen
Molecular Infectious Disease Research Center, Chang Gung Memorial Hospital, Taoyuan, Taiwan

Cheng-Hsun Chiu
Department of Pediatrics, Chang Gung Memorial Hospital, College of Medicine, Chang Gung University, Taoyuan, Taiwan
Molecular Infectious Disease Research Center, Chang Gung Memorial Hospital, Taoyuan, Taiwan
Graduate Institute of Clinical Medical Sciences, College of Medicine, Chang Gung University, Taoyuan, Taiwan

Pedro V. Baptista, Andreia Carvalho and Alexandra R. Fernandes
UCIBIO, Departamento de Ciências da Vida, Faculdade de Ciências e Tecnologia, Universidade Nova de Lisboa, Caparica, Portugal

Matthew P. McCusker
School of Food Science and Environmental Health, College of Sciences and Health, Dublin Institute of Technology, Dublin, Ireland

Daniela A. Ferreira and Marta Martins
Department of Microbiology, Moyne Institute of Preventive Medicine, Schools of Genetics and Microbiology, Trinity College Dublin, University of Dublin, Dublin, Ireland

Niamh M. Mohan
Department of Microbiology, Moyne Institute of Preventive Medicine, Schools of Genetics and Microbiology, Trinity College Dublin, University of Dublin, Dublin, Ireland
Nuritas Limited, Dublin, Ireland

Xiao-Qing Zhu, Yi-Yun Liu, Renjie Wu, Haoliang Xun, Jian Sun and Jian-Hua Liu
College of Veterinary Medicine, Guangdong Provincial Key Laboratory of Veterinary Pharmaceutics Development and Safety Evaluation, Key Laboratory of Zoonosis of Ministry of Agricultural and Rural Affairs, National Risk Assessment Laboratory for Antimicrobial Resistance of Microorganisms in Animals, South China Agricultural University, Guangzhou, China
Guangdong Laboratory for Lingnan Modern Agriculture, Guangzhou, China

Jian Li
Biomedicine Discovery Institute and Department of Microbiology, School of Biomedical Sciences, Monash University, Clayton, VIC, Australia

Yaoyu Feng
Guangdong Laboratory for Lingnan Modern Agriculture, Guangzhou, China
College of Veterinary Medicine, Center for Emerging and Zoonotic Diseases, South China Agricultural University, Guangzhou, China

Vinod Kumar, Piyush Agrawal, Rajesh Kumar, Salman Sadullah Usmani and Gajendra P. S. Raghava
Center for Computational Biology, Indraprastha Institute of Information Technology, Okhla, India
Bioinformatics Centre, CSIR-Institute of Microbial Technology, Sector-39A, Chandigarh, India

Sherry Bhalla
Center for Computational Biology, Indraprastha Institute of Information Technology, Okhla, India

Grish C. Varshney
Cell Biology and Immunology, CSIR-Institute of Microbial Technology, Sector-39A, Chandigarh, India

Debajyoti Dutta
Department of Biochemistry, Faculty of Medicine and Dentistry, University of Alberta, Edmonton, AB, Canada

Wenhao Wu
Department of Infectious Diseases, Zhejiang Provincial People's Hospital, People's Hospital of Hangzhou Medical College, Hangzhou, China
Medical College, Qingdao University, Qingdao, China

Lingling Lu
Adicon Clinical Laboratories, Hangzhou, China

Wenjia Fan and Hongying Pan
Department of Infectious Diseases, Zhejiang Provincial People's Hospital, People's Hospital of Hangzhou Medical College, Hangzhou, China

Chun Chen
Department of Pneumology, Zhejiang Provincial People's Hospital, People's Hospital of Hangzhou Medical College, Hangzhou, China

Dazhi Jin and Xi Li
Centre of Laboratory Medicine, Zhejiang Provincial People's Hospital, People's Hospital of Hangzhou Medical College, Hangzhou, China

Rajashree Bhalchandra Patwardhan
Department of Microbiology, Haribhai V. Desai College of Arts, Science and Commerce, Pune University, Pune, India

Prashant Kamalakar Dhakephalkar
Bioenergy Group, Agharkar Research Institute, Pune, India

Balu Ananda Chopade
Department of Microbiology, Savitribai Phule Pune University, Aurangabad, India

Dilip D. Dhavale
Department of Chemistry, Savitribai Phule Pune University, Pune, India

Ramesh R. Bhonde
School of Regenerative Medicine - Manipal Academy of Higher Education, Bengaluru, India

Juan Xu
School of Public Health, Hangzhou Medical College, Hangzhou, China

Zhongliang Zhu, Yanmin Chen, Weizhong Wang and Fang He
Department of Clinical Laboratory, Zhejiang Provincial People's Hospital, People's Hospital of Hangzhou Medical College, Hangzhou, China

Sanjay Chhibber, Jasjeet Kaur and Sandeep Kaur
Department of Microbiology, Panjab University, Chandigarh, India

Mansura S. Mulani, Ekta E. Kamble, Shital N. Kumkar, Madhumita S. Tawre and Karishma R. Pardesi
Department of Microbiology, Savitribai Phule Pune University, Pune, India

Baomo Liu
State Key Laboratory of Respiratory Disease, The First Affiliated Hospital of Guangzhou Medical University, Guangzhou, China
Department of Respiratory Medicine, The First Affiliated Hospital of Sun Yat-sen University, Guangzhou, China

Yingyi Guo, Ningjing Liu, Jiong Wang, Feifeng Li, Likang Yao and Chao Zhuo
State Key Laboratory of Respiratory Disease, The First Affiliated Hospital of Guangzhou Medical University, Guangzhou, China

Samsher Singh and Inshad A. Khan
Clinical Microbiology Division, Indian Institute of Integrative Medicine (CSIR), Jammu, India
Academy of Scientific and Innovative Research (AcSIR), Indian Institute of Integrative Medicine (CSIR), Jammu, India

Nitin P. Kalia
Clinical Microbiology Division, Indian Institute of Integrative Medicine (CSIR), Jammu, India

Prashant Joshi and Sandip B. Bharate
Academy of Scientific and Innovative Research (AcSIR), Indian Institute of Integrative Medicine (CSIR), Jammu, India
Medicinal Chemistry Division, Indian Institute of Integrative Medicine (CSIR), Jammu, India

Ajay Kumar
Cancer Pharmacology Division, Indian Institute of Integrative Medicine (CSIR), Jammu, India

Parduman R. Sharma and Ashok Kumar
Academy of Scientific and Innovative Research (AcSIR), Indian Institute of Integrative Medicine (CSIR), Jammu, India
Cancer Pharmacology Division, Indian Institute of Integrative Medicine (CSIR), Jammu, India

Baoyue Zhang and Wei Zhou
CAS Key Laboratory of Special Pathogens and Biosafety, Center for Biosafety Mega-Science, Wuhan Institute of Virology, Chinese Academy of Sciences, Wuhan, China
University of Chinese Academy of Sciences, Beijing, China

Bing Yu
Department of Pathogen Biology, School of Basic Medicine, Tongji Medical College, Huazhong University of Science and Technology, Wuhan, China

Yue Wang and Ziyong Sun
Department of Laboratory Medicine, Tongji Hospital, Tongji Medical College, Huazhong University of Science and Technology, Wuhan, China

Xiaojun Wu
Department of Respiratory and Critical Medicine, Renmin Hospital of Wuhan University, Wuhan, China

Shiyun Chen and Yangbo Hu
CAS Key Laboratory of Special Pathogens and Biosafety, Center for Biosafety Mega-Science, Wuhan Institute of Virology, Chinese Academy of Sciences, Wuhan, China

Ming Ni
Department of Infectious Diseases, Tongji Hospital, Tongji Medical College, Huazhong University of Science and Technology, Wuhan, China

Leron Khalifa, Daniel Gelman, Axel Lionel Dessal, Shunit Coppenhagen-Glazer and Ronen Hazan
Faculty of Dental Sciences, Hadassah School of Dental Medicine, Hebrew University of Jerusalem, Jerusalem, Israel

Mor Shlezinger and Nurit Beyth
Faculty of Dental Sciences, Hadassah School of Dental Medicine, Hebrew University of Jerusalem, Jerusalem, Israel
Department of Prosthodontics, Hadassah School of Dental Medicine, Hebrew University of Jerusalem, Jerusalem, Israel

Index